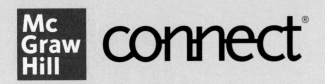 
Instructors: Student Success Starts with You

Tools to enhance your unique voice

Want to build your own course? No problem. Prefer to use our turnkey, prebuilt course? Easy. Want to make changes throughout the semester? Sure. And you'll save time with Connect's auto-grading too.

65%
Less Time Grading

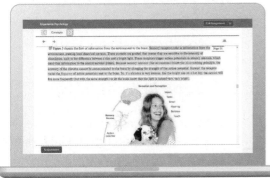

Laptop: McGraw Hill; Woman/dog: George Doyle/Getty Images

Study made personal

Incorporate adaptive study resources like SmartBook® 2.0 into your course and help your students be better prepared in less time. Learn more about the powerful personalized learning experience available in SmartBook 2.0 at **www.mheducation.com/highered/connect/smartbook**

Affordable solutions, added value

Make technology work for you with LMS integration for single sign-on access, mobile access to the digital textbook, and reports to quickly show you how each of your students is doing. And with our Inclusive Access program you can provide all these tools at a discount to your students. Ask your McGraw Hill representative for more information.

Padlock: Jobalou/Getty Images

Solutions for your challenges

A product isn't a solution. Real solutions are affordable, reliable, and come with training and ongoing support when you need it and how you want it. Visit **www.supportateverystep.com** for videos and resources both you and your students can use throughout the semester.

Checkmark: Jobalou/Getty Images

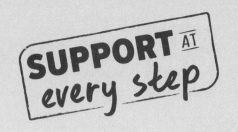

Students: Get Learning that Fits You

Effective tools for efficient studying

Connect is designed to make you more productive with simple, flexible, intuitive tools that maximize your study time and meet your individual learning needs. Get learning that works for you with Connect.

Study anytime, anywhere

Download the free ReadAnywhere app and access your online eBook or SmartBook 2.0 assignments when it's convenient, even if you're offline. And since the app automatically syncs with your eBook and SmartBook 2.0 assignments in Connect, all of your work is available every time you open it. Find out more at **www.mheducation.com/readanywhere**

> *"I really liked this app—it made it easy to study when you don't have your text-book in front of you."*
>
> - Jordan Cunningham,
>   Eastern Washington University

Calendar: owattaphotos/Getty Images

Everything you need in one place

Your Connect course has everything you need—whether reading on your digital eBook or completing assignments for class, Connect makes it easy to get your work done.

Learning for everyone

McGraw Hill works directly with Accessibility Services Departments and faculty to meet the learning needs of all students. Please contact your Accessibility Services Office and ask them to email accessibility@mheducation.com, or visit **www.mheducation.com/about/accessibility** for more information.

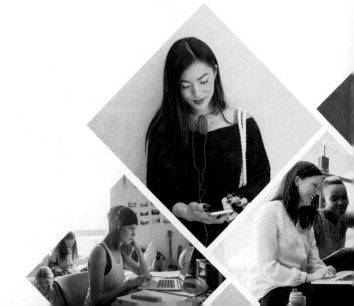

Top: Jenner Images/Getty Images, Left: Hero Images/Getty Images, Right: Hero Images/Getty Images

cultural anthropology

APPRECIATING CULTURAL DIVERSITY

NINETEENTH EDITION

Conrad Phillip Kottak
University of Michigan

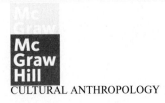

CULTURAL ANTHROPOLOGY

Published by McGraw Hill LLC, 1325 Avenue of the Americas, New York, NY 10121. Copyright © 2022 by McGraw Hill LLC. All rights reserved. Printed in the United States of America. No part of this publication may be reproduced or distributed in any form or by any means, or stored in a database or retrieval system, without the prior written consent of McGraw Hill LLC, including, but not limited to, in any network or other electronic storage or transmission, or broadcast for distance learning.

Some ancillaries, including electronic and print components, may not be available to customers outside the United States.

This book is printed on acid-free paper.

1 2 3 4 5 6 7 8 9 LWI 26 25 24 23 22 21

ISBN 978-1-260-59811-7
MHID 1-260-59811-X

Cover Image: *Rodrigo A Torres/Glow Images*

mheducation.com/highered

contents in brief

contents

PART 1   INTRODUCTION TO ANTHROPOLOGY

1   What Is Anthropology?   1

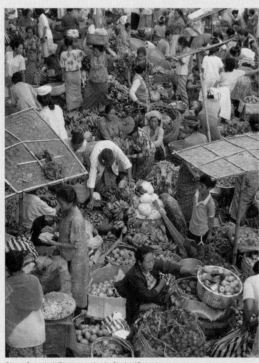

Steve Satushek/Photographer's Choice/Getty Images

2 Culture 18

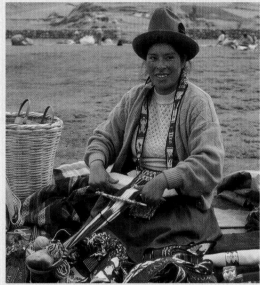

Danita Delimont/Alamy Images

3 Method and Theory in Cultural Anthropology 36

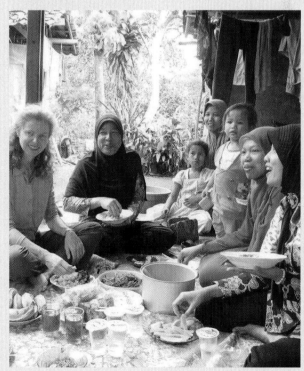

Courtesy Dr. Priscilla Magrath

4 Applying Anthropology *61*

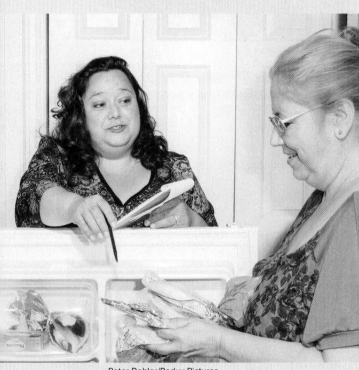

Peter Bohler/Redux Pictures

5 Language and Communication 80

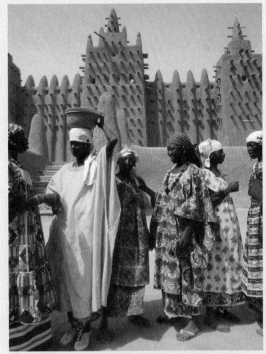

Glen Allison/Getty Images

6 Ethnicity and Race 101

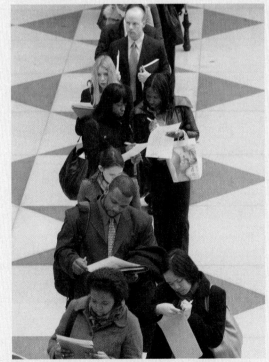

Don Emmert/Getty Images

7 Making a Living 132

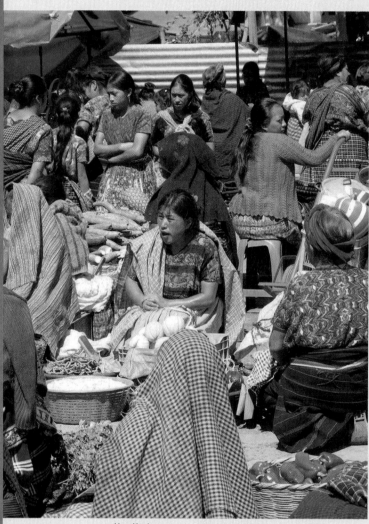

Lissa Harrison

8 Political Systems 155

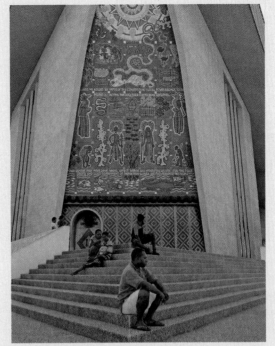

imageBROKER/Alamy Stock Photo

9 Gender 177

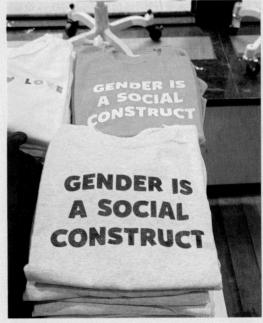

Ira Berger/Alamy Stock Photo

10 Families, Kinship, and Descent 199

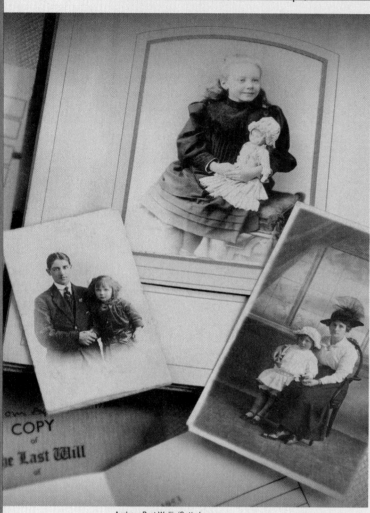

Andrew Bret Wallis/Getty Images

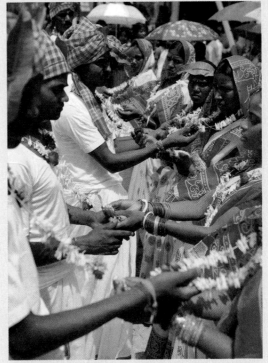

Diptendu Dutta/Getty Images

12 Religion 237

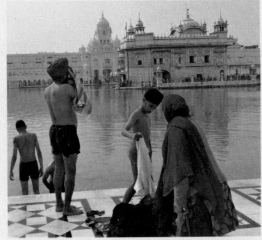

Conrad P. Kottak

13 Arts, Media, and Sports *259*

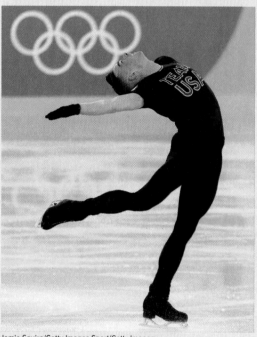

Jamie Squire/Getty Images Sport/Getty Images

14 The World System, Colonialism, and Inequality *281*

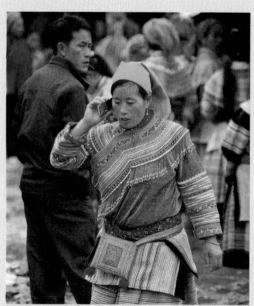

Jamie Marshall - Tribaleye Images/Photolibrary/Getty Images

15 Anthropology's Role in a Globalizing World *303*

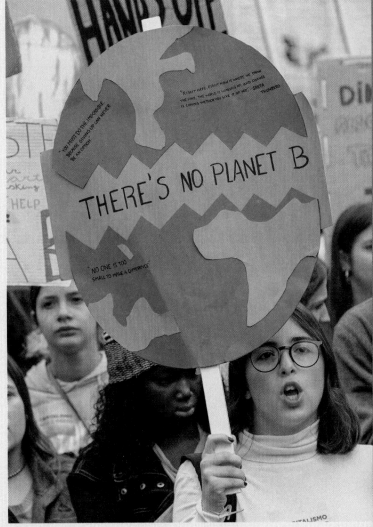

Horacio Villalobos/Getty Images

list of boxes

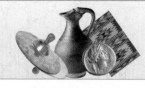

appreciating ANTHROPOLOGY

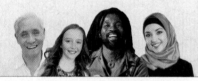

appreciating DIVERSITY

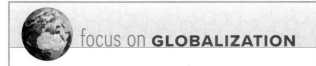

focus on GLOBALIZATION

RECAP

about the author

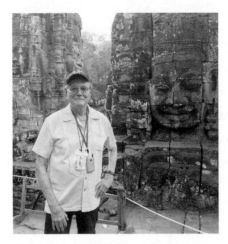

Conrad Phillip Kottak

The author at Bayon temple, Angkor Thom, Cambodia in February 2018.

Courtesy Isabel Wagley Kottak

Conrad Phillip Kottak (A.B. Columbia College, Ph.D. Columbia University) is the Julian H. Steward Collegiate Professor Emeritus of Anthropology at the University of Michigan, where he served as anthropology department chair from 1996 to 2006. He has been honored for his undergraduate teaching by the university and the state of Michigan and by the American Anthropological Association. He is an elected member of the American Academy of Arts and Sciences and the National Academy of Sciences, where he chaired Section 51, Anthropology from 2010 to 2013.

Professor Kottak has done ethnographic fieldwork in Brazil, Madagascar, and the United States. His general interests are in the processes by which local cultures are incorporated—and resist incorporation—into larger systems. This interest links his earlier work on ecology and state formation in Africa and Madagascar to his more recent research on globalization, national and international culture, and the mass media, including new media and social media.

Kottak's popular case study *Assault on Paradise: The Globalization of a Little Community in Brazil* (2006) describes his long-term and continuing fieldwork in Arembepe, Bahia, Brazil. His book *Prime-Time Society: An Anthropological Analysis of Television and Culture* (2009) is a comparative study of the nature and impact of television in Brazil and the United States.

Kottak's other books include *The Past in the Present: History, Ecology and Cultural Variation in Highland Madagascar; Researching American Culture: A Guide for Student Anthropologists;* and *Madagascar: Society and History.* The most recent editions (19th) of his texts *Anthropology: Appreciating Human Diversity* (this book) and *Cultural Anthropology: Appreciating Cultural Diversity* are published by McGraw-Hill. He also is the author of *Mirror for Humanity: A Concise Introduction to Cultural Anthropology* (12th ed., McGraw-Hill, 2020) and *Window on Humanity: A Concise Introduction to Anthropology* (9th ed., McGraw-Hill, 2020). With Kathryn A. Kozaitis, he wrote *On Being Different: Diversity and Multiculturalism in the North American Mainstream* (4th ed., McGraw-Hill, 2012).

Conrad Kottak's articles have appeared in academic journals, including *American Anthropologist, Journal of Anthropological Research, American Ethnologist, Ethnology, Human Organization,* and *Luso-Brazilian Review.* He also has written for popular journals, including *Transaction/SOCIETY, Natural History, Psychology Today,* and *General Anthropology.*

Kottak and his colleagues have researched television's impact in Brazil, environmental risk perception in Brazil, deforestation and biodiversity conservation in Madagascar, and economic development planning in northeastern Brazil. More recently, Kottak and his colleague Lara Descartes investigated how middle-class American families use various media in planning, managing, and evaluating the competing demands of work and family. That research is the basis of their book *Media and Middle Class Moms: Images and Realities of Work and Family* (Descartes and Kottak 2009). Professor Kottak currently is collaborating with Professor Richard Pace of Middle Tennessee State University and several graduate students on research investigating "The Evolution of Media Impact: A Longitudinal and Multi-Site Study of Television and New Electronic/Digital Media in Brazil."

Conrad Kottak appreciates comments about his books from professors and students. He can be reached by e-mail at the following address: **ckottak@bellsouth.net.**

a letter from the author

Welcome to the 19th Edition of *Cultural Anthropology: Appreciating Cultural Diversity!*

I wrote the first edition of this book during a time of rapid change in my favorite academic discipline—anthropology. My colleagues and I were excited about new discoveries and directions in all four of anthropology's subfields—biological anthropology, anthropological archaeology, sociocultural anthropology, and linguistic anthropology. My goal was to write a book that would capture that excitement, addressing key changes, while also providing a solid foundation of core concepts and the basics.

In preparing this edition, I benefited tremendously from both professors' and students' reactions to my book. Just as anthropology is a dynamic discipline that encourages new discoveries and explores the profound changes now affecting people and societies, this edition of *Cultural Anthropology* makes a concerted effort to keep pace with changes in the way students read and learn core content today. Our digital program, **Connect Anthropology,** includes assignable and assessable quizzes, exercises, and interactive activities, organized around course-specific learning objectives. Furthermore, **Connect** includes an interactive eBook; **LearnSmart,** which is an adaptive testing program; and **SmartBook,** the first and only truly adaptive reading experience. The tools and resources provided in **Connect Anthropology** are designed to engage students and enable them to improve their performance in the course. This 19th edition has benefited from feedback from thousands of students who have worked with these tools and programs while using the previous editions. We were able to flag and respond to specific areas of difficulty that students encountered, chapter by chapter. I used this extensive feedback to revise, rethink, and clarify my writing in almost every chapter. I started work on this 19th edition by once again reviewing how students had done on the probes and quizzes for each chapter in the previous edition. It became apparent that areas of difficulty reflected ambiguities both in the LearnSmart probes and in the textbook. Accordingly, I reviewed and, when necessary, rewrote every question for every chapter in the LearnSmart probes. I also wrote new probes for content new to this edition. I am eager to see, as students work with this new edition, whether my detailed work on both supplements and text enhances understanding and performance.

As I embark on each new edition, it becomes ever more apparent to me that while any competent and useful text must present anthropology's core, that text also must demonstrate anthropology's relevance to the 21st-century world we inhabit. Accordingly, each new edition contains thorough updating and substantial content changes as well as a series of features that examine our changing world. For example, several "Focus on Globalization" essays in this book examine topics as diverse as disease pandemics, world sports events (including the Olympics and the World Cup), and the expansion of international finance and branding. Several chapters contain discussions of new media, including social media. Many of the boxes titled "Appreciating Anthropology" and "Appreciating Diversity" (at least one per chapter) also present new discoveries and topics.

Each chapter begins with a discussion titled "Understanding Ourselves." These introductions, along with examples from popular culture throughout the book, show how anthropology relates to students' everyday lives. My overarching goal is to help students appreciate the field of cultural anthropology and the various kinds of diversity it studies. How do anthropologists think and work? Where do we go, and how do we interpret what we see? How do we step back, compare, and analyze? How does anthropology contribute to our understanding of the world? The "Appreciating Anthropology" boxes focus on the value and usefulness of anthropological research and approaches while the "Appreciating Diversity" boxes focus on various forms and expressions of human cultural diversity.

Most students who read this book will not go on to become anthropologists, or even anthropology majors. For those who do, this book should provide a solid foundation to build on. For those who don't—that is, for most of my readers—my goal is to instill a sense of appreciation: of human diversity, of anthropology as a field, and of how anthropology can build on, and help make sense of, the experience that students bring to the classroom. May this course and this text help students think differently about, and achieve greater understanding of, their own culture and its place within our globalizing world.

Conrad Phillip Kottak

preface

For over 40 years, students have found Conrad Kottak's Introductions to Anthropology and Cultural Anthropology thoughtful guides to the ever-changing discipline. His books are classics in the field offering undergraduates a comprehensive and robust set of materials that support and expand on the instruction they receive in the classroom or online. Students engage with rich content with an effective, efficient, and easy-to-use platform in Connect.

Connect is proven effective

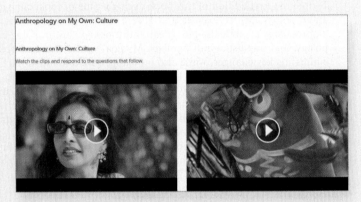

McGraw-Hill Connect® is a digital teaching and learning environment that improves performance over a variety of critical outcomes; it is easy to use; and it is proven effective. Connect® empowers students by continually adapting to deliver precisely what they need, when they need it, and how they need it, so your class time is more engaging and effective. Connect for *Anthropology* offers a wealth of interactive online content, including quizzes, exercises, and critical thinking questions, and "Applying Anthropology," "Anthropology on My Own," and "Anthropology on the Web" activities.

New to this edition, **Newsflash** activities bring in articles on current events relevant to anthropology with accompanying assessment. Topics include "Why Racism is Not Backed by Science" and "What Each of Facebook's 51 New Gender Options Means."

Connect also features these advanced capabilities

SMARTBOOK®   Available within Connect, **SmartBook®** makes study time as productive and efficient as possible by identifying and closing knowledge gaps. SmartBook is powered by the proven **LearnSmart®** engine, which identifies what an individual student knows and doesn't know based on the student's confidence level, responses to questions, and other factors. LearnSmart builds an optimal, personalized learning path for each student, so students spend less time on concepts they already understand and more time on those they don't. As a student engages with SmartBook, the reading experience continuously adapts by highlighting the most impactful content a student needs to learn at that moment in time. This ensures that every minute spent with SmartBook is returned to the student as the most value-added minute possible. The result? More confidence, better grades, and greater success.

New to this edition, SmartBook is now optimized for phones and tablets and accessible for students with disabilities using interactive features.

Culture Is Learned

The ease with which children absorb any cultural tradition rests on the uniquely elaborated human capacity to learn. Other animals may learn from experience; for example, they avoid fire after discovering that it hurts. Social animals also learn from other members of their group. Wolves, for instance, learn hunting strategies from other pack members. Such social learning is particularly important among monkeys and apes, our closest biological relatives. But our own *cultural learning* depends on the uniquely developed human capacity to use **symbols**, signs that have no necessary or natural connection to the things they signify or for which they stand.

On the basis of cultural learning, people create, remember, and deal with ideas. They grasp and apply specific systems of symbolic meaning. Anthropologist Clifford Geertz defines culture as ideas based on cultural learning and symbols. Cultures have been characterized as sets of "control mechanisms—plans, recipes, rules, instructions, what computer engineers call programs for the governing of behavior" (Geertz 1973, p. 44) These programs are absorbed by people through enculturation in particular traditions. People gradually internalize a previously established system of meanings and symbols. They use this cultural system to define their world, express their feelings, and make their judgments. This system helps guide their behavior and perceptions throughout their lives.

Every person begins immediately, through a process of conscious and unconscious learning and interaction with others, to internalize, or incorporate, a cultural tradition through the process of enculturation. Sometimes culture is taught directly, as when parents tell their children to say "thank you" when someone gives them something or does them a favor.

Practice « ← **22** / 546 → » A

Children learn to avoid fire by being told that it is dangerous while animals learn to avoid fire by discovering that it burns them. The difference between the two is that human cultural learning depends on

Click the answer you think is right.

primate tendencies.

evolutionary psychology.

the capacity to use symbols.

cultural diffusion.

Do you know the answer?   Read about this

I know it   Think so   Unsure   No idea

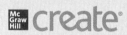 **Connect** INSIGHT   Connect Insight® is Connect's one-of-a-kind visual analytics dashboard—now available for both instructors and students—that provides at-a-glance information regarding student performance, which is immediately actionable. By presenting assignment, assessment, and topical performance results together with a time metric that is easily visible for aggregate or individual results, Connect Insight gives the user the capability to take a just-in-time approach to teaching and learning, which was never before available. Connect Insight presents data that empowers students and helps instructors improve class performance in a way that is efficient and effective.

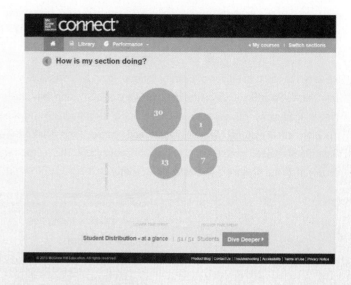

Your course, your way

McGraw-Hill Create® is a self-service website that allows you to create customized course materials using McGraw-Hill Education's comprehensive, cross-disciplinary content and digital products. You can even access third-party content such as readings, articles, cases, videos, and more.

- Select and arrange content to fit your course scope and sequence.
- Upload your own course materials.
- Select the best format for your students—print or eBook.
- Select and personalize your cover.
- Edit and update your materials as often as you'd like.

Experience how McGraw-Hill Education's Create empowers you to teach your students your way: **http://create.mheducation.com**.

Campus   **McGraw-Hill Campus®** is a groundbreaking service that puts world-class digital learning resources just a click away for all faculty and students. All faculty—whether or not they use a McGraw-Hill title—can instantly browse, search, and access the entire library of McGraw-Hill instructional resources and services, including eBooks, test banks, PowerPoint slides, animations, and learning objects—from any Learning Management System (LMS), at no additional cost to an institution. Users also have single sign-on access to McGraw-Hill digital platforms, including Connect, Create, and Tegrity, a fully automated lecture caption solution.

Instructor Resources

Instructor resources available through Connect for *Anthropology* include an Instructor's Manual, Test Bank, and PowerPoint presentation for each chapter.

Updates and Revisions—Informed by Student Data

Revisions to the 19th edition of *Cultural Anthropology* were extensively informed by student data, collected anonymously by McGraw-Hill Education's SmartBook. Using this data, we were able to graphically illustrate "hot spots," indicating content area students struggle with (see image below). This data provided feedback at the paragraph and even sentence level. Conrad Kottak relied on this data when making decisions about material to revise, update, and improve. Professor Kottak also reviewed and, when necessary, revised probes to make SmartBook an even more efficient and effective study tool. This revision was also informed by the many excellent reviews provided by faculty at 2- and 4-year schools across the country.

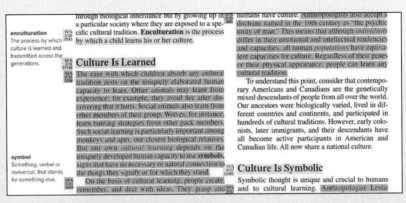

In addition to updated source research and statistical data, new photographs and illustrations, and newly titled "Think Like an Anthropologist" questions (formerly "Critical Thinking" questions) throughout the text, the following chapter-by-chapter changes have been made for the 19th edition:

CHAPTER 1: WHAT IS ANTHROPOLOGY?
- The chapter has been updated throughout, and the writing has been simplified in the section on the scientific method.

CHAPTER 2: CULTURE
- Recent studies of tool making by capuchin monkeys in Brazil and chimps in Guinea are discussed.
- President Trump's January 2020 threat to bomb Iranian cultural sites is used to frame the updated discussion of why heritage should be preserved and protected.
- There is new information on transnational communication in the section on globalization.

CHAPTER 3: METHOD AND THEORY IN CULTURAL ANTHROPOLOGY
- This chapter has been extensively updated, with revisions in writing to enhance clarity.

CHAPTER 4: APPLYING ANTHROPOLOGY
- The section on Urban Anthropology has been revised and updated.

CHAPTER 5: LANGUAGE AND COMMUNICATION
- The major section on "Sociolinguistics" has been reorganized, with new subheads added for clarity.
- The "Appreciating Diversity" box, "Words of the Year," has been updated and rewritten to reflect how the personal expression of gender identity (as in [my] pronouns and singular *they*) has become an increasing part of our shared discourse.
- A new "Focus on Globalization" box, "Naming a Pandemic: Do Geographic Names Stigmatize?" examines the naming of diseases, including the COVID-19 coronavirus.
- I streamlined the section on African American Vernacular English (AAVE).

CHAPTER 6: ETHNICITY AND RACE
- This chapter has been significantly updated, reorganized, and revised, with much new material. Specifics include:
- To the section "American Ethnic Groups," I have added the most recent changes in composition of racial and ethnic groups/categories in the United States.
- I have updated the section "Minority Groups and Stratification," with new data on the relation between poverty, income, and minority status.
- An updated discussion of "Race in the Census" describes the 2020 census form and its detailed questions on ethnicity, race, and national origins.
- A new discussion of biracial Japanese has been added.
- Recent election results now inform the "Backlash to Multiculturalism" section.
- The section "Ethnic Groups, Nations, and Nationalities" incorporates new data on ethnic diversity by country.
- Material formerly in the "Focus on Globalization" box on "The Gray and the Brown" has been moved into the text, as part of a new discussion of demographic projections for the United States through 2060, including significant growth in the dependency ratio.
- There are expanded discussions of the Bosnian and Rwandan genocides in the section on "Ethnic Conflict."

CHAPTER 7: MAKING A LIVING
- I updated the "Focus on Globalization" box, "Our Global Economy."
- A new "Appreciating Anthropology" box "To Give Is Good: Reciprocity and Human Survival" describes ongoing research by the Human Generosity Project, with a focus on recent fieldwork among the Ik of Uganda.
- I moved the old "Appreciating Anthropology" box on deindustrialization to Chapter 14.

CHAPTER 8: POLITICAL SYSTEMS
- To enhance clarity, I revised the discussions of bands, nomadic politics, and chiefdoms, offering clearer or more familiar examples.
- I updated the "Appreciating Anthropology" box, "The Illegality Industry: A Failed System of Border Control."

CHAPTER 9: GENDER

- I wrote a new "Appreciating Anthropology" box, "Patriarchy Today: Case Studies in Fundamentalist Communities," to replace the old one, which was dated. This one highlights Maxine Margolis's recent comparative study of female status in three fundamentalist religious communities.
- The section "Changes in Gendered Work" includes a revised and thoroughly updated discussion of labor force participation by gender.
- The section "Work and Happiness" contains an updated and expanded discussion of workforce participation and national feelings of wellbeing.
- The section titled "The Feminization of Poverty" has updated information on the relation between wealth and family structure.
- The "Beyond Male and Female" section has been revised substantially to clarify American gender categories in flux.

CHAPTER 10: FAMILIES, KINSHIP, AND DESCENT

- The section "Changes in North American Kinship" contains a revised and updated discussion of changing characteristics of American families, households, and children's living arrangements.
- There is a new discussion of "Relationships Queried in the 2020 Census."

CHAPTER 11: MARRIAGE

- I streamlined the section on "Divorce."
- The section on "The Online Marriage Market" has been substantially revised and updated.

CHAPTER 12: RELIGION

- I wrote a new "Appreciating Anthropology" box, "Rituals in a Pandemic's Shadow."
- In the section "Religion and Change," I added a new subsection on "Religious Change in the United States," informed by 2019 surveys and focusing on the shift to nonaffiliation.

CHAPTER 13: ARTS, MEDIA, AND SPORTS

- This chapter has been updated and streamlined throughout.
- There is a retitled, reorganized, and substantially rewritten section on "Online Access and Connectivity" in the major section "Media and Culture."

CHAPTER 14: THE WORLD SYSTEM, COLONIALISM, AND INEQUALITY

- The section "Wealth Distribution in the United States" has been revised and incorporates the latest available statistics on inequality, and its relation to political mobilization.
- Thoroughly revised and updated section on "Neoliberalism and NAFTA's Economic Refugees," including discussion of the USMCA trade pact revision.
- A new box for this chapter, "When the Mills Shut Down: An Anthropologist Looks at Deindustrialization," was moved here from Chapter 7.

CHAPTER 15: ANTHROPOLOGY'S ROLE IN A GLOBALIZING WORLD

- Two major sections: "Energy Consumption and Industrial Degradation" and "Global Climate Change" have been thoroughly revised, updated, and reorganized, including an updated Table 15.1, "Energy Consumption for the Top 12 Countries, 2018."
- In the section on "Emerging Diseases," there is a new discussion of the 2020 coronavirus, as well as a report on the Trump administration's termination of the USAID-supported PREDICT program, which searched for, identified, and catalogued potentially lethal zoonotic pathogens.

Acknowledgments

I'm grateful to many colleagues at McGraw-Hill Education. I offer particular thanks to product developer Bruce Cantley, who helped me plan and implement this revision, and worked with me to complete and submit the manuscript on schedule.

Bruce responded rapidly, efficiently, and encouragingly to my revisions, making helpful suggestions, and keeping track of all the changes I made chapter-by-chapter. Thanks, too, to Claire Brantley, portfolio manager; Dawn Groundwater, lead product developer; Elisa Odoardi, editorial coordinator; and to McGraw-Hill's entire team of sales reps and regional managers for the work they do in helping professors and students gain access to my books. I also acknowledge Michael Ryan, President of Higher Education.

As usual, Rick Hecker has done a great job as content project manager, guiding the manuscript through production and keeping everything moving on schedule. Sue Culbertson, buyer, worked with the printer to make sure everything came out right. Thanks, too, to Charlotte Goldman, freelance photo researcher. I also thank Amy Marks for copyediting, Marlena Pechan for proofreading, and Egzon Shaqiri for executing the design.

Carrie Burger also deserves thanks as content licensing specialist.

I'm also indebted to the reviewers who have evaluated this book and, through their comments, helped guide its development.

Their names are as follows:

AnnMarie Beasley, *American River College*
Beau Bowers, *Central Piedmont Community College*
Robert B. Chamberlain, *Eastern Florida State College*
Carolyn Coulter, *Atlantic Cape Community College*
Alexa Dietrich, *Wagner College*
Jennifer Elliott, *Estrella Mountain Community College*
Pam Frese, *College of Wooster*
Allison Harnish, *Albion College*
Ridge Harper, *Bainbridge State College*
John Henderson, *Cornell University*

Elizabeth Hoag, *Cuyahoga Community College*
Mary Hotvedt, *Western New Mexico University*
Kendi Howells Douglas, *Johnson University*
Danielle James, *Community College of Baltimore County*
Shepherd Jenks, *Central New Mexico Community College*
Priscilla LoForte, *Cosumnes River College*
Vincent Lyon-Callo, *Western Michigan University*
Ann Magennis, *Colorado State University*
Jose Martinez-Reyes, *University of Massachusetts, Boston*
Megan McCullen, *Alma College*

David Otto, *Centenary College*

Jason Pribilsky, *Whitman College*

Van Reidhead, *East Stroudsburg University*

Wayman Smith, *Georgia State University–Perimeter College*

Lisa Volle, *Central Texas College*

Deborah J. Wickering, *Aquinas College*

LaCretia Williams, *Alabama State University*

Andre Yefremian, *Chaffey College*

I'm also grateful to the reviewers of previous editions of this book and of my *Cultural Anthropology* text. Their names are as follows:

Julianna Acheson, *Green Mountain College*

Stephanie W. Alemán, *Iowa State University*

Mohammad Al-Madani, *Seattle Central Community College*

Maria Altemara, *West Virginia University, Robert Morris University*

Douglas J. Anderson, *Front Range Community College*

E. F. Aranyosi, *University of Washington*

Timi Lynne Barone, *University of Nebraska, Omaha*

Robert Bee, *University of Connecticut*

Joy A. Bilharz, *SUNY at Fredonia*

James R. Bindon, *University of Alabama*

Kira Blaisdell-Sloan, *Louisiana State University*

Kathleen T. Blue, *Minnesota State University*

Renée M. Bonzani, *University of Kentucky*

Daniel Boxberger, *Western Washington University*

Vicki Bradley, *University of Houston*

Lisa Kaye Brandt, *North Dakota State University*

Ethan M. Braunstein, *Northern Arizona University*

Ned Breschel, *Morehead State University*

Christopher A. Brooks, *Virginia Commonwealth University*

Peter J. Brown, *Emory University*

Margaret S. Bruchez, *Blinn College*

Vaughn M. Bryant, *Texas A&M University*

Andrew Buckser, *Purdue University*

Richard H. Buonforte, *Brigham Young University*

Karen Burns, *University of Georgia*

Richard Burns, *Arkansas State University*

Mary Cameron, *Auburn University*

Joseph L. Chartkoff, *Michigan State University*

Dianne Chidester, *University of South Dakota*

Stephen Childs, *Valdosta State University*

Inne Choi, *California Polytechnic State University–San Luis Obispo*

Bonny Christy, *Blinn College*

Wanda Clark, *South Plains College*

Jeffrey Cohen, *Penn State University*

Fred Conquest, *Community College of Southern Nevada*

Barbara Cook, *California Polytechnic State University–San Luis Obispo*

Maia Greenwell Cunningham, *Citrus College*

Sean M. Daley, *Johnson County Community College*

Karen Dalke, *University of Wisconsin–Green Bay*

Norbert Dannhaeuser, *Texas A&M University*

Michael Davis, *Truman State University*

Hillary Delprete, *Wagner College*

Paul Demers, *University of Nebraska–Lincoln*

Darryl de Ruiter, *Texas A&M University*

Robert Dirks, *Illinois State University*

William W. Donner, *Kutztown University*

William Doonan, *Sacramento City College*

Mary Durocher, *Wayne State University*

Paul Durrenberger, *Pennsylvania State University*

George Esber, *Miami University of Ohio*

Les W. Field, *University of New Mexico*

Grace Fraser, *Plymouth State College*

Todd Jeffrey French, *University of New Hampshire, Durham*

Richard H. Furlow, *College of DuPage*

Vance Geiger, *University of Central Florida*

Laurie Godfrey, *University of Massachusetts–Amherst*

Bob Goodby, *Franklin Pierce College*

Gloria Gozdzik, *West Virginia University*

Tom Greaves, *Bucknell University*

Mark Grey, *University of Northern Iowa*

Sharon Gursky, *Texas A&M University*

John Dwight Hines, *University of California, Santa Barbara*

Brian A. Hoey, *Marshall University*

Homes Hogue, *Mississippi State University*

Kara C. Hoover, *Georgia State University*

Charles W. Houck, *University of North Carolina–Charlotte*

Stevan R. Jackson, *Virginia Tech*

Alice James, *Shippensburg University of Pennsylvania*

Cara Roure Johnson, *University of Connecticut*

Kevin Keating, *Broward College*

Richard King, *Drake University*

Max Kirsch, *Florida Atlantic University*

Amy Kowal, *Florida State University*

Christine Kray, *Rochester Institute of Technology*

Eric Lassiter, *Ball State University*

Jill Leonard, *University of Illinois–Urbana-Champaign*

Kenneth Lewis, *Michigan State University*

David Lipset, *University of Minnesota*

Walter E. Little, *University at Albany, SUNY*

Jon K. Loessin, *Wharton County Junior College*

Brian Malley, *University of Michigan*

Jonathan Marks, *University of North Carolina–Charlotte*

Merri Mattison, *Red Rocks Community College*

Reece Jon McGee, *Texas State University*

Kare McManama-Kearin, *Weber State University*

H. Lyn Miles, *University of Tennessee at Chattanooga*

Barbara Miller, *George Washington University*

Richard G. Milo, *Chicago State University*

John Nass, Jr., *California University of Pennsylvania*

Andrew Nelson, *University of North Texas*

Frank Ng, *California State University–Fresno*

Constanza Ocampo-Raeder, *University of Maine (Orono)*

Divinity B. O'Connor DLR-Roberts, *Des Moines Area Community College*

Martin Ottenheimer, *Kansas State University*

De Ann Pendry, *University of Tennessee–Knoxville*

Holly Peters-Golden, *University of Michigan*

Leonard Plotnicov, *University of Pittsburgh*

Janet Pollak, *William Paterson University*

Christina Nicole Pomianek, *University of Missouri–Columbia*

Geoffrey G. Pope, *William Paterson University*

Howard Prince, *CUNY–Borough of Manhattan Community College*

Frances E. Purifoy, *University of Louisville*

Asa Randall, *University of Florida*

Mark A. Rees, *University of Louisiana at Lafayette*

Bruce D. Roberts, *Minnesota State University Moorhead*

Rita C. Rodabaugh, *Central Piedmont Community College*

Leila Rodriguez, *University of Cincinnati*

Steven Rubenstein, *Ohio University*

Robert Rubinstein, *Syracuse University*

Richard A. Sattler, *University of Montana*

Richard Scaglion, *University of Pittsburgh*

Mary Scott, *San Francisco State University*

Scott Sernau, *Indiana University South Bend*

James Sewastynowicz, *Jacksonville State University*

Brian Siegel, *Furman University*

Michael Simonton, *Northern Kentucky University*

Megan Sinnott, *University of Colorado–Boulder*

Esther Skirboll, *Slippery Rock University of Pennsylvania*

Alexia Smith, *University of Connecticut*

Wayman Smith, *Georgia State University–Perimeter College*

Gregory Starrett, *University of North Carolina–Charlotte*

Karl Steinen, *University of West Georgia*

Noelle Stout, *Foothill and Skyline Colleges*

Merrily Stover, *University of Maryland–University College*

Jessica Thompson, *Emory University*

Elizabeth A. Throop, *Eastern Kentucky University*

Ruth Toulson, *Brigham Young University*

Susan Trencher, *George Mason University*

Mark Tromans, *Broward Community College*

Christina Turner, *Virginia Commonwealth University*

Donald Tyler, *University of Idaho*

Daniel Varisco, *Hofstra University*

Albert Wahrhaftig, *Sonoma State University*

Heather Walder, *University of Wisconsin–La Crosse*

Joe Watkins, *University of New Mexico*

David Webb, *Kutztown University of Pennsylvania*

George Westermark, *Santa Clara University*

Donald A. Whatley, *Blinn College*

Nancy White, *University of South Florida*

Katharine Wiegele, *Northern Illinois University*

Mary S. Willis, *University of Nebraska–Lincoln*

Brent Woodfill, *University of Louisiana at Lafayette*

Very, very, special thanks as well to the thousands of students whose responses in SmartBook helped me pinpoint content and writing that needed clarification. Never have so many voices contributed to a revision as to this one.

Other professors and students regularly share their insights about this and my other texts via e-mail and so have contributed to this book. I'm especially grateful to my Michigan colleagues who use my books and have suggested ways of making them better. Thanks especially to a 101 team that has included Tom Fricke, Stuart Kirsch, Holly Peters-Golden, and Andrew Shryock. By now, I've benefited from the knowledge, help, and advice of so many friends, colleagues, teaching assistants, graduate student instructors, and students that I can no longer fit their names into a short acnowledgment. I hope they know who they are and accept my thanks.

As usual, my family offers me understanding, support, and inspiration during the preparation of this book. Dr. Nicholas Kottak, who, like me, holds a doctorate in anthropology, regularly shares his insights with me, as does my daughter, Dr. Juliet Kottak Mavromatis, and my wife, Isabel Wagley Kottak. Isabel has been my companion in the field and in life during my entire career in anthropology, and I can't imagine being without her. I renew my dedication of this book to the memory of my mother, Mariana Kottak Roberts, who kindled my interest in the human condition and provided many insights about people and society.

Over my many years of teaching anthropology, feedback from students has kept me up to date on the interests and needs of my readers, as does my ongoing participation in workshops on the teaching of anthropology. I hope this product of my experience will be helpful to others.

Conrad Phillip Kottak
Seabrook Island, South Carolina, and Decatur, Georgia
ckottak@bellsouth.net

What Is Anthropology?

▶ What distinguishes anthropology from other fields that study human beings?

▶ How do anthropologists study human diversity in time and space?

▶ Why is anthropology both scientific and humanistic?

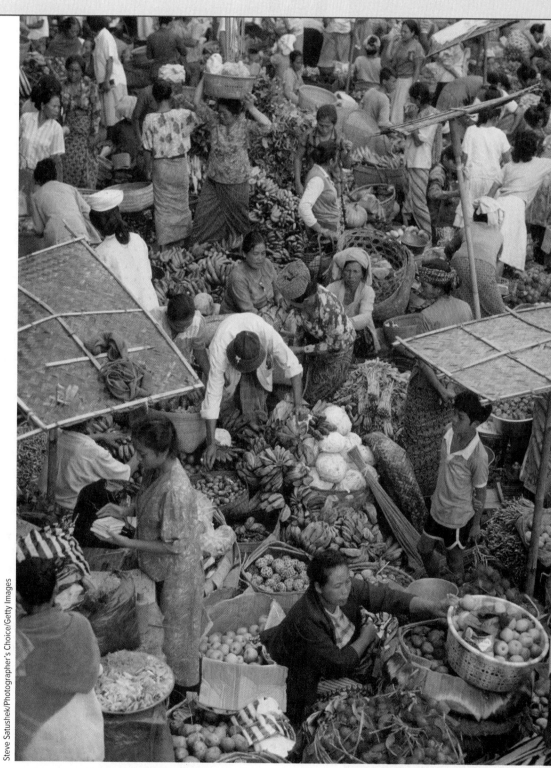

Steve Satushek/Photographer's Choice/Getty Images

A produce market in Ubud, Bali, Indonesia.

understanding OURSELVES

When you grew up, which sport did you appreciate the most— soccer, swimming, football, baseball, tennis, golf, or some other sport (or perhaps none at all)? Is this because of "who you are" or because of the opportunities you had as a child to practice and participate in this particular activity? Think about the phrases and sentences you would use to describe yourself in a personal ad or on a networking site—your likes and dislikes, hobbies, and habits. How many of these descriptors would be the same if you had been born in a different place or time?

When you were young, your parents might have told you that drinking milk and eating vegetables would help you grow up "big and strong." They probably didn't recognize as readily the role that culture plays in shaping bodies, personalities, and personal health. If nutrition matters in growth, so, too, do cultural guidelines. What is proper behavior for boys and girls? What kinds of work should men and women do? Where should people live? What are proper uses of their leisure time? What role should religion play? How should people relate to their family, friends, and neighbors? Although our genetic attributes provide a foundation for our growth and development, human biology is fairly plastic—that is, it is malleable. Culture is an environmental force that affects our development as much as do nutrition, heat, cold, and altitude. Culture also guides our emotional and cognitive growth and helps determine the kinds of personalities we have as adults.

Among scholarly disciplines, anthropology stands out as the field that provides the cross-cultural test. How much would we know about human behavior, thought, and feeling if we studied only our own kind? What if our entire understanding of human behavior were based on analysis of questionnaires filled out by college students in Oregon? Get in the habit of asking this question: What is the basis of any statement or generalization you may read or hear concerning what humans are like, individually or collectively? A primary reason anthropology can uncover so much about what it means to be human is that the discipline is based on the cross-cultural perspective. A single nation or culture simply cannot tell us everything we need to know about what it means to be human. We need to compare and contrast. Often culture is "invisible" (assumed to be normal, or just the way things are) until it is placed in comparison to another culture. For example, to appreciate how people use media, and the effects of such use, we need to consider not just contemporary North America but other places—and perhaps even other times. Right now, for example, I am part of a research team that is studying the evolution of media (including broadcast and streaming TV as well as social media) and its use in Brazil from the 1980s through the present. We will eventually compare this evolution with changes in media use and effects in the United States over a comparable period of time. The cross-cultural test is fundamental to the anthropological approach, which orients this textbook.

HUMAN DIVERSITY

Anthropologists study human beings and their products wherever and whenever they find them—in rural Kenya, a Turkish café, a Mesopotamian tomb, or a North American shopping center. Anthropology explores human diversity across time and space, seeking to understand as much as possible about the human condition. Of particular interest is the diversity that comes through human adaptability.

Humans are among the world's most adaptable animals. In the Andes of South America, people wake up in villages 16,000 feet above sea level and then trek 1,500 feet higher to work in tin mines. In the Australian outback, people worship animals and discuss philosophy. Humans survive malaria in the tropics. A dozen men have walked on the moon. The model of the USS *Enterprise* in Washington's Smithsonian Institution symbolizes the desire to "seek out new life and civilizations, to boldly go where no one has gone before." Wishes to know the unknown, control the uncontrollable, and create order out of chaos find expression among all peoples. Creativity, adaptability, and flexibility are basic human attributes, and human diversity is the subject matter of anthropology.

Students often are surprised by the breadth of **anthropology,** which is the study of humans around the world and through time. Anthropology is a uniquely comparative and **holistic** science. *Holism* refers to the study of the whole of the human condition: past, present, and future; biology, society, language, and culture. Most people think that anthropologists study fossils and nonindustrial, non-Western cultures, and many of them do. But anthropology is much more than the study of nonindustrial peoples: It is a comparative field that examines all societies, ancient and modern, simple and complex, local and global. The other social sciences tend to focus on a single society, usually their own nation, such as the United States or Canada. Anthropology, however, offers a unique cross-cultural perspective by constantly comparing the customs of one society with those of others.

People share **society**—organized life in groups—with other animals, including monkeys, apes, wolves, mole rats, and even ants. **Culture,** however, is more distinctly human. Cultures are traditions and customs, transmitted through learning, that form and guide the beliefs and behavior of the people exposed to them. Children learn such a tradition by growing up in a particular society, through a process called enculturation. Cultural traditions include customs and opinions, developed over the generations, about proper and improper behavior. These traditions answer such questions as: How should we do things? How do we make sense of the world? How do we distinguish between what is right, and what is wrong? A culture produces a degree of consistency in behavior and thought among the people who live in a particular society.

The most critical element of cultural traditions is their transmission through learning rather than through biological inheritance. Culture is not itself biological, but it rests on certain features of human biology. For more than a million years, humans have possessed at least some of the biological capacities on which culture depends. These abilities are to learn, to think symbolically, to use language, and to make and use tools.

Anthropology confronts and ponders major questions about past and present human existence. By examining ancient bones and tools, we unravel the mysteries of human origins. When did our ancestors separate from those of the apes? Where and when did *Homo sapiens* originate?

society
Organized life in groups; shared with humans by monkeys, apes, wolves, mole rats, and ants, among other animals.

culture
Traditions and customs transmitted through learning.

anthropology
The study of the humans around the world and through time.

holistic
Encompassing past, present, and future; biology, society, language, and culture.

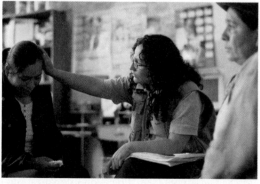
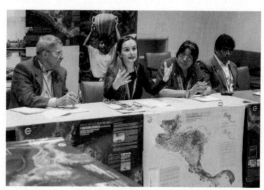

Today's anthropologists work in varied roles and settings. Nory Condor Alarcon (left photo) is an anthropologist who works for the Forensic Laboratory of the Public Ministry of Ayacucho, Peru. Here she comforts a young woman as she confirms that the lab's forensic team has identified the remains of several of her close relatives. In the photo on the right, a group of experts including anthropologist Mac Chapin (left), hold a press conference at UN Headquarters in New York introducing a new high-tech map of Indigenous Peoples of Central America.
(left): Robin Hammond/IDRC/Panos Pictures/Redux Pictures; (right): EDUARDO MUNOZ ALVAREZ/Stringer/Getty Images

FORM OF ADAPTATION	TYPE OF ADAPTATION	EXAMPLE
Technology	Cultural	Pressurized airplane cabin with oxygen masks
Genetic adaptation (occurs over generations)	Biological	Larger "barrel chests" of native highlanders
Long-term physiological adaptation (occurs during growth and development of the individual organism)	Biological	More efficient respiratory system, to extract oxygen from "thin air"
Short-term physiological adaptation (occurs spontaneously when the individual organism enters a new environment)	Biological	Increased heart rate, hyperventilation

How has our species changed? What are we now, and where are we going? How have social and cultural changes influenced biological change? Our genus, *Homo,* has been changing for more than one million years. Humans continue to adapt and change both biologically and culturally.

Adaptation, Variation, and Change

Adaptation refers to the processes by which organisms cope with environmental forces and stresses. How do organisms change to fit their environments, such as dry climates or high mountain altitudes? Like other animals, humans have biological means of adaptation. But humans also habitually rely on cultural means of adaptation. Recap 1.1 summarizes some of the cultural and biological ways in which humans adapt to high altitudes.

Mountainous terrains pose particular challenges, those associated with altitude and oxygen deprivation. Consider four ways (one cultural and three biological) in which humans may cope with low oxygen pressure at high altitudes. Illustrating cultural (technological) adaptation would be a pressurized airplane cabin equipped with oxygen masks. There are three ways of adapting biologically to high altitudes: genetic adaptation, long-term physiological adaptation, and short-term physiological adaptation. First, native populations of high-altitude areas, such as the Andes of Peru and the Himalayas of Tibet and Nepal, seem to have acquired certain genetic advantages for life at very high altitudes. The Andean tendency to develop a voluminous chest and lungs probably has a genetic basis. Second, regardless of their genes, people who grow up at a high altitude become physiologically more efficient there than genetically similar people who have grown up at sea level would be. This illustrates long-term physiological adaptation during the body's growth and development. Third, humans also have the capacity for short-term or

food production

An economy based on plant cultivation and/or animal domestication.

immediate physiological adaptation. Thus, when lowlanders arrive in the highlands, they immediately increase their breathing and heart rates. Hyperventilation increases the oxygen in their lungs and arteries. As the pulse also increases, blood reaches their tissues more rapidly. These varied adaptive responses—cultural and biological—all fulfill the need to supply an adequate amount of oxygen to the body.

As human history has unfolded, the social and cultural means of adaptation have become increasingly important. In this process, humans have devised diverse ways of coping with the range of environments they have occupied in time and space. The rate of cultural adaptation and change has accelerated, particularly during the last 10,000 years. For millions of years, hunting and gathering of nature's bounty—*foraging*—was the sole basis of human subsistence. However, it took only a few thousand years for **food production** (the cultivation of plants and domestication of animals), which originated some 12,000–10,000 years ago, to replace foraging in most areas. Between 6000 and 5000 B.P. (before the present), the first civilizations arose. These were large, powerful, and complex societies, such as ancient Egypt, that conquered and governed large geographic areas.

Much more recently, the spread of industrial production has profoundly affected human life. Throughout human history, major innovations have spread at the expense of earlier ones. Each economic revolution has had social and cultural repercussions. Today's global economy and communications link all contemporary people, directly or indirectly, in the modern world system. Nowadays, even remote villagers experience world forces and events (see "Focus on Globalization"). The study of how local people adapt to global forces poses new challenges for anthropology: "The cultures of world peoples need to be constantly rediscovered as these people reinvent them in changing historical circumstances" (Marcus and Fischer 1986, p. 24).

focus on GLOBALIZATION

World Events

People everywhere—even remote villagers—now participate in world events, especially through the mass media. The study of global–local linkages is a prominent part of modern anthropology. What kinds of events generate global interest? Disasters provide one example. Think of missing airplanes, nuclear plant meltdowns, and the earthquakes and tsunamis that have ravaged Thailand, Indonesia, and Japan. In July 2018, the world was riveted to the plight of Thai kids trapped in a cave and their daring rescue. Think, too, of space—the final frontier: As many as 600 million people may have watched the first (Apollo 11) moon landing in 1969—a huge audience in the early days of global television.

Consider, too, the British royal family, especially the photogenic ones. The wedding of Prince William and Catherine Middleton attracted 161 million viewers—twice the population of the United Kingdom. A generation earlier, millions of people had watched Lady Diana Spencer marry England's Prince Charles. Her funeral also attracted a global audience. In 2020, Prince Harry and his wife Meghan Markle, Duke and Duchess of Sussex, fled with their son Archie to Canada. To escape global media attention, the Sussexes were willing to give up their royal duties and titles.

And, of course, think of sports: Billions of people watched at least some of the last Summer Olympics. Consider the FIFA World Cup (soccer), also held every four years. In 2006, an estimated 320 million people tuned in to the tournament's final game. This figure almost tripled to 909 million in 2010, and more than one billion viewers saw Germany defeat Argentina in the 2014 final. Four years later, more than 3.5 billion people, half the world's population, watched at least

some of the 2018 World Cup. Once again, more than a billion people (1.12) tuned in the for the final, in which France beat Croatia 4-2. The World Cup generates huge global interest because it truly is a "world series," with 32 countries and five continents competing. Similarly, the Cricket World Cup, held every four years (most recently in 2019), is the world's third most watched event: Only the Summer Olympics and the FIFA World Cup exceed it. Live coverage of the 2019 Cricket World Cup attracted a cumulative audience of 1.6 billion people in over 200 countries.

It's rather arrogant to call American baseball's ultimate championship "The World Series" when only one non-U.S. team, the Toronto Blue Jays, can play in it. (The title dates back to 1903, a time of less globalization and more American provincialism.) Baseball is popular in the United States (including Puerto Rico), Canada, Japan, Cuba, Mexico, Venezuela, and the Dominican Republic. South Korea, Taiwan, and China have professional leagues. Elsewhere the sport has little mass appeal (see Gmelch and Nathan 2017).

Even so, when we focus on the players in American baseball we see a multiethnic world in miniature. With its prominent Latino and Asian players, American baseball is more ethnically diverse than American football or basketball. Consider the finalists for the major MLB (Major League Baseball) awards (Most Valuable Player, Cy Young, Rookie of the Year) for the years 2018 and 2019. Those finalists included players from Canada, Cuba, the Dominican Republic, Japan, Puerto Rico, South Korea, the United States, and Venezuela. Can you think of a sport as ethnically diverse as baseball? What's the last world event that drew your attention?

Cultural Forces Shape Human Biology

Anthropology's comparative, biocultural perspective recognizes that cultural forces constantly mold human biology. (**Biocultural** refers to using and combining both biological and cultural perspectives and approaches to analyze and understand a particular issue or problem.) As we saw in "Understanding Ourselves," culture is a key environmental force in determining how human bodies grow and develop. Cultural traditions promote certain activities and abilities, discourage others, and set standards of physical well-being and attractiveness. Consider how this works in sports. North American girls are encouraged to pursue, and therefore do well in, competition involving figure skating, gymnastics, track and field, swimming, diving, and many other sports. Brazilian girls, although excelling in the team sports of basketball and volleyball, haven't fared nearly as

well in individual sports as have their American and Canadian counterparts. Why are people encouraged to excel as athletes in some nations but not others? Why do people in some countries invest so much time and effort in competitive sports that their bodies change significantly as a result? Why do Americans engage in combat sports such as football, which can cause irreversible damage to brains and bodies.

Cultural standards of attractiveness and propriety influence participation and achievement in sports. Americans run or swim not just to compete but also to keep trim and fit. Brazil's beauty standards traditionally have accepted more fat, especially in female buttocks and hips. Brazilian men have had significant international success in swimming and running, but it is less common to see Brazilian women excelling in those sports. One reason why Brazilian women are underrepresented in competitive swimming may be that sport's

biocultural
Combining biological and cultural approaches to a given problem.

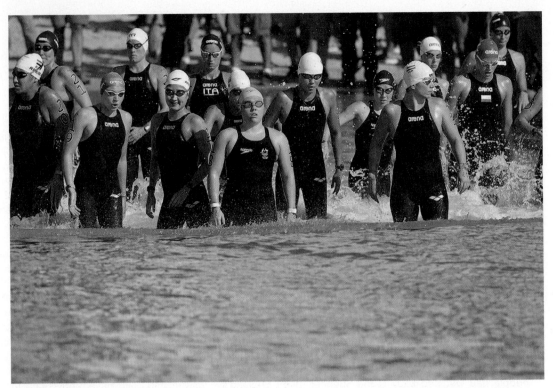

Athletes primed for the start of the 10 kilometer women's marathon swim at the 2016 Summer Olympics in Rio de Janeiro. Years of swimming sculpt a distinctive physique—an enlarged upper torso and neck, and powerful shoulders and back.

Tim de Waele/Getty Images

effects on the body. Years of swimming sculpt a distinctive physique: an enlarged upper torso, a massive neck, and powerful shoulders and back. Successful female swimmers tend to be big, strong, and bulky. The countries that have produced them most consistently are the United States, Canada, Australia, Germany, the Scandinavian nations, the Netherlands, the former Soviet Union, and (more recently) China, where this body type isn't as stigmatized as it is in Latin countries. For women, Brazilian culture prefers more ample hips and buttocks to a more muscled upper body. Many young female swimmers in Brazil choose to abandon the sport rather than their culture's "feminine" body ideal.

general anthropology
Anthropology as a whole: cultural, archaeological, biological, and linguistic anthropology.

GENERAL ANTHROPOLOGY

The academic discipline of anthropology, also known as **general anthropology** or "four-field" anthropology, includes

Early American anthropology was especially concerned with the history and cultures of Native North Americans. Ely S. Parker, or Ha-sa-noan-da, was a Seneca Indian who made important contributions to early anthropology. Parker also served as commissioner of Indian affairs for the United States.

National Archives and Records Administration

four main subdisciplines or subfields. They are sociocultural anthropology, anthropological archaeology, biological anthropology, and linguistic anthropology. (From here on, I'll use the shorter term *cultural anthropology* as a synonym for "sociocultural anthropology.") Cultural anthropology focuses on societies of the present and recent past. Anthropological archaeology reconstructs lifeways of ancient and more recent societies through analysis of material remains. Biological anthropology studies human biological variation through time and across geographic space. Linguistic anthropology examines language in its social and cultural contexts. Of the four subfields, cultural anthropology has the largest membership. Most departments of anthropology teach courses in all four subfields. (Note that general anthropology did not develop as a comparable field of study in most European countries, where the subdisciplines tend to exist separately.)

There are historical reasons for the inclusion of the four subfields in a single discipline in North America. The origin of anthropology as a scientific field, and of American anthropology in particular, can be traced back to the 19th century. Early American anthropologists were concerned especially with the history and cultures of the indigenous peoples of North America. Interest in the origins and diversity of Native Americans (called First Nations in Canada) brought together studies of customs, social life, language, and physical traits. Anthropologists still are pondering such questions as these: Where did Native Americans come from? How many waves of migration brought them to the New World? What are the linguistic, cultural, and biological links among Native Americans and between them and Asians?

There also are logical reasons for including anthropology's four subfields in the same academic discipline. Answers to key questions in anthropology often require an understanding of both human biology and culture and of both the past and the present. Each subfield considers variation in time and space (that is, in different geographic areas). Cultural anthropologists and anthropological archaeologists study (among many other topics) changes in social life and customs. Archaeologists have used studies of living societies and behavior patterns to imagine what life might have been like in the past. Biological anthropologists examine evolutionary changes in physical form, for example, anatomical changes that might have been associated with the origin of tool use or language. Linguistic anthropologists may reconstruct the basics of ancient languages by studying modern ones.

The subdisciplines influence each other as members of the different subfields talk to each other, share books and journals, and associate in departments and at professional meetings. General anthropology explores the basics of human biology, society, and culture and considers their interrelations. Anthropologists share certain key assumptions. Perhaps the most fundamental is the idea that we cannot reach sound conclusions about "human nature" by studying a single nation, society, or cultural tradition. A comparative, cross-cultural approach is essential.

THE SUBDISCIPLINES OF ANTHROPOLOGY

Cultural Anthropology

Cultural anthropology, the study of human society and culture, is the subfield that describes, analyzes, interprets, and explains social and cultural similarities and differences. To study and interpret cultural diversity, cultural anthropologists

engage in two kinds of activity: ethnography (based on fieldwork) and ethnology (based on cross-cultural comparison). **Ethnography** provides an account of a particular group, community, society, or culture. During ethnographic fieldwork, the ethnographer gathers data that he or she organizes, describes, analyzes, and interprets to build and present that account, which may be in the form of a book, an article, or a film. Traditionally, ethnographers lived in small communities, where they studied local behavior, beliefs, customs, social life, economic activities, politics, and religion. Today, any ethnographer will recognize that external forces and events have an increasing influence on such settings.

An anthropological perspective derived from ethnographic fieldwork often differs radically from that of economics or political science. Those fields focus on national and official organizations and policies and often on elites. However, the groups that anthropologists traditionally have studied usually have been relatively poor and powerless. Ethnographers often observe discriminatory practices directed toward such people, who experience food and water shortages, dietary deficiencies, and other aspects of poverty. Political scientists tend to study programs that national planners develop, whereas anthropologists discover how these programs work on the local level.

Communities and cultures are less isolated today than ever before. In fact, as the anthropologist Franz Boas (1940/1966) noted many years ago, contact between neighboring tribes has always existed and has extended over enormous areas. "Human populations construct their cultures in interaction with one another, and not in isolation" (Wolf 1982, p. ix). Villagers increasingly participate in regional, national, and world events. Exposure to external forces comes through the mass media, migration, and modern transportation. (This chapter's "Appreciating Anthropology" box examines the role of a residential school in eastern India in bridging barriers between cultures.) City, nation, and world increasingly invade local communities with the arrival of tourists, development agents, government and religious officials, and political candidates. Such linkages are prominent components of regional, national, and global systems of politics, economics, and information. These larger systems increasingly affect the people and places anthropology traditionally has studied. The study of such linkages and systems is part of the subject matter of modern anthropology.

Ethnology examines, interprets, and analyzes the results of ethnography—the data gathered in different societies. It uses such data to compare and contrast and to generalize about society and culture. Looking beyond the particular to the more general, ethnologists attempt to identify and

ethnography
Fieldwork in a particular cultural setting.

cultural anthropology
The comparative, cross-cultural study of human society and culture.

ethnology
The study of sociocultural differences and similarities.

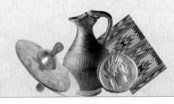

appreciating ANTHROPOLOGY

School of Hope

A school is one kind of community in which culture is transmitted—a process known as enculturation. A boarding school where students reside for several years is fully comparable as a enculturative setting to a village or other local community. You've all heard of Hogwarts. Although fictional, is it not a setting in which enculturation takes place?

Often, schools serve as intermediaries between one cultural tradition and another. As students are exposed to outsiders, they inevitably change. In today's world, opportunities to become bilingual and bicultural—that is, to learn more than one language and to participate in more than one cultural tradition—are greater than ever before.

The Kalinga Institute of Social Sciences (KISS) is a boarding school in Bhubaneswar, India, whose mission is to instill in indigenous students a "capacity to aspire" to a better life (Finnan 2016). KISS is the world's largest residential school for tribal children. Located in Odisha, one of India's poorest states, KISS supports 25,000 students from first grade through graduate training. Its students represent 62 of India's tribal groups. Children as young as age 6 travel to KISS by bus or train, sometimes from hundreds of miles away. They leave their

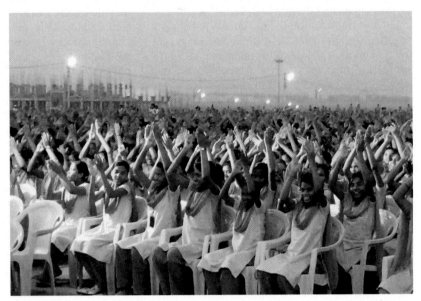

KISS students at an assembly for visiting foreign dignitaries. KISS officials use such events not only to showcase the school to visitors but also to help build solidarity among students.
Courtesy Christine Finnan

families for up to 10 months at a time, returning to their villages only during the summer.

During six months of research at KISS in 2014–2015, anthropologist Christine Finnan gathered stories and personal accounts about the school and its effects. Working with three Indian research partners, she interviewed 160 people: students, former students, parents, staff, teachers, administrators, and visitors. Her team observed classes, meals, celebrations, and athletic competitions. They also visited several tribal villages to find out why parents send their children so far away to school. Finnan wanted to determine what children gained and lost from growing up at KISS.

explain cultural differences and similarities, to test hypotheses, and to build theory to enhance our understanding of how social and cultural systems work. (See the section "The Scientific Method" later in this chapter.) Ethnology gets its data for

comparison not just from ethnography but also from the other subfields, particularly from archaeology, which reconstructs social systems of the past. (Recap 1.2 summarizes the main contrasts between ethnography and ethnology.)

RECAP 1.2	Ethnography and Ethnology—Two Dimensions of Cultural Anthropology
ETHNOGRAPHY	**ETHNOLOGY**
Requires fieldwork to collect data	Uses data collected by a series of researchers
Often descriptive	Usually synthetic
Group/community specific	Comparative/cross-cultural

(For a fuller account of the research described here, see Finnan [2016] at www.sapiens.org.)

Acceptance to KISS is based on need, so that the poorest of the poor are chosen to attend. The school offers cost-free room and board, classes, medical care, and vocational and athletic training to all its students. The value system at KISS encourages responsibility, orderliness, and respect. Children learn those behaviors not only from KISS employees but also from each other—especially from older students. Students are repeatedly reminded that they are special, that they can rise out of poverty and become change agents for their communities. Many students hope to return to their villages as teachers, doctors, or nurses.

KISS receives no government support. Most of its funding comes from its profitable sister institution, the Kalinga Institute of Industrial Technology (KIIT), a respected private university. By targeting indigenous children, KISS meets an educational need that is unmet by the government. In India's tribal villages, the presence of teachers is unreliable, even when there are village schools. At KISS, in sharp contrast, teachers don't just instruct; they also serve in loco parentis, living in the dormitories or in nearby housing, and viewing many of their students as family members.

During her fieldwork, Finnan found attitudes about KISS among all parties to be overwhelmingly positive. Students contrasted their KISS education with the poor quality of their village schools. Teachers mentioned their shared commitment to poverty reduction. Parents were eager for their children to be admitted. Although KISS encourages students to take pride in their native language and culture, both students and parents understand that change is inevitable. Students will adopt new beliefs, values, and behaviors, and they will learn Odia, the state language used at KISS. They will become bilingual and bicultural.

When Finnan began her research, she was aware of the now-notorious boarding schools for indigenous students that were established during the 19th and 20th centuries in the United States, Canada, and Australia. Children were forcibly removed from their families, required to speak English and accept Christianity, and taught that their own cultures were inferior. The educational style was authoritarian, and its goal was forced assimilation. Finnan found KISS's positive educational philosophy and respect for indigenous cultures to be very different from those archaic institutions.

To fully evaluate KISS's success in meeting its goals, Finnan has retained her connection with KISS. In 2018 she received data indicating that their promise of improved employment opportunities is being realized. A survey of 10,023 former students indicates that approximately 85 percent have jobs that are likely a result of their KISS education. In addition, while over 80 percent of tribal students drop out of district schools before completing tenth grade, only about 20 percent of KISS students do so. Those who stay at KISS score higher than the state average on state-mandated tests, and considerably higher than averages for tribal children. KISS also can point to a series of successful scholars, ambassadors, and athletes among its graduates. Each year, 5 percent of its graduating class is admitted tuition-free to KIIT. At that highly selective university, students can study engineering, medicine, and law, among other subjects.

Later in this chapter, we examine applied anthropology—how anthropological data, perspectives, theory, and methods can be used to identify, assess, and solve contemporary social problems. Think about whether Finnan's research is academic or applied, and whether there is a sharp distinction between these two dimensions of anthropology. Even if Finnan did not intend her work to be applied anthropology, her findings certainly suggest educational lessons that can be applied beyond this case. What are some of those lessons?

Anthropological Archaeology

Anthropological archaeology (or, more simply, archaeology) reconstructs, describes, and interprets human behavior and cultural patterns through material remains. At sites where people live or have lived, archaeologists find artifacts, material items that humans have made, used, or modified, such as tools, weapons, campsites, buildings, and garbage. Plant and animal remains and garbage tell stories about consumption and activities. Wild and domesticated grains have different characteristics, which allow archaeologists to distinguish between the gathering and the cultivation of plants. Animal bones reveal the age and sex of slaughtered animals, providing other information useful in determining whether species were wild or domesticated.

Analyzing such data, archaeologists answer several questions about ancient economies. Did the group get its meat from hunting, or did it domesticate and breed animals, killing only those of a certain age and sex? Did plant food come from wild plants or from sowing, tending, and harvesting crops? Did the residents make, trade for, or buy particular items? Were raw materials available locally? If not, where did they come from? From such information, archaeologists reconstruct patterns of production, trade, and consumption.

Archaeologists have spent much time studying *potsherds,* fragments of earthenware. Potsherds are more durable than many other artifacts, such as textiles and wood. The quantity of pottery fragments allows estimates of population size and

anthropological archaeology
The study of human behavior through material remains.

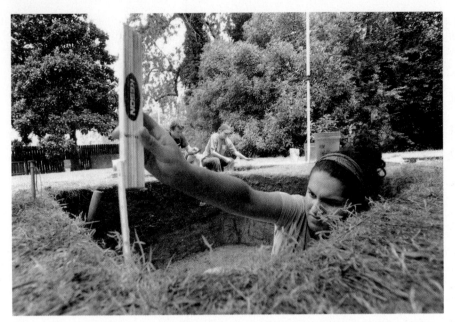

Sabrina Shirazi, a sophomore at University of Maryland, measures the elevation of the unit she has dug at an archaeological site called "The Hill" in Easton, Maryland. This site may be the oldest settlement of free African-Americans in the United States.

Kenneth K. Lam/Getty Images

places where people came to attend ceremonies. Others were burial sites; still others were farming communities.

Archaeologists also reconstruct behavior patterns and lifestyles of the past by excavating. This involves digging through a succession of levels at a particular site. In a given area, through time, settlements may change in form and purpose, as may the connections between settlements. Excavation can document changes in economic, social, and political activities.

Although archaeologists are best known for studying prehistory, that is, the period before the invention of writing, they also study the cultures of historical and even living peoples. Studying sunken ships off the Florida coast, underwater archaeologists have been able to verify the living conditions on the vessels that brought ancestral African Americans to the New World as enslaved people. In a research project begun in 1973 in Tucson, Arizona, archaeologist William Rathje launched a long-term study of modern garbage disposal practices. The value of "garbology," as Rathje called it, is that it provides "evidence of what people did, not what they think they did, what they think they should have done, or what the interviewer thinks they should have done" (Harrison, Rathje, and Hughes 1994, p. 108). What people report may contrast strongly with their real behavior as revealed by garbology. For example, the garbologists discovered that the three Tucson neighborhoods that reported the lowest beer consumption actually had the highest number of discarded beer cans per household (Podolefsky and Brown 1992, p. 100)! Findings from garbology also have challenged common misconceptions about the kinds and quantities of trash found in landfills: Although most people thought that styrofoam containers and disposable diapers were major waste problems, they were actually relatively insignificant compared with plastic, and especially paper (Rathje and Murphy 2001; Zimring 2012).

density. The discovery that potters used materials unavailable locally suggests systems of trade. Similarities in manufacture and decoration at different sites may be proof of cultural connections. Groups with similar pots may share a common history. They might have common cultural ancestors. Perhaps they traded with each other or belonged to the same political system.

Many archaeologists examine paleoecology. *Ecology* is the study of interrelations among living things in an environment. The organisms and environment together constitute an ecosystem, a patterned arrangement of energy flows and exchanges. Human ecology studies ecosystems that include people, focusing on the ways in which human use "of nature influences and is influenced by social organization and cultural values" (Bennett 1969, pp. 10–11). *Paleoecology* looks at the ecosystems of the past.

In addition to reconstructing ecological patterns, archaeologists may infer cultural transformations, for example, by observing changes in the size and type of sites and the distance between them. A city develops in a region where only towns, villages, and hamlets existed a few centuries earlier. The number of settlement levels (city, town, village, hamlet) in a society is a measure of social complexity. Buildings offer clues about political and religious features. Temples and pyramids suggest that an ancient society had an authority structure capable of marshaling the labor needed to build such monuments. The presence or absence of certain structures, like the pyramids of ancient Egypt and Mexico, reveals differences in function between settlements. For example, some towns were

biological anthropology

The study of human biological variation through time and as it exists today.

Biological Anthropology

Biological anthropology is the study of human biological diversity through time and as it exists in the world today. There are five specialties within biological anthropology:

1. Human biological evolution as revealed by the fossil record (paleoanthropology)

2. Human genetics

3. Human growth and development

4. Human biological plasticity (the living body's ability to change as it copes with environmental conditions, such as heat, cold, and altitude)

5. Primatology (the study of monkeys, apes, and other nonhuman primates)

A common thread that runs across all five specialties is an interest in biological variation among humans, including their ancestors and their closest animal relatives (monkeys and apes).

These varied interests link biological anthropology to other fields: biology, zoology, geology, anatomy, physiology, medicine, and public health. Knowledge of osteology—the study of bones—is essential for anthropologists who examine and interpret skulls, teeth, and bones, whether of living humans or of our fossilized ancestors. *Paleontologists* are scientists who study fossils. *Paleoanthropologists* study the fossil record of human evolution. Paleoanthropologists often collaborate with archaeologists, who study artifacts, in reconstructing biological and cultural aspects of human evolution. Fossils and tools often are found together. Different types of tools provide information about the habits, customs, and lifestyles of the ancestral humans who used them.

More than a century ago, Charles Darwin noticed that the variety that exists within any population permits some individuals (those with the favored characteristics) to do better than others at surviving and reproducing. Genetics, which developed after Darwin, enlightens us about the causes and transmission of the variety on which evolution depends. However, it isn't just genes that cause variety. During any individual's lifetime, the environment works along with heredity to determine biological features. For example, people with a genetic tendency to be tall will be shorter if they have poor nutrition during childhood. Thus, biological anthropology also investigates the influence of environment on the body as it grows and matures. Among the environmental factors that influence the body as it develops are nutrition, altitude, temperature, and disease, as well as cultural factors, such as the standards of attractiveness that were discussed previously.

Biological anthropology (along with zoology) also includes *primatology*. The primates include our closest relatives—apes and monkeys. *Primatologists* study their biology, evolution, behavior, and social life, often in their natural environments. Primatology assists paleoanthropology, because primate behavior and social organization may shed light on early human behavior and human nature.

Linguistic Anthropology

We don't know (and probably never will know) when our ancestors started speaking, although biological anthropologists have looked to the anatomy of the face and the skull to speculate about the origin of language. As well, primatologists have described the communication systems of monkeys and apes. We do know that well-developed, grammatically complex languages have existed for thousands of years. Linguistic anthropology offers further illustration of anthropology's interest in comparison, variation, and change. **Linguistic anthropology** studies language in its social and cultural context, throughout the world and over time. Some linguistic anthropologists also make inferences about universal features of language, linked perhaps to uniformities in the human brain. Others reconstruct ancient languages by comparing their contemporary descendants and in so doing make discoveries about history. Still others study linguistic differences to discover varied perceptions and patterns of thought in different cultures.

Historical linguistics considers variation over time, such as the changes in sounds, grammar, and vocabulary between Middle English (spoken from approximately 1050 to 1550 C.E.) and modern English. **Sociolinguistics** investigates relationships between social and linguistic variation. No language is a homogeneous system in which everyone speaks just like everyone else. How do different speakers use a given language? How do linguistic features correlate with social factors, including class and gender differences? One reason for variation is geography, as in regional dialects and accents. Linguistic variation also is expressed in the bilingualism of ethnic groups. Linguistic and cultural anthropologists collaborate in studying links between language and many other aspects of culture, such as how people reckon kinship and how they perceive and classify colors.

APPLIED ANTHROPOLOGY

What sort of man or woman do you envision when you hear the word *anthropologist*? Although anthropologists have been portrayed as quirky and eccentric, bearded and bespectacled, anthropology is not a science of the exotic carried on by quaint scholars in ivory towers. Rather, anthropology has a lot to tell the public. Anthropology's foremost professional organization, the American Anthropological Association (AAA), has formally acknowledged a public service role by recognizing that anthropology has two dimensions: (1) academic anthropology and (2) practicing, or **applied anthropology.** The latter refers to the application of anthropological data, perspectives, theory, and methods to identify, assess, and solve contemporary social problems. As American anthropologist Erve Chambers (1987, p. 309) has stated, applied anthropology is "concerned with the relationships between anthropological knowledge and the uses of that knowledge in the world beyond anthropology." More and more anthropologists from the four subfields now work in "applied"

linguistic anthropology
The study of language and linguistic diversity in time, space, and society.

sociolinguistics
The study of language in society.

applied anthropology
The use of anthropology to solve contemporary problems.

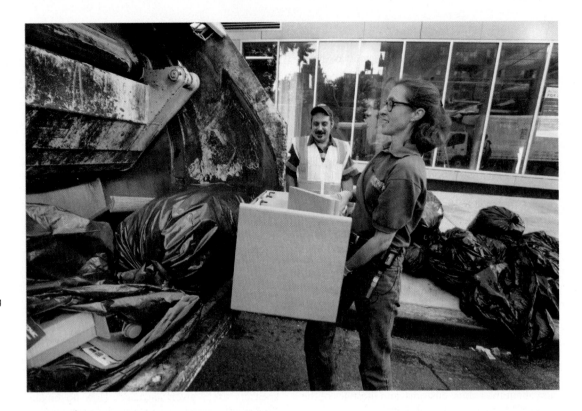

Applied anthropology in action. Professor Robin Nagle of New York University is also an anthropologist-in-residence at New York City's Department of Sanitation. Nagle studies curbside garbage as a mirror into the lives of New Yorkers. Here she accompanies sanitation worker Joe Damiano during his morning rounds in August 2015.
Richard Drew/AP Images

areas such as public health, family planning, business, market research, economic development, and cultural resource management.

Because of anthropology's breadth, applied anthropology has many applications. For example, applied medical anthropologists consider both the sociocultural and the biological contexts and implications of disease and illness. Perceptions of good and bad health, along with actual health threats and problems, differ among societies. Various ethnic groups recognize different illnesses, symptoms, and causes and have developed different health care systems and treatment strategies.

Applied archaeology, usually called *public archaeology,* includes such activities as cultural resource management, public educational programs, and historic preservation. Legislation requiring evaluation of sites threatened by dams, highways, and other construction activities has created an important role for public archaeology. To decide what needs saving, and to preserve significant information about the past when sites cannot be saved, is the work of **cultural resource management** (CRM). CRM involves not only preserving sites but also allowing their destruction if they are not significant. The *management* part of the term refers to the evaluation and decision-making process. Cultural resource managers work for federal, state, and county agencies and other clients. Applied cultural anthropologists sometimes work with public archaeologists, assessing the human problems generated by the proposed change and determining how they can be reduced.

science
A field of study that seeks reliable explanations, with reference to the material and physical world.

cultural resource management
Deciding what needs saving when entire archaeological sites cannot be saved.

ANTHROPOLOGY AND OTHER ACADEMIC FIELDS

As mentioned previously, one of the main differences between anthropology and the other fields that study people is holism, anthropology's unique blend of biological, social, cultural, linguistic, historical, and contemporary perspectives. Paradoxically, while distinguishing anthropology, this breadth also is what links it to many other disciplines. Techniques used to date fossils and artifacts have come to anthropology from physics, chemistry, and geology. Because plant and animal remains often are found with human bones and artifacts, anthropologists collaborate with botanists, zoologists, and paleontologists.

Anthropology is a **science**—a "systematic field of study or body of knowledge that aims, through experiment, observation, and deduction, to produce reliable explanations of phenomena, with reference to the material and physical world" (*Webster's New World Encyclopedia,* p. 937). This book presents anthropology as a *humanistic science* devoted to discovering, describing, understanding, appreciating, and explaining similarities and differences in time and space among humans and our ancestors. Clyde Kluckhohn (1944) described anthropology as "the science of human similarities and differences" (p. 9). His statement of the need for such a field still stands: "Anthropology provides a scientific basis for dealing with the crucial dilemma of the world today: how can peoples of different appearance, mutually unintelligible languages, and dissimilar ways of life get along peaceably together?" (p. 9). Anthropology has compiled an impressive body of knowledge, which this textbook attempts to encapsulate.

Besides its links to the natural sciences (e.g., geology, zoology) and social sciences (e.g., sociology, psychology), anthropology also has strong links to the humanities. The humanities include English, comparative literature, classics, folklore, philosophy, and the arts. These fields study languages, texts, philosophies, arts, music, performances, and other forms of creative expression. Ethnomusicology, which studies forms of musical expression on a worldwide basis, has close links to anthropology. Also linked is folklore, the systematic study of tales, myths, and legends from a variety of cultures. One can make a strong case that anthropology is one of the most humanistic of all academic fields because of its fundamental respect for human diversity. Anthropologists listen to, record, and represent voices from a multitude of nations, cultures, times, and places. Anthropology values local knowledge, diverse worldviews, and alternative philosophies. Cultural anthropology and linguistic anthropology in particular bring a comparative and non-elitist perspective to forms of creative expression, including language, art, narratives, music, and dance, viewed in their social and cultural context.

Cultural Anthropology and Sociology

Sociology is probably the discipline that is closest to anthropology, specifically to cultural anthropology. Like cultural anthropologists, sociologists study society—consisting of human social behavior, social relations, and social organization. Key differences between sociology and anthropology reflect the kinds of societies traditionally studied by each discipline. Sociologists typically have studied contemporary, Western, industrial societies. Anthropologists, by contrast, have focused on nonindustrial and non-Western societies. Sociologists and anthropologists developed different methods to study these different kinds of society. To study large-scale, complex nations, sociologists have relied on surveys and other means of gathering quantifiable data. Sociologists use sampling and statistical techniques to collect and analyze such data, and statistical training has been fundamental in sociology. Working in much smaller societies, such as a village, anthropologists can get to know almost everyone and have less need for sampling and statistics. However, because anthropologists today are working increasingly in modern nations, use of sampling and statistics is becoming more common in cultural anthropology.

Traditionally, ethnographers (field workers in cultural anthropology) studied small and nonliterate (without writing) populations and developed methods appropriate to that context. An ethnographer participates directly in the daily life of another culture and must be an attentive, detailed observer of what people do and say. The focus is on a real, living population, not just a sample of a population. During ethnographic fieldwork, the anthropologist takes part in the events she or he is *observing,* describing, and analyzing. Anthropology, we might say, is more personal and less formal than sociology.

In today's interconnected world, however, the interests and methods of cultural anthropology and sociology are converging (becoming more similar), because they are studying some of the same topics and areas. For example, many sociologists now work in non-Western countries, smaller communities, and other settings that used to be mainly within the anthropological orbit. As industrialization and urbanization have spread across the globe, anthropologists now work increasingly in industrial nations and cities, rather than villages. Among the many topics studied by contemporary sociocultural anthropologists are rural–urban and transnational (from one country to another) migration, urban adaptation, inner-city life, ethnic diversity and conflict, crime, and warfare. Cultural anthropologists today may be as likely as sociologists are to study issues of globalization and inequality.

Anthropology and Psychology

Psychologists, like sociologists, typically do their research in only one—their own—society. Anthropologists know, however, that statements about "human" psychology cannot rely solely on observations made in a single society. Cross-cultural comparison suggests that certain psychological patterns may indeed be universal. Others occur in some but not all societies, while still others are confined to one or very few cultures. *Psychological anthropology* studies cross-cultural similarities and differences in psychological traits and conditions (see Church 2017; Matsumoto and Juang 2019). During the 1920s, 1930s, and 1940s, several prominent anthropologists, including Bronislaw Malinowski (1927) and Margaret Mead (1935/1950; 1928/1961), described how particular cultures create distinctive adult personality types by inculcating in their children specific values, beliefs, and behavior patterns. Anthropologists have provided needed cross-cultural perspectives on aspects of developmental and cognitive psychology (Boyer 2018; Brekhus and Ignatow 2019; Fox 2020), psychoanalytic interpretations (Paul 1989), and psychiatric conditions (Bures 2016; Dos Santos and Pelletier 2018; Khan 2017).

Anthropologists are familiar, for example, with an array of *culturally specific syndromes.* These are patterns of unusual, aberrant, or abnormal behavior confined to a single culture or a group of related cultures (see Bures 2016; Khan 2017). One example is *koro,* the East Asian term for intense anxiety arising from the fear that one's sexual organs will recede into one's body and cause death. A distinctive Latin American syndrome is *susto,* or soul loss, whose symptoms are extreme sadness, lethargy, and listlessness. The victim typically falls prey to susto after experiencing a personal tragedy, such as the death of a loved one. A milder malady is *mal de ojo* ("evil eye"), most typically found in Mediterranean countries. Symptoms of evil eye, which mainly affects children, include fitful sleep, crying, sickness, and fever. Western cultures, too, have distinctive psychiatric syndromes (e.g., anorexia nervosa), some of which appear now to be spreading internationally through globalization (see Watters 2010).

THE SCIENTIFIC METHOD

Anthropology, remember, is a science, although a very humanistic one. Any science aims for reliable explanations that *predict* future occurrences. Accurate predictions stand up to tests designed to disprove (falsify) them. Scientific explanations rely on data, which can come from experiments, observation, and other systematic procedures. Scientific causes are material, physical, or natural (e.g., viruses) rather than supernatural (e.g., ghosts).

Theories, Associations, and Explanations

In their 1997 article "Science in Anthropology," Melvin Ember and Carol R. Ember describe how scientists test hypotheses in order to provide explanations. A **hypothesis** is a *proposed* explanation for something. Until it is *tested*, it is merely hypothetical. If the test confirms the hypothesis, then we have an explanation. An *explanation* shows how and why one variable causes or is closely associated with another variable. An **association** means that the variables

hypothesis
A suggested but as yet unverified explanation.

association
An observed relationship between two or more variables.

theory
A set of ideas formulated to explain something.

covary: when one variable changes, the other one also changes. A **theory** is a framework of logically connected ideas that helps us explain not just one, but many, associations. As an example, Darwinian evolutionary theory is used to explain giraffes' long necks and other adaptive features in multiple species.

We *generalize* when we say that something usually follows (or is usually associated with) something else. Some generalizations turn out to be laws. A *law* is a *generalization* that applies to and explains *all* instances of an association. An example of a law is the statement "water freezes at 32 degrees Fahrenheit." This law states a uniform association between two variables: the state of the water (whether liquid or ice) and the air temperature. We confirm the truth of the statement by repeated observations of freezing and by the fact that water does not solidify at higher temperatures. The existence of laws makes the world a more predictable place, helping us to understand the past and predict the future. Yesterday ice formed at 32 degrees F, and tomorrow it will still form at 32 degrees F.

The social sciences have few, if any, absolute laws of the water-freezing sort. "Laws" in social science tend to be imperfect generalizations, and explanations in social science tend to be probable rather than certain. They usually have exceptions; that is, sometimes the explanation does not hold. Does that mean such explanations are useless? Not at all. Imagine a law that said that water freezes at 32 degrees 83 percent of the time. Although we cannot make an exact prediction based on such a generalization, it still tells us something useful, even if there are exceptions. Most of the time, we would predict correctly that water was going to freeze. To take a real example from social science, we can generalize that "conflict tends to increase as a group's population size increases." Even if this statement applies only 83 percent of the time, it still is useful. In the social sciences, including anthropology, the variables of interest only *tend* to be associated in a predictable way; there are always exceptions. Recap 1.3 summarizes the key terms used in this section: association, hypothesis, explanation, theory, generalization, and law.

Case Study: Explaining the Postpartum Taboo

One classic cross-cultural study revealed a strong (but not 100 percent) association, or correlation, between a sexual restriction and a type of diet. A long postpartum sex taboo (a ban on sexual intercourse between husband and wife for a year or more after the birth of a child) tended to occur in societies where the diet was low in protein (Whiting 1964).

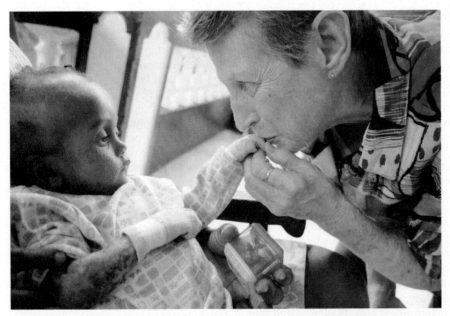

The Kwashiorkor Rehabilitation Facility in Jeremie, Haiti, is a residential treatment center for severely malnourished children. Kwashiorkor, caused by a severe protein deficiency, kills 15 percent of Haitian children before their fifth birthday. Shown here, Sheila Marshall, a nurse and full-time volunteer, comforts a young patient. The name *kwashiorkor* comes from a West African word meaning "one-two." Some cultures abruptly wean one infant when a second one is born.

Avital Greener/Newscom

This association was confirmed by cross-cultural data (ethnographic information from a randomly chosen sample of several societies). How might one explain why the *dependent variable* (the thing to be explained, in this case the postpartum sex taboo) is related to the *predictor variable* (a low-protein diet). A likely explanation is that, when there is too little protein in their diets, babies can develop and die from a protein-deficiency disease called kwashiorkor. If the mother delays her next pregnancy, her current baby gets to breast-feed longer, thereby getting protein from the mother and enhancing its survival chances. Having another baby too soon—forcing early weaning—would jeopardize the survival of the previous one. The postpartum taboo thus enhances infant survival. When the taboo becomes institutionalized as a cultural expectation, people are more likely to comply, and less likely to succumb to momentary temptation.

Theories suggest patterns and relationships, and they generate additional hypotheses. Based, for example, on the theory that the postpartum taboo exists because it reduces infant mortality when the diet is low in protein, one could hypothesize that changes in the conditions that favor the taboo might cause it to disappear. By adopting birth control, for instance, families could space births without avoiding intercourse. The taboo might also disappear if babies started receiving protein supplements, which would reduce the threat of kwashiorkor.

Recap 1.4 summarizes the main steps in using the scientific method. In hypothesis testing, the

RECAP 1.3　Theories and Associations

Key question: How do you explain associations?

ASSOCIATION	A systematic relationship between variables, so that when one variable changes (varies), the other does, too (covaries). **Example:** When temperatures fall, water solidifies.
HYPOTHESIS	A proposed explanation for an association; must be tested—may be confirmed or not. **Example:** Conflict will increase along with population size.
EXPLANATION	Reasons how and why a particular association exists. **Example:** Giraffes with longer necks have higher rates of survival and more surviving offspring than do shorter-necked giraffes, because they can feed themselves better when food is scarce.
THEORY	An explanatory framework of logically interconnected ideas used to explain multiple phenomena. **Example:** Darwinian evolutionary theory used to explain giraffes' long necks and other adaptive features in multiple species.
GENERALIZATION	A statement that change in one variable tends to follow or be associated with change in another variable. **Example:** When societies have low-protein diets, they tend to have longer postpartum taboos than when the diet is richer in protein.
LAW	A generalization that is universally valid. **Example:** When temperature reaches 32 degrees F, water turns from liquid to solid (ice).

RECAP 1.4　Steps in the Scientific Method

Have a research question.	Why do some societies have long postpartum taboos?
Construct a hypothesis.	Delaying marital sex reduces infant mortality when diets are low in protein.
Posit a mechanism.	Babies get more protein when they nurse longer; nursing is not a reliable method of contraception.
Get data to test your hypothesis.	Use a (random) sample of cross-cultural data (data from several societies; such data sets exist for cross-cultural research).
Devise a way of measuring.	Code societies 1 when they have a postpartum taboo of one year or longer, 0 when they do not; code 1 when diet is low in protein, 0 when it is not.
Analyze your data.	Notice patterns in the data: Long postpartum taboos generally are found in societies with low-protein diets, whereas societies with better diets tend to lack those taboos. Use appropriate statistical methods to evaluate the strength of these associations.
Draw a conclusion.	In most cases, the hypothesis is confirmed.
Derive implications.	Such taboos tend to disappear when diets improve or new reproductive technologies become available.
Contribute to larger theory.	Cultural practices can have adaptive value by enhancing the survival of offspring.

relevant variables should be clearly defined (e.g., "height in centimeters" or "weight in kilograms" rather than "body size") and measured reliably. The strength and significance of the results should be evaluated using legitimate statistical methods (Bernard 2018; Bernard, Wutich, and Ryan 2017). Scholars should be careful to avoid a common mistake in generalizing–citing only cases that confirm their hypothesis, while ignoring negative ones. The best procedure is random selection of cases from a wide sample of societies, not all of which are likely to fit the hypothesis.

The Value, and Limitations, of Science

Science is one way–an excellent way–of understanding the world, but it certainly is not the only way. Indeed, the work of many prominent anthropologists has more in common with the humanities than with a strictly scientific approach. Many cultural anthropologists prefer to analyze and interpret aspects of culture, rather than trying to explain them scientifically. Accordingly, anthropological approaches that are interpretive, qualitative, and humanistic are considered in this book, along with those that are quantitative and scientific.

for REVIEW

summary

1. Anthropology is the holistic and comparative study of humanity. It is the systematic exploration of human biological and cultural diversity. Examining the origins of, and changes in, human biology and culture, anthropology provides explanations for similarities and differences. The four subfields of general anthropology are sociocultural anthropology, anthropological archaeology, biological anthropology, and linguistic anthropology. All consider variation in time and space. Each also examines adaptation–the process by which organisms cope with environmental stresses.

2. Cultural forces mold human biology, including our body types and images. Societies have particular standards of physical attractiveness. They also have specific ideas about what activities–for example, various sports–are appropriate for males and females.

3. Cultural anthropology explores the cultural diversity of the present and the recent past. Anthropological archaeology reconstructs cultural patterns, often of prehistoric populations. Biological anthropology documents variety, involving fossils, genetics, growth and development, bodily responses, and nonhuman primates. Linguistic anthropology considers diversity among languages. It also studies how speech changes in social situations and over time. Anthropology has two dimensions:

academic and applied. Applied anthropology is the use of anthropological data, perspectives, theory, and methods to identify, assess, and solve contemporary social problems.

4. Concerns with biology, society, culture, and language link anthropology to many other fields—sciences and humanities. Anthropologists study art, music, and literature across cultures. But their concern is more with the creative expressions of common people than with arts designed for elites. Anthropologists examine creators and products in their social context. Sociologists traditionally study Western industrial societies, whereas anthropologists have focused on rural, nonindustrial peoples. Psychological anthropology views human psychology in the context of social and cultural variation.

5. Ethnologists attempt to identify and explain cultural differences and similarities and to build theories about how social and cultural systems work. Scientists strive to improve understanding by testing hypotheses—suggested explanations. Explanations rely on associations and theories. An association is an observed relationship between variables. A theory is an explanatory framework capable of explaining many associations. The scientific method characterizes any anthropological endeavor that formulates research questions and gathers or uses systematic data to test hypotheses.

key terms

1. How might a *biocultural* approach help us understand the complex ways in which human populations adapt to their environments?

2. What themes and interests unify the subdisciplines of anthropology? In your answer, refer to historical reasons for the unity of anthropology. Are these historical reasons similar in all places where anthropology developed as a discipline?

3. If, as Franz Boas illustrated early on in American anthropology, cultures are not isolated, how can ethnography provide an account of a particular community, society, or culture? *Note:* There is no easy answer to this question! Anthropologists continue to deal with it as they define their research questions and projects.

4. The American Anthropological Association has formally acknowledged a public service role by recognizing that anthropology has two dimensions: (1) academic anthropology and (2) practicing, or applied, anthropology. What is applied anthropology? Based on your reading of this chapter, identify examples from current events in which an anthropologist could help identify, assess, and solve contemporary social problems.

5. In this chapter, we learn that anthropology is a science, although a very humanistic one. What do you think this means? What role does hypothesis testing play in structuring anthropological research? What are the differences between theories, laws, and hypotheses?

think like an anthropologist

Design Elements: Understanding Ourselves: muha/123RF (rock paintings); Focus on Globalization: janrysavy/Getty Images (globe); Appreciating Diversity (left to right): Floresco Productions/age footstock; Hero/Corbis/Glow Images, Hill Street Studios/Blend Images, Billion Photos/Shutterstock; Understanding Ourselves: Hemera Technologies/Alamy (Cymbal), LACMA - Los Angeles County Museum of Art (Trefoil Oinochoe), Ingram Publishing/SuperStock (Coin), ChuckSchugPhotography/Getty Images (Rug).

credits

Culture

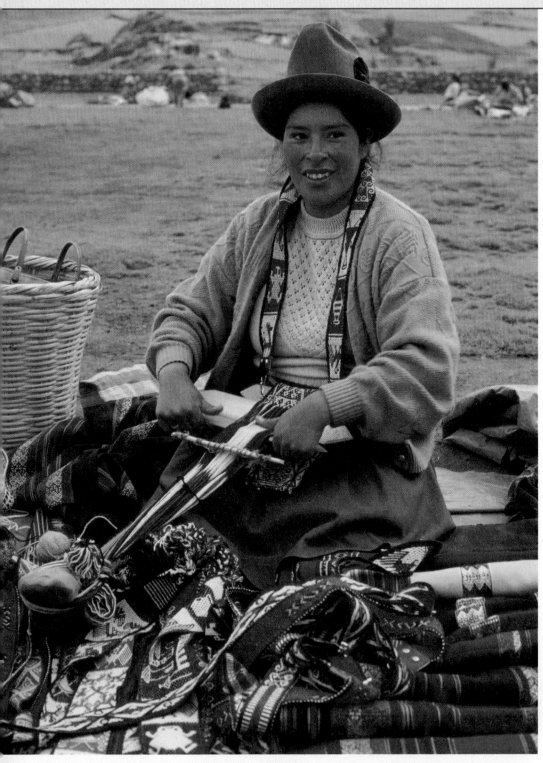

▶ What is culture and why do we study it?

▶ What is the relation between culture and the individual?

▶ How does culture change— especially with globalization?

Danita Delimont/Alamy Images

This Peruvian Quechua woman weaves while offering handwoven textiles for sale in an outdoor market in Peru's Urubamba Valley. People learn and share beliefs and practices as members of cultural groups.

understanding OURSELVES

How special are you? To what extent are you "your own person" and to what extent are you a product of your particular culture? How much does your cultural background influence your actions and decisions? Americans may not fully appreciate the power of culture because of the value their culture assigns to "the *individual.*" Americans like to regard everyone as unique in some way. Yet individualism itself is a distinctive *shared* value, a feature of American culture, transmitted constantly in our daily lives. In the media, count how many stories focus on individuals versus groups. Agents of enculturation, ranging from TV personalities to our parents, grandparents, and teachers, continually insist that we all are "someone special." That we are individuals first and members of groups second is the opposite of this chapter's lesson about culture. To be sure, we have distinctive features because we are individuals, but we have other distinct attributes because we belong to cultural groups.

For example, a comparison of the United States with Brazil, Italy, or virtually any Latin nation reveals striking contrasts between a national culture (American) that tends to discourage physical affection and national cultures in which the opposite is true. Brazilians touch, embrace, and kiss one another much more frequently than North Americans do. Such behavior reflects years of exposure to particular cultural traditions. Middle-class Brazilians teach their kids—both boys and girls—to kiss (on the cheek, two or three times, coming and going) every adult relative they see. Given the size of Brazilian extended families, this can mean hundreds of people. Women continue kissing all those people throughout their lives. Until they are adolescents, boys kiss all adult relatives. Men typically continue to kiss female relatives and friends, as well as their fathers and uncles, throughout their lives.

Do you kiss your father? Your uncle? Your grandfather? How about your mother, aunt, or grandmother? The answers to these questions may differ between men and women, and for male and female relatives. Culture can help us to make sense of these differences. In America, a cultural homophobia (fear of homosexuality) may prevent American men from engaging in displays of affection with other men; similarly, American girls typically are encouraged to show affection, while American boys typically are not. It's important to note that these cultural explanations rely on example and expectation, and that no cultural trait exists because it is natural or right. *Ethnocentrism* is the error of viewing one's own culture as superior and applying one's own cultural values in judging people from other cultures. How easy is it for you to see beyond the ethnocentric blinders of your own experience? Do you have an ethnocentric position regarding displays of affection?

WHAT IS CULTURE?

The concept of culture is fundamental in anthropology. A century and a half ago, in his book *Primitive Culture,* the British anthropologist Sir Edward Tylor proposed that cultures—systems of human behavior and thought—obey natural laws and therefore can be studied scientifically. Tylor's definition of culture still offers an overview of the subject matter of anthropology, and it is widely quoted: "Culture . . . is that complex whole which includes knowledge, belief, arts, morals, law, custom, and any other capabilities and habits acquired by man as a member of society"

(Tylor 1871/1958, p. 1). The crucial phrase here is "acquired . . . as a member of society." Tylor's definition focuses on attributes that people acquire not through biological inheritance but by growing up in a particular society where they are exposed to a specific cultural tradition. **Enculturation** is the process by which a child learns his or her culture.

enculturation
The process by which culture is learned and transmitted across the generations.

symbol
Something, verbal or nonverbal, that stands for something else.

Culture Is Learned

The ease with which children absorb any cultural tradition rests on the uniquely elaborated human capacity to learn. Other animals may learn from experience; for example, they avoid fire after discovering that it hurts. Social animals also learn from other members of their group. Wolves, for instance, learn hunting strategies from other pack members. Such social learning is particularly important among monkeys and apes, our closest biological relatives. But our own *cultural learning* depends on the uniquely developed human capacity to use **symbols,** signs that have no necessary or natural connection to the things they signify or for which they stand.

Through cultural learning, people create, remember, and deal with ideas. They understand and apply specific systems of symbolic meaning. Anthropologist Clifford Geertz (1973) described cultures as sets of "control mechanisms—plans, recipes, rules, instructions" and likens them to computer programs that govern human behavior (Geertz 1973, p. 44). During enculturation, people gradually absorb and internalize their particular culture—a previously established system of meanings and symbols that helps guide their behavior and perceptions throughout their lives.

Every child begins immediately, through a process of conscious and unconscious learning and interaction with others, to internalize, or incorporate, a cultural tradition through the process of enculturation. Sometimes culture is taught directly, as when parents tell their children to say "thank you" when someone gives them something or does them a favor.

We also acquire culture through observation. Children pay attention to the things that go on around them. They modify their behavior not only because other people tell them to do so, but also because of their own observations and growing awareness of what their culture considers right and wrong. Many aspects of culture are absorbed unconsciously. North Americans acquire their culture's notions about how far apart people should stand when they talk not by being told directly to maintain a certain distance but through a gradual process of observation, experience, and conscious and unconscious behavior modification. No one tells Latins to stand closer together than North Americans do, but they learn to do so anyway as part of their cultural tradition.

Anthropologists agree that cultural learning is uniquely elaborated among humans and that all humans have culture. Anthropologists also agree that although *individuals* differ in their emotional and intellectual tendencies and capacities, all human *populations* have equivalent capacities for culture. Regardless of their genes or their physical appearance, people can learn any cultural tradition.

To understand this point, consider that contemporary North Americans are the genetically mixed descendants of people from all over the world. Our ancestors lived in different countries and continents and participated in hundreds of cultural traditions. However, early colonists, later immigrants, and their descendants have all become active participants in American or Canadian life. All now share a national culture.

Culture Is Symbolic

Symbolic thought is unique and crucial to humans and to cultural learning. Anthropologist Leslie White defined culture as

> dependent upon symbolling. . . . Culture consists of tools, implements, utensils, clothing, ornaments, customs, institutions, beliefs, rituals, games, works of art, language, etc. (White 1959, p. 3)

For White, culture originated when our ancestors acquired the ability to use symbols, that is, to originate and bestow meaning on a thing or an event, and, correspondingly, to grasp and appreciate such meanings (White 1959, p. 3).

A symbol is something verbal or nonverbal, within a particular language or culture, that comes to stand for something else. There is no obvious, natural, or necessary connection between the symbol and the thing that it symbolizes. A pet that barks is no more naturally a *dog* than a *chien, Hund,* or *mbwa,* to use the words for the animal we call "dog" in French, German, and Swahili. Language is one of the distinctive possessions of *Homo sapiens.* No other animal has developed anything approaching the complexity of language.

There also is a rich array of nonverbal symbols. Flags, for example, stand for countries, as arches do for a hamburger chain. Holy water is a potent symbol in Roman Catholicism. As is true of all symbols, the association between water and what it stands for (holiness) is arbitrary and conventional. Water is not intrinsically holier than milk, blood, or other natural liquids. Nor is holy water chemically different from ordinary water. Holy water is a symbol within Roman Catholicism, which is part of an international cultural system. A natural thing has been arbitrarily associated with a particular meaning for Catholics, who share common beliefs and experiences that are based on learning and that are transmitted across the generations. Our cultures immerse us in a world of symbols that are both linguistic and nonverbal. Particular items and brands of clothing, such as jeans, shirts,

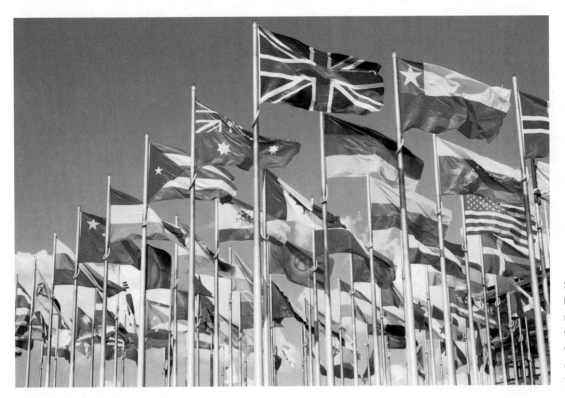

Some symbols are linguistic. Others are nonverbal, such as these colorful flags, which stand for countries.
TommL/Getty Images

or shoes, can acquire symbolic meanings, as can our gestures, posture, and body decoration and ornamentation.

For hundreds of thousands of years, humans have possessed the abilities on which culture rests. These abilities are to learn, to think symbolically, to manipulate language, and to use tools and other cultural products in organizing their lives and coping with their environments. Every contemporary human population has the ability to use symbols and thus to create and maintain culture. Our nearest relatives—chimpanzees and gorillas—have rudimentary cultural abilities. No other animal, however, has elaborated cultural abilities—to learn, to communicate, and to store, process, and use information—to the extent that *Homo* has.

Culture Is Shared

Culture is an attribute not of individuals per se but of individuals as members of *groups.* Culture is transmitted in society. We learn our culture by observing, listening, talking, and interacting with many other people. Shared beliefs, values, memories, and expectations link people who grow up in the same culture. Enculturation unifies people by providing us with common experiences. Today's parents were yesterday's children. If they grew up in North America, they absorbed certain values and beliefs transmitted over the generations. People become agents in the enculturation of their children, just as their parents were for them. Although a culture changes constantly, certain fundamental beliefs, values,

worldviews, and child-rearing practices endure. One example of enduring shared enculturation is the American emphasis on self-reliance and independent achievement.

Despite characteristic American notions that people should "make up their own minds" and "have a right to their opinion," little of what we think is original or unique. We share our opinions and beliefs with many other people—nowadays not just in person but also via new media. Think about how often (and with whom) you share information or an opinion via texting, Snapchat, Instagram, Facebook, Pinterest, Twitter, or WhatsApp. Illustrating the power of shared cultural background, we are most likely to agree with and feel comfortable with people who are socially, economically, and culturally similar to ourselves. This is one reason Americans abroad tend to socialize with each other, just as French and British colonists did in their overseas empires. Birds of a feather flock together, but for people, the familiar plumage is culture.

Culture and Nature

Culture takes the natural biological urges we share with other animals and teaches us how to express them in particular ways. People have to eat, but culture teaches us what, when, and how. In many cultures, people have their main meal at noon, but most North Americans prefer a large dinner. English people may eat fish for breakfast, while North Americans may prefer hot cakes and cold cereals. Brazilians put hot milk into strong coffee, whereas

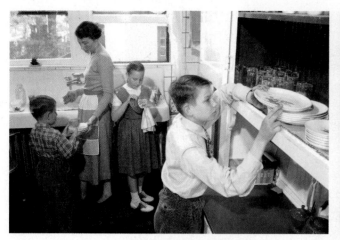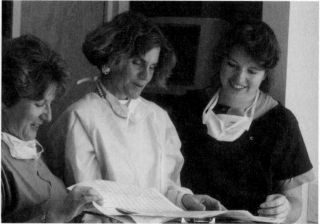

Cultures are integrated systems. When one behavior pattern changes, others also change. During the 1950s, most American women expected to have careers as wives, mothers, and domestic managers. As more and more women have entered the workforce, attitudes toward work and family have changed. In the earlier photo, a 1950s mom and kids do the dishes. In the recent photo, a doctor and two nurses examine a patient's record. What do you imagine these three women do when they get home?

(left): Steven Gottlieb/Getty Images; (right): Tom Tracy Photography/Alamy Stock Photo

North Americans pour cold milk into a weaker brew. Midwesterners dine at 5 or 6 P.M., Spaniards at 10 P.M.

Culture molds "human nature" in many directions. People have to eliminate wastes from their bodies. But some cultures teach people to defecate squatting, while others tell them to do it sitting down. A generation ago, in Paris and other French cities, it was customary for men to urinate almost publicly, and seemingly without embarrassment, in barely shielded *pissoirs* located on city streets. Our "bathroom" habits, including waste elimination, bathing, and dental care, are parts of cultural traditions that have converted natural acts into cultural customs.

Our culture—and cultural changes—affect the ways in which we perceive nature, human nature, and "the natural." Through science, invention, and discovery, cultural advances have overcome many "natural" limitations. We prevent and cure diseases, such as polio and smallpox, that felled our ancestors. We can use pills to restore and enhance sexual potency. Through cloning, scientists have altered the way we think about biological identity and the meaning of life itself. Culture, of course, has not freed us from natural disasters. Hurricanes, earthquakes, tsunamis, and other natural forces regularly challenge our efforts to modify the environment through building, development, and expansion.

Culture Is All-Encompassing

For anthropologists, culture includes much more than refinement, taste, sophistication, education, and appreciation of the fine arts. Not only college graduates but all people are "cultured." The most interesting and significant cultural forces are those that affect people every day of their lives, particularly those that influence children during enculturation. *Culture,* as defined anthropologically,

encompasses features that sometimes are considered trivial or unworthy of serious study, such as "popular" culture. To understand contemporary North American culture, however, we must consider social media, cell phones, the Internet, television, fast-food restaurants, sports, and games. As a cultural manifestation, a rock star may be as interesting as a symphony conductor, a comic book as significant as a book-award winner.

Culture Is Integrated

Cultures are not haphazard collections of customs and beliefs. Cultures are integrated, patterned systems. If one part of the system (e.g., the economy) changes, other parts also change. For example, during the 1950s, most American women planned domestic careers as homemakers and mothers. Since then, an increasing number of American women, including wives and mothers, have entered the workforce. Only 32 percent of married American women worked outside the home in 1960, compared to about 60 percent today. By December 2019, women outnumbered men in the U.S. workforce, holding 50.04 percent of all payroll jobs–a trend that is likely to continue (Siegel 2020).

Economic changes have social repercussions. Attitudes and behavior about marriage, family, and children have changed. Late marriage, "living together," and divorce have become commonplace. Work may compete with marriage and family responsibilities, reducing time spent at home and interfering with child care. Recognizing this, employers increasingly make it possible for workers to work remotely from home.

Cultures are integrated not simply by their dominant economic activities and related social patterns but also by sets of values, ideas, symbols, and judgments. Cultures train their individual members to share certain personality traits. A set of **core values** (key, basic, or central values) integrates each culture and helps distinguish it from others. For instance, the work ethic and individualism are core values that have integrated American culture for generations. Different sets of dominant values exist in other cultures.

Culture Is Instrumental, Adaptive, and Maladaptive

Culture is the main reason for human adaptability and success. Other animals rely on biological means of adaptation (such as fur or blubber, which are adaptations to cold). Humans also adapt biologically—for example, by shivering when we get cold or sweating when we get hot. People, however, also have cultural ways of adapting. To cope with environmental stresses, we habitually use technology, or tools. We hunt cold-adapted animals and use their fur coats as our own. We turn the thermostat up in the winter and down in the summer. In summer we have a cold drink, jump in a pool, or travel to someplace cooler. In winter we have hot chocolate, seek out a sauna, or vacation in warmer climes. People use culture instrumentally, that is, to fulfill their basic biological needs for food, drink, shelter, comfort, and reproduction.

People also use culture to fulfill psychological and emotional needs, such as friendship, companionship, approval, and sexual desirability. People seek informal support—help from people who care about them—as well as formal support from associations and institutions. To these ends, individuals cultivate ties with others based on common experiences, political interests, aesthetic sensibilities, or personal attraction. Increasingly, people use such Internet platforms as Facebook, Google+, and LinkedIn to create and maintain social or professional connections.

On one level, cultural traits (e.g., air conditioning) are adaptive because they help individuals cope with environmental stresses. On a different level, however, such traits can also be *maladaptive.* For example, emissions from our machines have environmental effects that can harm humans and other life forms. Many modern cultural patterns may be maladaptive in the long run. Examples of maladaptive aspects of culture include policies that encourage overpopulation, poor food-distribution systems, overconsumption, and environmental degradation.

CULTURE'S EVOLUTIONARY BASIS

The human capacity for culture has an evolutionary basis that extends back perhaps 3 million years, to the date of the earliest evidence of tool manufacture in the archaeological record. Toolmaking by our distant ancestors may extend even farther back, based on observations of tool manufacture by chimpanzees in their natural habitats (Mercader, Panger, and Boesch 2002; Schaik 2016).

Similarities between humans and apes, our closest relatives, are evident in anatomy, brain structure, genetics, and biochemistry. Most closely related to us are the African great apes: chimpanzees and gorillas. *Hominidae* is the zoological family that includes fossil and living humans. Also included as **hominids** are chimps and gorillas. The term **hominins** is used for the group that leads to humans but not to chimps and gorillas and that encompasses all the human species that ever have existed.

Many human traits reflect the fact that our primate ancestors lived in the trees. These traits include grasping ability and manual dexterity (especially opposable thumbs), depth and color vision, learning ability based on a large brain, substantial parental investment in a limited number of offspring, and tendencies toward sociality and cooperation. Like other primates, humans have flexible, five-fingered hands and *opposable thumbs:* Each thumb can touch all the other fingers on the same hand. Like monkeys and apes, humans also have excellent depth and color vision. Our eyes are located forward in the skull and look directly ahead, so that their fields of vision overlap. Depth perception, impossible without overlapping visual fields, proved adaptive—for judging distance, for example—in the trees. Having color and depth vision also facilitates the identification of various food sources, as well as mutual grooming, picking out burrs, insects, and other small objects from hair. Such grooming is one way of forming and maintaining social bonds.

The combination of manual dexterity and depth perception allows monkeys, apes, and humans to pick up small objects, hold them in front of their eyes, and appraise them. Our ability to thread a needle reflects an intricate interplay of hands and eyes that took millions of years of primate evolution to achieve. Such dexterity, including the opposable thumb, confers a tremendous advantage in manipulating objects and is essential to a major human adaptive capacity: toolmaking. In primates, and especially in humans, the ratio of brain size to body size exceeds that of most mammals. Even more important, the brain's outer layer—concerned with memory, association, and integration—is relatively larger. Monkeys, apes, and humans store an array of images in their memories, which permits them to learn more. Such a capacity for learning is a tremendous adaptive

Primates have five-digited feet and hands, well suited for grasping. Flexible hands and feet that could encircle branches were important features in the early primates' arboreal life. In adapting to bipedal (two-footed) locomotion, hominins eliminated most of the foot's grasping ability—illustrated here by the chimpanzee.
Kenneth Garrett/ National Geographic Creative

advantage. Like most other primates, humans usually give birth to a single offspring rather than a litter. Receiving greater parental attention, that one infant has enhanced learning opportunities. The need for longer and more attentive care of offspring places a selective value on support by a social group. Humans have developed considerably the primate tendency to be social animals, living and interacting regularly with other members of their species.

What We Share with Other Primates

There is a substantial gap between primate *society* (organized life in groups) and fully developed human *culture,* which is based on symbolic thought. Nevertheless, studies of nonhuman primates reveal many similarities with humans, such as the ability to learn from experience and change behavior as a result. Apes and monkeys, like humans, learn throughout their lives. In one group of Japanese macaques (land-dwelling monkeys), for example, a 3-year-old female started washing sweet potatoes before she ate them. First her mother, then her age peers, and finally the entire troop began washing sweet potatoes as well. The ability to benefit from experience confers a tremendous adaptive advantage, permitting the avoidance of fatal mistakes. Faced with environmental change, humans and other primates don't have to wait for a genetic or physiological response. They can modify learned behavior and social patterns instead.

Although humans do employ tools much more than any other animal does, tool use also turns up among several nonhuman species, including birds, beavers, sea otters, and especially apes. Nor are humans the only animals that make tools with a specific purpose in mind. It is well-known that capuchin monkeys in South America use rocks to pound shells off nuts, which they then eat. Recent excavations show that they have not only hammered and dug with carefully chosen stones for the last 3,000 years, but they also have selected pounding tools of varying sizes and weights over time. Before 2,500 B.P. (Before the Present), the monkeys used small pounders on tiny foods such as seeds or fruits; by 600 B.P., they were using larger pounders on hard-shelled fruits and nuts, and by 100 years ago, they had turned to downsized pounders to crack cashew nuts. Similar change over time in pounding-tool usage has also been established for chimpanzees (Bower 2019).

Chimpanzees living in the Tai forest of Ivory Coast make and use stone tools to break open hard, golf-ball-sized nuts (Mercader et al. 2002). At specific sites, the chimps gather nuts, place them on stumps or flat rocks, which are used as anvils, and pound the nuts with heavy stones. The chimps must select hammer stones suited to smashing the nuts and carry them to where the nut trees grow. Nut cracking is a learned skill, with mothers showing their young how to do it. Chimpanzees at Bossou, Guinea (West Africa) systematically use sticks to gather algae floating in ponds. They stand at the edge of a pond, each chimp holding a stalk or stick, which they carefully place in the water. Then they slowly lift the sticks covered with algae to their mouths (Matsuzawa 2019).

In 1960, Jane Goodall began observing wild chimps—including their tool use and hunting behavior—at Gombe Stream National Park in Tanzania, East Africa (see Goodall 2010). The most studied form of ape toolmaking involves "termiting," in which chimps make tools to probe termite hills. They choose twigs, which they modify by removing leaves and peeling off bark to expose the underlying sticky surface. They carry the twigs to termite hills, dig holes with their fingers, and insert the twigs. Finally, they pull out the twigs and dine on termites that have been attracted to the sticky surface. Given what we know about ape tool use and manufacture, it is almost certain that early hominins shared this ability, although the first evidence for hominin stone toolmaking dates back only about 3 million years. Upright bipedalism would have permitted the carrying and use of tools and weapons against predators and competitors.

The apes have other abilities essential to culture. Wild chimps and orangs aim and throw objects. Gorillas build nests, and they throw branches, grass, vines, and other objects. Hominins have elaborated the capacity to aim and throw, without which we never would have developed projectile technology and weaponry—or baseball.

As with toolmaking, anthropologists used to regard hunting as a distinctive human activity not shared with the apes. Again, however, primate research shows that other primates, especially chimpanzees, are habitual hunters. For example, in Uganda's Kibale National Park, chimps form large hunting parties, including an average of 26 individuals (adult and adolescent males). Most hunts (78 percent) result in at least one prey item being caught—a much higher success rate than that among lions (26 percent), hyenas (34 percent), or cheetahs (30 percent). Chimps' favored prey in Kibale is the red colobus monkey (Mitani et al. 2012).

It is likely that human ancestors were doing some hunting by at least 3 million years ago, based on the existence of early stone tools designed to cut meat. Given our current understanding of chimp hunting and toolmaking, we can infer that hominids may have been hunting much earlier than the first archaeological evidence attests. Because chimps typically devour the monkeys they kill, leaving few remains, we may never find archaeological evidence for the first hominin hunt, especially if it proceeded without stone tools.

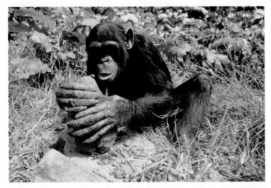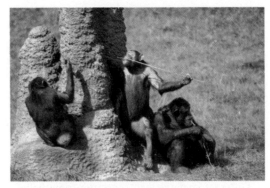

These two photos show different forms of tool use by chimps. Liberian chimps, like the one on the left, use hammer stones to crack palm nuts. On the right, chimps use prepared twigs to "fish" for termites from a termite hill.

(left): Clive Bromhall/Oxford Scientific/Getty Images; (right): Stan Osolinski/Oxford Scientific/Getty Images

How We Differ from Other Primates

Although chimps often share meat from a hunt, apes and monkeys (except for nursing infants) tend to feed themselves individually. Cooperation and sharing are much more characteristic of humans. Until fairly recently (12,000 to 10,000 years ago), all humans were hunter-gatherers who lived in small groups called bands. In some world areas, the hunter-gatherer way of life persisted into recent times, permitting study by ethnographers. In such societies, men and women take resources back to the camp and share them. Everyone shares the meat from a large animal. Nourished and protected by younger band members, elders live past reproductive age and are respected for their knowledge and experience. Humans are among the most cooperative of the primates—in the food quest and other social activities. In addition, the amount of information stored in a human band is far greater than that in any other primate group.

Another difference between humans and other primates involves mating. Among baboons and chimps, most mating occurs when females enter estrus, during which they ovulate. In estrus, the vaginal area swells and reddens, and receptive females form temporary bonds with, and mate with, males. Human females, by contrast, lack a visible estrus cycle, and their ovulation is concealed. Not knowing when ovulation is occurring, humans maximize their reproductive success by mating throughout the year. Human pair bonds for mating are more exclusive and more durable than are those of chimps. Related to our more constant sexuality, all human societies have some form of marriage. Marriage gives mating a reliable basis and grants to each spouse special, though not always exclusive, sexual rights to the other.

Marriage creates another major contrast between humans and nonhuman primates: exogamy and kinship systems. Most cultures have rules of exogamy requiring marriage outside one's kin or local group. Coupled with the recognition of kinship, exogamy confers adaptive advantages. It creates ties between the spouses' different groups of origin. Their children have relatives, and therefore allies, in two kin groups rather than just one. The key point here is that ties of affection and mutual support between members of different local groups tend to be absent among primates other than *Homo*. Other primates tend to disperse at adolescence. Among chimps and gorillas, females tend to migrate, seeking mates in other groups. Humans also choose mates from outside the natal group, and usually at least one spouse moves. However, *humans maintain lifelong ties with sons and daughters.* The systems of kinship and marriage that preserve these links provide a major contrast between humans and other primates (see Martin 2019).

UNIVERSALITY, GENERALITY, AND PARTICULARITY

In studying human diversity in time and space, anthropologists distinguish among the universal, the generalized, and the particular. Certain biological, psychological, social, and cultural features are **universal,** found in every culture. Others are merely **generalities,** common to several but not all human groups. Still other traits are **particularities,** unique to certain cultural traditions.

Universals and Generalities

Biologically based universals include a long period of infant dependency, year-round (rather than seasonal) sexuality, and a complex brain that enables us to use symbols, languages, and tools. Among the social universals is life in groups and in some kind of family. Generalities occur in certain times and places but not in all cultures. They may be widespread, but they are not universal. One cultural generality that is present in many but not all societies is the nuclear family, a kinship group consisting of parents and children. Many middle-class Americans still view the "traditional" nuclear family, consisting

universal
Something that exists in every culture.

generality
Culture pattern or trait that exists in some but not all societies.

particularity
Distinctive or unique culture trait, pattern, or integration.

of a married man and woman and their children, as a proper and "natural" group. This view persists despite the fact that nuclear families now comprise only about 20 percent of contemporary American households. Cross-culturally, too, this kind of "traditional" family is far from universal. Consider the Nayars, who live on the Malabar Coast of India. Traditionally, the Nayars lived in female-headed households, and husbands and wives did not live together. In many other societies, the nuclear family is submerged in larger kin groups, such as extended families, lineages, and clans.

Different societies can share the same beliefs and customs because of borrowing or through (cultural) inheritance from a common cultural ancestor. Speaking English is a generality shared by North Americans and Australians because both countries had English settlers. Another reason for generalities is domination, as in colonial rule, when a more powerful nation imposes its customs and procedures on another group. In many countries, use of the English language reflects colonial history. More recently, English has spread through diffusion (cultural borrowing) to many other countries, as it has become the world's foremost language for business, travel, and the Internet.

Particularity: Patterns of Culture

A cultural particularity is a trait or feature of culture that is not generalized or widespread; rather, it is confined to a single place, culture, or society. Yet because of cultural borrowing and exchanges, which have accelerated with globalization, traits that once were limited in their distribution have

become more widespread. Traits that are useful, that have the capacity to please large audiences, and that don't clash with the cultural values of potential adopters are more likely to spread than are others. Nevertheless, certain cultural particularities persist. One example is a particular food dish (e.g., pork barbeque with a mustard-based sauce available in South Carolina, or the pastie—beef stew baked in pie dough—characteristic of Michigan's Upper Peninsula). Besides diffusion, which, for example, has spread McDonald's food outlets, once confined to San Bernardino, California, across the globe, there are other reasons cultural particularities are increasingly rare. Many cultural traits are shared as cultural universals or because of independent invention. Facing similar problems, people in different places have come up with similar solutions.

At the level of the individual cultural trait or element (e.g., bow and arrow, hot dog, HBO), particularities may be getting rarer. At a higher level, however, particularity is more obvious. Different cultures emphasize different things. *Cultures are integrated and patterned differently and display tremendous variation and diversity.* When cultural traits are borrowed, they are modified to fit the culture that adopts them. They are reintegrated—patterned anew—to fit their new setting. The television show *Big Brother* in Germany or Brazil isn't at all the same thing as Big Brother in the United States. As was stated in the section "Culture Is Integrated" earlier in the chapter, patterned beliefs, customs, and practices lend distinctiveness to particular cultural traditions.

Consider universal life-cycle events, such as birth, puberty, marriage, parenthood, and death, which many cultures observe and celebrate. The occasions

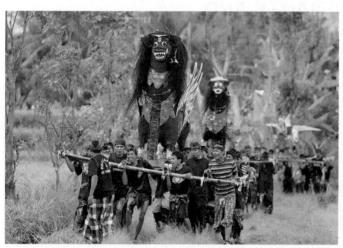 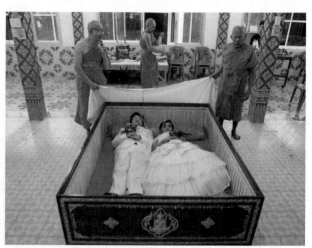

Cultures use rituals to mark such universal life-cycle events as birth, puberty, marriage, parenthood, and death. But particular cultures differ as to which events merit special celebration and in the emotions expressed during their rituals. Compare the Balinese cremation ceremony (Left) with the Thai wedding (Right). In the cremation ceremony, participants celebrate the life of the deceased as they carry a body (underneath each creature) to be burned and released from worldly ties. In this Thai Buddhist wedding ceremony, a groom, age 40, and bride, age 26, temporarily lie down in a coffin. This custom is believed to banish bad luck and bring happiness. How would you describe the emotions suggested by the photos?

(left): Tuul & Bruno Morandi/Getty Images (right): Chaiwat Subprasom/Newscom

(e.g., marriage, death) may be the same and universal, but the patterns of ceremonial observance may be dramatically different. Cultures vary in just which events merit special celebration. Americans, for example, regard expensive weddings as more socially appropriate than lavish funerals. However, the Betsileo of Madagascar take the opposite view. The marriage ceremony there is a minor event that brings together just the couple and a few close relatives. However, a funeral is a measure of the deceased person's social position and lifetime achievement, and it may attract a thousand people. Why use money on a house, the Betsileo say, when one can use it on the tomb where one will spend eternity in the company of dead relatives? How unlike contemporary Americans' dreams of home ownership and preference for quick and inexpensive funerals. Cremation, an increasingly common option in the United States, would horrify the Betsileo, for whom ancestral bones and relics are important ritual objects.

Cultures vary tremendously in their beliefs, practices, integration, and patterning. By focusing on and trying to explain alternative customs, anthropology forces us to reappraise our familiar ways of thinking. In a world full of cultural diversity, contemporary American culture is just one cultural variant, more powerful perhaps, but no more natural, than the others.

CULTURE AND THE INDIVIDUAL

Generations of anthropologists have theorized about the relationship between the "system" on one hand and the "person" or "individual" on the other. *System* can refer to various concepts, including culture, society, social relations, or social structure. Individual human beings always make up, or constitute, the system. Within that system, however, humans also are constrained (to some extent, at least) by its rules and by the actions of other individuals. Cultural rules provide guidance about what to do and how to do it, but people don't always do what the rules say should be done. People use their culture actively and creatively, rather than blindly following its dictates. Cultures are dynamic and constantly changing. People learn, interpret, and manipulate the same rule in different ways—or they emphasize different rules (or "alternative facts") that better suit their interests. Culture is contested: Different groups in society struggle with one another over whose ideas, values, goals, and beliefs will prevail. Even common symbols may have radically different meanings to different individuals and groups in the same culture. Golden arches may cause one person to salivate, while someone else plots a vegetarian protest. Different people may wave the same flag to support or oppose a particular war or political candidate. Behavior as the U.S. national anthem is played at an NFL game may symbolically pledge allegiance or protest police brutality.

Even when they agree about what should and should not be done, people don't always do as their culture directs or as other people expect. Many rules are violated, some very often (e.g., automobile speed limits). Some anthropologists find it useful to distinguish between ideal culture and real culture. The *ideal culture* consists of what people say they should do and what they say they do. *Real culture* refers to their actual behavior as observed by the anthropologist.

Culture is both public and individual, both in the world and in people's minds. Anthropologists are interested not only in public and collective behavior but also in how *individuals* think, feel, and act. As Roy D'Andrade (1984) has noted, the individual and culture are linked because human social life is a process in which individuals internalize the meanings of *public* (i.e., cultural)

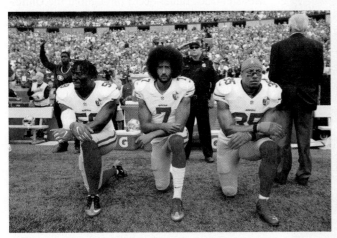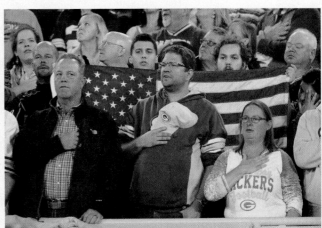

Symbolic acts at a public event, such as an NFL game, may be used to convey very different messages. In the photo on the left, as the national anthem is played, players Eli Harold #58, Colin Kaepernick #7, and Eric Reid #35 take a knee to protest racism and brutality against African Americans. In the photo on the right, hearing the same music, fans display the American flag and stand with hands over heart.

(left): Michael Zagaris/Getty Images Sport/Getty Images; (right): Jonathan Daniel/Getty Images Sport/Getty Images

international culture
Cultural traditions that extend beyond national boundaries.

subcultures
Different cultural traditions associated with subgroups in the same complex society.

national culture
Cultural features shared by citizens of the same nation.

messages. Then, alone and in groups, people influence culture by converting their private (and often divergent) understandings into public expressions.

Conventionally, culture has been seen as social glue transmitted across the generations, binding people through their common past, rather than as something being continually created and reworked in the present. The tendency to view culture as an entity rather than a process is changing. Contemporary anthropologists now emphasize how day-to-day action, practice, or resistance can make and remake culture (Gupta and Ferguson 1997b). *Agency* refers to the actions that individuals take, both alone and in groups, in forming and transforming cultural identities.

The approach to culture known as *practice theory* (Ortner 1984) recognizes that individuals within a society or culture have diverse motives and intentions and different degrees of power and influence. Such contrasts may be associated with gender, age, ethnicity, class, and other social variables. Practice theory focuses on how such varied individuals—through their ordinary and extraordinary actions and practices—manage to influence, create, and transform the world they live in. Practice theory appropriately recognizes a reciprocal relation between culture (the system) and the individual. The system shapes the way individuals experience and respond to external events, but individuals also play an active role in the way society functions and changes. Practice theory recognizes both constraints on individuals and the flexibility and changeability of cultures and social systems.

Levels of Culture

We can distinguish levels of culture, which vary in their membership and geographic extent. **National culture** encompasses those beliefs, learned behavior

patterns, values, and institutions shared by citizens of the same nation. **International culture** is the term for cultural traditions that extend beyond and across national boundaries. Because culture is transmitted through learning rather than genetically, cultural traits can spread through borrowing, or *diffusion,* from one group to another.

Many cultural traits and patterns have become international in scope. For example, Roman Catholics in many different countries share beliefs, symbols, experiences, and values transmitted by their church. The contemporary United States, Canada, Great Britain, and Australia share cultural traits they have inherited from their common linguistic and cultural ancestors in Great Britain. The World Cup is an international cultural event, as people in many countries know the rules of, play, and follow soccer.

Cultures also can be smaller than nations. Although people who live in the same country partake in a national cultural tradition, all nations also contain diversity. Individuals, families, communities, regions, classes, and other groups within a culture have different learning experiences as well as shared ones. **Subcultures** are different symbol-based patterns and traditions associated with particular groups within the same society. In a large nation like the United States or Canada, subcultures originate in region, ethnicity, language, class, and religion. The backgrounds of Christians, Jews, and Muslims—and the diverse branches of those religions—create subcultural differences among them. While sharing a common national culture, U.S. northerners and southerners also differ in aspects of their beliefs, values, and customary behavior. Italian Americans have ethnic traditions different from those of Irish, Polish, Latino, or African Americans. Using sports and foods, Table 2.1 gives some examples of international culture, national culture, and subculture. Soccer and basketball are played internationally. Monster-truck rallies occur throughout the United States. Bocci is a bowling-like sport from Italy still played in some Italian–American neighborhoods.

Nowadays, many anthropologists are reluctant to use the term *subculture.* They feel that the prefix "sub-" is offensive because it means "below."

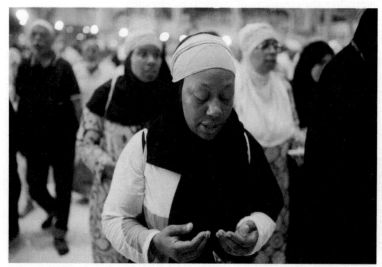

Illustrating the international level of culture (a world religion), an African-American Muslim woman circles the Kaaba, the cubic building at the Grand Mosque in Mecca, Saudi Arabia. Each year, millions of Muslims from around the world make the pilgrimage (haj) to Islam's holiest city.

Mosa'ab Elshamy/AP Images

TABLE 2.1 Levels of Culture, with Examples from Sports and Foods

LEVEL OF CULTURE	SPORTS EXAMPLES	FOOD EXAMPLES
International	Soccer, basketball	Pizza
National	Monster-truck rallies	Apple pie
Subculture	Bocci	Big Joe Pork Barbeque (South Carolina)

"Subcultures" may thus be perceived as "less than" or somehow inferior to a dominant, elite, or national culture. In this discussion of levels of culture, I intend no such implication. My point is simply that nations may contain many different culturally defined groups. As mentioned earlier, culture is contested. Various groups may and do strive to promote the correctness and value of their own practices, values, and beliefs in comparison with those of other groups or of the nation as a whole.

Ethnocentrism, Cultural Relativism, and Human Rights

Ethnocentrism is the tendency to view one's own culture as superior and to use one's own standards and values in judging outsiders. We witness ethnocentrism when people consider their own cultural beliefs to be truer, more proper, or more moral than those of other groups. However, fundamental to anthropology, as the study of human diversity, is the fact that what is alien (even disgusting) to us may be normal, proper, and prized elsewhere (see the discussion of cultural particularities, including burial customs, in the section "Particularity: Patterns of Culture"). The fact of cultural diversity calls ethnocentrism into question, as anthropologists have shown all kinds of reasons for unfamiliar practices. During a course like this, anthropology students often reexamine their own ethnocentric beliefs. Sometimes as the strange becomes familiar, the familiar seems a bit stranger and less comfortable. One goal of anthropology is to show the value in the lives of others. But how far is too far? What happens when cultural practices, values, and rights come into conflict with human rights?

Several societies in Africa and the Middle East have customs requiring female genital modification. *Clitoridectomy* is the removal of a girl's clitoris. *Infibulation* involves sewing the lips (labia) of the vagina to constrict the vaginal opening. Both procedures reduce female sexual pleasure and, it is believed in some societies, the likelihood of adultery. Although traditional in the societies where they occur, such practices, characterized as female genital mutilation, have been opposed by human rights advocates, especially women's rights groups. The idea is that the custom infringes on a basic human right: disposition over one's body and one's sexuality. Indeed, such practices are fading because of worldwide attention to the problem and changing sex/gender roles. Some African countries have banned or otherwise discouraged the procedures, as have Western nations that receive immigration from such cultures. Similar issues arise with circumcision and other male genital operations. Is it right to require adolescent boys to undergo collective circumcision to fulfill cultural traditions, as has been done traditionally in parts of Africa and Australia? Is it right to circumcise a baby boy without his permission, as has been done routinely in the United States and as is customary among Jews and Muslims? (A 2011 initiative aimed at banning circumcision in San Francisco, California, failed to make it to the ballot.)

According to an idea known as **cultural relativism,** it is inappropriate to use outside standards to judge behavior in a given society. We should evaluate such behavior with reference to the culture in which it occurs. Anthropologists employ cultural relativism not as a moral belief but as a methodological position: In order to understand another culture fully, we must try to understand how the people in that culture see things. What motivates them—what are they thinking when they do those things? Such an approach does not preclude making moral judgments. In the female genital mutilation example, we can best understand the motivations for the practice by considering the perspective of those who engage in it. Having done this, one then faces the moral question of what, if anything, to do about it.

We also should recognize that different people and groups within the same society—for example,

ethnocentrism
Judging other cultures using one's own cultural standards.

cultural relativism
The idea that behavior should be evaluated not by outside standards but in the context of the culture in which it occurs.

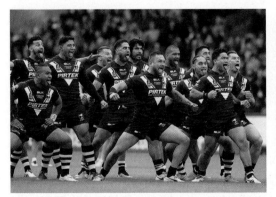 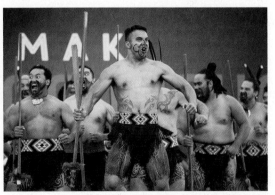

Left: A Maori haka. Maori men dressed as warriors perform their traditional haka during a festival celebrating Maori heritage in January 2016 in Auckland, New Zealand. Right: Illustrating cultural appropriation, members of New Zealand's Kiwis rugby team enact their version of the haka prior to an October 2016 match against England. The notion of indigenous property rights states that any society has a fundamental right to preserve and manage its cultural base. Does the rugby team have the right to perform the haka?

(left): Hannah Peters/Getty Images News/Getty Images; (right): Jan Kruger/Getty Images Sport/Getty Images

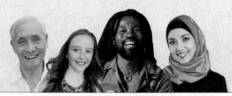
Preserving Cultural Heritage

On January 5, 2020 American President Donald Trump issued a tweet threatening to target 52 Iranian sites, including cultural sites, should Iran retaliate against the United States for killing top General Qassem Soleimani. Trump may have been unaware that the 1954 Hague Convention for the Protection of Cultural Property in the Event of Armed Conflict found the targeting of cultural sites to be a war crime. In 2017, the U.N. Security Council unanimously passed a resolution condemning the destruction of heritage sites. That resolution was largely in response to acts of heritage destruction in Syria and Iraq (see below) by the Islamic State. UNESCO, the United Nations' cultural agency, has reminded governments that cultural sites are off limits according to international law. Two days later, Defense Secretary Mike Esper distanced the Pentagon from Trump's threat, declaring that the United States would follow the laws of armed conflict, which include a prohibition on targeting cultural sites.

Heritage refers to something that has been passed on from previous generations. *Cultural heritage*—the culture, values, and traditions of a particular group—includes not only such material things as artifacts, artwork, and buildings but also intangibles such as language, music, dances, and stories. Every human group has a shared heritage. Members of that group are its proper guardians. Heritage becomes a matter of international concern when one group seizes it from another, or destroys it for political, military, or religious purposes.

For centuries, heritage items have been collected, purchased, and stolen from indigenous people for museums and private collections. Often they were sold by people (e.g., explorers or colonial officials) who had no right to sell them. Among the world's most famous items of cultural heritage are the Parthenon Sculptures, also known as the Elgin Marbles, on display at—and one of the most prized possessions of—London's famed British Museum. Lord Elgin, the British ambassador to the Ottoman empire, acquired these sculptures in the early 19th century in Athens, Greece. Their ownership remains a point of contention between Greece and the United Kingdom.

Some items are recognized as important to the shared history and heritage of humanity as a whole. This is what UNESCO (the United Nations Educational, Scientific and Cultural Organization) has in mind when it designates sites as having "*World* Heritage" value. Their significance extends beyond their particular geographic location. The disappearance or destruction of such sites would deprive future generations of key aspects of our shared history. Surveying the globe, UNESCO has designated (as of this writing) 1,121 World Heritage sites (see http://whc.unesco.org/en/list/). Of those, 213 were chosen because of their natural resources, such as waterfalls, glaciers, rivers, flora, and fauna. However, the overwhelming majority (869 sites) are cultural heritage sites, so chosen because of their archaeological or historical value. The final 39 sites are mixed cultural and natural, such as the Tikal National Park in Guatemala, which is an archaeological site in a rainforest. Fifty-three of the World Heritage sites are currently considered endangered. Many of those are in areas of war and instability, including six sites in Syria, five in Libya, and three each in Iraq and Mali (see http://whc.unesco.org/en/danger/).

In 2012, Islamic extremists occupied and wreaked havoc on Timbuktu, Mali, one of those endangered sites, where they destroyed mausoleums and other heritage items, which they considered to be objects of idolatry. One of the perpetrators, Ahmad al-Faqi al-Mahdi, was successfully prosecuted in 2016 by the International Criminal Court, where he pleaded guilty and was sentenced to nine years in prison.

In 2015, members of the Islamic State (known variously as ISIS, IS, ISIL, and Daesh)

---

human rights
Rights based on justice and morality beyond and superior to particular countries, cultures, andreligions.

cultural rights
Rights vested in religious and ethnic minorities and indigenous societies.

women versus men or old versus young—can have very different opinions about what is proper, necessary, and moral. When there are power differentials in a society, a particular practice may be supported by some people more than others (e.g., old men versus young women). In trying to understand the meaning of a practice or belief within any cultural context, we should ask who benefits from that custom, and who does not.

The idea of **human rights** invokes a realm of justice and morality beyond and superior to particular countries, cultures, and religions. Human rights, usually seen as vested in individuals, include the right to speak freely, to hold religious beliefs without persecution, and not to be murdered, injured, enslaved, or imprisoned without charge. These rights are not ordinary laws that particular governments make and enforce. Human rights are seen as *inalienable* (nations cannot abridge or terminate them) and international (larger than and superior to individual nations and cultures). Four United Nations documents describe nearly all the human rights that have been internationally recognized. Those documents are the UN Charter; the Universal Declaration of Human Rights; the Covenant on Economic, Social and Cultural Rights; and the Covenant on Civil and Political Rights.

Alongside the human rights movement has arisen an awareness of the need to preserve cultural rights. Unlike human rights, **cultural rights**

destroyed architectural ruins—and murdered a prominent Syrian archaeologist—at Palmyra, Syria, a major cultural center of the ancient world and another endangered UNESCO World Heritage site. The structures destroyed included Palmyra's almost 2,000-year-old Arch of Triumph and Temple of Baalshamin. In both these cases, items of cultural heritage were intentionally destroyed, in violation of the Hague Convention.

Responding to ongoing threats to cultural preservation, local activists, cultural historians, anthropologists, and others have taken various steps to ensure that indigenous groups maintain or recover items of cultural heritage (see Marshall 2020). The United Nations has enacted a number of measures, including those mentioned previously, as well as the 1972 Convention Concerning the Protection of the World Cultural and Natural Heritage and its 2007 Declaration on the Rights of Indigenous Peoples. Both affirm that indigenous peoples have the right to keep, control, protect, and develop their particular cultural heritage, traditional knowledge, and cultural expressions. An American example is the Native

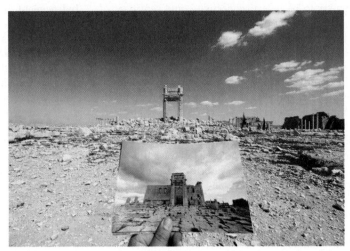

On March 31, 2016, in Palmyra, Syria, a photographer holds up his photo of the Temple of Bel taken two years earlier. Members of ISIS destroyed this historic temple in September 2015.

Joseph Eid/AFP/Getty Images

American Graves Protection and Repatriation Act (NAGPRA), which affirms that Native American remains belong to Native Americans. NAGPRA requires American museums to return remains and artifacts to any tribe that requests them and can prove a "cultural affiliation" between itself and the remains or artifact.

We see that different groups may value cultural heritage sites, artifacts, and remains for different reasons. Anthropologists value an ancient skeleton they have dubbed "Kennewick Man" because of its scientific importance—what this early fossil from Oregon can tell us about the peopling of North America. Native American tribes in Oregon, by contrast, value Kennewick Man as "the Ancient One," an ancestor whose remains needed to be buried in a culturally appropriate manner. For Lord Elgin, the Parthenon friezes were a valuable commodity that he could (and did) sell to the British government. For the British Museum, the Elgin Marbles are prized works of art proudly displayed in a chamber far from their point of origin. Athenians value the Marbles as a creation of their classic civilization that should be returned to Greece, where descendants of their makers can determine their use. Khaled al-Asaad, an 81-year-old Syrian archaeologist known for his work in preservation, died in Palmyra at the hands of ISIS, who regard ancient buildings as objects of idolatry, but who also see ancient artifacts as commodities that can be traded for money. Cultural heritage items, then, can be viewed in multiple ways—as a source of identity, as a commodity, or as a threat to be destroyed.

are vested not in individuals but in groups, including indigenous peoples and religious and ethnic minorities. Cultural rights include a group's ability to raise its children in the ways of its forebears, to continue its language, and not to be deprived of its economic base by the nation in which it is located. Many countries have signed pacts endorsing, for cultural minorities within nations, such rights as self-determination; some degree of home rule; and the right to practice the group's religion, culture, and language. The related notion of indigenous intellectual property rights (**IPR**) has arisen in an attempt to conserve each society's cultural base—its core beliefs and principles. IPR are claimed as a cultural right, allowing indigenous groups to control who may know and use their collective knowledge and its applications. Much traditional cultural knowledge has commercial value. Examples include ethnomedicine (traditional medical knowledge and techniques), cosmetics, cultivated plants, foods, folklore, arts, crafts, songs, dances, costumes, and rituals. According to the IPR concept, a particular group may determine how its indigenous knowledge and the products of that knowledge are used and distributed, and the level of compensation required. (This chapter's "Appreciating Diversity" discusses the related concept of "cultural heritage.")

The notion of cultural rights recalls the previous discussion of cultural relativism, and the issue raised

IPR

Intellectual property rights; an indigenous group's collective knowledge and its applications.

there arises again. What does one do about cultural rights that interfere with human rights? I believe that anthropology, as the scientific study of human diversity, should strive to present accurate accounts and explanations of cultural phenomena. Most ethnographers try to be objective, accurate, and sensitive in their accounts of other cultures. However, using objectivity, sensitivity, and a cross-cultural perspective doesn't mean that anthropologists have to ignore international standards of justice and morality. The anthropologist doesn't have to approve customs such as infanticide, cannibalism, and torture to recognize their existence and determine their causes and the motivations behind them. Each anthropologist has a choice about where he or she will do fieldwork. Some anthropologists choose not to study a particular culture because they discover in advance or early in fieldwork that behavior they consider morally repugnant is practiced there. When confronted with such behavior, each anthropologist must make a judgment about what, if anything, to do about it. What do you think?

MECHANISMS OF CULTURAL CHANGE

Why and how do cultures change? One way is through **diffusion,** or the borrowing of traits between cultures. Such exchange of information and products has gone on throughout human history because cultures never have been truly isolated. Contact between neighboring groups has always existed and has extended over vast areas (Boas 1940/1966). Diffusion is *direct* when two cultures trade, intermarry, or wage war on one another. Diffusion is *forced* when one culture subjugates another and imposes its customs on the dominated group. Diffusion is *indirect* when items move from group A to group C via group B without any firsthand contact between A and C. In this case, group B might consist of traders or merchants who take products from a variety of places to new markets. Or group B might be geographically situated between A and C, so that what it gets from A eventually winds up in C, and vice versa. In today's world, much transnational diffusion is due to the spread of the mass media and advanced information technology.

Acculturation, a second mechanism of cultural change, is the exchange of cultural features that results when groups have continuous firsthand contact. This contact may change the cultures of either group or both groups, but each group remains distinct. In situations of continuous contact, cultures may exchange and blend foods, recipes, music, dances, clothing, tools, technologies, and languages.

One example of acculturation is a *pidgin,* a mixed language that develops to ease communication between members of different societies in contact. This usually happens in situations of trade or colonialism. Pidgin English, for example,

is a simplified form of English that blends English grammar with the grammar of a locally spoken language. Pidgin English first developed to facilitate commerce in Chinese ports. Similar pidgins developed later in Papua New Guinea and West Africa.

Independent invention—the process by which humans innovate, creatively finding solutions to problems—is a third mechanism of cultural change. Faced with similar problems and challenges, people in different societies have innovated and changed in similar ways, which is one reason cultural generalities exist. One example is the independent invention of agriculture in the Middle East and Mexico. Often a major invention, such as agriculture, triggers a series of subsequent interrelated changes. Thus, in both Mexico and the Middle East, agriculture led to many social, political, and legal changes, including notions of property and distinctions in wealth, class, and power.

GLOBALIZATION: ITS MEANING AND ITS NATURE

The term **globalization** encompasses a series of processes that work transnationally to promote change in a world in which nations and people are increasingly interlinked and mutually dependent (see Spooner 2015). The forces of globalization include international commerce and finance, travel and tourism, transnational migration, and the media—including the Internet and other high-tech information flows (see Haugerud, Stone, and Little 2011). New economic unions (which have met considerable resistance in their member nations) have been created through the World Trade Organization (WTO), the International Monetary Fund (IMF), and the European Union.

It's important to distinguish between two different meanings of the term *globalization.* As used in this book, the primary meaning of globalization is *worldwide connectedness.* Modern systems of production, distribution, consumption, finance, transportation, and communication are global in scope. A second meaning of globalization is *political* and has to do with ideology, policy, and free trade (see Kotz 2015). In this more limited sense, globalization refers to efforts by international financial powers to create a global *free market* for goods and services. This second, political, meaning of globalization has generated, and continues to generate, significant opposition. In this book, *globalization* is a neutral term for the fact of global connectedness and linkages, rather than any kind of political position (see also Eriksen 2014; Ervin 2014).

The media play a key role in globalization. Long-distance communication is faster and easier than ever, and now it covers most of the globe. The media help fuel a transnational culture of consumption by spreading information about products, events, lifestyles, and the perceived benefits

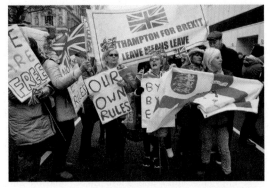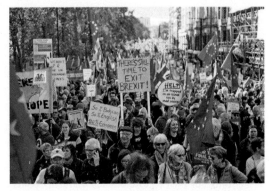

On June 23, 2016, the United Kingdom voted 52-48 percent to leave the European Union (EU). The opposing sides are shown here. On the left, Pro-Brexit supporters wave Union Jack flags while standing on an EU flag in London's Parliament Square. On the right, Anti-Brexit demonstrators march to that same square, in response to Prime Minister Boris Johnson's address to the House of Commons on his new Brexit deal.

(left): Jeff J Mitchell/Getty Images; (right): Victoria Jones/Getty Images

(and sometimes costs) of globalization. Emigrants transmit information and resources transnationally, as they maintain their ties with home (phoning, texting, or e-mailing; visiting; sending money; watching satellite TV). The Internet is a vital resource for communication within and across national boundaries. As of 2019, WhatsApp is the most popular messenger app worldwide with approximately 1.6 billion monthly users, outranking Facebook Messenger at 1.3 billion and WeChat at 1.1 billion users. Following Facebook and YouTube, it is also the third most popular social network worldwide. People increasingly live their lives across borders, maintaining connections with more than one nation-state (see Lugo 1997; Staudt 2018).

The Internet and cell phones have made possible the very rapid global transmission of money, resources, and information. Transactions that once involved face-to-face contact now proceed across vast distances. For example, when you order something using the Internet, the only human being you might speak to is the delivery driver, and a drone may soon replace that human. The computers that process your order from Amazon can be on different continents, and the products you order can come from a warehouse anywhere. The average food product travels 1,300 miles and changes hands a dozen times before it reaches an American consumer (Lewellen 2010).

The effects of globalization are broad and often unwelcome. An army of outsiders and potential change agents now intrudes on people everywhere. Tourism has become the world's number one industry. Airbnb, VRBO, and other short-term rental sites are transforming residential neighborhoods in many cities. Economic development agents and the media promote the idea that work should be for cash rather than mainly for subsistence. Local people have devised various strategies to deal with threats to their autonomy, identity, and livelihood (Maybury-Lewis, Macdonald, and

Maybury-Lewis, 2009). New forms of cultural expression and political mobilization, including the rights movements discussed previously, are emerging from the interplay of local, regional, national, and international cultural forces (see Ong and Collier 2005).

Multinational corporations lay off workers in their home country when they automate, move, or outsource their operations to places where labor and materials are cheaper. Automation and the globalization of labor create unemployment "back home." Financial globalization means that nations have less control over their own economies. Such institutions as the World Bank, the IMF, the European Union, and the European Central Bank routinely constrain and dictate the national economic policies of countries like Greece and Spain.

Sovereign nations resist. The successful campaign for British withdrawal from the European Union ("Brexit") is one example of political mobilization against globalization, as are regular protests at meetings of the principal agencies concerned with international trade. Demonstrators continue to show their disapproval of policies of the WTO, the IMF, and the World Bank. Anti-globalization activists fault those organizations for policies that, they say, promote corporate wealth at the expense of farmers, workers, and others at or near the bottom of the economy. Protesters also include environmentalists seeking tougher environmental regulations and trade unionists advocating global labor standards. Related to these protests was the 2011 Occupy movement, which spread quickly from Wall Street to other American (and Canadian) cities. That movement protested growing inequality—between the top 1 percent and everyone else (see Hickel 2017). Similar sentiments motivated the 2016 and 2020 presidential campaigns of Vermont senator Bernie Sanders. In a related vein, anti-globalization sentiment helped elect Donald Trump as the 45th President of the United States.

summary

1. Although cultures change constantly, certain fundamental beliefs, values, worldviews, and child-rearing practices endure across the generations in any culture. What are some examples from your own culture of such enduring beliefs or practices?

2. Culture, which is distinctive to humanity, refers to customary behavior and beliefs that are transmitted through enculturation. Culture rests on the human capacity for cultural learning. Culture encompasses rules for conduct internalized in human beings, which lead them to think and act in characteristic ways.

3. Although other animals learn, only humans have cultural learning, dependent on symbols. Humans think symbolically—arbitrarily bestowing meaning on things and events. By convention, a symbol stands for something with which it has no necessary or natural relation. Symbols have special meaning for people who share memories, values, and beliefs because of common enculturation. People absorb cultural lessons consciously and unconsciously.

4. Cultural traditions mold biologically based desires and needs in particular directions. Everyone is cultured, not just people with elite educations. Cultures may be integrated and patterned through economic and social forces, key symbols, and core values. Cultural rules don't rigidly dictate our behavior. There is room for creativity, flexibility, diversity, and disagreement within societies. Cultural means of adaptation have been crucial in human evolution. Aspects of culture also can be maladaptive.

5. The human capacity for culture has an evolutionary basis that extends back at least 3 million years—to early toolmakers whose products survive in the archaeological record (and most probably even farther back—based on observation of tool use and manufacture by apes). Humans share with monkeys and apes such traits as manual dexterity (especially opposable thumbs), depth and color vision, learning ability based on a large brain, substantial parental investment in a limited number of offspring, and tendencies toward sociality and cooperation.

6. Many hominin traits are foreshadowed in other primates, particularly in the African apes, which, like us, belong to the hominid family. The ability to learn, basic to culture, is an adaptive advantage available to monkeys and apes. Chimpanzees make tools for several purposes. They also hunt and share meat. Sharing and cooperation are more developed among humans than among the apes, and only humans have systems of kinship and marriage that permit us to maintain lifelong ties with relatives in different local groups.

7. Using a comparative perspective, anthropology examines biological, psychological, social, and cultural universals and generalities. There also are unique and distinctive aspects of the human condition (cultural particularities). North American cultural traditions are no more natural than any others. Levels of culture can be larger or smaller than a nation. Cultural traits may be shared across national boundaries. Nations also include cultural differences associated with ethnicity, region, and social class.

8. Ethnocentrism describes judging other cultures by using one's own cultural standards. Cultural relativism, which anthropologists may use as a methodological position rather than a moral stance, is the idea of avoiding the use of outside standards to judge behavior in a given society. Human rights are those based on justice and morality beyond and superior to particular countries, cultures, and religions. Cultural rights are vested in religious and ethnic minorities and indigenous societies, and IPR, or intellectual property rights, apply to an indigenous group's collective knowledge and its applications.

9. Diffusion, migration, and colonialism have carried cultural traits and patterns to different world areas. Mechanisms of cultural change include diffusion, acculturation, and independent invention.

10. Globalization describes a series of processes that promote change in a world in which nations and people are interlinked and mutually dependent. There is a distinction between globalization as fact (the primary meaning of globalization in this book) and globalization as contested ideology and policy (international efforts to create a global free market for goods and services).

key terms

1. Our culture—and cultural changes—affect how we perceive nature, human nature, and "the natural." This theme continues to fascinate science fiction writers. Recall a recent science fiction book, movie, or TV program that creatively explores the boundaries between nature and culture. How does the story develop the tension between nature and culture to craft a plot?

2. In American culture today, the term *diversity* is used in many contexts, usually referring to some positive attribute of our human experience, something to appreciate, to maintain, and even to increase. In what contexts have you heard the term used? To what precisely does the term refer?

3. What are some issues about which you find it hard to be culturally relativistic? If you were an anthropologist with the task of investigating these issues in real life, can you think of a series of steps that you would take to design a project that would, to the best of your ability, practice methodological cultural relativism? (You may want to review the use of the scientific method in an anthropological project presented in Chapter 1.)

4. What are the mechanisms of cultural change described in this chapter? Can you come up with additional examples of each mechanism? Also, recall the relationship between culture and the individual. Can individuals be agents of cultural change?

think like an anthropologist

credits

Method and Theory in Cultural Anthropology

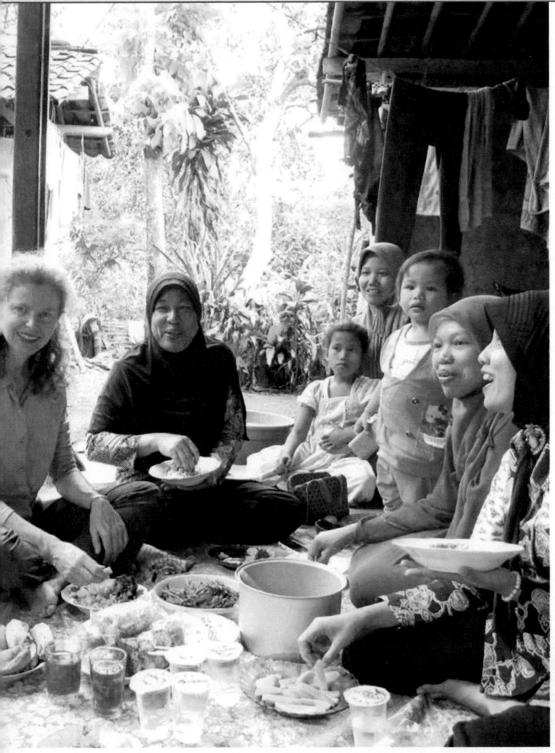

▶ Where and how do cultural anthropologists do fieldwork?

▶ What are some ways of studying modern societies?

▶ What theories have guided anthropologists over the years?

Anthropologist Priscilla Magrath of the University of Arizona does ethnographic fieldwork in Indonesia.

Courtesy Dr. Priscilla Magrath

understanding OURSELVES

To many people, the word *anthropology* evokes an image of archaeological digs. Remember, however, that anthropology has four subfields, only two of which (archaeology and biological anthropology) require much digging—in the ground, at least. To be sure, cultural anthropologists "dig out" information about lifestyles, just as linguistic anthropologists do about the features of languages. Traditionally, cultural anthropologists have done a variant on the *Star Trek* theme of seeking out, if not new, at least different "life" and "civilizations," sometimes boldly going where no scientist has gone before.

Despite globalization, the cultural diversity under anthropological scrutiny right now may be as great as ever before, because the anthropological universe has expanded to modern nations. Today's cultural anthropologists are as likely to be studying artists in Miami or bankers in Beirut as indigenous Australians in the outback or Polynesians in outrigger canoes. Still, we can't forget that anthropology did originate in non-Western, nonindustrial societies. Its research techniques, especially

those subsumed under the label *ethnography,* were developed to deal with small populations. Even when working in modern nations, anthropologists still consider ethnography with small groups to be an excellent way of learning about how people live their lives and make decisions.

For the general public, biological anthropologists and archaeologists tend to be better known than cultural anthropologists because of what they study. One cultural anthropologist was an extremely important public figure when (and before and after) I was in college. Margaret Mead, famed for her work on teen sexuality in Samoa and gender roles in New Guinea, may well be the most famous anthropologist who ever lived. Mead, one of my own professors at Columbia University, appeared regularly on NBC's *The Tonight Show*. In all her venues, including teaching, museum work, TV, anthropological films, popular books, and magazines, Mead helped Americans appreciate the relevance of anthropology to understanding their daily lives. Her work is featured here and elsewhere in this book.

ETHNOGRAPHY: ANTHROPOLOGY'S DISTINCTIVE STRATEGY

Traditionally, the process of becoming a cultural anthropologist has required a field experience in another society. Early ethnographers studied small-scale, relatively isolated societies with simple technologies and economies and little social differentiation (see Hewitt 2020; Konopinski 2014; Moore 2019). Ethnographers typically try to understand the whole of a particular culture (or,

more realistically, as much as they can, given limitations of time and perception). To pursue this goal, ethnographers adopt a free-ranging research strategy, moving from setting to setting, person to person, and place to place to discover the totality and interconnectedness of social life. By expanding our knowledge of the range of human diversity, ethnography provides a foundation for generalizations about human behavior and social life. Ethnographers draw on varied techniques to piece together a picture of otherwise alien lifestyles (see Bernard 2018; Bernard and Gravlee 2014; Bloomaert and Jie 2020; Gmelch and Gmelch 2018;

chapter outline

Kirner and Mills 2020; Vivanco 2017). We turn now to a consideration of those techniques.

Observation and Participant Observation

participant observation

Taking part in community life, participating in the events one is observing, describing, and analyzing.

Ethnographers must pay attention to hundreds of details of daily life, seasonal events, and unusual happenings. They should record what they see as they see it. Things never again will seem quite as strange as they do during the first few weeks in the field. Often anthropologists experience culture shock—a creepy and profound feeling of alienation—on arrival at a new field site (see Cohen 2015). Although anthropologists study human diversity, the actual field experience of diversity takes some getting used to. The ethnographer eventually grows accustomed to, and accepts as normal, cultural patterns that initially were alien. Staying a bit more than a year in the field allows the ethnographer to repeat the season of his or her arrival, when certain events and processes may have been missed because of initial unfamiliarity and culture shock.

Many ethnographers record their impressions in a personal *diary,* which is kept separate from more formal *field notes.* Later, this record of early impressions will help point out some of the most basic aspects of cultural diversity. Such aspects include distinctive smells, noises people make, how they cover their mouths when they eat, and how they gaze at others. These patterns, which are so basic as to seem almost trivial, are part of what Bronislaw Malinowski called "the imponderabilia of native life and of typical behavior" (Malinowski 1922/1961, p. 20). These aspects of culture are so fundamental that people take them for granted. They are too

basic even to talk about, but the unaccustomed eye of the fledgling ethnographer picks them up. Thereafter, becoming familiar, they fade to the edge of consciousness. I mention my initial impressions of some such imponderabilia of northeastern Brazilian culture in this chapter's "Appreciating Diversity."

Ethnographers strive to establish *rapport,* a good, friendly working relationship based on personal contact, with their hosts. Fundamental to ethnography is **participant observation**—taking part in community life, participating in the events one is observing. As human beings living among others, ethnographers cannot be totally impartial and detached observers. By participating, ethnographers may learn why people find various events meaningful, as they see how those events are organized and conducted.

In Arembepe, Brazil, I learned about fishing by sailing on the Atlantic with local fishers. I gave Jeep rides to malnourished babies, to pregnant women, and once to a teenage girl possessed by a spirit. All those people needed to consult specialists outside the village. I danced on Arembepe's festive occasions, drank libations commemorating new births, and became a godfather to a village girl. Most anthropologists have similar field experiences. The common humanity of the student and the studied, the ethnographer and the research community, makes participant observation inevitable (see Hewitt 2020).

Conversation, Interviewing, and Interview Schedules

Participating in local life means that ethnographers constantly talk to people and ask questions. As their knowledge of the local language and culture increases, they understand more. There are several stages in learning a field language. First is the naming phase—asking name after name of the objects around us. Later we are able to pose more complex questions and understand the replies. We begin to understand simple conversations between two villagers. If our language expertise proceeds far enough, we eventually become able to comprehend rapid-fire public discussions and group conversations.

One data-gathering technique I have used in both Arembepe and Madagascar involves an ethnographic survey that includes an interview schedule. During my second summer of fieldwork in Arembepe, my fellow field workers and I attempted to complete an interview schedule in each of that community's 160 households. We entered almost every household (fewer than 5 percent refused to participate) to ask a set of questions on a printed form. Our results provided us with a census and basic information about the village. We wrote down the name, age, and gender of each household member. We gathered data on family type, religion, present and previous jobs, income, expenditures, diet, possessions, and many other items on our eight-page form.

A month after the devastating Indian Ocean earthquake and tsunami of December 2004, Thai anthropologist Narumon Hinshiranan (left) helped guide the relief effort among the Moken, a maritime people who live on the Surin Islands along Thailand's Andaman coast. Hinshiranan had done prior fieldwork among the Moken people and speaks their language.

Aroon Thaewchatturat/Alamy Stock Photo

Although we were doing a survey, our approach differed from the survey research done by sociologists and other social scientists working in large, industrial nations. That survey research, discussed later in this chapter, involves *sampling* (choosing a small, manageable study group from a larger population). We did not select a partial sample from Arembepe's total population. Instead, we tried to interview in all households (i.e., to have a total sample). We used an interview schedule rather than a questionnaire. With the **interview schedule,** the ethnographer talks face-to-face with people, asks the questions, and writes down the answers. **Questionnaire** procedures tend to be more impersonal; often the respondent fills in the form. Think of how many times in the past month you have been asked to fill out some kind of the survey, usually online, perhaps using a service known as Survey Monkey. Calls to customer service frequently lead to a request that a survey be completed at the end of the call. The ostensible purpose of such surveys is to improve customer service. During the survey process, however, no one ever sees another human being.

In contrast, our goal as ethnographers to obtain a total sample allowed us to meet almost everyone in the village and helped us establish rapport. Decades later, Arembepeiros still talk warmly about how we were interested enough in them to visit their homes and ask them questions. We stood in sharp contrast to the other outsiders the villagers had known, who considered them too poor and backward to take seriously.

Like other survey research, however, our interview schedule did gather comparable quantifiable information. It gave us a basis for assessing patterns and exceptions in village life. Our schedules included a core set of questions that were posed to everyone. However, some interesting side issues often came up during the interview, which we would pursue then or later. We followed such leads into many dimensions of village life. One woman, for instance, a midwife, became our go-to person for detailed information about local childbirth. Another woman had done an internship in an Afro-Brazilian religious center (*candomblé*) in the city. She still went there regularly to study, dance, and get possessed. She became our candomblé expert.

Thus, our interview schedule provided a structure that *directed but did not confine* us as researchers. It enabled our ethnography to be both quantitative and qualitative. The quantitative part consisted of the basic information we gathered and later analyzed statistically. The qualitative dimension came from our follow-up questions, open-ended discussions, pauses for gossip, and work with key consultants.

The Genealogical Method

Many of us learn about our ancestry and relatives by tracing our genealogies. Computer programs, websites, and DNA testing services allow us to fill in our "family trees." The **genealogical method** is a well-established ethnographic technique. Kinship is a prominent building block in the social organization of nonindustrial societies, where people live and work each day with their close kin. Anthropologists need to collect genealogical data to understand current social relations and to reconstruct history. In many nonindustrial societies, links through kinship and marriage form the core of social life. Anthropologists even call such cultures "kin-based societies." Everyone is related and spends most of his or her time with relatives. Rules of behavior associated with particular kin relations are basic to everyday life. Marriage also is crucial in organizing such societies, because strategic marriages between villages, tribes, and clans create political alliances.

Key Cultural Consultants

The term **cultural consultants,** or *informants,* refers to individuals the ethnographer gets to know in the field, the people who teach him or her about their culture. Every community has people who by accident, experience, talent, or training can provide the most complete or useful information about particular aspects of life. These people are **key cultural consultants,** also called *key informants.* In Ivato, the Betsileo village in Madagascar where I lived for about a year, a man named Rakoto was particularly knowledgeable about village history. However, when I asked him to work with me on a genealogy of the 50 to 60 people buried in the village tomb, he called in his cousin Tuesdaysfather, who knew more about that subject. Tuesdaysfather had survived an epidemic of influenza

genealogical method
The use of diagrams and symbols to record kin connections.

interview schedule
A form (guide) used to structure a formal, but personal, interview.

questionnaire
A form used by sociologists to obtain comparable information from respondents.

cultural consultants
People who teach an ethnographer about their culture.

key cultural consultants
Experts on a particular aspect of local life.

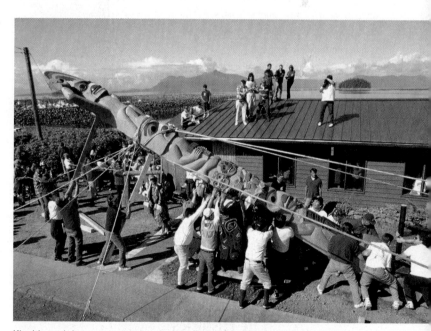

Kinship and descent are vital social building blocks in nonindustrial cultures. Without writing, genealogical information may be preserved in material culture, such as this totem pole being raised in Metlakatla, Alaska.

Lawrence Migdale/Science Source

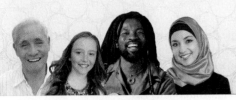

appreciating DIVERSITY

Even Anthropologists Get Culture Shock

My first field experience in Arembepe (Brazil) took place between my junior and senior years at New York City's Columbia College, where I was majoring in anthropology. I went to Arembepe as a participant in a now defunct program designed to provide undergraduates with experience doing ethnography—firsthand study of an alien society's culture and social life.

Brought up in one culture, intensely curious about others, anthropologists nevertheless experience culture shock, particularly on their first field trip. *Culture shock* refers to the whole set of feelings about being in an alien setting, and the ensuing reactions. It is a chilly, creepy feeling of alienation, of being without some of the most ordinary, trivial (and therefore basic) cues of one's culture of origin.

As I planned my departure for Brazil that year, I could not know just how naked I would feel without the cloak of my own language and culture. My sojourn in Arembepe would be my first trip outside the United States. I was an urban boy who had grown up in Atlanta, Georgia, and New York City. I had little experience with rural life in my own country, none with Latin America, and I had received only minimal training in the Portuguese language.

New York City direct to Salvador, Bahia, Brazil. Just a brief stopover in Rio de Janeiro; a longer visit

would be a reward at the end of fieldwork. As our prop jet approached tropical Salvador, I couldn't believe the whiteness of the sand. "That's not snow, is it?" I remarked to a fellow field team member. . . .

My first impressions of Bahia were of smells—alien odors of ripe and decaying mangoes, bananas, and passion fruit—and of swatting the

ubiquitous fruit flies I had never seen before, although I had read extensively about their reproductive behavior in genetics classes. There were strange concoctions of rice, black beans, and gelatinous gobs of unidentifiable meats and floating pieces of skin. Coffee was strong and sugar crude, and every tabletop had containers

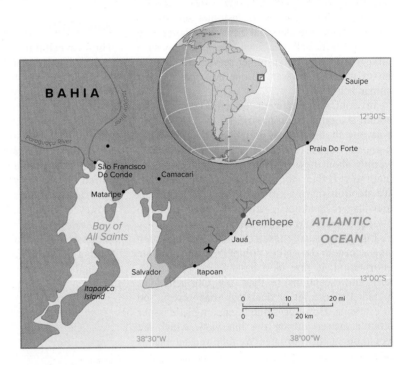

FIGURE 3.1 Location of Arembepe, Bahia, Brazil.

life history

Of a key consultant; a personal portrait of someone's life in a culture.

that ravaged Madagascar, along with much of the world, in 1918-19. Immune to the disease himself, Tuesdaysfather had the grim job of burying his kin as they died. He kept track of everyone buried in the tomb. Tuesdaysfather helped me with the tomb genealogy. Rakoto joined him in telling me personal details about the deceased villagers.

Life Histories

In nonindustrial societies as in our own, individual personalities, interests, and abilities vary. Some villagers prove to be more interested in the

ethnographer's work and are more helpful, interesting, and pleasant than others are. Anthropologists develop likes and dislikes in the field as we do at home. Often, when we find someone unusually interesting, we collect his or her **life history.** This recollection of a lifetime of experiences provides a more intimate and personal cultural portrait than would be possible otherwise. Life histories, which may be audio- or video-recorded for later review and analysis, reveal how specific people perceive, react to, and contribute to changes that affect their lives. Such accounts can illustrate diversity, which exists within any community, because the

for toothpicks and for manioc (cassava) flour to sprinkle, like Parmesan cheese, on anything one might eat. I remember oatmeal soup and a slimy stew of beef tongue in tomatoes. At one meal a disintegrating fish head, eyes still attached, but barely, stared up at me as the rest of its body floated in a bowl of bright orange palm oil. . . .

I only vaguely remember my first day in Arembepe [Figure 3.1]. Unlike ethnographers who have studied remote tribes in the tropical forests of interior South America or the highlands of Papua New Guinea, I did not have to hike or ride a canoe for days to arrive at my field site. Arembepe was not isolated relative to such places, only relative to every other place I had ever been. . . .

I do recall what happened when we arrived. There was no formal road into the village. Entering through southern Arembepe, vehicles simply threaded their way around coconut trees, following tracks left by automobiles that had passed previously. A crowd of children had heard us coming, and they pursued our car through the village streets until we parked in front of our house, near the central square. Our first few days in Arembepe were spent with children following us everywhere. For weeks we had few moments of privacy. Children watched our every move through our living room window. Occasionally one made an incomprehensible remark. Usually they just stood there. . . .

The sounds, sensations, sights, smells, and tastes of life in northeastern Brazil, and in Arembepe, slowly grew familiar. . . . I grew accustomed to this world without Kleenex, in which globs of mucus habitually drooped from the noses of village children whenever a cold passed through Arembepe. A world where, seemingly without effort, women . . . carried 18-liter kerosene cans of water on their heads, where boys sailed kites and sported at catching houseflies in their bare hands, where old women smoked pipes, storekeepers offered cachaça (common rum) at nine in the morning, and men played dominoes on lazy afternoons when there was no fishing. I was visiting a world where human life was oriented toward water—the sea, where men fished, and the lagoon, where women communally washed clothing, dishes, and their own bodies.

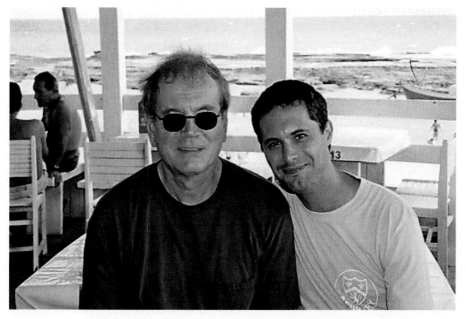

Conrad Kottak, with his Brazilian nephew, Guilherme Roxo, on a revisit to Arembepe in 2004.
Conrad P. Kottak

SOURCE: This description is adapted from my ethnographic study *Assault on Paradise: The Globalization of a Little Community in Brazil,* 4th ed., New York, NY: McGraw-Hill, 2006.

focus is on how different people interpret and deal with some of the same problems. Many ethnographers include the collection of life histories as an important part of their research strategy.

Problem-Oriented Ethnography

Although anthropologists remain interested in the totality of people's lives in a particular community or society, it is impossible to study everything. As a result, contemporary ethnographic fieldwork generally is aimed at investigating one or more specific topics or problems (see Murchison 2010; Sunstein and Chiseri-Strater 2012). Topics that an ethnographer might choose to investigate include marriage practices, gender roles, religion, and economic change. Examples of problem-oriented research include various impact studies done by anthropologists, such as the impact of television, the Internet, education, drought, a hurricane, or a change in government on a particular community or society.

In researching a specific problem, today's anthropologists often need to look beyond local people for relevant data. Government agencies or international organizations may have gathered information on such matters as climate and weather conditions, population density, and settlement patterns. Often, however, depending on the problem they are investigating, anthropologists have to do their own measurements of such variables as field size, yields, dietary quantities, or time allocation. Information of interest to ethnographers extends well beyond what local people can and do tell us. In an increasingly interconnected and complicated world, local people lack knowledge of and control over many factors that may affect their lives—for example, global pandemics, trade policies, international terrorism, warfare, or the exercise of power from regional, national, and international centers (see Koonings et al. 2019; Sanjek 2014).

Longitudinal Studies, Team Research, and Multisited Ethnography

Geography limits anthropologists much less now than in the past, when it could take months to reach a field site and return visits were rare. Modern transportation systems allow anthropologists

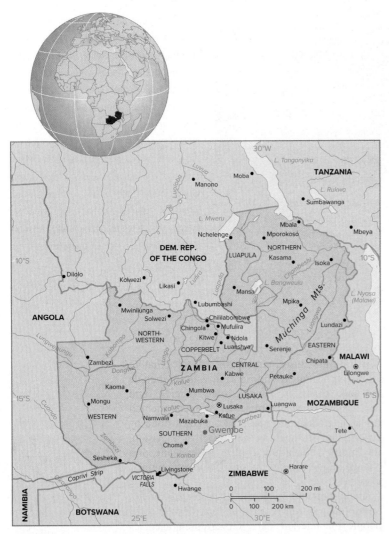

FIGURE 3.2 Location of Gwembe in Zambia.

to return to the field repeatedly. Ethnographic reports now routinely include data from two or more field stays. We can even follow the people we study as they move from village to city, cross the border, or travel internationally. **Longitudinal research** is the long-term study of an area or a population, usually based on repeated visits.

One example is the study of Gwembe District, Zambia (see Figure 3.2). This study, designed as a longitudinal project by Elizabeth Colson and Thayer Scudder in 1956, continued with Colson, Scudder, and their associates and successors of various nationalities. As is often the case with longitudinal research, the Gwembe study also illustrates *team research*—coordinated research by multiple ethnographers (Scudder and Colson 1980; see also Thomas and Harris 2018). Researchers studied four villages in different areas for decades. Periodic censuses provided basic data on population, economy, kinship, and religious behavior. Censused people who had moved were traced and interviewed to see how their lives compared with those of people who stayed behind. The initial focus of study was the impact of a large hydroelectric dam, which subjected the Gwembe people to forced resettlement. Thereafter, Scudder and Colson (1980) examined how education brought new opportunities, even as it also widened a social gap between people with different educational levels. The anthropologists next focused on a change in brewing and drinking patterns, including a rise in alcoholism (Colson and Scudder 1988). When Colson, who died in 2016 at the age of 99, retired from the University of California at Berkeley, she moved to Gwembe district, where she spent her last days and is buried.

As mentioned, longitudinal research often is team research. My own field site of Arembepe, Brazil, first entered the world of anthropology as a field-team village in the 1960s. It was one of four sites for the now-defunct Columbia-Cornell-Harvard-Illinois Summer Field Studies Program in Anthropology. For at least three years, that program sent a total of about 20 undergraduates annually, the author included, to do summer research abroad. The teams were stationed in rural communities in four countries: Brazil, Ecuador, Mexico, and Peru. Since my wife, Isabel Wagley Kottak, and I began studying it in 1962, Arembepe has become a longitudinal field site. Generations of researchers have monitored various aspects of change and development. The community has changed from a village into a town and illustrates the process of globalization at the local level. Its economy, religion, and social life have been transformed (see Kottak 2018).

Brazilian and American researchers worked with us on team research projects during the 1980s (on the impact of television) and the 1990s (on ecological awareness and environmental risk perception). Students from various universities have drawn on our baseline information from the 1960s in their recent studies in Arembepe. Their topics have included standards of physical attractiveness, family planning, conversion to Protestantism, changing food habits, and the influence of the Internet and social media. Arembepe is thus a site where various field workers have worked as members of a longitudinal, multigenerational team. The more recent researchers have built on prior contacts and findings to increase knowledge about how local people meet and manage new circumstances. As of this writing (2020), researchers are continuing fieldwork in Arembepe and other Brazilian communities, updating our study of media impact, which began during the 1980s.

Traditional ethnographic research focused on a single community or "culture," treated as more or less isolated and unique in time and space. In recent years, ethnography has shifted toward studies of change and of contemporary flows of people, technology, images, and information. Reflecting today's world, fieldwork must be more flexible and on a larger scale. Ethnography increasingly is *multitimed* and *multisited.* That is, it studies people through time and in multiple places. Malinowski could focus on Trobriand culture and spend most of his field time in a particular community (see Galman 2019). Nowadays we cannot afford to ignore, as Malinowski did, the outside forces that increasingly impinge on the places we study. Integral to our analyses now are the external entities and factors (e.g., governments, corporations, nongovernmental organizations, new social movements, the drug trade, pandemics) that interact with and influence local communities throughout the world.

Anthropologists increasingly study people in motion. Examples include people living on or near national borders, nomads, seasonal migrants, homeless and displaced people, immigrants, and refugees (see Andersson 2014; Lugo 1997, 2008). As fieldwork changes, with less and less of a spatially set field, what can we take from traditional ethnography? Gupta and Ferguson (1997*a*) correctly cite the "characteristically anthropological emphasis on daily routine and lived experience" (p. 5). The treatment of communities as discrete entities may be a thing of the past. However, "anthropology's traditional attention to the close observation of particular lives in particular places" has an enduring importance (Gupta and Ferguson 1997*b,* p. 25). The method of close observation helps distinguish cultural anthropology from sociology and survey research, which we examine later in this chapter.

ETHNOGRAPHIC PERSPECTIVES

Emic and Etic

One goal of ethnography is to discover local (native) views, beliefs, and perceptions, which may be compared with the ethnographer's own observations and conclusions. In the field, ethnographers typically combine two perspectives, the emic (native-oriented) and the etic (scientist-oriented). These terms, derived from linguistics, have been applied to ethnography by various anthropologists. Marvin Harris (1968/2001*b*) popularized the following meanings of the terms: An **emic** perspective is concerned with how local people think. How do they perceive, categorize, and explain things? What are their rules for behavior? What has meaning for them? The ethnographer seeks to understand the "native viewpoint," relying on local people to explain things and to say whether something is significant or not.

With the **etic** perspective, the focus shifts from local observations, categories, explanations, and interpretations to those of the anthropologist. Members of a culture often are too involved in what they are doing to interpret their culture impartially. Operating etically, the ethnographer emphasizes what he or she (the observer) notices and considers important. As a trained scientist, the ethnographer should try to bring an objective and comprehensive viewpoint to the study of other cultures. Of course, the ethnographer, like any other scientist, is also a human being with cultural blinders that prevent complete objectivity. As in other sciences, proper training can reduce, but not totally eliminate, the observer's bias. But anthropologists do have special training to compare behavior in different societies.

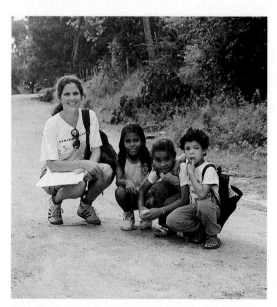

Janet Dunn, one of many anthropologists who have worked in Arembepe. Her study focused on family planning and female reproductive strategies. Where is Arembepe, and what kinds of research have been done there?

Christopher M. O'Leary

emic
A research strategy focusing on local explanations and meanings.

etic
A research strategy emphasizing the ethnographer's explanations and categories.

What are some examples of emic versus etic perspectives? Consider our holidays. For North Americans (emically), Thanksgiving Day is our own unique holiday that commemorates particular historical events. But a wider, etic, perspective sees Thanksgiving as just one more example of the postharvest festivals held in many societies. Consider another example illustrating emic versus etic: Local people (including many Americans) may believe that chills and drafts cause colds, which scientists know are caused by germs. In cultures that lack the germ theory of disease, illnesses are emically explained by various causes, ranging from spirits to ancestors to witches. *Illness* refers to a culture's (emic) perception and explanation of bad health, whereas *disease* refers to the scientific (etic) explanation of poor health, involving known pathogens.

Ethnographers typically combine emic and etic perspectives in their fieldwork. The statements, perceptions, categories, and opinions of local people help ethnographers understand how cultures work. Local beliefs also are interesting and valuable in themselves. However, people often fail to admit, or even recognize, certain causes and consequences of their behavior. This is as true of North Americans as it is of people in other societies.

Online Ethnography

A distinguishing feature of anthropology is that it encompasses a wide range of times, spaces, and places. Anthropologists have even ventured into virtual worlds and their online communities. Tom Boellstorff, Bonnie Nardi, Celia Pearce, and T. L. Taylor have written a handbook for ethnographic fieldwork in cyberspace (2012). All four have researched gaming-oriented online environments, including *Second Life, World of Warcraft, Dreamscape,* and *Myst Online: Uru Live.* Ethnographers use varied techniques to study these virtual worlds. Most important has been participant observation: Researchers become skilled players as they observe the online environment and interactions within it (see Boellstorff 2015; Nardi 2010; Pearce 2009).

Each virtual world has its own culture, which includes rules and governance, customary practices and events, social roles and modes of interaction, and power differentials. When *Uru Live* was discontinued in 2008, Uru refugees moved on to other virtual worlds, where they created and maintained an Uru ethnic identity. Although software designers create the virtual environments, the ordinary people who enter and thrive in these worlds can innovate within the constraints set by "the system"—either the software program or other participants. Within these worlds, the online ethnographers have observed and described various forms of play, performance, creativity, and ritual.

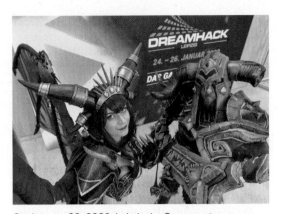

On January 22, 2020, in Leipzig, Germany, two cosplayers present themselves as World-Of-Warcraft characters "Alextrasza" and "T10 Warrior" in a run-up to a gaming festival.

Hendrik Schmidt/Getty Images

Virtual worlds have been heavily influenced by works of science fiction and fantasy. Early games owed a debt to the imaginary world of Middle Earth created by J. R. R. Tolkien, of *The Hobbit* and *The Lord of the Rings* fame. Online worlds contain their own species, artifacts, characters, and customs. The avatar is the representation of self in a virtual world. For example, Bonnie Nardi (2010) describes her "life as an Elf Priest" in the *World of Warcraft.* Online, people can have multiple identities, which often contrast—in gender, for example—with their real-world identities.

Online ethnographers sometimes move offline to visit players in their real-world setting (e.g., a home or an Internet café). In some cases, ethnographers have traveled abroad to see how a given game is played in different countries and how real-world culture influences participation in the virtual world. There are virtual-world fan conventions, which the ethnographer may attend. Interviews can be conducted online and/or offline in a participant's virtual- or real-world home. Informal conversations online reveal what players are thinking about as they play. To understand the social organization of their virtual field site, ethnographers may draw diagrams of social relations, similar to genealogies drawn during real-world fieldwork. Timelines are useful for understanding the succession of virtual events such as dances, festivals, or auctions. Brief online drop-ins can be used to respond to instant messages, keep up with announcements, and find out when players typically log in. Virtual research offers various means of record keeping, note taking, and recording typical of the online environment. These include chat logs and screenshots, as well as audio- and video-recording.

This section has summarized some features of online research as discussed by Boellstorff and his colleagues in their handbook *Ethnography and Virtual Worlds* (2012; see also Hammersley and Atkinson 2019).

SURVEY RESEARCH

As anthropologists work increasingly in large-scale societies, they have developed innovative ways of blending ethnography and survey research (Fricke 1994; Kottak 2009; Pace and Hinote 2013). Before examining such combinations of field methods, let's consider survey research and the main differences between survey research and ethnography. Working mainly in large, populous nations, sociologists, political scientists, and economists have developed and refined the **survey research** design, which involves sampling, impersonal data collection, and statistical analysis. Survey research usually draws a **sample** (a manageable study group) from a much larger population. By studying a properly selected and representative sample, social scientists can make accurate inferences, or at least good guesses, about the larger population.

In smaller-scale societies and communities, ethnographers get to know most of the people. Given the greater size and complexity of nations, survey research can't help being more impersonal. Survey researchers call the people they study *respondents*. These are people who respond to questions during a survey. Sometimes survey researchers interview their respondents directly—in person or by phone. Respondents may be asked to fill out a questionnaire, written or online. A survey may be mailed or e-mailed to randomly selected sample members. In a **random sample,** all members of the population have an equal statistical chance of being chosen for inclusion. A random sample is selected by randomizing procedures, such as tables of random numbers, which are found in many statistics textbooks.

Probably the most familiar example of sampling is political polling. An ever increasing number of organizations gather information designed to estimate outcomes and to determine what kinds of people voted for which candidates. During sampling, researchers gather information about age, gender, education, religion, occupation, income, and political party preference. These characteristics (**variables**—attributes that vary among members of a sample or population) are known to influence political decisions. Polling then leads to pronouncements about the voting tendencies and behavior of such categories as "soccer moms," college-educated women, and blue-collar men.

Many more variables affect social identities, experiences, behavior, and opinions in a modern nation than in the small communities where ethnography grew up. In contemporary North America, hundreds of factors influence our behavior and attitudes. These social predictors include our religion; where we grew up or live now; and our parents' professions, ethnic origins, political leanings, and income levels.

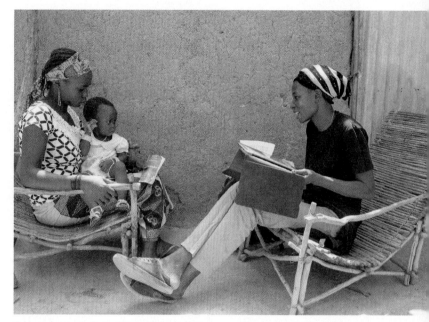

Survey research: Sally Belem (right) questions a mother about child nutrition in a village in the Yako province, Burkina Faso, Africa, as part of a two-year study. Sometimes the research settings and procedures of survey researchers and anthropologists can be very similar.

Mike Goldwater/Alamy Stock Photo

Ethnography can be used to supplement and fine-tune survey research. Anthropologists can transfer the personal, firsthand techniques of ethnography to a variety of settings. A combination of survey research and ethnography can provide new perspectives on life in **complex societies** (large and populous societies with social stratification and central governments). Preliminary ethnography can help develop culturally appropriate questions for inclusion in surveys. Recap 3.1 contrasts traditional ethnography with survey research.

In any complex society, many predictor variables (*social indicators*) influence behavior and opinions. Because we must be able to detect, measure, and compare the influence of social indicators, many contemporary anthropological studies have a statistical foundation. Even in rural fieldwork, anthropologists increasingly use samples, gather quantitative data, and use statistics to interpret them (see Bernard 2013, 2018; Bernard and Gravlee 2014). Statistical analysis can support and round out an ethnographic account of local social life.

However, in the best studies, the hallmark of ethnography remains: Anthropologists enter the community and get to know the people. They participate in local activities, networks, and associations. They watch the effects of national and international policies on local life. The ethnographic method and the emphasis on personal relationships in social research are valuable gifts that cultural anthropology brings to the study of any society.

survey research
The study of society through sampling, statistical analysis, and impersonal data collection.

sample
A smaller study group chosen to represent a larger population.

random sample
A sample in which all population members have an equal statistical chance of inclusion.

variables
Attributes that differ from one person or case to the next.

complex societies
Large, populous societies (e.g., nations) with social stratification and central governments.

ETHNOGRAPHY (TRADITIONAL)	SURVEY RESEARCH
Studies whole, functioning communities	Studies a small sample of a larger population
Usually is based on firsthand fieldwork, during which information is collected after rapport, based on personal contact, is established	Often is conducted with little or no personal contact between study subjects and researchers, as interviews are frequently conducted in printed form, over the phone, or online
Traditionally is interested in all aspects of local life (holistic)	Usually focuses on a small number of variables (e.g., factors that influence voting) rather than on the totality of people's lives
Traditionally has been conducted in nonindustrial, small-scale societies, where people often do not read and write	Typically is carried out in modern nations, where most people are literate, permitting respondents to fill in their own questionnaires
Makes little use of statistics, because the communities being studied tend to be small, with little diversity besides that based on age, gender, and individual personality variation	Depends heavily on statistical analyses to make inferences regarding a large and diverse population, based on data collected from a small subset of that population

DOING ANTHROPOLOGY RIGHT AND WRONG: ETHICAL ISSUES

The anthropologist Clyde Kluckhohn (1944) saw a key public service role for anthropology. It could provide a "scientific basis for dealing with the crucial dilemma of the world today: how can peoples of different appearance, mutually unintelligible languages, and dissimilar ways of life get along peaceably together?" Many anthropologists never would have chosen their profession if they doubted that anthropology had the capacity to enhance human welfare. Because we live in a world that contains unpredictable leaders, pandemics, unrest, war, and terrorism, we must consider the proper role of anthropologists in studying such phenomena.

Science exists in society and in the context of law and ethics. Anthropologists can't study things simply because they happen to be interesting or of value to science. We must consider ethics as well (see Gonzalez-Ruibal 2018; Radin 2018). Anthropologists typically have worked abroad, outside their own society. In the context of international contacts and cultural diversity, different ethical codes and value systems will meet, and often compete (Castellanos 2019).

Anthropologists must be sensitive to such cultural differences, and aware of procedures and standards in the host country (the place where the research takes place). Researchers must *inform* officials and colleagues about the purpose, funding, and likely results of their research. **Informed consent** should be obtained from anyone who provides information or who might be affected by the research.

Anthropologists should try to (1) include host country colleagues in their research planning, (2) establish collaborative relationships with host country institutions, (3) include host country colleagues in dissemination, including publication, of the research results, and (4) ensure that something is "given back" to the host country. For example, research equipment stays in the host country, or funding is sought for host country colleagues to do research, attend international meetings, or visit foreign institutions.

The Code of Ethics

The Code of Ethics of the American Anthropological Association (AAA) recognizes that anthropologists have obligations to their scholarly field, to the wider society, and to the human species, other species, and the environment (see Piemmons and Barker 2015). The anthropologist's primary obligation is to *do no harm* to the people being studied (see Borofsky and Hutson 2016). The stated aim of the AAA code is to offer guidelines and to promote discussion and education, rather than to investigate possible misconduct. Two of the code's key points are as follows: (1) anthropologists should inform all parties affected by their research about its nature, goals, procedures, potential impacts, and source(s) of funding (and obtain their consent based on the information provided), and (2) researchers should establish proper relationships with the countries and communities where they work. The most recent version of the AAA Code of Ethics can be found at the following website: http://ethics.americananthro.org/category/statement/.

informed consent
An agreement to take part in research—after having been informed about its purpose, nature, procedures, and possible impacts.

Anthropologists and Terrorism

The AAA has deemed it of "paramount importance" that anthropologists study the causes of terrorism and violence. But how should such studies be conducted (see Koonings 2019)? What ethical issues might arise? What should not be done?

As an example of ethically problematic research consider the Pentagon's Human Terrain System (HTS) program. Launched in February 2007 and ended in September 2014, HTS embedded anthropologists and other social scientists in military teams in Iraq and Afghanistan (see Jaschik 2015; Sims 2016; Weston and Djohari 2020). In October 2007, the AAA issued a statement of disapproval of HTS—outlining how HTS violates the AAA Code of Ethics. (See http://www.americananthro.org/ConnectWithAAA/Content.aspx?ItemNumber=1626.) HTS placed anthropologists, as contractors with the U.S. military, in war zones, where they were expected to collect cultural and social data for use by the military. The AAA identified the following as some of the ethical concerns raised by these activities:

1. Anthropologists in war zones may be unable to identify themselves as anthropologists, as distinct from military personnel. This constrains their ethical responsibility to disclose who they are and what they are doing.

2. HTS anthropologists may be asked to negotiate relations among several groups, including local populations and the military units in which they are embedded. Their responsibilities to their units might conflict with their obligations to the local people they study or consult. This could interfere with the obligation, stipulated in the AAA Code of Ethics, to do no harm.

3. In an active war zone, it is difficult for local people to give informed consent without feeling coerced to provide information. As a result, "voluntary informed consent" (as stipulated in the AAA Code of Ethics) is compromised.

4. HTS anthropologists might supply information that could be used to target specific groups for military action. Such use of fieldwork-derived information would violate the AAA Code of Ethics stipulation to do no harm to people.

5. Identification of anthropology and anthropologists with the U.S. military might indirectly (through suspicion of guilt by association) endanger the research, and even the personal safety, of other anthropologists and their consultants throughout the world.

What do you think about anthropologists' proper role in studying terrorism and war?

THEORY IN ANTHROPOLOGY OVER TIME

Anthropology has various fathers and mothers. The fathers include Lewis Henry Morgan, Sir Edward Burnett Tylor, Franz Boas, and Bronislaw Malinowski. The mothers include Ruth Benedict and Margaret Mead. Some of the fathers might be classified better as grandfathers, because one of them, Franz Boas, was the intellectual father of Mead and Benedict. Furthermore, what is known now as Boasian anthropology arose mainly in opposition to the 19th-century evolutionism of Morgan and Tylor.

My goal in the remainder of this chapter is to survey the major theoretical perspectives that have characterized anthropology since its emergence in the second half of the 19th century (see also Erickson and Murphy 2017; McGee and Warms 2017; Moberg 2019; Moore 2019). Evolutionary perspectives, especially those associated with Morgan and Tylor, dominated 19th-century anthropology. The early 20th century witnessed various reactions to 19th-century evolutionism. In Great Britain, functionalists such as Malinowski and Alfred Reginald Radcliffe-Brown abandoned the speculative historicism of the evolutionists and instead did studies of living societies. In the United States, Boas and his followers rejected the search for evolutionary stages in favor of a historical approach that traced borrowing and the spread of culture traits across geographic areas. Functionalists and Boasians alike saw cultures as integrated and patterned.

Nineteenth-Century Evolutionism

Let's begin this survey of anthropology's history with Morgan (United States) and Tylor (Great Britain), both of whom wrote classic books during the 19th century. Lewis Henry Morgan, although an important founder of anthropology, was not himself a professionally trained anthropologist. Rather, he was a lawyer in upper New York state who was fond of visiting a nearby Seneca reservation and learning about the tribe's history and customs. He wrote about the Seneca and other Iroquois tribes in his book *League of the Ho-dé-no-sau-nee or Iroquois* (1851/1966). This work, anthropology's earliest ethnography, was based on occasional rather than protracted fieldwork. Through his fieldwork, and his friendship with Ely Parker, an educated Iroquois man, Morgan was able to describe the social, political, religious, and economic principles of Iroquois life, including the history of their confederation. He laid out the structural principles on which Iroquois society was based. Morgan also used his skills as a lawyer to help the Iroquois in their fight with the Ogden Land Company, which was attempting to seize their lands.

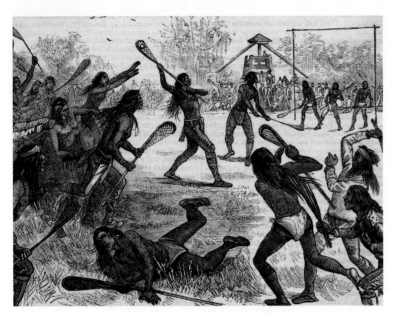

The early American anthropologist Lewis Henry Morgan described lacrosse (shown here) as one of the six games played by the tribes of the Iroquois nation, whose League he described in a famous book (1851/1966).

Bettmann/Corbis

Morgan's second influential book, *Ancient Society* (1877/1963), was a theoretical treatise rather than an ethnography. *Ancient Society* is a key example of 19th-century evolutionism applied to society. Morgan assumed that human society had evolved through a series of stages, which he named savagery, barbarism, and civilization. He subdivided savagery and barbarism into three substages each: lower, middle, and upper savagery and lower, middle, and upper barbarism. In Morgan's scheme, the earliest humans lived in lower savagery, with subsistence based on fruits and nuts. In middle savagery, people started fishing and gained control over fire. Upper savagery was marked by the invention of the bow and arrow. Lower barbarism began when humans started making pottery. Middle barbarism in the Old World depended on the domestication of plants and animals, and in the Americas on irrigated agriculture. Iron smelting and the use of iron tools ushered in upper barbarism. Civilization, finally, came about with the invention of writing.

Morgan's evolutionism is known as **unilinear evolutionism,** because he assumed there was one line or path along which all societies evolved. Any society in upper barbarism, for example, had to include in its history, in order, periods of lower, middle, and upper savagery, and then lower and middle barbarism. Furthermore, Morgan believed that the indigenous societies that had managed to survive into the 19th century could be viewed as, in a sense, "living fossils," which could be placed in the various stages. Some had not advanced beyond upper savagery. Others had made it to middle barbarism, while others had attained civilization.

unilinear evolutionism

The (19th-century) idea of a single line or path of cultural development.

Morgan's critics have disputed various elements of his scheme, including such loaded terms as *savagery* and *barbarism,* and the particular criteria he used for each stage. Also, Morgan erred in assuming that societies could follow only one evolutionary path. In fact, societies have followed multiple developmental paths.

Like Morgan, Sir Edward Burnett Tylor came to anthropology through personal experience rather than formal training. In 1855, he left England to travel to Mexico and Central America, where he began what turned out to be a lifelong investigation of unfamiliar cultures. Returning to England, Tylor continued his study of the customs and beliefs of non-Western peoples—both contemporary and prehistoric. He wrote a series of books that established his reputation, leading to his eventual appointment as the first professor of anthropology at Oxford University.

In his two-volume work, *Primitive Culture* (1871/1958), Tylor offered an influential and enduring definition of culture (see Chapter 2 in this book) and proposed it as a topic to be studied scientifically. The second volume of *Primitive Culture,* titled *Primitive Religion,* offered an evolutionary approach to the anthropology of religion. Like Morgan, Tylor proposed a unilinear path—from animism to polytheism, then monotheism, and finally science. In Tylor's view, religion would retreat when science provided better explanations. Both Tylor and Morgan were interested in *survivals,* practices that survive in contemporary society from earlier evolutionary stages. The belief in ghosts today, for example, would represent a survival from the stage of animism—the belief in spiritual beings. Survivals were taken as evidence that a particular society had passed through earlier evolutionary stages.

Historical Particularism

Franz Boas is the founder of American four-field anthropology. Most of his career was spent at Columbia University, where he trained dozens of influential anthropologists, now remembered as the Boasians. Boas contributed to cultural, biological, and linguistic anthropology. His book *Race, Language, and Culture* (1940/1966) is a collection of essays on those key topics. His biological studies of European immigrants to the United States revealed and measured phenotypical plasticity. The children of immigrants differed physically from their parents not because of genetic change but because they had grown up in a different environment. Boas showed that human biology was plastic. It could be changed by the environment, including cultural forces. Boas and his students worked hard to demonstrate that biology (including race) did not determine cultural achievements. In her important book, *Race, Science, and Politics,* Ruth Benedict (1940) stressed the idea that people of many races have contributed to major historical advances.

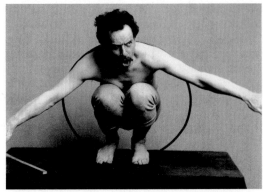

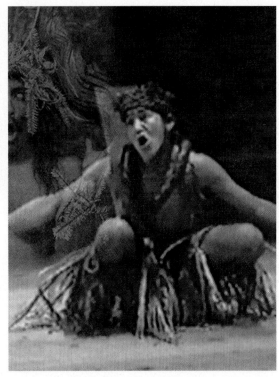

Franz Boas, founder of American four-field anthropology, studied the Kwakwaka'wakw, or Kwakiutl, in British Columbia (BC), Canada. The photo above shows Boas posing for a museum model of a Kwakiutl dancer. The photo on the right is a still from a film by anthropologist Aaron Glass titled In *Search of the Hamat'sa: A Tale of Headhunting* (DER distributor). It shows a real Kwakiutl dancer, Marcus Alfred, performing the same Hamat'sa (or "Cannibal Dance"), which is a vital part of an important Kwakiutl ceremony. The U'mista Cultural Centre in Alert Bay, BC (www.umista.org) owns the rights to the video clip of the Hamat'sa featuring Marcus Alfred.

(left): Science Source; (right): Used with permission of Dr. Aaron Glass and U'mista Cultural Centre in Alert Bay, BC

In his ethnographic fieldwork, Boas studied language and culture among Native Americans, most notably the Kwakiutl (also known as Kwakwaka'wakw) of the North Pacific coast of North America. Boas took issue with 19th-century evolutionism on many counts, including the idea of a single, preordained evolutionary path. He argued that a particular cultural feature, for example, totemism, did not follow a single path of development but could arise for many reasons. His position was one of **historical particularism.** Because the particular histories of totemism in societies A, B, and C had each been different, those forms of totemism had different causes. Totemism might look the same in all these cases, but each case was actually unique, because it had its own, separate and distinct, history. Any cultural form, from totemism to clan organization, could develop, Boas believed, for all sorts of reasons.

To explain *cultural generalities* (cultural traits that are shared by some but not all societies), 19th-century evolutionists had stressed independent invention: People in many areas had come up with the same cultural solution to a common problem. Agriculture, for example, was invented several times. Boas and his students, while not denying independent invention, stressed the importance of diffusion, or borrowing, among cultures. The analytic units they used to study diffusion were the culture trait, the trait complex, and the culture area. A culture trait was something like a bow and arrow. A trait complex was the hunting pattern that went along with it. A culture area was based on the diffusion of traits and trait complexes

across a particular geographic area, such as the Plains, the Southwest, or the North Pacific coast of North America. Such areas often had environmental boundaries that limited the spread of culture traits beyond that area. Historical particularism and diffusion were seen as complementary. As culture traits diffused, they developed their particular histories as they entered and moved through particular societies.

Historical particularism rejected comparison and generalization in favor of an individuating historical approach. In this rejection, historical particularism stands in contrast to most of the approaches that have followed it (see Candea 2019; Salzman 2012).

Functionalism

Another challenge to evolutionism (as well as to historical particularism) came from Great Britain. **Functionalism** abandoned the search for origins (whether through evolution or through diffusion) and instead focused on the role that cultural traits and social practices play in contemporary society. The two main strands of functionalism are associated, respectively, with Bronislaw Malinowski, a Polish anthropologist who taught mainly in Great Britain, and the British anthropologist Alfred Reginald Radcliffe-Brown.

Malinowski
Both Malinowski and Radcliffe-Brown focused on present-day societies rather than history. Malinowski did pioneering fieldwork among living

historical particularism
(Boas) The idea that histories are not comparable; diverse paths can lead to the same cultural result.

functionalism
An approach that focuses on the role (function) of sociocultural practices in social systems.

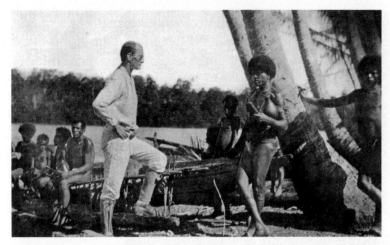

Bronislaw Malinowski (1884–1942), who was born in Poland but spent most of his professional life in England, did fieldwork in the Trobriand Islands from 1914 to 1918. Malinowski is generally considered to be the father of ethnography. Does this photo suggest anything about his relationship with Trobriand villagers?

Chronicle/Alamy Stock Photo

synchronic
(Studying societies) at one time.

diachronic
(Studying societies) across time.

people. Usually considered the father of ethnography because of his years of fieldwork in the Trobriand Islands, Malinowski was a functionalist in two senses. In the first, rooted in his ethnography, he believed that all customs and institutions in society were integrated and interrelated, so that if one changed, others would change as well. Each, then, was a *function* of the others. A corollary of this belief was that an ethnographer could begin anywhere and eventually get at the rest of the culture. Thus, a study of Trobriand fishing eventually would lead the ethnographer to study the entire economic system, the role of magic and religion, myth, trade, and kinship. The second strand of Malinowski's functionalism is known as *needs functionalism.* Malinowski (1944) believed that humans had a set of universal biological needs, and that customs developed to fulfill those needs. The function of any practice was the role it played in satisfying those universal biological needs, such as the need for food, sex, shelter, and so on.

Radcliffe-Brown and Structural Functionalism

According to Radcliffe-Brown (1962/1965), although history is important, anthropologists could never hope to discover the histories of people without writing. He trusted neither evolutionary nor diffusionist reconstructions. Viewing all historical statements about nonliterate peoples as merely conjectural, Radcliffe-Brown urged anthropologists to focus on the role that particular practices play in the life of societies today. For example, in a famous essay Radcliffe-Brown (1962/1965) examined the prominent role of the mother's brother among the Ba Thonga of Mozambique. An evolutionist priest previously had explained the special role of the mother's brother in this patrilineal society as a survival from a time when the descent rule had been matrilineal.

(In a patrilineal society, people belong to their father's group, whereas in a matrilineal society they belong to their mother's group. The unilinear evolutionists believed that all human societies had passed through a matrilineal stage before becoming patrilineal.) Radcliffe-Brown rejected that idea as unproven, conjectural history. He instead explained the special role of the mother's brother with reference to the institutions of present rather than past Ba Thonga society. Radcliffe-Brown advocated that anthropology be a **synchronic** rather than a **diachronic** science, that is, that it study societies as they exist today (synchronic, at one time) rather than across time (diachronic).

The term *structural functionalism* is associated with Radcliffe-Brown and Edward Evan Evans-Pritchard, another prominent British social anthropologist. The latter is famous for many books, including *The Nuer* (1940), an ethnographic classic that laid out very clearly the structural principles that organized Nuer society in what is now South Sudan. According to structural functionalism, customs (social practices) function to preserve the social structure. In Radcliffe-Brown's view, the *function* of any practice is the role it plays in maintaining the system of which it is a part. That system has a structure whose parts work (function) to maintain the whole. Radcliffe-Brown saw social systems as comparable to anatomical and physiological systems. The function of organs and physiological processes is their role in keeping the body running smoothly. So, too, he thought, did customs, practices, social roles, and behavior function to keep the social system running smoothly. Given this suggestion of harmony, functionalist models have been criticized for a tendency to see things as functioning not just to maintain the system but to do so in the most optimal way possible, so that any deviation from the norm is viewed as detrimental.

The Manchester School

A group of British anthropologists working at the University of Manchester, dubbed the Manchester school, are well known for their research in African societies and their studies of conflict and its resolution. Manchester anthropologist Max Gluckman, for example, made conflict an important part of his analysis by focusing on rituals of rebellion and other expressions of discontent. However, Gluckman and his colleagues did not abandon functionalism totally. The Manchester anthropologists examined how rebellion and conflict were dissipated and resolved, thus maintaining the system.

Contemporary Functionalism

A form of functionalism persists today in the widely accepted view that there are social and cultural systems and that their elements, or constituent parts, are functionally related (are functions of each other) so that they covary: When one part changes, others also change. Also enduring is the idea that some elements—often the economic ones—are more important than others are. Few would deny, for example, that significant economic changes, such as the increasing cash employment of women, have led to changes in family and household organization and in related variables such as age at marriage and frequency of divorce. Changes in work and family arrangements then affect other variables, such as frequency of church attendance, which has declined in the United States and Canada.

Configurationalism

Two of Boas's best-known students, Benedict and Mead, developed an approach to culture that has been called **configurationalism.** This is related to functionalism in the sense that culture is seen as integrated. We've seen that the Boasians traced the geographic distribution of culture traits. Boas recognized, however, that diffusion wasn't automatic. Traits might not spread if they met environmental barriers, or if they were not accepted by a particular culture. There had to be a fit between the culture and the trait diffusing in, and borrowed traits would be *indigenized*—modified to fit the culture adopting them. Although traits can diffuse in from various directions, Benedict stressed that culture traits—indeed, whole cultures—are uniquely patterned or integrated. Her best-selling book *Patterns of Culture* (1934/1959) described such culture patterns.

Mead, who is best known for her focus on child-rearing practices, also found patterns in the cultures she studied, including Samoa, Bali, and Papua New Guinea. Mead was particularly interested in different patterns of enculturation. Stressing the plasticity of human nature, she saw culture as a powerful force that created almost endless possibilities. Even among neighboring societies, different patterns of enculturation could mold children into very different kinds of adults. Neighboring cultures could therefore have very different personality types and cultural configurations. Mead's best-known—albeit controversial (see Dresser 2020)—book is *Coming of Age in Samoa* (1928/1961). As a young woman, she traveled to Samoa to study female adolescence there in order to compare it with the same period of life in the United States. Suspicious of biologically determined universals, she assumed that Samoan adolescence would differ from the same period in the United States and that this would affect adult personality. Using her Samoan ethnographic findings, Mead contrasted the apparent sexual freedom there with the greater repression of adolescent sexuality in the United States. Her findings supported the Boasian view that culture, not biology, determines variation in human behavior and personality. Mead's later fieldwork among the Arapesh, Mundugumor, and Tchambuli of New

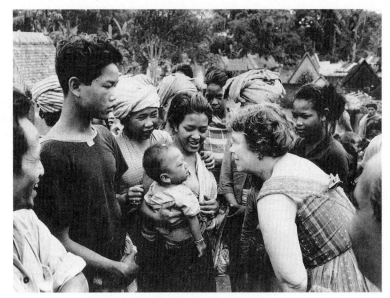

Margaret Mead in the field in Bali, Indonesia, in 1957.
Associated Press/AP Images

Guinea resulted in *Sex and Temperament in Three Primitive Societies* (1935/1950). She offered that book, which documented significant variation in male and female personality traits and behavior in three nearby societies, as further support for cultural determinism.

Evolutionism Returns

Around 1950, with the end of World War II and a growing anticolonial movement, anthropologists renewed their interest in culture change and even evolution. The American anthropologists Leslie White and Julian Steward complained that the Boasians had inappropriately thrown the baby (evolution) out with the bath water (the particular flaws of 19th-century evolutionary schemes). In his book *The Evolution of Culture* (1959), White claimed to be returning to the same concept of cultural evolution used by Tylor and Morgan, now better informed by a century of archaeological discoveries and a much larger ethnographic record. White's approach has been called *general evolution,* the idea that over time and through the archaeological, historical, and ethnographic records, we can see the evolution of culture as a whole. For example, human economies have evolved from Paleolithic foraging, through early farming and herding, to intensive forms of agriculture, to industrialism. Socially and politically, too, there has been evolution, from bands and tribes to chiefdoms and states. There can be no doubt, White argued, that culture has evolved. But unlike the unilinear evolutionists of the 19th century, White realized that particular cultures might not evolve in the same direction.

White considered energy capture to be the main engine of cultural evolution. Cultural advance, he

configurationalism
The view of culture as integrated and patterned.

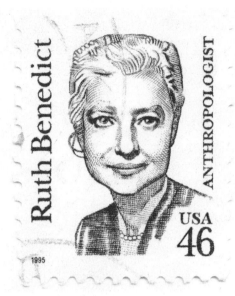
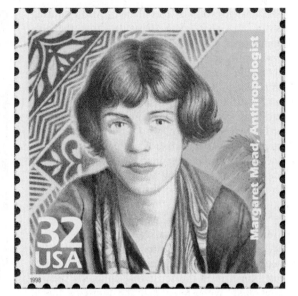

Two U.S. stamps commemorating anthropologists. The 46-cent stamp, issued in 1995, honors Ruth Fulton Benedict (1887–1948), best known for her widely read book *Patterns of Culture*. In 1998, the U.S. Postal Service issued this 32-cent Margaret Mead (1901–1978) stamp as part of its "Celebrate the Century" commemorative series. The stamp shows a young Dr. Mead against a Samoan background.

(left): Solodov Alexey/Shutterstock; (right): catwalker/Shutterstock

thought, could be measured by the amount of energy harnessed per capita per year in a society. In this view, Canada and the United States would rank among the world's most advanced nations because of the amount of energy they use per capita. White's notion that social advance can be measured by energy expenditure seems strange today, because it views societies that use the most fossil fuel per capita as being more advanced than those that have taken measures to reduce their dependence on finite energy sources.

Julian Steward, in his influential book *Theory of Culture Change* (1955), proposed a different evolutionary model, which he called *multilinear evolution*. He showed how cultures have followed several different evolutionary paths. For example, he recognized different paths to statehood (e.g., those followed by irrigated versus nonirrigated societies). Steward also was a pioneer in a field of anthropology he called *cultural ecology,* today generally known as *ecological anthropology,* which pays particular attention to the relationships between cultures and their environments. Steward looked to technology and the environment as the main causes of culture change. The environment and the technology available to exploit it were seen as part of what he called the *culture core*—the combination of environmental and economic factors that determined the overall configuration of any society.

Cultural Materialism

In proposing **cultural materialism** as a theoretical paradigm, Marvin Harris drew on models of determinism associated with White and Steward.

Harris (1979/2001*a*) thought that any society had three parts: infrastructure, structure, and superstructure. The *infrastructure,* similar to Steward's culture core, consisted of technology, economics, and demography—the systems of production and reproduction without which societies could not survive. Growing out of infrastructure was *structure*—social relations, forms of kinship and descent, and patterns of distribution and consumption. The third layer was *superstructure:* religion, ideology, and play—aspects of culture farthest away from the meat and bones that enable cultures to survive. Harris's key belief, shared with White, Steward, and Karl Marx, was that in the final analysis infrastructure determines structure and superstructure. Harris therefore took issue with theorists (he called them "idealists"), such as Max Weber (see Chapter 12), who argued for the prominent role of religion (an aspect of superstructure) in changing society. Like most of the anthropologists discussed so far, Harris insisted that anthropology is a *science.* For Harris, as for White and Steward, the primary goal of anthropology, as a science, is to seek explanations—relations of cause and effect.

Cultural Determinism: Culturology, the Superorganic, and Social Facts

In this section we consider three prominent early anthropologists (White, Kroeber, and Durkheim) who stressed the importance of culture and the role it plays in determining individual behavior. Leslie White, although an avowed evolutionist, was also a strong believer in the power of culture. White saw cultural anthropology as a distinctive

cultural materialism

(Harris) The idea that cultural infrastructure determines structure and superstructure.

science, which he named *culturology*. The cultural forces studied by that science were so powerful, White believed, that individuals made little difference. White disputed what was then called the "great man theory of history," the idea that particular individuals were responsible for great discoveries and epochal changes. White looked instead to the constellation of cultural forces that produced great individuals. During certain historical periods, such as the Renaissance, conditions were right for the expression of creativity and greatness, and individual genius blossomed. At other times and places, there may have been just as many great minds, but the culture did not encourage their expression. As proof of this theory, White pointed to the *simultaneity of discovery*. Several times in human history, when culture was ready, people working independently in different places have come up with the same revolutionary idea or achievement at the same time. Examples include the formulation of the theory of evolution through natural selection by Charles Darwin and Alfred Russel Wallace, the independent rediscovery of Mendelian genetics by three scientists in 1917, and the independent invention of flight by the Wright brothers in the United States and Alberto Santos-Dumont in Brazil.

The prolific Boasian anthropologist Alfred Kroeber (1952/1987) also stressed the need for a new and distinctive science focusing on culture, perceived as a distinctive realm, which he called the **superorganic.** Its study, he thought, was just as important as the study of the organic (biology) and the inorganic (chemistry and physics). In his studies of fashion, such as variations in women's hemlines from year to year, Kroeber (1944) attempted to show the power of culture over the individual. People had little choice, he thought, but to follow the styles and trends of their times.

In France, Émile Durkheim had taken a similar approach, calling for a new social science to be based in what he called, in French, the *conscience collectif*. The usual translation of this as "collective consciousness" does not convey adequately the similarity of this notion to Kroeber's superorganic and White's culturology. This new science, Durkheim proposed, would be based on the study of *social facts,* which were analytically distinct from facts about individuals. Psychologists study individuals; anthropologists study individuals as representative of something more. It is those larger systems, which consist of social positions—statuses and roles—and which are perpetuated across the generations through enculturation, that anthropologists should study.

Of course, sociologists also study such social systems, and Durkheim was a prominent early figure in both anthropology and sociology. He wrote about religion in Native Australia as readily as about suicide rates in modern societies. Durkheim (1897/1951, 1912/2001) analyzed suicide rates and religion as collective phenomena. Individuals commit suicide for all sorts of reasons, but the variation in rates (which apply only to collectivities) can and should be linked to social phenomena, such as a sense of general social alienation at particular times and in particular places.

Symbolic and Interpretive Anthropology

Victor Turner was a prominent British social anthropologist who taught successively at the Universities of Manchester, Chicago, and Virginia. Turner wrote several important works on ritual and symbols. *The Forest of Symbols* (1967) is a collection of essays about symbols and rituals among the Ndembu of Zambia, where Turner did his major fieldwork. In that book, Turner examines how symbols and rituals are used to regulate, anticipate, and avoid conflict. He also examines a hierarchy of meanings of symbols, from their social meanings and functions to their internalization within individuals.

Along with anthropologist Mary Douglas (1970a), Turner founded the field of **symbolic anthropology**—the study of symbols in their social and cultural context. Turner saw important links among symbolic anthropology, social psychology, psychology, and psychoanalysis. The study of symbols is all-important in psychoanalysis, whose founder, Sigmund Freud, also recognized a hierarchy of symbols, from potentially universal ones to those that had meaning for particular individuals and emerged during the analysis and interpretation of their dreams. Turner's symbolic anthropology flourished at the University of Chicago, where another major advocate, David Schneider (1968), developed a symbolic approach to American culture in his book *American Kinship: A Cultural Account.*

Related to symbolic anthropology is **interpretive anthropology,** whose primary advocate was Clifford Geertz. Interpretive anthropology (Geertz 1973, 1983) approaches cultures as symbolic texts whose meanings must be deciphered in particular

Mary Douglas (1921–2007), a prominent symbolic anthropologist, who taught at University College, London, England, and Northwestern University, Evanston, Illinois. This photo shows her at an awards ceremony celebrating her receipt in 2003 of an honorary degree from Oxford.
Rob Judges

superorganic
(Kroeber) The special domain of culture, beyond the organic and inorganic realms.

symbolic anthropology
The study of symbols in their social and cultural context.

interpretive anthropology
(Geertz) The study of a culture as a system of meaning.

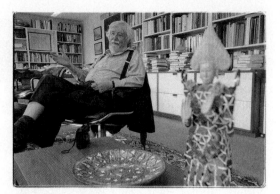

Anthropologist Clifford Geertz (1926–2006), who taught for many years at Princeton University.

Laura Pedrick/*The New York Times*/Redux Pictures

cultural and historical settings. Geertz's approach recalls Malinowski's belief that the ethnographer's primary task is "to grasp the native's point of view, his relation to life, to realize *his* vision of *his* world" (1922/1961, p. 25—Malinowski's italics). Since the 1970s, interpretive anthropology has focused on describing and interpreting that which is meaningful to the local people. According to Geertz (1973), anthropologists may choose anything in a culture that interests or engages them (such as a Balinese cockfight he interprets in a famous essay), fill in details, and elaborate to inform their readers about meanings in that culture. Meanings are carried by and expressed in public symbolic forms, including words, rituals, and customs.

Structuralism

In anthropology, structuralism mainly is associated with Claude Lévi-Strauss, a renowned and prolific French anthropologist, who died in 2009 at the age of 100. Lévi-Strauss's structuralism evolved over time, from his early interest in the structures of kinship and marriage systems to his later interest in the structure of the human mind. In this latter sense, Lévi-Straussian structuralism (1967) aims not at explaining relations, themes, and connections among aspects of culture but at discovering them.

Structuralism rests on Lévi-Strauss's belief that human minds have certain universal characteristics, which originate in common features of the *Homo sapiens* brain. These common mental structures lead people everywhere to think similarly regardless of their society or cultural background. Among these universal mental characteristics are the need to classify: to impose order on aspects of nature, on people's relation to nature, and on relations between people.

According to Lévi-Strauss, a universal aspect of classification is opposition, or contrast. Although many phenomena are continuous rather than discrete, the mind, because of its need to impose order, treats them as being more different than

agency
The actions of individuals, alone and in groups, that create and transform culture.

they are. One of the most common means of classifying is by using binary opposition. Good and evil, white and black, old and young, high and low are oppositions that, according to Lévi-Strauss, reflect the universal human need to convert differences of degree into differences of kind.

Lévi-Strauss applied his assumptions about classification and binary opposition to myths and folk tales. He showed that these narratives have simple building blocks—elementary structures or "mythemes." Examining the myths of different cultures, Lévi-Strauss shows that one tale can be converted into another through a series of simple operations—for example, by doing the following:

1. Converting the positive element of a myth into its negative

2. Reversing the order of the elements

3. Replacing a male hero with a female hero

4. Preserving or repeating certain key elements

Through such operations, two apparently dissimilar myths can be shown to be variations on a common structure. One example is Lévi-Strauss's (1967) analysis of "Cinderella," a widespread tale whose elements vary between neighboring cultures. Through reversals, oppositions, and negations, as the tale is told, retold, diffused, and incorporated within the traditions of successive societies, "Cinderella" becomes "Ash Boy," along with a series of other oppositions (e.g., stepfather versus stepmother) related to the change in gender from female to male.

Processual Approaches

Agency
Anthropologists traditionally have viewed culture as a kind of social glue transmitted across the generations, binding people through their common past—cultural traditions. More recently, anthropologists have come to see culture as something that is continually created and reworked in the present. Contemporary anthropologists now emphasize how the day-to-day actions of individuals can make and remake culture (Gupta and Ferguson 1997). **Agency** refers to the actions that individuals take, both alone and in groups, in forming and transforming culture.

Practice Theory
The approach to culture known as *practice theory* (Ortner 1984) recognizes that individuals within a society vary in their motives and intentions and in the amount of power and influence they have. Such contrasts may be associated with gender, age, ethnicity, class, and other social variables. Practice theory focuses on how these varied individuals—through their actions and practices—influence and transform the world they live in. Practice theory appropriately recognizes a reciprocal relation

between culture and the individual. Culture shapes how individuals experience and respond to events, but individuals also play an active role in how society functions and changes. Practice theory recognizes both constraints on individuals and the flexibility and changeability of cultures and social systems. Well-known practice theorists include Sherry Ortner, an American anthropologist, and Pierre Bourdieu and Anthony Giddens, French and British social theorists, respectively.

Edmund Leach

Some of the germs of practice theory can be traced to the British anthropologist Edmund Leach, who wrote the influential book *Political Systems of Highland Burma* (1954/1970). Leach focused on how individuals work to achieve power and how their actions can transform society. In the Kachin Hills of Burma, now Myanmar, Leach identified three forms of political organization, which he called *gumlao, gumsa,* and Shan. Leach made a tremendously important point by taking a regional rather than a local perspective. The Kachins participated in a regional system that included all three forms of organization. Those three forms coexist and interact, as possibilities known to everyone, in the same region. Leach showed how Kachins creatively use power struggles to transform society—for example, to convert *gumlao* into *gumsa* organization. He made the study of *process* central to social anthropological analysis. By focusing on power and how individuals get and use it, he showed the creative role of the individual in transforming culture.

World-System Theory and Political Economy

Leach's regional perspective and interest in power was not all that different from another development at the same time. Julian Steward, discussed previously for his work on multilinear evolution and cultural ecology, joined the faculty of Columbia University in 1946. He worked there with a group of graduate students including Eric Wolf and Sidney Mintz, who would go on to become prominent anthropologists themselves. Steward and his students planned and conducted a team research project in Puerto Rico, described in Steward's volume *The People of Puerto Rico* (1956). This project exemplified a post–World War II turn of anthropology away from "primitive" and nonindustrial societies, assumed to be somewhat isolated and autonomous, to contemporary societies recognized as forged by colonialism and participating fully in the modern world system. The team, which included Mintz and Wolf, studied communities in different parts of Puerto Rico. The field sites were chosen to sample major events and adaptations, such as the sugar plantation, in the island's history. The approach emphasized economics, politics, and history.

Wolf and Mintz retained their interest in history throughout their careers. Wolf wrote the modern classic *Europe and the People without History* (1982), which viewed local people, such as Native Americans, in the context of world-system events, such as the fur trade. Wolf focused on how such "people without history"— that is, nonliterate people, those who lacked written histories of their own—participated in and were transformed by the world system and the spread of capitalism.

Mintz's *Sweetness and Power* (1985) is another example of historical anthropology that focuses on **political economy** (the web of interrelated economic and power relations). Mintz traces the domestication and spread of sugar, its transformative role in England, and its impact on the New World, where it became the basis for slave-based

political economy
The web of interrelated economic and power relations in society.

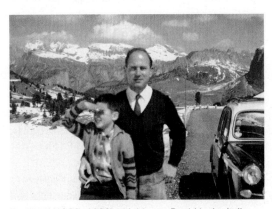

Eric Wolf (1923–1999) with his son David in the Italian Alps, one of Eric Wolf's research sites; he also worked in and wrote about Mexico and Puerto Rico.

Courtesy Sydel Silverman

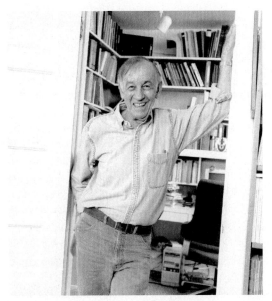

Sidney Mintz (1922–2015) at his office at Johns Hopkins University. Mintz was an anthropologist known best for his studies of the Caribbean, the anthropology of food, and Afro-Caribbean traditions.

Jay VanRensselaer/homewoodphoto.jhu.edu

plantation economies in the Caribbean and Brazil. Such works in political economy illustrate a movement of anthropology toward interdisciplinarity, drawing on other academic fields, most notably history. Such approaches have been criticized, however, for overstressing the influence of outsiders, and for paying insufficient attention to the transformative actions of "the people without history" themselves. Recap 3.2 summarizes anthropology's major theoretical perspectives and key works associated with them.

Culture, History, Power

More recent approaches in historical anthropology, while sharing an interest in power and inequality with the world-system theorists, have focused more on local agency, the transformative actions of individuals and groups within colonized societies. Archival work has been prominent in recent historical anthropology, particularly in areas, such as Indonesia, for which colonial and postcolonial archives contain valuable information on relations between colonizers and colonized (see Roque and Wagner 2011). Studies of culture, history, and power have drawn heavily on the work of European social theorists such as Antonio Gramsci and Michel Foucault.

Gramsci (1971) developed the concept of *hegemony* to describe a stratified social order in which subordinates comply with domination by internalizing their rulers' values and accepting domination as "natural." Both Pierre Bourdieu (1977) and Foucault (1979) contend that it is easier to dominate people in their minds than to try to control their bodies. Contemporary societies have devised various forms of social control

RECAP 3.2	Timeline and Key Works in Anthropological Theory

THEORETICAL APPROACH	KEY AUTHORS AND WORKS
Culture, history, power	Ann Stoler, *Carnal Knowledge and Imperial Power* (2002); Frederick Cooper and Ann Stoler, *Tensions of Empire* (1997)
Crisis of representation/postmodernism	Jean-François Lyotard, *The Postmodern Explained* (1993); George Marcus and Michael Fischer, *Anthropology as Cultural Critique* (1986)
Practice theory	Sherry Ortner, "Theory in Anthropology since the Sixties" (1984); Pierre Bourdieu, *Outline of a Theory of Practice* (1977)
World-system theory/political economy	Sidney Mintz, *Sweetness and Power* (1985); Eric Wolf, *Europe and the People without History* (1982)
Feminist anthropology (see Chapter 9, on gender, later in this book)	Rayna Reiter, *Toward an Anthropology of Women* (1975); Michelle Rosaldo and Louise Lamphere, *Women, Culture, and Society* (1974)
Cultural materialism	Marvin Harris, *Cultural Materialism* (1979/2001a), *The Rise of Anthropological Theory* (1968/2001b)
Interpretive anthropology	Clifford Geertz, *The Interpretation of Cultures* (1973)*
Symbolic anthropology	Mary Douglas, *Purity and Danger* (1970b); Victor Turner, *The Forest of Symbols* (1967)*
Structuralism	Claude Lévi-Strauss, *Structural Anthropology* (1967)*
Twentieth-century evolutionism	Leslie White, *The Evolution of Culture* (1959); Julian Steward, *Theory of Culture Change* (1955)
Manchester school and Leach	Victor Turner, *Schism and Continuity in an African Society* (1957/1996); Edmund Leach, *Political Systems of Highland Burma* (1954/1970)
Culturology	Leslie White, *The Science of Culture* (1949)*
Configurationalism	Alfred Kroeber, *Configurations of Cultural Growth* (1944); Margaret Mead, *Sex and Temperament in Three Primitive Societies* (1935/1950); Ruth Benedict, *Patterns of Culture* (1934/1959)
Structural functionalism	A. R. Radcliffe-Brown, *Structure and Function in Primitive Society* (1962/1965)*; E. E. Evans-Pritchard, *The Nuer* (1940)
Functionalism	Bronislaw Malinowski, *A Scientific Theory of Culture* (1944)*, *Argonauts of the Western Pacific* (1922/1961)
Historical particularism	Franz Boas, *Race, Language, and Culture* (1940/1966)*
Nineteenth-century evolutionism	Lewis Henry Morgan, *Ancient Society* (1877/1963); Sir Edward Burnett Tylor, *Primitive Culture* (1871/1958)

*Includes essays written at earlier dates.

in addition to physical violence. These include techniques of persuading, coercing, and managing people and of monitoring and recording their beliefs, behavior, movements, and contacts. Anthropologists interested in culture, history, and power, such as Ann Stoler (2002, 2009, 2013), have examined systems of power, domination, accommodation, and resistance in various contexts, including colonies, postcolonies, and other stratified contexts.

ANTHROPOLOGY TODAY

Early American anthropologists typically contributed to more than one of the four subfields. If there has been a single dominant trend in anthropology since the 1960s, it has been one of increasing specialization. During the 1960s, graduate students at Columbia University (where I studied) had to pass examinations in all four subfields. This has changed. There are still strong four-field anthropology departments, but many excellent departments lack one or more of the subfields. Even in four-field departments, graduate students now are expected to specialize in a particular subfield. In Boasian anthropology, all four subfields shared a single theoretical assumption about human plasticity. Today, following specialization, the theories that guide the subfields differ. Evolutionary paradigms of various sorts still dominate biological anthropology and remain strong in archaeology as well. Within cultural anthropology, it has been many decades since evolutionary approaches dominated.

Ethnography, too, has grown more specialized. Cultural anthropologists now head for the field with a specific problem in mind, rather than with the goal of producing a holistic ethnography—a complete account of a given culture—as Morgan and Malinowski intended when they studied, respectively, the Iroquois and the Trobriand Islanders. Boas, Malinowski, and Mead went somewhere and stayed there for a while, studying the local culture. Today "the field" that anthropologists study has expanded—inevitably and appropriately—to include regional and national systems and the movement of people, such as immigrants and diasporas, across national boundaries. Border theory (see Lugo 1997) is an emerging field that examines social relations at the margins of a society, contexts in which members of different groups increasingly meet and interact. Border research can occur on the boundaries of nation-states, such as the U.S–Mexican border (De Leon 2015; Lugo 2008), as well as in places within a nation where diverse groups come into regular contact (see Castellanos 2019). Many anthropologists now follow the flows of people, information, finance, and media to multiple sites. Such movement—and the anthropologist's ability to study it—has been made possible by advances in transportation and communication.

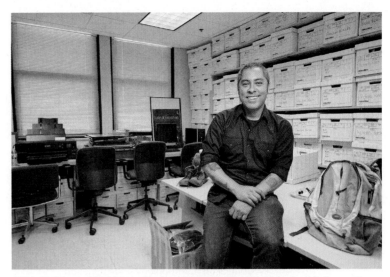

Jason DeLeon's 2016 book, *The Land of Open Graves: Living and Dying on the Migrant Trail,* is based on six years of ethnographic, archaeological, and forensic research on undocumented migration between Latin America and the United States. Dr. De Leon is shown here in his former lab at the University of Michigan. He is now a Professor at UCLA.

Reflecting the trend toward specialization, the American Anthropological Association now has all sorts of active and vital subgroups. In its early years, there were just anthropologists within the AAA. Now there are groups based on specialization in biological anthropology, archaeology, and linguistic, cultural, and applied anthropology. The AAA also includes dozens of groups formed around particular interests (e.g., psychological anthropology, urban anthropology, culture and agriculture) and identities (e.g., midwestern or southeastern anthropologists, anthropologists in community colleges or small programs). The AAA also includes units representing senior anthropologists, LGBT anthropologists, Latino and Latina anthropologists, and so on. Table 3.1 lists the 40 specialized sections of the American Anthropological Association as of this writing.

Anthropology also has witnessed a *crisis in representation,* including questions about the ethnographer's impartiality, and even the validity of ethnographic accounts. Some critics challenge the value of science itself, pointing out that all scientists come from particular individual and cultural backgrounds, which interfere with objectivity. What are we to do if we, as I do, continue to share Margaret Mead's view of anthropology as a humanistic science of unique value in understanding and improving the human condition? We must try, I think, to stay aware of our biases and our inability to escape them totally. The best scientific choice would seem to be to combine the perpetual goal of objectivity with skepticism about our capacity to achieve it.

TABLE 3.1   The 40 Sections of the American Anthropological Association as of 2018

American Ethnological Society	National Association of Student Anthropologists
Archaeology Division	Society for Anthropological Sciences
Association of Latina and Latino Anthropologists	Society for Anthropology in Community Colleges
Anthropology & Environment Society	Society for Cultural Anthropology
Association for Africanist Anthropology	Society for East Asian Anthropology
Association for Feminist Anthropology	Society for Economic Anthropology
Association for Political and Legal Anthropology	Society for Humanistic Anthropology
Association for Queer Anthropology	Society for Latin American and Caribbean Anthropology
Association for the Anthropology of Policy	Society for Linguistic Anthropology
Association of Black Anthropologists	Society for Linguistic Anthropology
Association of Indigenous Anthropologists	Society for Medical Anthropology
Association of Senior Anthropologists	Society for Psychological Anthropology
Biological Anthropology Section	Society for the Anthropology of Consciousness
Central States Anthropological Society	Society for the Anthropology of Europe
Council for Museum Anthropology	Society for the Anthropology of Food and Nutrition
Council on Anthropology and Education	Society for the Anthropology of North America
Culture and Agriculture	Society for the Anthropology of Religion
Evolutionary Anthropology Society	Society for the Anthropology of Work
General Anthropology Division	Society for Urban, National, and Transnational/Global Anthropology
Middle East Section	
National Association for the Practice of Anthropology	Society for Visual Anthropology

SOURCE: http://www.americananthro.org/ParticipateAndAdvocate/SJDList.aspx?navItemNumber=593.

for REVIEW

summary

1. Ethnographic methods include observation, rapport building, participant observation, interviewing, genealogies, work with key consultants, life histories, problem-oriented research, longitudinal research, and team research. Ethnographers do not systematically manipulate their subjects or conduct experiments. Rather, they work in actual communities and form personal relationships with local people as they study their lives.

2. An interview schedule is a form that an ethnographer completes as he or she visits a series of households. The schedule organizes and guides each interview, ensuring that comparable information is collected from everyone. Key cultural consultants teach about particular areas of local life. Life histories dramatize the fact that culture bearers are individuals. Such case studies document personal experiences with culture and culture change. Genealogical information is particularly useful in societies in which principles of kinship and marriage organize social and political life. Emic approaches focus on native perceptions and explanations. Etic approaches give priority to the ethnographer's own observations

and conclusions. Longitudinal research is the systematic study of an area or a site over time. Anthropological research may be done by teams and at multiple sites. Outsiders, flows, linkages, and people in motion are now included in ethnographic analyses. Anthropologists also have developed techniques of doing online ethnography in studying virtual worlds.

3. Traditionally, anthropologists worked in small-scale societies; sociologists, in modern nations. Different techniques were developed to study such different kinds of societies. Social scientists working in complex societies use survey research to sample variation. Anthropologists do their fieldwork in communities and study the totality of social life. Sociologists study samples to make inferences about a larger population. The diversity of social life in modern nations and cities requires survey procedures. However, anthropologists add the intimacy and direct investigation characteristic of ethnography.

4. Because science exists in society, and in the context of law and ethics, anthropologists can't study things simply because they happen to be

interesting or of scientific value. Anthropologists have obligations to their scholarly field, to the wider society and culture (including that of the host country), and to the human species, other species, and the environment. The AAA Code of Ethics offers ethical guidelines for anthropologists. Ethical problems often arise when anthropologists work for governments, especially the military.

5. Evolutionary perspectives, especially those of Morgan and Tylor, dominated early anthropology, which emerged during the latter half of the 19th century. The early 20th century witnessed various reactions to 19th-century evolutionism. In the United States, Boas and his followers rejected the search for evolutionary stages in favor of a historical approach that traced borrowing between cultures and the spread of culture traits across geographic areas. In Great Britain, functionalists such as Malinowski and Radcliffe-Brown abandoned conjectural history in favor of studies of present-day living societies. Functionalists and Boasians alike saw cultures as integrated and patterned. The functionalists especially viewed societies as systems in which various parts worked together to maintain the whole. A form of functionalism persists in the widely accepted view that there are social and cultural systems whose constituent parts are functionally related, so that when one part changes, others change as well.

6. In the mid-20th century, following World War II and as colonialism was ending, there was a revived interest in change, including evolutionary approaches. Some anthropologists developed symbolic and interpretive approaches to uncover patterned symbols and meanings within cultures. By the 1980s, anthropologists had grown more interested in the relation between culture and the individual, as well as the role of human action (agency) in transforming culture. There also was a resurgence of historical approaches, including those that viewed local cultures in relation to colonialism and the world system.

7. Contemporary anthropology is marked by increasing specialization, based on special topics and identities. Reflecting this specialization, some universities have moved away from the holistic, biocultural view of anthropology that is reflected in this book. However, this Boasian view of anthropology as a four-subfield discipline—including biological, archaeological, cultural, and linguistic anthropology—continues to thrive at many universities as well.

key terms

agency 54

complex societies 45

configurationalism 51

cultural consultants 39

cultural materialism 52

diachronic 50

emic 43

etic 43

functionalism 49

genealogical method 39

historical particularism 49

informed consent 46

interpretive anthropology 53

interview schedule 39

key cultural consultants 39

life history 40

longitudinal research 42

participant observation 38

political economy 55

questionnaire 39

random sample 45

sample 45

superorganic 53

survey research 45

symbolic anthropology 53

synchronic 50

unilinear evolutionism 48

variables 45

think like an anthropologist

1. What do you see as the strengths and weaknesses of ethnography compared with survey research? Which provides more accurate data? Might one be better for finding questions, while the other is better for finding answers? Or does it depend on the context of research?

2. In what sense is anthropological research comparative? How have anthropologists approached the issue of comparison? What do they compare (what are their units of analysis)?

3. In your view, is anthropology a science? How have anthropologists historically addressed this question? Should anthropology be a science?

4. Historically, how have anthropologists studied culture? What are some contemporary trends in the study of culture, and how have they changed the way anthropologists carry out their research?

5. Do the theories examined in this chapter relate to ones you have studied in other courses? Which courses and theories? Are those theories more scientific or humanistic, or somewhere in between?

CHAPTER 4

Applying Anthropology

▸ Can change be bad and, if so, how?

▸ How can anthropology be applied to medicine, education, and business?

▸ How does the study of anthropology fit into a career path?

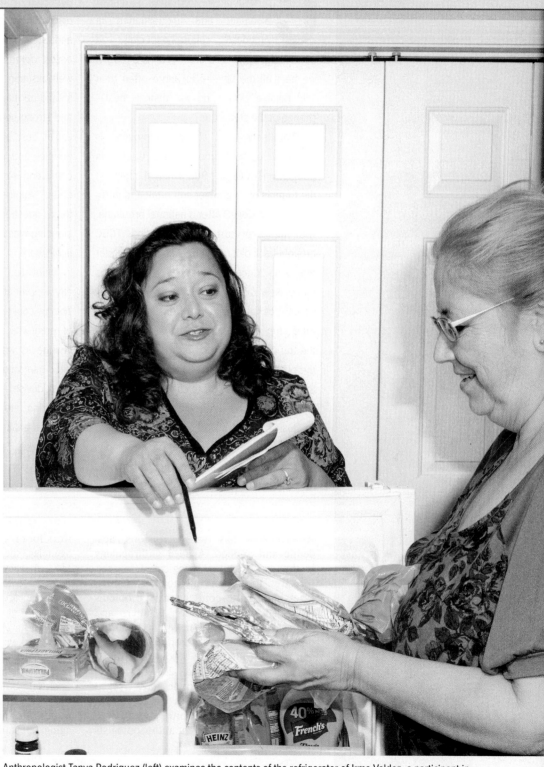

Peter Bohler/Redux Pictures

Anthropologist Tanya Rodriguez (left) examines the contents of the refrigerator of Irma Valdez, a participant in Rodriguez's applied research. Rodriguez has studied American food trends for Hormel Foods for over a decade.

understanding OURSELVES

Can change be bad? The idea that innovation is desirable is almost axiomatic and unquestioned in American culture—especially in advertising. "New and improved" is a slogan we hear all the time—a lot more often than "old reliable." Which do you think is best—change or the status quo?

That "new" isn't always "improved" is a painful lesson learned by the Coca-Cola Company (TCCC) in 1985 when it changed the formula of its premier soft drink and introduced "New Coke." After a national brouhaha, with hordes of customers protesting, TCCC brought back old, familiar, reliable Coke under the name "Coca-Cola Classic," which thrives today. New Coke, now history, offers a classic case of how not to treat consumers. TCCC tried a *top-down change* (a change initiated at the top of a hierarchy rather than inspired by the people most affected by the change). Customers didn't ask TCCC to change its product; executives made that decision.

Business executives, like public policy makers, run organizations that provide goods and services to people. The field of market research, which employs a good number of anthropologists, is based on the need to appreciate what actual and potential customers do, think, and want. Smart planners study and listen to people to try to determine *locally based demand*. In general, what's working well (assuming it's not discriminatory or illegal) should be maintained, encouraged, tweaked, and strengthened. If something's wrong, how can it best be fixed? What changes do the people—and which people—want? How can conflicting wishes and needs be accommodated? Applied anthropologists help answer these questions, which are crucial in understanding whether change is needed, and how it will work.

Innovation succeeds best when it is culturally appropriate. This axiom of applied anthropology could guide the international spread of programs aimed at social and economic change as well as of businesses. Each time an organization expands to a new nation, it must devise a culturally appropriate strategy for fitting into the new setting. In their international expansion, companies as diverse as McDonald's, Starbucks, and Ford have learned that more money can be made by fitting in with, rather than trying to Americanize, local habits.

Anthropology has two dimensions: academic and applied. **Applied anthropology** is the use of anthropological data, perspectives, theory, and methods to identify, assess, and solve contemporary problems (see Pelto 2013; Wasson, Butler, and Copeland-Carson 2012). Applied anthropologists help make anthropology relevant and useful to the world beyond anthropology (see Beck and Maida 2013). Medical anthropologists, for example, have worked as cultural interpreters in public health programs, helping such programs fit into local culture. Development anthropologists work for or with international development agencies, such as the World Bank and the U.S. Agency for International Development (USAID). The findings of garbology, the archaeological study of waste, are relevant to the U.S. Environmental Protection Agency, the paper industry, and packaging and trade associations. Archaeology also is applied in cultural resource management and historic preservation. Biological anthropologists apply their expertise in programs aimed at public health, nutrition, genetic counseling, aging, substance abuse, and mental health.

ANTHROPOLOGY'S SUBFIELDS (ACADEMIC ANTHROPOLOGY)	EXAMPLES OF APPLICATION (APPLIED ANTHROPOLOGY)
Cultural anthropology	Development anthropology
Archaeological anthropology	Cultural resource management (CRM)
Biological anthropology	Forensic anthropology
Linguistic anthropology	Study of linguistic diversity in classrooms

Forensic anthropologists work with the police, medical examiners, the courts, and international organizations to identify victims of crimes, accidents, wars, and terrorism. Linguistic anthropologists have studied physician–patient speech interactions and have shown how dialect differences influence classroom learning. Most applied anthropologists seek humane and effective ways of helping local people (see Nahm and Hughes Rinker 2016). Recap 4.1 gives examples of applied anthropology in the four subdisciplines.

The ethnographic method is a particularly valuable tool in applying anthropology (see Vannini 2019). Remember that ethnographers study societies firsthand, living with, observing, and learning from ordinary people. Nonanthropologists working in social-change programs often are content to converse with officials, read reports, and copy statistics. However, the applied anthropologist's likely early request is some variant of "take me to the local people." Anthropologists know that people must play an active role in the changes that affect them and that "the people" have information that "the experts" lack.

Anthropological theory, the body of findings and generalizations of the four subfields, also guides applied anthropology. Just as theory aids practice, application fuels theory (see Pink, Fors, and O'Dell 2017). As we compare social-change programs, our understanding of cause and effect increases. We add new generalizations about culture change to those discovered in traditional and ancient cultures.

THE ROLE OF THE APPLIED ANTHROPOLOGIST

Early Applications

Anthropology is, and has long been, the main academic discipline that focuses on non-Western cultures. One example is the role that anthropologists played as agents of and advisors to colonial regimes during the first half of the 20th century. Under colonialism, some anthropologists worked as administrators in the colonies or held lower level positions as government agents, researchers, or advisors. Other anthropologists who supported colonialism were university professors who offered advice to colonial regimes. The main European

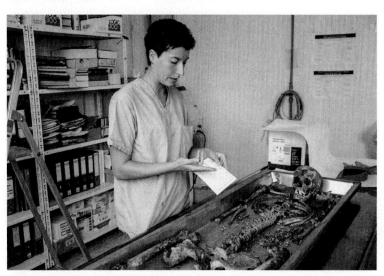

In Tuzla, Bosnia and Herzegovina, forensic anthropologist Dragana Vucetic displays human bones that have been cut for sampling in the DNA identification process. Vucetic is helping to identity victims of the 1995 Srebrenica genocide. Forensic anthropologists work with the police, medical examiners, the courts, and international organizations to identify victims of crimes, accidents, wars, terrorism, and genocide.

David Bathgate/Getty Images

colonial powers at that time—Britain, France, Portugal, and the Netherlands—all employed anthropologists. When those colonial empires began to collapse after World War II, as the former colonies gained independence, many anthropologists continued to offer advice to government agencies about the areas and cultures they knew the best.

In the United States, American anthropologists have worked extensively with the subjugated Native American populations within its borders. The 19th-century American anthropologist Lewis Henry Morgan studied the Seneca Iroquois tribe, Native Americans living in New York state, not far from his home in Rochester. Morgan was also a lawyer who represented the Iroquois in their disputes with a company that wanted to seize some of their land. Just as Morgan worked on behalf of the Seneca, there are anthropologists today who work on behalf of the non-Western groups they have studied. Other anthropologists, however, working as government employees and agents, have helped to establish and enforce policies developed by ruling classes and aimed at local populations.

applied anthropology
The use of anthropology to solve contemporary problems.

Bronislaw Malinowski, a Polish-born scholar who spent most of his career teaching in England, was one of the most prominent cultural anthropologists of the early 20th century. Malinowski is well known for his ethnographic fieldwork with the Trobriand Islanders of the South Pacific and for his role in establishing ethnographic field methods. He also is recognized as one of the founders of applied anthropology, which he called "practical anthropology" (Malinowski 1929). Like many other anthropologists of his time, Malinowski worked *with* colonial regimes, rather than opposing the European subjugation of non-Western peoples.

Malinowski, who focused on Britain's African colonies, intended his "practical anthropology" to support and facilitate colonial rule. He believed that anthropologists could help European colonial officials to effectively administer non-Western societies. Anthropologists could help answer questions like the following: How was contact with European settlers and colonial officials affecting tribal societies? How much taxation and forced labor could "the natives" tolerate without resisting? Anthropologists could study local land ownership and use in order to determine how much of their own land "natives" could keep and how much Europeans could take from them. Malinowski did not question the right of Europeans to rule the societies they had conquered. For him, the anthropologist's job was not to question colonial rule, but to make it work as harmoniously as possible. Other colonial-era anthropologists offered similar advice to the French, Portuguese, and Dutch regimes (see also Duffield and Hewitt 2009; Lange 2009).

During World War II, American anthropologists applied anthropology by trying to gain insights about the motivations and behavior of the enemies of the United States—principally Germany and Japan. Margaret Mead (1977) estimated that during the 1940s, 95 percent of U.S. anthropologists were engaged in the war effort. For example, Ruth Benedict (1946) wrote an influential study of Japanese national culture not by doing fieldwork in Japan, but by studying Japanese literature, movies, and other cultural products and by interviewing Japanese in the United States. She called her approach "the study of culture at a distance." After World War II, American anthropologists worked to promote local-level cooperation with American policies on several Pacific islands that had been under Japanese control and were now administered by the United States.

Many of the early applications of anthropology described in this section were problematic because they aided and abetted the subjugation and control of non-Western cultures by militarily stronger societies. Contemporary applied anthropologists see their work as radically removed from colonial-era applied anthropology and as more of a helping profession, designed to assist local people (see Kirsch 2018).

Academic and Applied Anthropology

The U.S. baby boom, which began in 1946 and peaked in 1957, fueled a tremendous expansion of the American educational system. New junior, community, and four-year colleges opened, and anthropology became a standard part of the college curriculum. During the 1950s and 1960s, most American anthropologists were college professors, although some still worked in agencies and museums.

Most anthropologists still worked in colleges and museums during the 1970s and 1980s. However, an increasing number of anthropologists were finding jobs in international organizations, governments, businesses, hospitals, and schools. Today, applied anthropologists work in varied contexts, including economic development organizations, government agencies, nongovernmental organizations (NGOs) and nonprofit organizations, international policy bodies, and private entities, such as unions, social movements, and increasingly businesses and corporations. The American Anthropological Association estimates that well over half of anthropology PhDs today seek nonacademic employment. This shift toward application has benefited the profession. It has forced anthropologists to consider the wider social value and implications of their research.

Applied Anthropology Today

Although poverty (and its alleviation) has been a key focus of applied anthropology, applied anthropologists also engage with clients who are neither poor nor powerless. An applied anthropologist working as a market researcher may be asked to discover effective ways to increase sales of a particular product. Such commercial goals can pose ethical dilemmas, which also may arise in cultural resource management (CRM). The CRM anthropologist helps decide how to preserve significant remains when development threatens sites. The client that hires a CRM firm may be seeking to build a road or a factory. That client may have a strong interest in a CRM finding that no sites need protection, and the client may pressure the CRM firm in that direction. Among the ethical questions that arise in applied anthropology are these: To whom does the researcher owe loyalty? What problems might be involved in sticking to the truth? What happens when applied anthropologists don't create the policies they have to implement? How does one criticize programs in which one has participated? Anthropology's professional organizations have addressed such questions by establishing codes of ethics and ethics committees.

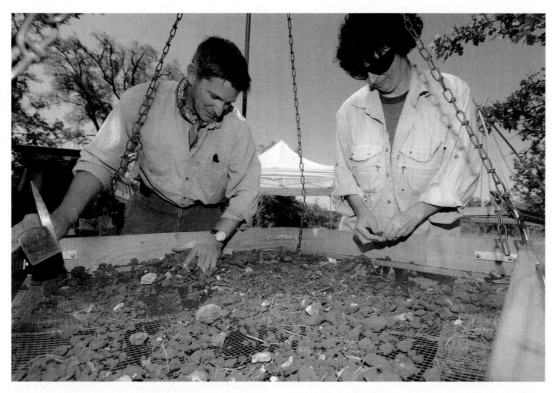

Archaeologists Tim Griffith, left, and Ginny Hatfield of Fort Hood's (Texas) Cultural Resources Management Program, sift through sediment collected from an archaeological site. This CRM program manages resources representing more than 10,000 years of occupation of the land around Fort Hood.

Scott Gaulin/AP Images

Anthropologists study, understand, and respect diverse cultural values. Because of this knowledge of human problems and social change, anthropologists are highly qualified to suggest, plan, and implement policies affecting people. Proper roles for applied anthropologists include (1) identifying needs for change that local people perceive, (2) collaborating with those people to design culturally appropriate and socially sensitive change, and (3) working to protect local people from harmful policies and projects that may threaten them.

For decades, applied anthropologists have collaborated directly with communities to achieve community-directed change. Applied anthropologists not only work collaboratively with local people, but they may even be hired by such communities to advocate on their behalf. One example is Barbara Rose Johnston's (2005) research on behalf of Guatemalan communities that were adversely affected by the construction of the Chixoy Dam. Johnston's reports documented the dam's long-term impact on these communities. She also offered recommendations and a plan for reparations (see also Kirsch 2018).

DEVELOPMENT ANTHROPOLOGY

Development anthropology is the branch of applied anthropology that focuses on social issues in, and the cultural dimension of, economic development. Development anthropologists don't just carry out development policies planned by others; they also plan and guide policy. (For more detailed discussions of issues in development anthropology, see Colbourne and Anderson 2020; Crewe and Axelby 2013; Mosse 2011; Mathur 2019.)

Still, ethical dilemmas often confront development anthropologists (Escobar 2012; Venkatesan and Yarrow 2014). Foreign aid, including funds for economic development, usually does not go where need and suffering are greatest. Rather, such aid tends to support political, economic, and strategic priorities that are set by international donors, political leaders, and powerful interest groups. The goals and interests of the planners may ignore or conflict with the best interests of the local people. Although the stated aim of most development projects is to enhance the quality of life, living standards often decline in the affected area.

Equity

One oft-stated goal of development projects has been to promote equity. **Increased equity** entails (1) reducing poverty and (2) evening out the distribution of wealth. Projects should not benefit only the "haves," but also the "have nots." If people who are already doing well get most of the benefits of a project, then it has not increased equity.

If projects are to increase equity, they must have the support of reform-minded governments. Wealthy and powerful people typically resist projects that offer more to the "have nots" than to the "haves." Often, they will actively oppose a project that threatens the status quo.

development anthropology
A field that examines the sociocultural dimensions of economic development.

increased equity
Reduction in absolute poverty, with a more even distribution of wealth.

Negative Equity Impact

Some projects not only fail to promote equity, but they actually widen the gap between the "haves" and "have nots." In this case, we say they have a *negative equity impact*. I observed firsthand an example of negative equity impact in Arembepe, Bahia, Brazil, a fishing community on the Atlantic Ocean (see Kottak 2018). A development initiative there offered loans to buy motors for fishing boats, but only people who already owned boats ("haves") could get these loans. Nonowners ("have nots") did not qualify. After getting the loans, the boat owners, in order to pay off their debt, increased the percentage of the catch they took from the men who fished in their boats. Their rising profits allowed them to eventually buy larger and more expensive boats. They cited their increased capital expense as a reason to pay their workers less. Over the years, the gap between "haves" and "have nots" widened substantially. The eventual result was socioeconomic stratification—the creation of social classes in a community that had been egalitarian. In the past, Arembepe's fishing boats had been simple sailboats, relying only on wind power, and any enterprising young fisher could hope eventually to own one of his own. In the new economy, the larger motorized boats were so expensive that ambitious young men, who once would have sought careers in fishing, no longer could afford to buy a boat of their own. They sought wage labor on land instead. To avoid this kind of negative equity impact, credit-granting agencies must seek out and invest in enterprising young fishers, rather than giving loans only to owners and established businesspeople. A lesson here is that the stated goal of increased equity is easier said than done. Because

overinnovation
Trying to achieve too much change.

the "haves" tend to have better connections than the "have nots," they are more likely to find out about and take advantage of new programs. They also tend to have more clout with government officials, who often decide who will benefit from a particular program.

STRATEGIES FOR INNOVATION

Development anthropologists should work collaboratively and proactively with local people, especially the "have nots," to assess, and help them realize, their own wishes and needs for change. Too many true local needs cry out for a solution to waste money funding projects in area A that are inappropriate there but are needed in area B, or that are unnecessary anywhere. Development anthropology can help sort out the needs of the As and Bs and fit projects accordingly. Projects that put people first by consulting with them and responding to their expressed needs must be identified (Cernea 1991). To maximize social and economic benefits, projects must (1) be culturally compatible, (2) respond to locally perceived needs, (3) involve men and women in planning and carrying out the changes that affect them, (4) harness traditional organizations, and (5) be flexible (see Kottak 1990*b*, 1991).

Consider the following example of a development initiative that failed because it ignored local culture. Working in Afghanistan after the fall of the Taliban, ethnographer Noah Coburn (2011) studied Istalif, a village of potters. During his fieldwork there, Coburn discovered that an NGO had spent $20,000 on an electric kiln that could have greatly enhanced the productivity of local potters. The only problem was that the kiln was donated to a women's center that men could not enter. The misguided donors ignored the fact that Istalif's men did the work—pot-making and firing—that a kiln could facilitate. Women's role in pottery came later—in glazing and decorating.

Overinnovation

Policies and projects aimed at social change are most likely to succeed when they avoid the fallacy of **overinnovation** (too much change). People usually are willing to change just enough to maintain, or slightly improve on, what they already have. Motives for modifying behavior come from the traditional culture and the small concerns of ordinary life. Peasants' values are not such abstract ones as "learning a better way," "progressing," "increasing technical know-how," "improving efficiency," "adopting modern techniques," or "structural change." Rather, their objectives are down-to-earth and specific. People want to grow and harvest their crops, amass resources for a ceremony, get a child through school, or have enough cash to pay

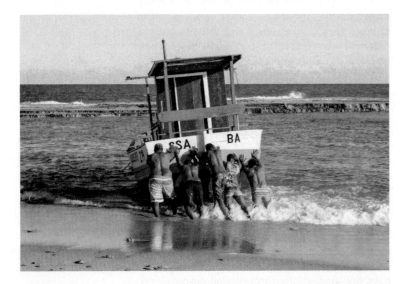

In Arembepe, Bahia, Brazil, on September 18, 2019, five men push a fishing boat into the harbor. A boat owner gets a loan to buy a motor. To repay it, he increases the share of the catch he takes from his crew. Later, he uses his rising profits to buy a more expensive boat (like the one shown here) and takes even more from his crew. Can a more equitable solution be found?

Helissa Grundemann/Shutterstock

bills. The goals and values of people who farm and fish for their own subsistence differ from those of people who work for cash, just as they differ from those of development planners.

Development projects that fail usually do so because they are either economically or culturally incompatible (or both). For example, one South Asian project tried to get farmers to start growing onions and peppers, expecting these cash crops to fit into the existing system of rice cultivation—the main local subsistence crop. However, it turned out that the labor peaks for these new cash crops coincided with those for rice, to which the farmers naturally gave priority. This project failed because it was overinnovative. It promoted too much change, introducing unfamiliar crops that conflicted with, rather than building on and complementing, an existing system. The planners should have realized that cultivation of the new crops would conflict with that of the main subsistence crop in the area. A good anthropologist could have told them as much.

Recent development efforts in Afghanistan also illustrate the problematic nature of overinnovation. Reporting on social change efforts in Afghanistan after the fall of the Taliban, anthropologists Noah Coburn (2011) and Thomas Barfield (2010) criticize various top-down initiatives that proved incompatible with local culture. Coburn suggests that the best strategy to maintain peace in the Afghan countryside is to work with existing resources, drawing on local beliefs and social organization. To be avoided are overinnovative plans from outside, whether from the national government or foreign donors. Destined for failure, according to Coburn, are attempts to create impersonal bureaucracies based on merit. Also doomed are attempts to impose liberal beliefs about gender at the village level. These are Western ideas that are particularly incompatible in rural areas. Barfield also cites the futility of direct attempts to change rural Afghans' beliefs about such entrenched matters as religion and gender equality. A better strategy, he suggests, is for change agents to work first in urban areas, where innovation is more welcome, and then let those changes spread gradually to the countryside.

In 2014, Afghanistan elected an anthropologist as its president. Ashraf Ghani, who received his doctorate in anthropology from Columbia University in New York, had worked for the World Bank as a development anthropologist. Let us hope that Ghani's background in anthropology and development will encourage more culturally appropriate development strategies in the still troubled nation he continued to lead in 2020.

Underdifferentiation

The fallacy of **underdifferentiation** is planners' tendency to view "the less-developed countries" (LDCs) as more alike than they are. Often

development agencies have ignored huge cultural contrasts (e.g., between Brazil and Botswana) and adopted a uniform approach to deal with very different societies. Planners often try to impose incompatible property concepts and social units. Most often, the faulty social design assumes either (1) units of production that are privately owned by an individual or a couple and worked by a nuclear family or (2) cooperatives based at least partially on models from the former Eastern bloc and Socialist countries.

One example of using an inappropriate First World model (the individual and the nuclear family) was a West African project designed for an area where the extended family was the basic social unit. The project succeeded despite its faulty social design because the participants used their traditional extended family networks to attract additional settlers. Eventually, twice as many people as planned benefited as extended family members flocked to the project area. In this case, the settlers used their traditional social organization to modify the project design that planners had tried to impose on them.

The second dubious foreign social model that is common in development planning is the cooperative. In a comparative study of rural development projects, new cooperatives tended to succeed only when they harnessed preexisting local-level communal institutions. This is a corollary of a more general rule: Participants' groups are most effective when they are based on traditional social organization or on a socioeconomic similarity among members (Kottak 1990*b*, 1991).

underdifferentiation
Seeing less-developed countries as all the same; ignoring cultural diversity.

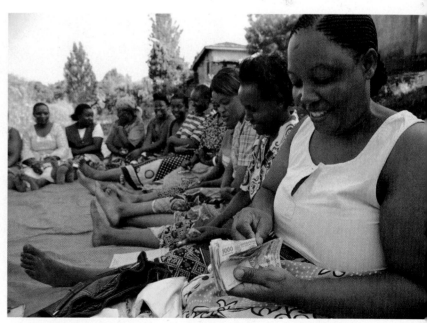

Rural women attend a BRAC microfinance meeting in Tanzania's Kilimanjaro region. BRAC, the world's largest development NGO, provides affordable financial services, including credit, to the poor in many countries (see www.brac.net).

Majority World/Universal Images Group/Getty Images

An alternative to such foreign models is needed: greater use of indigenous social models in economic development. These are traditional social units, such as the clans, lineages, and other extended kin groups of Africa, Oceania, and many other nations, with their communally held estates and resources. The most humane and productive strategy for change is to base the social design for innovation on traditional social forms in each target area.

Indigenous Models

Many governments are not genuinely, or realistically, committed to improving the lives of their citizens. Interference by major powers also has kept governments from enacting needed reforms. Occasionally, however, a government does act as an agent of and for its people. One historic example is Madagascar, whose people, the Malagasy, were organized into descent groups prior to indigenous state formation in the 18th century. The Merina, creators of the major precolonial state of Madagascar, wove descent groups into its structure, making members of important groups advisers to the king and thus giving them authority in government. The Merina state made provisions for the people it ruled. It collected taxes and organized labor for public works projects. In return, it redistributed resources to peasants in need. It also granted them some protection against war and slave raids and allowed them to cultivate their rice fields in peace. The government maintained the water works for rice cultivation. It opened to ambitious peasant boys the chance of becoming, through hard work and study, state bureaucrats.

Throughout the history of the Merina state—and continuing to some extent in postcolonial Madagascar—there have been strong relationships between the individual, the descent group, and the state. Local Malagasy communities, where residence is based on descent, are more cohesive and homogeneous than are communities in Latin America or North America. Madagascar gained political independence from France in 1960. Its new government implemented an economic development policy aimed at increasing the ability of the Malagasy to feed themselves. Government policy emphasized increased production of rice, a subsistence crop, rather than cash crops. Furthermore, local communities, with their traditional cooperative patterns and solidarity based on kinship and descent, were treated as partners in, not obstacles to, the development process.

In a sense, the descent group (see Chapter 10) is preadapted to equitable national development. In Madagascar, descent groups pooled their resources to educate their most ambitious members. Once educated, these men and women gained economically secure positions in the nation. They then shared the advantages of their new positions with their kin. For example, they gave room and board to rural cousins attending school and helped them find jobs.

This Madagascar example suggests that when government officials are of "the people" (rather than the elites) and have strong personal ties to common folk, they are more likely to promote democratic economic development. In Latin America, by contrast, leaders and followers too often have been from different socioeconomic strata, with no connections based on kinship, descent, marriage, or common background. When elites rule, elites usually prosper. Recently, however, Latin America has elected some non-elite leaders. Brazil's lower class (indeed the entire nation) benefited socioeconomically when one of its own was elected president. Luiz Inácio da Silva, aka Lula, a former factory worker with only a fourth-grade education, served two terms (ending in 2011) as one of the Western Hemisphere's most popular leaders. Lula's better educated successor, Dilma Rousseff, from the same Workers' Party, became one of Brazil's least popular presidents and was impeached in 2016. Brazil's most recently elected president is Jair Bolsonaro, a right-wing former army captain and practicing Evangelical, whose substantial victory in the 2018 elections reflected populist disgust with established politicians and corruption.

Compatible and successful development projects promote change but

Social stratification is marked—economically, socially, and residentially—in Brazil. Shown here, in Rio de Janeiro, residents of Rocinha, the largest favela, or urbanized slum, in Brazil, gaze down on one of Rio's wealthiest neighborhoods with its high-rise condos and apartments.

Viviane Moos/Getty Images

not overinnovation. Many changes are possible if the aim is to preserve things while making them work better. Successful economic development projects respect, or at least don't attack, local cultural patterns. Effective development draws on indigenous cultural practices and social structures. As nations become more tied to the world capitalist economy, it is not inevitable that indigenous forms of social organization will break down into nuclear family organization, impersonality, and alienation. Descent groups, with their traditional communalism and solidarity, have important roles to play in economic development.

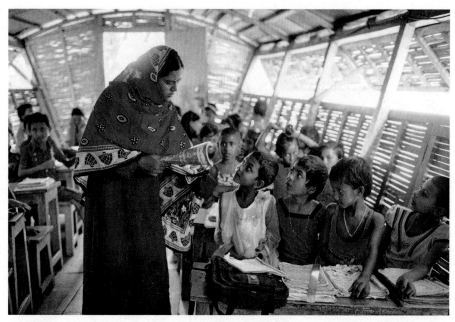

The NGO Shidhulai Swanirvar Sangstha operates a multi-vessel fleet of floating one-room elementary schools in flood-prone areas of Bangladesh. Here we see a teacher and students in one of those classrooms. Each schoolboat docks every day to pick up and let off about 30 students. The boats have solar panels that power an Internet-linked laptop, library, and electronic resources.

Jonas Gratzer/LightRocket/Getty Images

ANTHROPOLOGY AND EDUCATION

Attention to culture also is fundamental to **anthropology and education,** a field whose research extends from classrooms into homes, neighborhoods, and communities (see Anderson-Levitt 2012; Anderson-Levitt and Rockwell 2017; Levinson and Pollock 2011). In classrooms, anthropologists have observed interactions among teachers, students, parents, and visitors. Jules Henry's classic account of the American elementary school classroom (1955; see also Henry 1972) shows how students learn to conform to and compete with their peers. Anthropologists view children as total cultural creatures whose enculturation and attitudes toward education belong to a context that includes family and peers (see also Kontopodis, Wulf, and Fichtner 2011; Reagan 2018; Reyhner 2015).

Sociolinguists and cultural anthropologists have worked side by side in education research. In one classic study of Puerto Rican seventh graders in the urban Midwest (Hill-Burnett 1978), anthropologists uncovered some key misconceptions held by teachers. The teachers mistakenly had assumed that Puerto Rican parents valued education less than did non-Hispanics, but in-depth interviews revealed that the Puerto Rican parents valued it more. The anthropologists also identified certain practices that were preventing Hispanics from being adequately educated. For example, the teachers' union and the board of education had agreed to teach "English as a foreign language." However, they had provided no bilingual teachers to work with Spanish-speaking students. The school was assigning all students (including non-Hispanics) with low reading scores and behavior problems to the English-as-a-foreign-language classroom. This educational disaster brought together in the classroom a teacher who spoke no Spanish, children who barely spoke English, and a group of English-speaking students with reading and behavior problems. The Spanish speakers were falling behind not just in reading but in all subjects. They could at least have kept up in the other subjects if a Spanish speaker had been teaching them science, social studies, and math until they were ready for English-language instruction in those areas.

URBAN ANTHROPOLOGY

In today's world, media-transmitted images and information play an important role in attracting people to cities. Often, people move to cities for economic reasons, because jobs are scarce at home. Cities also attract people who want to be where the action is. Rural Brazilians routinely cite *movimento,* urban activity and excitement, as something to be valued. International migrants tend to settle in large cities, where a lot is going on and where they can feel at home in ethnic enclaves. Three-quarters of immigrants to Canada, for example, settle in Toronto, Vancouver, or Montreal. It is estimated that by 2036 immigrants (mostly from Asia) will constitute as much as 30 percent of Canada's population, compared with 21 percent in 2011 (Morency et al. 2017).

More than half (55 percent) of Earth's people now live in cities. That figure first surpassed 50 percent in 2008 and is projected to rise to 68 percent by 2050. Only about 3 percent of people were city dwellers in 1800, compared with 13 percent in

anthropology and education
The study of students in the context of their family, peers, and enculturation.

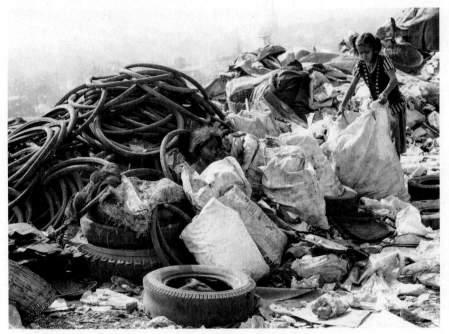

In Kolkata (formerly Calcutta), India, girls scavenge garbage for useful artifacts to sell. Almost a third of Kolkata's population live in slums, and an additional 70,000 are homeless.

Samir Hussein/Getty Images

Nonini 2014; Schwanhäusser, ed. 2016; Zukin, Kasinitz, and Chen 2016). Urban anthropologists explore a range of topics including rural-urban and transnational migration, ethnicity, poverty, class, and urban violence (Nonini and Susser 2020, Vigil 2010).

In any nation, urban and rural represent different social systems. However, cultural diffusion, or borrowing, occurs as people, products, images, and messages move from one to the other. Migrants bring rural practices and beliefs to cities and take urban patterns back home. The experiences and social forms of the rural area affect adaptation to city life. City folk also develop new institutions to meet specific urban needs.

An applied anthropology approach to urban planning begins by identifying key social groups in *specific* urban contexts—avoiding the fallacy of underdifferentiation. After identifying those groups, the anthropologist might elicit their wishes for change, convey those needs to funding agencies, and work with agencies and local people to realize those goals. In Africa, relevant urban groups might include ethnic associations, occupational groups, social clubs, religious groups, and burial societies. Through membership in such groups, urban Africans maintain wide networks of personal contacts and support. The groups provide cash support and urban lodging for their rural relatives. Members may call one another "brother" and "sister." As in an extended family, richer members help their poorer relatives. A member's improper behavior, however, can lead to expulsion—an unhappy fate for a migrant in a large, ethnically heterogeneous city.

1900, 40 percent in 1980, and 55 percent today. The number of urban residents worldwide has risen rapidly from 751 million in 1950 to 4.3 billion in 2020. Asia contains 54 percent of those city dwellers, followed by Europe and Africa, with 13 percent each (United Nations 2018a).

The degree of urbanization (about 30 percent) in the less-developed countries (LDCs) is well below the world average (55 percent). Even in the LDCs, however, the urban growth rate now exceeds the rural growth rate. By 2030, the percentage of city dwellers in the LDCs is projected to rise to 41 percent. The world had only 16 cities with more than a million people in 1900, versus more than 500 today, including over 100 such cities in China alone (United Nations 2014, 2018b). In 2018, 1.7 billion people—23 percent of the world's population—lived in a city with at least 1 million inhabitants. This figure is projected to rise to 28 percent by 2030 (United Nations 2018b).

More than one billion people now live in urban slums, mostly without reliable water, sanitation, public services, and legal security. If current trends continue, urban population increase and the concentration of people in slums will continue to be accompanied by rising rates of crime, along with water, air, and noise pollution. These problems will be most severe in the LDCs.

As industrialization and urbanization spread globally, anthropologists increasingly study these processes and the social problems they create. **Urban anthropology,** which has theoretical (basic research) and applied dimensions, is the cross-cultural and ethnographic study of urbanization and life in cities (see Jaffe and De Koning 2016;

medical anthropology
The comparative, biocultural study of disease, health problems, and health care systems.

urban anthropology
The anthropological study of cities and urban life.

MEDICAL ANTHROPOLOGY

Medical anthropology is the comparative, biocultural study of disease, health problems, and health care systems (see Wiley and Allen 2017). Medical anthropology includes anthropologists from all four subfields, and it is both academic and applied (see Brown and Closser 2016; Manderson, Cartwright, and Hardon 2016; Lock and Nguyen 2018; Singer et al. 2020). Medical anthropology emerged out of applied work done in public health and international development (Foster and Anderson 1978). Current medical anthropology continues to have clear policy applications, partly because it so often deals with pressing human problems that cry out for solutions. Medical anthropologists examine such questions as which diseases and health conditions affect particular populations (and why) and how illness is socially constructed, diagnosed, managed, and treated in various societies (Lupton 2012; Lerman et al. 2017).

Disease refers to a scientifically identified health threat caused genetically or by a bacterium, virus, fungus, parasite, or other pathogen. **Illness** is a condition of poor health perceived or felt by an individual within a particular culture. Particular cultures and ethnic groups recognize different illnesses, symptoms, and causes and have developed different health care systems and treatment strategies.

The incidence and severity of disease vary as well (see Baer, Singer, and Susser 2013). Group differences are evident in the United States. Consider, for example, health status indicators in relation to U.S. census categories: white, Black, Hispanic, American Indian or Alaska Native, and Asian or Pacific Islander. African Americans' rates for six indicators (total mortality, heart disease, lung cancer, breast cancer, stroke, and homicide) range from 2.5 to 10 times greater than those of the other groups. Other ethnic groups have higher rates for suicide (white Americans) and motor vehicle accidents (American Indians and Alaskan Natives). Overall, Asians have the longest lifespans.

Reviewing the health conditions of the world's surviving indigenous populations (about 400 million people), anthropologists Claudia Valeggia and Josh Snodgrass (2015) found their health indicators to be uniformly low. Compared with nonindigenous people, indigenous groups tend to have shorter and riskier lives. Mothers are more likely to die in childbirth; infants and children have lower survival chances. Malnutrition stunts their growth, and they suffer more from infectious diseases. Reflecting their increasing exposure to global forces, they have rising rates of cardiovascular and other chronic diseases, as well as depression and substance abuse. They also have limited access to medical care. An increasing number of anthropologists are working in global health programs at academic and research institutions. This presence should increase understanding of the health concerns of indigenous peoples—but more is needed. Valeggia and Snodgrass (2015) urge medical anthropologists to involve themselves more in community outreach, which could help bring better health care to indigenous populations.

In many areas, the world system and colonialism have worsened the health of indigenous peoples by spreading diseases, warfare, servitude, and other stressors. Traditionally and in ancient times, hunter-gatherers, because of their small numbers, mobility, and relative isolation from other groups, lacked most of the epidemic infectious diseases that affect agrarian and urban societies (Cohen and Armelagos 2013; Singer 2015). Epidemic diseases such as cholera, typhoid, and bubonic plague thrive in dense populations, and thus among farmers and city dwellers. The spread of malaria has been linked to population growth and deforestation associated with food production.

Disease-Theory Systems

The kinds and incidence of disease vary among societies, and cultures perceive and treat illness differently (see Lupton 2012). Still, all societies have what George Foster and Barbara Anderson call "disease-theory systems" to identify, classify, and explain illness. Foster and Anderson (1978) identified three basic theories about the causes of illness: personalistic, naturalistic, and emotionalistic. *Personalistic disease theories* blame illness on agents, such as sorcerers, witches, ghosts, or ancestral spirits.

Naturalistic disease theories explain illness in impersonal terms. One example is Western medicine, or biomedicine, which aims to link illness to scientifically demonstrated agents that bear no personal malice toward their victims (see Lock and Nguyen 2018). Thus, Western medicine attributes illness to organisms (e.g., bacteria, viruses, fungi, or parasites), accidents, toxic materials, or genes. Other naturalistic systems blame poor health on unbalanced body fluids. Many Latin cultures classify food, drink, and environmental conditions as "hot" or "cold." People believe their health suffers when they eat or drink hot or cold substances together or under inappropriate conditions. For example, one shouldn't drink something cold after a hot bath or eat a pineapple (a cold fruit) when one is menstruating (a hot condition).

Emotionalistic disease theories assume that emotional experiences cause illness (see Kohrt and Mendenhall 2015). For example, Latin Americans may develop *susto,* an illness brought on by anxiety, fright, or tragic news. Its symptoms (lethargy, vagueness, distraction) are similar to those of "soul loss," a diagnosis of similar symptoms made by people in Madagascar.

All societies have **health care systems** consisting of beliefs, customs, specialists, and techniques aimed at ensuring health and diagnosing and curing illness. A society's illness-causation theory is important for treatment. When illness has a personalistic cause, magicoreligious specialists may be effective curers. They draw on varied techniques (occult and practical), which constitute their special expertise. A shaman may cure soul loss by enticing the spirit back into the body. Shamans may ease difficult childbirths by asking spirits to travel up the birth canal to guide the baby out (Lévi-Strauss 1967). A shaman may cure a cough by counteracting a curse or removing a substance introduced by a sorcerer.

If there is a "world's oldest profession" besides hunter and gatherer, it is **curer,** often a shaman. The curer's role has some universal features (Foster and Anderson 1978). Thus, a curer emerges through a culturally defined process of selection (parental prodding, inheritance of the role, visions, dream instructions) and training (apprentice shamanship, medical school). Eventually, the curer is certified by older practitioners and acquires a

disease
A scientifically identified health threat caused by a known pathogen.

illness
A condition of poor health perceived or felt by an individual within a particular culture.

health care systems
Beliefs, customs, and specialists concerned with preventing and curing illness.

curer
One who diagnoses and treats illness.

professional image. Patients believe in the skills of the curer, whom they consult and compensate. Health interventions always have to fit into local cultures. When Western medicine is introduced, people usually preserve many of their old methods while also accepting new ones. Native curers may go on treating certain conditions (e.g., spirit possession), while physicians deal with others. The native curer may get as much credit as the physician for a cure.

Scientific Medicine versus Western Medicine

We should not lose sight, ethnocentrically, of the difference between scientific medicine and Western medicine per se. **Scientific medicine** relies on advances in technology, genomics, molecular biology, neuroscience, pathology, surgery, diagnostics, and applications. Scientific medicine surpasses tribal treatment in many ways. Although medicines such as quinine, coca, opium, ephedrine, and rauwolfia were discovered in nonindustrial societies, thousands of effective drugs are available today to treat myriad diseases. Today's surgical procedures are much safer and more effective than those of traditional societies. These are strong benefits of scientific medicine, even if they are not always successful.

Western medicine refers to the practice of medicine in a particular modern Western nation, such as the United States. Of course, the practice of medicine and the quality and availability of heath care vary among Western nations. Some make free or low-cost health care available to all citizens, while other countries are not so generous.

scientific medicine
A health care system based on scientific knowledge and procedures.

Millions of Americans, for example, remain uninsured. Western medicine has both "pros" and "cons." The strongest pro of Western medicine is that it incorporates scientific medicine and its many benefits. Cons associated with Western medicine include overprescription of drugs (e.g., opioids and antibiotics), unnecessary surgeries, and the impersonality and inequality of the physician–patient relationship. Overuse of antibiotics seems to be triggering an explosion of resistant microorganisms. Another con associated with Western medicine is that it tends to draw a rigid line between biomedical and psychological causation. Non-Western theories usually lack this sharp distinction, recognizing that poor health has intertwined physical, emotional, and social causes (see also Brown and Closser 2016; Joralemon 2010; White 2017).

Treatment strategies that emulate the more personal non-Western curer–patient–community relationship might benefit Western systems. Physician–patient encounters too often are rushed and truncated. Those who perform a surgical procedure or diagnose a condition often include specialists (e.g., radiologists and lab technicians) whom the patient will never see. Surgeons are not renowned for their "bedside manner." Efforts are being made to improve physician–patient relationships. A recent trend in the United States is the rise of "concierge medicine," in which a physician charges an annual fee to each patient, limits the practice to a certain number of patients, and has ample time to spend with each patient because of the reduced caseload. To an extent, the Internet has empowered patients, who now have access to all kinds of medical information that used to be

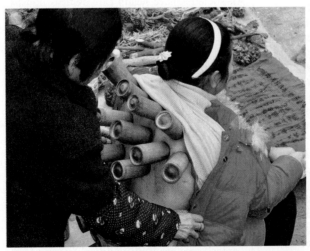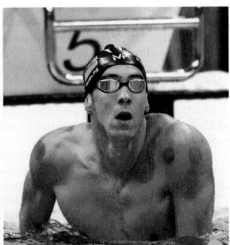

Left: At a market in Yangshuo, China, a woman undergoes a moxibustion treatment, in which mugwort, a small, spongy herb, is burned to facilitate healing. Right: Cupping is a similar ancient Chinese healing and recovery technique that has been adopted by international athletes, most prominently swimmer Michael Phelps at the 2016 Summer Olympics in Rio de Janeiro. Practitioners place specialized cups on the skin, then use either heat or an air pump to suck the skin slightly up and away from the underlying muscles. This causes the capillaries just beneath the surface to rupture, creating circular purple bruises. Note the marks on Phelps's upper body as he celebrates his victory in the Men's 200m Butterfly and his 20th Olympic Gold medal in Rio.

(left): agefotostock/Alamy Stock Photo; (right): Ian MacNicol/Getty Images

the sole property of physicians. This access, however, has its drawbacks. Information can make patients more informed as health care consumers, but it also prompts more questions than a physician usually can answer during a brief appointment.

Industrialization, Globalization, and Health

Despite the advances in scientific medicine, industrialization and globalization have spawned many significant health problems. Certain diseases, and physical conditions such as obesity, have spread with economic development and globalization (Inhorn and Wentzell 2012). Schistosomiasis, or bilharzia (liver flukes), is a dangerous and rapidly spreading parasitic threat. People get schistosomiasis from snails living in ponds, lakes, and waterways, often those created by irrigation projects. The applied anthropology approach to reducing such diseases is to see if local people perceive a connection between the vector (e.g., snails in the water) and the disease. If not, local organizations, schools, and the media, including social media, can help spread the relevant information.

HIV/AIDS, one of the deadliest global pandemics of our times, has been spread through international travel within the modern world system. The world's highest rates of HIV infection and AIDS-related deaths have been in Africa, especially southern Africa. Sexually transmitted infections are spread through prostitution as young men from rural areas seek wage work in cities, labor camps, and mines, often across national borders. When the men return home, they infect their wives (see Baer et al. 2013). As it kills productive adults, AIDS leaves behind dependent children and seniors. Cultural factors affect the spread of HIV, which is less likely to spread when men are circumcised.

Other problems of our times include nutritional decline, dangerous machinery, impersonal work, isolation, poverty, homelessness, substance abuse, and pollution (see McElroy and Townsend 2014). With industrialization and globalization, people turn from subsistence work, usually alongside family and neighbors, to cash employment in more impersonal settings such as factories. Rather than living in villages where everyone knows everyone else, people increasingly live in cities—and often in slums, where they tend to have poorer diets, and more exposure to pathogens and crime, poor sanitation, and polluted air. We all remember the scares caused by Ebola, H1N1, Zika, coronavirus, and other emergent viruses. Such pathogens, however, are not the only, or perhaps even the primary, cause of health problems associated with

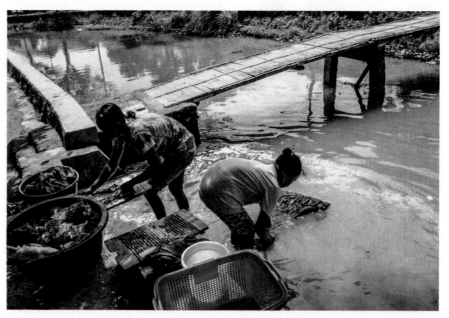

A mother and daughter wash their clothes in polluted canal water in Tangerang, Indonesia. Lack of access to clean water forces residents to rely on river water contaminated with household waste. What are some of the health risks associated with polluted water?

Garry Andrew Lotulung/Pacific Press/LightRocket/Getty Images

industrialization and globalization. Other stressors that endanger our health are economic (e.g., poverty), social (e.g., crowding, homelessness, crime), political (e.g., terrorism, corruption), and cultural (e.g., ethnic conflict). Poverty contributes to many illnesses, including arthritis, heart conditions, back problems, and hearing and vision impairment.

In the United States and other developed countries, good health has become something of an ethical imperative (Foucault 1990). Individuals are expected to regulate their behavior so as to achieve bodies in keeping with new medical knowledge. Those who do so acquire the status of sanitary citizens—people with modern understanding of the body, health, and illness. Such citizens practice hygiene and look to health care professionals when they are sick. People who act differently (e.g., smokers, overeaters, those who avoid doctors) are stigmatized and blamed for their own health problems (Briggs 2005; Foucault 1990).

Nowadays, even getting an epidemic disease such as cholera may be viewed as a moral failure, because people did not take proper precautions. It's assumed that people who act rationally can avoid "preventable" diseases. Individuals are expected to follow scientifically based imperatives (e.g., boil water, don't smoke). People (e.g., smokers, veterans, the homeless) can become objects of avoidance and discrimination simply by belonging to a group seen as having a greater risk of poor health.

Medical anthropology also studies the impact of new scientific and medical techniques on ideas about life, death, and personhood (what it means to be a person). For decades, disagreements about personhood—such as about when life begins and

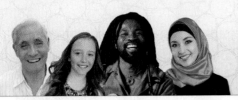

Culturally Appropriate Marketing

Innovation succeeds best when it is culturally appropriate. This axiom of applied anthropology could guide the international spread not only of development projects but also of businesses, including fast food. Each time McDonald's, KFC, or Starbucks expands to a new nation, it must devise a culturally appropriate strategy for fitting into the new setting.

McDonald's has been very successful internationally. More than half of its current annual revenue comes from sales outside the United States. As a highly successful global restaurant chain, McDonald's has about 37,000 restaurants in some 120 countries. One place where McDonald's has expanded successfully is Brazil, where 100 million middle-class people, most living in densely packed cities, provide a concentrated market for a fast-food chain. Still, it took McDonald's some time to find the right marketing strategy for Brazil.

In 1980 when I visited Brazil after a seven-year absence, I first noticed, as a manifestation of Brazil's growing participation in the world economy, the appearance of two McDonald's restaurants in Rio de Janeiro. There wasn't much difference between Brazilian and North American McDonald's. The restaurants looked alike. The menus were more or less the same, as was the taste of the quarter-pounders. I picked up an artifact, a white paper bag with yellow lettering, exactly like the take-out bags then used in American McDonald's. An advertising device, it carried several messages about how Brazilians could bring McDonald's into their lives. However, it seemed to me that McDonald's Brazilian ad campaign was missing some important points about how fast food should be marketed in a culture that valued large, leisurely lunches.

The bag proclaimed, "You're going to enjoy the [McDonald's] difference," and listed several "favorite places where you can enjoy McDonald's products." This list confirmed that the marketing people were trying to adapt to Brazilian middle-class culture, but they were making some mistakes. "When you go out in the car with the kids" transferred the uniquely developed North American cultural combination of highways, affordable cars, and suburban living to the very different context of urban Brazil. A similar suggestion was "traveling to the country place." Even Brazilians who owned country places could not find McDonald's, still confined to the cities, on the road. The ad creator had apparently never attempted to drive up to a fast-food restaurant in a neighborhood with no parking spaces.

Several other suggestions pointed customers toward the beach, where *cariocas* (Rio natives) do spend much of their leisure time. One could eat McDonald's products "after a dip in the ocean," "at a picnic at the beach," or "watching the surfers." These suggestions ignored the Brazilian custom of consuming cold things, such as beer, soft drinks, ice cream, and ham and cheese sandwiches, at the beach. Brazilians don't consider a hot, greasy hamburger proper beach food. They view the sea as "cold" and hamburgers as "hot"; they avoid hot foods at the beach. Also culturally dubious was the suggestion to eat McDonald's hamburgers "lunching at the office." Brazilians prefer their main meal at midday, often eating at a leisurely pace with business associates. Many firms serve ample lunches to their employees. Other workers take advantage of a two-hour lunch break to go home to eat with the spouse and children.

ends—have been part of political and religious discussions of contraception, abortion, and assisted suicide. Recent technological and scientific advances have raised new debates about personhood associated with stem cells, "harvested" embryos, assisted reproduction, genetic screening and editing, cloning, and life-prolonging medical treatments.

Kaufman and Morgan (2005) emphasize the contrast between what they call low-tech and high-tech births and deaths. A desperately poor young mother dies of AIDS in Africa, while half a world away an American child of privilege is born as the result of a $50,000 in-vitro fertilization procedure. Medical anthropologists increasingly are concerned with how the boundaries of life and death are being questioned and negotiated in our globalized world.

ANTHROPOLOGY AND BUSINESS

As David Price (2000) has noted, activities encompassed under the label "applied anthropology" are extremely diverse, ranging from research for activist NGOs to workplace studies commissioned by and for management. For decades, anthropologists have used ethnographic procedures to understand organizations and business settings in North America and abroad (Briody and Trotter 2008; Cefkin 2009; Ferraro

Nor did it make sense to suggest that children should eat hamburgers for lunch, since most kids attend school for half-day sessions and have lunch at home. Two other suggestions—"waiting for the bus" and "in the beauty parlor"—did describe common aspects of daily life in a Brazilian city. However, these settings have not proved especially inviting to hamburgers or fish filets.

The homes of Brazilians who can afford McDonald's products have cooks and maids to do many of the things that fast-food restaurants do in the United States. The suggestion that McDonald's products be eaten "while watching your favorite television program" is culturally appropriate, because Brazilians watch TV a lot. However, Brazil's consuming classes can ask the cook to make a snack when hunger strikes. Indeed, much televiewing occurs during the light dinner served when the husband gets home from the office.

Most appropriate to the Brazilian lifestyle was the suggestion to enjoy McDonald's "on the cook's day off." Throughout Brazil, Sunday is that day. The Sunday pattern for middle-class families who live on the coast is a trip to the beach, liters of beer, a full midday meal around 3 P.M., and a light evening snack.

McDonald's found its niche in the Sunday evening meal, when families flock to the fast-food restaurant.

McDonald's has expanded rapidly in Brazilian cities, suburbs, and shopping malls. As McDonald's outlets appeared in urban neighborhoods, Brazilian teenagers used them for after-school snacks, while families had evening meals there. As an anthropologist could have predicted, the fast-food industry has not revolutionized Brazilian food and meal customs.

Rather, McDonald's is succeeding because it has adapted to preexisting Brazilian cultural patterns.

The main contrast with North America is that the Brazilian evening meal is lighter. McDonald's in Brazil caters to the evening meal as much as, or more than, to lunch. Once McDonald's realized that more money could be made by fitting in with, rather than trying to Americanize, Brazilian meal habits, it started aiming its advertising at that goal. Today, McDonald's has more than 1,000 outlets in Brazil.

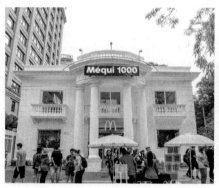 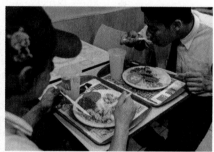

On the left, in São Paulo, Brazil's largest city, McDonald's celebrates the opening of its 1,000th Brazilian restaurant (November 2019). Méqui is McDonald's nickname in Brazilian Portuguese. On the right, we see how McDonald's has learned to indigenize its offerings to fit Brazilian culture. The chain now offers rice and beans as a meal option.

(left) Vinicius Bacarin/Shutterstock; (right) Paulo Fridman/Getty Images

and Briody 2017; A. Jordan 2013; B. Jordan 2013; McCabe 2017). Ethnographic research in an automobile factory, for example, might view line workers, managers, and executives as different social categories participating in a common system. Each group has its own characteristic attitudes and behavior patterns. The free-ranging nature of ethnography allows the anthropologist to move across levels and microcultures—from worker through management and back. Having learned the entire system by crossing and recrossing its internal boundaries, the anthropologist can become an effective "cultural broker," translating managers' goals or workers' concerns to the other group. A free-ranging ethnographer can be a perceptive oddball in settings where information

and decisions typically move through a rigid hierarchy. When allowed to observe and interact with all types and levels of personnel, the anthropologist gains a unique perspective on organizational conditions and problems (see Garsten and Nyqvist 2013).

Business executives, like public policy makers, run organizations that provide goods and services *for people*. The field of market research, which employs an increasing number of anthropologists, is based on the need to know what actual and potential customers do, think, and want. Smart planners study and listen to people to understand what they desire in a product or service and how they use it—the meaningful role it plays in their lives.

Ethnographers can help a business to rethink faulty preconceptions and assumptions about their clients' service needs or purchasing habits, and to *discover* what those clients really are seeking (see Graber and Atkinson 2012). Ethnography relies on in-depth observation of people as they lead their everyday lives. Applying ethnographic techniques, business anthropologists shadow actual and potential customers at home and at work. Researchers observe how those people interact with other people and products. They take notes and video-record behavior and interactions. Eventually, they draw conclusions and make recommendations (see Ha n.d.).

Consider a few case studies illustrating the value of anthropology to business. In an article titled "An Anthropologist Walks into a Bar," Christian Madsbjerg and Mikkel Rasmussen (2014) describe a study commissioned by a beer company, which they call BeerCo. A team of anthropologists studied a dozen bars in Finland and the United Kingdom. The researchers immersed themselves in the life of each bar or pub, observing and getting to know owners, staff, and regulars. The team analyzed 150 hours of video, thousands of still photographs, and massive field notes. Their findings convinced BeerCo to abandon its previous "one-size-fits-all" approach and to launch a more differentiated and targeted campaign. BeerCo started customizing its promotional materials for different types of bars and bar owners. It trained its salesforce to understand and treat each bar owner as an individual. It enhanced loyalty to the brand by offering taxi service for wait staff who had to work

late. BeerCo's pub and bar sales increased. This case illustrates once again the value of knowing the local culture, and for businesses, of targeting products and services accordingly. (This chapter's "Appreciating Diversity" provides yet another example of the value of cultural understanding for business expansion.)

Paco Underhill (2009) is a "retail anthropologist" whose influential book *Why We Buy: The Science of Shopping* has been translated into 27 languages. His market research company, Envirosell, specializes in the study of shopping habits (see also Malefyt and McCabe 2020). Researchers follow shoppers around stores, recording their interactions with merchandise. Underhill's team noted that Americans, on entering a store, tend to gravitate to the right, replicating a pattern used in driving and walking. Australians and Britons, who drive on the left, do the opposite. Based on this observation, Underhill recommended that North American stores place their best merchandise on the right side of the store. He also recommended that stores and departments that cater primarily to women need to give men a place to sit and something to do. (I would add the additional recommendation that Wi-Fi should be easily available, since nowadays "something to do" typically involves a smartphone.) Another Underhill recommendation is that products designed for older people should be placed above the bottom shelf, which gets harder to reach as customers age. Finally, he stresses the key role of the dressing room, as the place where most buying decisions are finalized. Dressing rooms should be clean and well-lit, with places to sit and for children to play (see Green 1999).

One common approach in market research is to assemble a focus group (a small group of people guided by a researcher as they discuss a topic). A limitation of focus groups, surveys, and other common market research techniques is that they elicit only what people *say*, report, or write down, rather than observing real-time, real-life behavior, as anthropologists do. Focus groups also face the danger of group think, when one or two very vocal members unduly influence (or hijack) the entire group. A limitation of surveys is that people want to answer the questions as quickly as possible. They have limited patience and imperfect recall. Their answers will be more accurate and complete when they are interviewed in person and probed for additional information.

The ethnographic market research firm Ethnographic Solutions provides qualitative research, including a variety of ethnographic approaches, that has benefited numerous pharmaceutical,

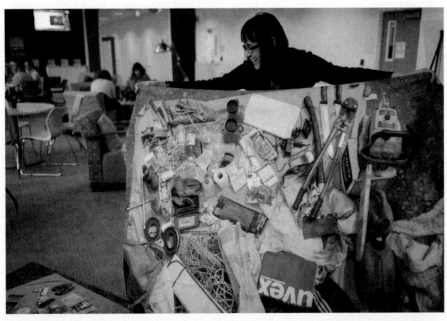

Business anthropology in action: At the Intel Corporation in Hillsboro, Oregon, anthropologist Alexandra Zafiroglu displays a blanket with a huge photograph of the contents of one automobile. Zafiroglu was part of an Intel team directed by anthropologist Genevieve Bell studying objects stored in cars. This research provided insights about how drivers use hand-held mobile devices in conjunction with technology built into their cars.

LEAH NASH/*The New York Times*/Red/Redux Pictures

biotech, and medical device companies. The firm's website describes the value of several techniques, including *physician–patient dialogue research*. The goal is to understand how physicians and patients decide together to initiate and navigate a course of treatment, including the products to be used. Conducted in physicians' offices, physician–patient dialogue research combines on-site interviewing and observation with later analysis of field notes and video-recorded interactions. The resulting perspective goes beyond traditional market research, which typically takes place in an artificial setting, such as a research facility or via a survey, and which relies on imperfect recall.

Key features of anthropology that are of value to business include (1) ethnography and observation as ways of gathering data, (2) a focus on diversity, and (3) cross-cultural expertise. Businesses have heard that anthropologists are specialists on cultural diversity and the observation of behavior. Hallmark Cards has hired anthropologists to observe parties, holidays, and celebrations of ethnic groups to improve its ability to design cards for targeted audiences (see Denny and Sunderland 2014).

PUBLIC AND APPLIED ANTHROPOLOGY

Many academic anthropologists, myself included, occasionally work as applied anthropologists. Often, our role is to consult and advise about the direction of change in places where we originally did "academic" research. In my case, this has meant policy-relevant work on environmental preservation in Madagascar and poverty reduction in northeastern Brazil.

Other academics, while not doing applied anthropology per se, have urged the field of anthropology as a whole to engage more in what they call **public anthropology** (Beck and Maida 2015; Borofsky 2000; Vannini 2019) or *public interest anthropology* (Sanday 2003). Suggested ways of making anthropology more visible and relevant to the public include nonacademic publishing; testifying at government hearings; consulting; acting as an expert witness; and engaging in citizen activism, electoral campaigns, and political administrations (Sanjek 2004). The stated goals of public anthropology are to engage with public issues by opposing policies that promote injustice and by working to reframe discussions of key social issues in the media and by public officials. As Rylko-Bauer and her colleagues (2006) point out, there is, as well, a long tradition of work guided by such goals in applied anthropology.

New media are helping to disseminate anthropological knowledge to a wider public. The complete world of cyberspace, including the blogosphere, constantly grows richer in the resources and communication opportunities available to anthropologists.

Some of the most widely read anthropological blogs include the following:

Anthrodendum (formerly Savage Minds), a group blog

https://anthrodendum.org/

Living Anthropologically, by Jason Antrosio

http://www.livinganthropologically.com

Among other resources, Living Anthropologically offers a detailed list of anthropology blogs. Worth visiting as well is the website of the American Anthropological Association, which is anthropology's largest and most inclusive professional organization: https://www.americananthro.org/

Anthropologists also participate in various listservs and networking groups (e.g., on LinkedIn and Research Gate). A bit of googling on your part will take you to anthropologists' personal websites, as well as research project websites.

CAREERS AND ANTHROPOLOGY

Many college students find anthropology interesting and consider majoring in it. However, their parents or friends may discourage them by asking, "What kind of job are you going to get with an anthropology degree?" The first step in answering that question is to consider the more general question "What do you do with any college major?" The answer is "Not much, without a good bit of effort, thought, and planning." A survey of graduates of the University of Michigan's literary college showed that few had jobs that were clearly linked to their majors. Most professions, including medicine and law, require advanced degrees. Although many colleges offer bachelor's degrees in engineering, business, accounting, and social work, master's degrees often are needed to get the best jobs in those fields. Anthropologists, too, need an advanced degree, usually a PhD, to find gainful employment as an anthropologist.

A broad college education, and even a major in anthropology, can be an excellent foundation for success in many fields (see Golub 2017). One survey of women executives showed that most had majored not in business but in the social sciences or humanities. Only after graduating from college did they study business, leading to an MBA, a master's degree in business administration. These executives felt that the breadth of their college educations had contributed to their business careers. Anthropology majors go on to medical, law, and business schools and find success in many professions that often have little explicit connection to anthropology.

Anthropology's breadth provides knowledge and an outlook on the world that are useful in many kinds of work. For example, an anthropology major combined with a master's degree in business

public anthropology
Efforts to extend anthropology's visibility beyond academia and to demonstrate its public policy relevance.

is excellent preparation for work in international business. Breadth is anthropology's hallmark. Anthropologists study people biologically, culturally, socially, and linguistically, across time and space, in various countries, in simple and complex settings. Most colleges offer anthropology courses that compare cultures, along with others that focus on particular world areas, such as Latin America, Asia, Africa, or Oceania. The knowledge of foreign areas acquired in such courses can be useful in many jobs. Anthropology's comparative outlook and its focus on diverse lifestyles combine to provide an excellent foundation for overseas employment (see Dominguez and French 2020; Ellick and Watkins 2011; Nolan 2017; Omohundro 2001).

For work in modern North America, anthropology's focus on culture is increasingly relevant. Every day we hear about cultural differences and about problems whose solutions require a multicultural viewpoint—an ability to recognize and reconcile ethnic differences. Government, schools, hospitals, and businesses constantly deal with people from different social classes, ethnic groups,

and cultural backgrounds. Physicians, attorneys, social workers, police officers, judges, teachers, and students can all do a better job if they understand cultural differences in a nation that is one of the most ethnically diverse in history.

Knowledge of the traditions and beliefs of the groups that make up a modern nation is important in planning and carrying out programs that affect those groups. Experience in planned social change—whether community organization in North America or economic development overseas—shows that a proper social study should be done before a project or policy is implemented. When local people want the change and it fits their lifestyle and traditions, it has a better chance of being successful, beneficial, and cost effective.

People with anthropology backgrounds do well in many fields. Even if one's job has little or nothing to do with anthropology in a formal or obvious sense, a background in anthropology provides a useful orientation when we work with our fellow human beings. For most of us, this means every day of our lives.

for REVIEW

summary

1. Anthropology has two dimensions: academic and applied. Applied anthropology uses anthropological perspectives, theory, methods, and data to identify, assess, and solve problems. Applied anthropologists have a range of employers. Examples are government agencies; development organizations; NGOs; tribal, ethnic, and interest groups; businesses; social service and educational agencies. Applied anthropologists come from all four subfields. Ethnography is one of applied anthropology's most valuable research tools.

2. Development anthropology focuses on social issues in, and the cultural dimension of, economic development. Not all governments seek to increase equity and end poverty. Resistance by elites to reform is typical and hard to combat. At the same time, local people rarely cooperate with projects requiring major and risky changes in their daily lives. Many projects seek to impose inappropriate property notions and incompatible social units on their intended beneficiaries. The best strategy for change is to base the social design for innovation on traditional social forms in each target area.

3. Anthropology and education researchers work in classrooms, homes, and other settings relevant to education. Such studies may lead to policy recommendations. Both academic and applied anthropologists study migration from rural areas to cities and across national boundaries. North America has become a popular arena for urban anthropological research on migration, ethnicity, poverty, and related topics. Although rural and urban are different social systems, there is cultural diffusion from one to the other.

4. Medical anthropology is the cross-cultural, biocultural study of health problems and conditions, disease, illness, disease theories, and health care systems. Medical anthropology includes anthropologists from all four subfields and has theoretical (academic) and applied dimensions. In a given setting, the characteristic diseases reflect diet, population density, the economy, and social complexity. Native theories of illness may be personalistic, naturalistic, or emotionalistic. In applying anthropology to business, the key features are (1) ethnography

and observation as ways of gathering data, (2) cross-cultural expertise, and (3) a focus on cultural diversity. Public anthropology describes efforts to extend anthropological knowledge of social problems and issues to a wider and more influential audience.

5. A broad college education, including anthropology and foreign-area courses, offers excellent background for many fields. Anthropology's comparative outlook and cultural relativism provide an excellent basis for overseas employment. Even for work in North America, a focus on culture and cultural diversity is valuable. Anthropology majors attend medical, law, and business schools and succeed in many fields, some of which have little explicit connection with anthropology.

think like an anthropologist

1. This chapter discusses the problematic association between early anthropology and colonialism to illustrate some of the dangers of early applied anthropology. We also learned how American anthropologists studied Japanese "culture at a distance" in an attempt to predict the behavior of the enemies of the United States during World War II. Political and military conflicts with other nations and cultures continue today. What role, if any, could and/or should applied anthropologists play in these conflicts?

2. What roles could an applied anthropologist play in the design and implementation of a development project? Based on past experience and research on this topic, what could an applied anthropologist focus on avoiding and/or promoting?

3. This chapter describes some of the applications of anthropology in educational settings. Think back to your grade school or high school classroom. Were there any social issues that might have interested an anthropologist? Were there any problems that an applied anthropologist might have been able to help solve? How so?

4. Indicate your career plans, if known, and describe how you might apply the knowledge learned through introductory anthropology in your future vocation. If you have not yet chosen a career, pick one of the following: economist, engineer, diplomat, architect, or elementary school teacher. Why is it important to understand the culture and social organization of the people who will be affected by your work?

credits

Design Elements: Understanding Ourselves: muha/123RF (rock paintings); Focus on Globalization: janrysavy/Getty Images (globe); Appreciating Diversity (left to right): Floresco Productions/age footstock; Hero/Corbis/Glow Images, Hill Street Studios/Blend Images, Billion Photos/Shutterstock; Understanding Ourselves: Hemera Technologies/Alamy (Cymbal), LACMA - Los Angeles County Museum of Art (Trefoil Oinochoe), Ingram Publishing/SuperStock (Coin), ChuckSchugPhotography/Getty Images (Rug).

Language and Communication

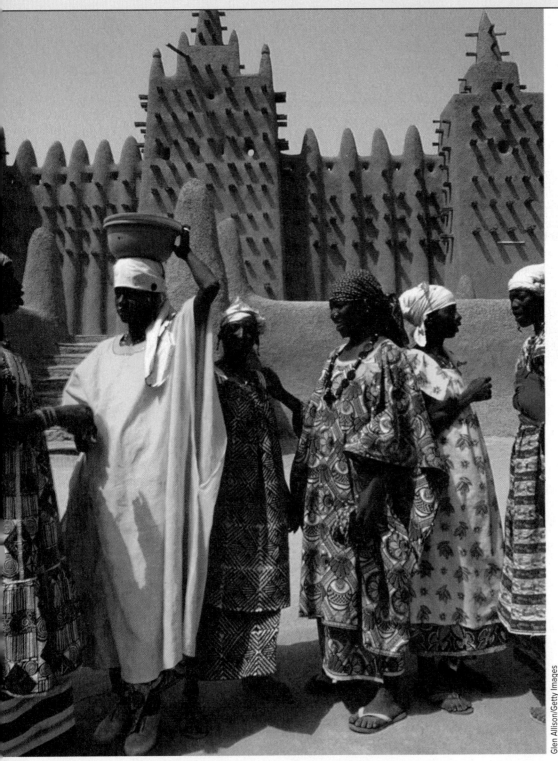

Glen Allison/Getty Images

Women converse in front of the Great Mosque of Djenné, Mali. The ancient pilgrimage city of Djenné, accessible only by ferry, stands between two rivers in central Mali, a predominantly Muslim West African country.

▶ What makes language different from other forms of communication?

▶ How do anthropologists and linguists study language in general and specific languages in particular?

▶ How does language change over short and long time periods?

understanding OURSELVES

Can you recognize anything distinctive or unusual in the way you talk? If you're from Canada, Virginia, or Savannah, you may say "oot" instead of "out." A southerner may request a "soft drink" rather than the New Yorker's "soda." How might a "Valley girl" or "surfer dude" talk? Take this dialect quiz from *The New York Times* to see how accurately it places you with respect to where you grew up: https://www.nytimes.com/interactive/2014/upshot/dialect-quiz-map.html?_r=0.

Usually when we pay attention to how we talk, it's because someone comments on our speech. It may be only when students move from one state or region to another that they appreciate how much of a regional accent they have. I moved as a teenager from Atlanta to New York City. Previously I hadn't realized I had a southern accent, but teachers in my new high school did. They put me in a speech class, pointing out linguistic flaws I never knew I had. One was my "dull s," particularly in terminal consonant clusters, as in the words "tusks" and "breakfasts." Apparently I didn't pronounce all three consonants at the ends of those words. Later it occurred to me that these weren't words I used very often. As far as I know, I've never conversed about tusks or proclaimed, "I ate seven breakfasts last week."

Unlike grammarians, linguists and anthropologists are interested in what people do

say, rather than what they should say. Speech differences are associated with, and tell us a lot about, social variation, such as region, education, ethnic background, and gender. Men and women talk differently. I'm sure you can think of examples based on your own experience, although you probably never realized that women tend to peripheralize their vowels (think of the sounds in *weasel* and *whee*), whereas men tend to centralize them (think of *rough* and *ugh*). Men are more likely to speak "ungrammatically" than women are. Men and women also show differences in their sports and color terminologies. Men typically know more terms related to sports, make more distinctions among them (e.g., "runs" versus "points"), and try to use the terms more precisely than women do.

Correspondingly, women use more color terms and attempt to use them more specifically than men do. To make this point when I lecture, I bring an off-purple shirt to class. Holding it up, I first ask women to say aloud what color the shirt is. The women rarely answer with a uniform voice, as they try to distinguish the actual shade (mauve, lilac, lavender, wisteria, or some other purplish hue). I then ask the men, who consistently answer as one, "PURPLE." Rare is the man who on the spur of the moment can imagine the difference between fuchsia and magenta or grape and aubergine.

WHAT IS LANGUAGE?

Linguistic anthropology illustrates anthropology's characteristic interests in diversity, comparison, and change—but here the focus is on language (see Ahearn 2017; Bonvillain 2016; Garcia, Flores and Spotti 2017; Tusting 2020). **Language,** whether spoken (*speech*)

or written (*writing*—which has existed for less than 6,000 years), is our primary means of communication. We can define language more broadly as a communication system based on meaningful signs, sounds, gestures, or marks (e.g., words, letters, and punctuation marks). Like culture in general, of which language is a part, language is transmitted through learning. Language is based on arbitrary, learned associations between words and the things they stand for. Unlike the communication systems of other animals, language allows us to discuss the past and future, share our experiences with others, and benefit from their experiences.

Anthropologists study language in its social and cultural context (see Bonvillain 2020; Salzmann et al. 2015). Some linguistic anthropologists reconstruct ancient languages by comparing their contemporary descendants. Others study languages to discover how worldviews and patterns of thought vary from culture to culture. Sociolinguists examine dialects and styles in a single language to show how speech reflects social differences. Linguistic anthropologists also explore the role of language in colonization, the world system, and globalization (Borjian 2017; Wang 2020).

NONHUMAN PRIMATE COMMUNICATION

Call Systems

Only humans speak. No other animal has anything approaching the complexity of language. The natural communication systems of other primates (monkeys and apes) are **call systems.** These vocal systems consist of a limited number of sounds—*calls*—that are produced only when particular environmental stimuli are encountered. Such calls may be varied in intensity and duration, but they are much less flexible than language because they are automatic and can't be combined. When primates encounter food and danger simultaneously, they can make only one call. They can't combine the calls for food and danger into a single utterance, indicating that both are present (for example, "There are lots of bananas here, but also snakes."). At some point in human evolution, however, our ancestors began to combine calls and to understand the combinations. The number of calls also expanded, eventually becoming too great to be transmitted even partly through the genes. Communication came to rely almost totally on learning.

Although wild primates use call systems, the vocal tract of apes is not suitable for speech. Until the 1960s, attempts to teach spoken language to apes suggested that they lack linguistic abilities. In the 1950s, a couple raised a chimpanzee, Viki, as a member of their family and systematically tried to teach her to speak. However, Viki learned only four words ("mama," "papa," "up," and "cup").

Sign Language

More recent experiments have shown that apes can learn to use, if not speak, true language (see Hanzel 2017). Several apes have learned to converse with people through means other than speech. One such communication system is American Sign Language,

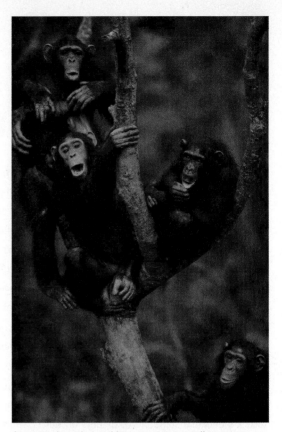

Apes, such as these chimpanzees, use call systems to communicate in the wild. Their vocal systems consist of a limited number of sounds—calls—that are produced only when particular environmental stimuli are encountered. What might they be signaling here?
Michael Nichols/*National Geographic*/Getty Images

or ASL, which is widely used by deaf Americans. ASL employs a limited number of basic gesture units that are analogous to sounds in spoken language. These units combine to form words and larger units of meaning.

The first chimpanzee to learn ASL was Washoe, a female who died in 2007 at the age of 42. Captured in West Africa, Washoe was acquired by R. Allen Gardner and Beatrice Gardner, scientists at the University of Nevada in Reno, in 1966, when she was a year old. Four years later, she moved to Norman, Oklahoma, to a converted farm that had become the Institute for Primate Studies. Washoe revolutionized the discussion of the language-learning abilities of apes (Carey 2007). At first she lived in a trailer and heard no spoken language. The researchers always used ASL to communicate with each other in her presence. The chimp gradually acquired a vocabulary of more than 100 signs representing English words (Gardner et al. 1989). At the age of 2, Washoe began to combine as many as five signs into rudimentary sentences such as "you, me, go out, hurry."

The second chimp to learn ASL was Lucy, Washoe's junior by one year. Lucy died, or was murdered by poachers, in 1986, after having been introduced to "the wild" in Africa in 1979 (Carter

1988). From her second day of life until her move to Africa, Lucy lived with a family in Norman, Oklahoma. Roger Fouts, a researcher from the nearby Institute for Primate Studies, came two days a week to test and improve Lucy's knowledge of ASL. During the rest of the week, Lucy used ASL to converse with her foster parents. After acquiring language, Washoe and Lucy exhibited several human traits: swearing, joking, telling lies, and trying to teach language to others (Fouts 1997).

When irritated, Washoe called her monkey neighbors at the institute "dirty monkeys." Lucy insulted her "dirty cat." On arrival at Lucy's place, Fouts once found a pile of excrement on the floor. When he asked the chimp what it was, she replied, "dirty, dirty," her expression for feces. Asked whose "dirty, dirty" it was, Lucy named Fouts's coworker, Sue. When Fouts refused to believe her about Sue, the chimp blamed the excrement on Fouts himself.

A fundamental attribute of language is its **cultural transmission** through learning. People talk to you and around you, and you learn. Washoe, Lucy, and other chimps have tried to teach ASL to other animals. Washoe taught gestures to other institute chimps, including her son Sequoia, who died in infancy (Gardner et al. 1989).

Because of their size and strength as adults, gorillas are less likely subjects than chimps for such experiments. Psychologist Francine "Penny" Patterson's work with gorillas at Stanford University therefore seems more daring than the chimp experiments. Patterson raised the female gorilla Koko (1971–2018) in a trailer next to a Stanford museum. Koko's vocabulary eventually surpassed that of any chimp. She learned more than 1,000 signs, of which she regularly used over 800. She also recognized at least 2,000 spoken words in English when she heard them. Video clips and other documentation of Patterson's work with Koko and Michael, a male gorilla who also learned sign language, are available at http://www.koko.org/sign-language.

Koko and the chimps also show that apes share still another linguistic ability with humans: **productivity.** Speakers routinely use the rules of their language to produce entirely new expressions that are comprehensible to other native speakers. I can, for example, create "baboonlet" to refer to a baboon infant. I do this by analogy with English words in which the suffix *-let* designates the young of a species. Anyone who speaks English immediately understands the meaning of my new word. Koko, Washoe, Lucy, and others have shown that apes also are able to use language productively. Lucy used gestures she already knew to create "drinkfruit" for watermelon. Washoe, seeing a swan for the first time, coined "waterbird." Koko, who knew the gestures for "finger" and "bracelet," formed "finger bracelet" when she was given a ring.

Chimps and gorillas have a rudimentary capacity for language. They may never have invented a meaningful gesture system in the wild. However, given such a system, they can learn and use it. Of

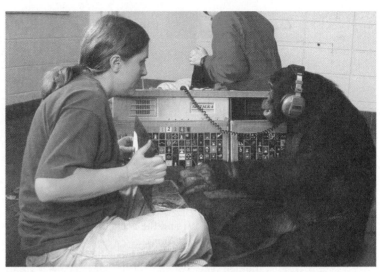

Kanzi, a male bonobo, identifies an object he has just heard named through headphone speakers. At a young age, Kanzi learned to understand simple human speech and to communicate by using lexigrams, abstract symbols that represent objects and actions. A keyboard of lexigrams is pictured in the background.
Michael Nichols/National Geographic Creative

course, language use by apes is a product of human intervention and teaching. The experiments mentioned here do not suggest that apes can invent language (nor are human children ever faced with that task). However, young apes have managed to learn the basics of gestural language. They can employ it productively and creatively, although not with the sophistication of human ASL users.

Apes also have demonstrated linguistic **displacement.** Absent in call systems, this is a key ingredient in language. Normally, a call is tied to a particular environmental stimulus and is uttered only when that stimulus is present. Displacement means that humans can talk about things that are not present. We can discuss the past and future, share our experiences with others, and benefit from theirs.

Patterson has described several examples of Koko's capacity for displacement (Patterson 1978, 1999). The gorilla once expressed sorrow about having bitten Penny three days earlier. Koko has used the sign "later" to postpone doing things she doesn't want to do. Recap 5.1 summarizes the contrasts between language, whether sign or spoken, and the call systems that primates use in the wild.

Certain scholars doubt the linguistic abilities of chimps and gorillas (Hess 2008; Sebeok and Umiker-Sebeok 1980; Terrace 1979). These people contend that Koko and the chimps are comparable to trained circus animals and don't really have linguistic ability. However, in defense of Patterson and the other researchers (Hill 1978; Van Cantfort and Rimpau 1982), only one of their critics has worked with an ape. This was Herbert Terrace, whose experience teaching a chimp sign language lacked the continuity and personal involvement that have contributed so much to Patterson's success with Koko. (For more on Terrace and his ill-fated chimp, Nim Chimpsky, see Hess [2008],

cultural transmission
Transmission through learning, basic to language.

displacement
Describing things and events that are not present; basic to language.

productivity
Creating new expressions that are comprehensible to other speakers.

HUMAN LANGUAGE	PRIMATE CALL SYSTEMS
Has the capacity to speak (or gesture) of things and events that are not present (displacement)	Are stimuli dependent; the food call will be made only in the presence of food; it cannot be faked
Has the capacity to generate new expressions by combining other expressions (productivity)	Consist of a limited number of calls that cannot be combined to produce new calls
Is group specific in that all humans have the capacity for language, but each linguistic community has its own language, which is culturally transmitted	Tend to be species specific, with little variation among communities of the same species for each call

Terrace [2019] and the acclaimed 2011 documentary film *Project Nim.*)

No one denies the huge difference between human language and gorilla signs. There is surely a major gap between the ability to write a book or say a prayer and an ape's use of signs. Apes may not be people, but they aren't just animals, either. Let us remember how Koko once expressed it: When asked by a reporter whether she was a person or an animal, Koko signed "fine animal gorilla" (Patterson 1978). Koko died in her sleep at the age of 46 on June 19, 2018, at the Gorilla Foundation's preserve in Woodside, California. Her legacy continues at http://www.koko.org.

The Origin of Language

Although the capacity to remember and combine linguistic symbols appears to be latent in the apes, human evolution was needed for this seed to sprout into language. A mutated gene known as *FOXP2* helps explain why humans speak and chimps don't (Paulson 2005). The key role of *FOXP2* in speech came to light in a study of a British family, identified only as KE, half of whose members had a severe inherited deficit in speech (Trivedi 2001). The same variant form of *FOXP2* that is found in chimpanzees causes this disorder in humans. Those with the non-speech version of the gene can't make the tongue and lip movements necessary for clear speech, and their speech is unintelligible (Trivedi 2001). Genomic analysis suggests that the speech-friendly form of *FOXP2* may have taken hold in humans around 150,000 years ago (Paulson 2005). We know now, however, that other genes and a series of anatomical changes were necessary for fully evolved human speech. It would be an oversimplification to call *FOXP2* "the language gene," as was done initially in the popular press, because other genes also determine language development.

Whatever its genetic underpinnings, language confers a tremendous adaptive advantage on *Homo sapiens.* Language permits the information stored by a human society to exceed by far that of any nonhuman group. Language is a uniquely effective vehicle for learning. Because we can speak of things we have never experienced, we can anticipate responses before we encounter the stimuli. Adaptation can occur more rapidly in *Homo* than in the other primates because our adaptive means are much more flexible.

NONVERBAL COMMUNICATION

Language is our principal means of communicating, but it isn't the only one we use. We communicate whenever we transmit information about ourselves to others and receive information from them. Our facial expressions, bodily stances, gestures, and movements, even if unconscious, convey information. Deborah Tannen (1990, 2017) discusses differences in the communication styles of American men and women. She notes that American girls and women tend to look directly at each other when they talk, whereas American boys and men do not. Males are more likely to look straight ahead rather than turn and make eye contact with someone, especially another man, seated beside them. Also, in conversational groups, American men tend to relax and sprawl out. Consider the phenomenon known as "manspreading"—the tendency for men using public transportation to open their legs and thus take up more than one place. American

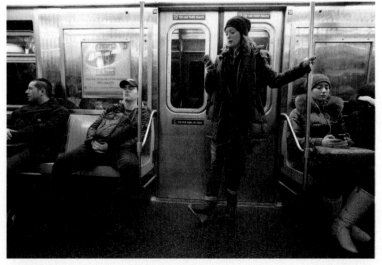

Manspreading on a New York subway. Why do you think the woman is standing?

Hiroko Masuike/*The New York Times*/Redux Pictures

women may relax their posture in all-female groups, but when they are with men, they tend to draw in their limbs and assume a tighter stance.

Kinesics is the study of communication through body movements, stances, gestures, and facial expressions. Linguists pay attention not only to what is said but to how it is said, and to features besides language itself that convey meaning. A speaker's enthusiasm is conveyed not only through words but also through facial expressions, gestures, and other signs of animation. We use gestures, such as a jab of the hand, for emphasis. We use verbal and nonverbal ways of communicating our moods: enthusiasm, sadness, joy, regret. We vary our intonation and the pitch or loudness of our voices. We communicate through strategic pauses, and even by being silent. An effective communication strategy may be to alter pitch, voice level, and grammatical forms, such as declaratives ("I am . . ."), imperatives ("Go forth . . ."), and questions ("Are you . . .?"). Culture teaches us that certain manners and styles should accompany certain kinds of speech. Our demeanor, verbal and nonverbal, when our favorite team is winning would be out of place at a funeral.

Much of what we communicate is nonverbal and reflects our emotional states and intentions. This can create problems when we use rapid means of communication such as texting and online messaging. People can use emoticons (coined from *emotion* and *icon*) to suggest what otherwise would be communicated by tone of voice, laughter, or facial expressions (see Baron 2009; Tannen and Trester 2013). Examples of emoticons are the following: ☺, ☹, :˜/ [confused], :˜0 ["hah!" no way!] and abbreviations: lol—laugh out loud; lmao—laugh my a** off; wtf—what the f***; omg—oh my gosh. While people still use emoticons, emojis have more recently taken on a similar and growing role in digital communication. An *emoji* is a digital image or pictograph, widely available on smartphones and tablets, used to express an idea or emotion, such as happiness or sadness.

Body movements communicate social differences. In Japan, bowing is a regular part of social interaction, but different bows are used depending on the social status of the people who are interacting. In Madagascar and Polynesia, people of lower status should not hold their heads above those of people of higher status. When one approaches someone older or of higher status, one bends one's knees and lowers one's head as a sign of respect. In Madagascar, one always does this, for politeness, when passing between two people.

THE STRUCTURE OF LANGUAGE

Descriptive linguistics—the scientific study of a spoken language—involves several interrelated areas of analysis: phonology, morphology, lexicon, and syntax (see Akmajian et al. 2017; McGregor 2015). **Phonology,** the study of speech sounds, considers which sounds are present and significant in a given language. **Morphology** studies how sounds combine to form *morphemes*—words and their meaningful parts. Thus, the word *cats* would be analyzed as containing two morphemes: *cat,* the name for a kind of animal, and -*s,* a morpheme indicating plurality. A morpheme, therefore, is a minimal unit of meaning. A language's **lexicon** is a dictionary containing all its morphemes and their meanings. **Syntax** refers to the arrangement and order of words in phrases and sentences. Syntactic questions include whether nouns usually come before or after verbs, and whether adjectives normally precede or follow the nouns they modify.

From the media, and from actually meeting foreigners, we know something about foreign accents and mispronunciations. We know that someone with a marked French accent doesn't pronounce *r* the same way an American does. But at least someone from France can distinguish between "craw" and "claw," which someone from Japan may not be able to do. The difference between *r* and *l* makes a difference in English and in French, but it doesn't in Japanese. In linguistics, we say that the difference between *r* and *l* is *phonemic* in English and French but not in Japanese; that is, *r* and *l* are phonemes in English and French but not in Japanese. A **phoneme** is a sound contrast that makes a difference, that differentiates meaning.

We find the phonemes in a given language by comparing *minimal pairs,* words that resemble each other in all but one sound. The words have totally different meanings, but they differ in just one sound. The contrasting sounds are therefore phonemes in that language. An example in English is the minimal pair *pit/bit.* These two words are distinguished by a single sound contrast between /p/ and /b/ (we enclose phonemes in slashes). Thus /p/ and /b/ are phonemes in English. Another example is the different vowel sounds of *bit* and *beat* (see Figure 5.1). This contrast serves to distinguish these two words and the two vowel phonemes written /I/ and /i/ in English.

Standard (American) English, the "region-free" dialect of TV network newscasters, has about 35 phonemes: at least 11 vowels and 24 consonants. The number of phonemes varies from language to language—from 15 to 60, averaging between 30 and 40. The number of phonemes also varies between dialects of a given language. In American English, for example, vowel phonemes vary noticeably from dialect to dialect. Readers should pronounce the words in Figure 5.1, paying attention to (or asking someone else) whether they distinguish each of the vowel sounds. Most Americans don't pronounce them all. My grandson Lucas thinks it's funny that I make a phonemic distinction he doesn't make. I pronounce words beginning with *wh* as though they began with *hw*. My personal set of phonemes includes both /hw/ and /w/.

phonology
The study of sounds used in speech in a particular language.

morphology
The (linguistic) study of morphemes and word construction.

kinesics
The study of communication through body movements and facial expressions.

lexicon
Vocabulary; all the morphemes in a language and their meanings.

syntax
The arrangement and order of words in phrases and sentences.

phoneme
The smallest sound contrast that distinguishes meaning.

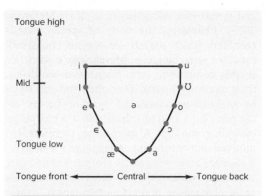

FIGURE 5.1 Vowel Phonemes in Standard American English.

The phonemes are shown according to height of tongue and tongue position at front, center, or back of mouth. Phonetic symbols are identified by English words that include them; note that most are minimal pairs.

SOURCE: Adaptation of excerpt and Figure 2-1 from Bolinger, Dwight and Donald A. Sears, *Aspects of Language,* 3rd ed. Cengage Learning, 1981.

[i]	as in *beat*	High front (spread)
[I]	as in *bit*	Lower high front (spread)
[e]	as in *bait*	Mid front (spread)
[ɛ]	as in *bet*	Lower mid front (spread)
[æ]	as in *bat*	Low front
[ə]	as in *butt*	Central
[a]	as in *pot*	Low back
[ɔ]	as in *bought*	Lower mid back (rounded)
[o]	as in *boat*	Mid back (rounded)
[ʊ]	as in *put*	Lower high back (rounded)
[u]	as in *boot*	High back (rounded)

This enables me to distinguish between *white* and *Wight* (as in the Isle of Wight) and between *where* and *wear.* Lucas pronounces all four of those words as though they begin with [w], so that he does not distinguish between *white* and *Wight* or between *where* and *wear.* How about you?

Phonetics is the study of speech sounds in general, what people actually say in various languages. **Phonemics** studies only the *significant* sound contrasts (phonemes) of a given language. In English, like /r/ and /l/ (remember *craw* and *claw*), /b/ and /v/ are also phonemes, occurring in minimal pairs like *bat* and *vat.* In Spanish, however, the contrast between [b] and [v] doesn't distinguish meaning, and they therefore are not phonemes (we enclose sounds that are not phonemic in brackets). Spanish speakers normally use the [b] sound to pronounce words spelled with either *b* or *v.*

In any language, a given phoneme extends over a phonetic range. In English, the phoneme /p/ ignores the phonetic contrast between the [pʰ] in *pin* and the [p] in *spin.* Most English speakers don't even notice that there is a phonetic difference: [pʰ] is aspirated, so that a puff of air follows the [p]; the [p] in *spin* is not. (To see the difference, light a match, hold it in front of your mouth, and watch the flame as you pronounce the two words.) The contrast between [pʰ] and [p] is phonemic in some languages, such as Hindi (spoken in India).

phonetics
The study of speech sounds—what people actually say.

phonemics
The study of significant sound contrasts (phonemes) in a language.

That is, there are words whose meaning is distinguished only by the contrast between an aspirated and an unaspirated [p].

Native speakers vary in their pronunciation of certain phonemes. This variation is important in the evolution of language. With no shifts in pronunciation, there can be no linguistic change. The "Sociolinguistics" section in this chapter considers phonetic variation and its relationship to social differences and the evolution of language.

LANGUAGE, THOUGHT, AND CULTURE

The well-known linguist Noam Chomsky (1957) has argued that the human brain contains a limited set of rules for organizing language, so that all languages have a common structural basis. (Chomsky calls this set of rules *universal grammar.*) The fact that people can learn foreign languages and that words and ideas can be translated from one language into another tends to support Chomsky's position that all humans have similar linguistic abilities and thought processes. Another line of support comes from creole languages. Such languages develop from pidgins, languages that form in situations of acculturation, when different societies come into contact and must devise a system of communication (see Adamou and Matras 2020; Lim and Ansaldo 2016; Velupillai 2015). Pidgins based on English and native languages developed in the context of trade and colonialism in China, Papua New Guinea, and West Africa (see Gu 2012; Rickford 2019). Eventually, after generations of being spoken, pidgins may develop into *creole languages.* These are more mature languages, with developed grammatical rules and native speakers (i.e., people who learn the language as their primary means of communication during enculturation). Creoles are spoken in several Caribbean societies. Gullah, which is spoken by African Americans on coastal islands in South Carolina and Georgia, is a creole language. Supporting the idea that creoles are based on universal grammar is the fact that they all share certain features. Syntactically, all creole languages use participles (e.g., *will, was*) to form future and past tenses, and multiple negation to deny or negate (e.g., "she don't got none"). Also, all form questions by changing inflection rather than by changing word order—for example, "You're going home for the holidays?" (with a rising tone at the end) rather than "Are you going home for the holidays?"

The Sapir-Whorf Hypothesis

Other linguists and anthropologists take a different approach to the relation between language and thought. Rather than seeking universal linguistic structures and processes, they believe that different languages produce different ways of thinking. This

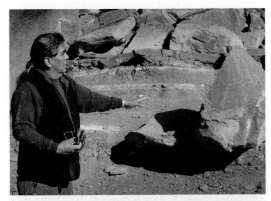

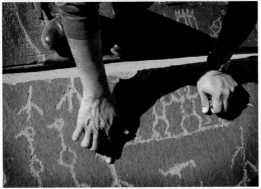

At the top, Lee Wayne Lomayestewa of the Hopi Cultural Preservation Office points out the site of the ancient Tutuveni petroglyphs near Tuba City, Arizona. This site, whose name means "newspaper rock," contains some 5,000 petroglyphs (rock engravings) of Hopi clan symbols. The photo on the bottom shows the petroglyphs up close.

Both: Pauline Arrillaga/AP Images

hypothetical events). Whorf argued that this difference causes Hopi speakers to think about time and reality in different ways than English speakers do. A similar example comes from Portuguese, which employs a future subjunctive verb form, introducing a degree of uncertainty into discussions of the future. In English, we routinely use the future tense to talk about something we think will happen. We don't feel the need to qualify "The sun'll come out tomorrow" by adding "if it doesn't go supernova." We don't hesitate to proclaim "I'll see you next summer," even when we can't be absolutely sure we will. The Portuguese future subjunctive qualifies the future event, recognizing that the future can't be certain. Our way of expressing the future as certain is so ingrained that we don't even think about it, just as the Hopi don't see the need to distinguish between present and past, both of which are real, while the future remains hypothetical. Contrary to Sapir-Whorf, however, it would seem that language does not tightly restrict thought, because cultural changes can produce changes in thought and in language, as we shall see in the next section (see McWhorter 2014).

Focal Vocabulary

A *lexicon* (vocabulary) is a language's dictionary, its set of names for things, events, actions, and qualities. Lexicon influences perception. Thus, Eskimos recognize, and have several distinct words for, types of snow that in English are all called *snow*. Most English speakers never notice the differences between these types of snow and might have trouble seeing them even if someone pointed them out. Similarly, the Nuer of South Sudan developed an elaborate vocabulary to describe cattle. Eskimos have several words for snow and Nuer have dozens for cattle because of their particular histories, economies, and environments (Robson 2013). When the need arises, English speakers also can elaborate their snow and cattle vocabularies. For example, skiers describe types of snow with words that are missing from the lexicons of Florida retirees. Similarly, the cattle vocabulary of a Texas rancher is much ampler than that of a salesperson in a New York City department store. Such specialized sets of terms and distinctions that are particularly important to certain groups (those with particular foci of experience or activity) are known as **focal vocabulary.**

Vocabulary is the area of language that changes most readily. New words and distinctions, when needed, appear and spread. For example, who would have "texted" or "e-mailed" anything 40 years ago? Names for items get simpler as they become common and important. A television has become a *TV,* an automobile a *car,* and a digital video disc a *DVD* (see this chapter's "Appreciating Diversity" for a discussion of recent changes in word use in English).

position is sometimes known as the **Sapir-Whorf hypothesis** after Edward Sapir (1931) and his student Benjamin Lee Whorf (1956), its prominent early advocates. Sapir and Whorf argued that the grammatical categories of different languages lead their speakers to think about things in particular ways. For example, the third-person singular pronouns of English (*he, she; him, her; his, hers*) distinguish gender, whereas those of the Palaung, a small tribe in Burma, do not (Burling 1970). Gender exists in English, although a fully developed noun-gender and adjective-agreement system, as in French and other Romance languages (*la belle fille, le beau fils*), does not. The Sapir-Whorf hypothesis therefore might suggest that English speakers can't help paying more attention to differences between males and females than do the Palaung and less than do French or Spanish speakers.

English divides time into past, present, and future. Hopi, a language of the Pueblo region of the Native American Southwest, does not. Rather, Hopi distinguishes between events that exist or have existed (what we use present and past to discuss) and those that don't or don't yet (our future events, along with imaginary and

Sapir-Whorf hypothesis
The theory that different languages produce different patterns of thought.

focal vocabulary
A set of words describing particular domains (foci) of experience.

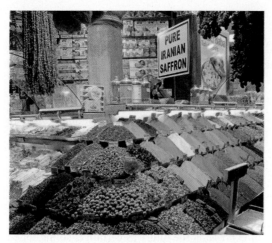

Spices galore, but what kinds? Merchants at this spice market in Istanbul, Turkey, have a much more elaborate focal vocabulary for what they sell than you or I do.

Conrad P. Kottak

for the causes, symptoms, and cures of disease; ethnobotany—native classification of plant life; and ethnoastronomy.

Anthropologists have discovered that certain lexical domains and vocabulary items evolve in a determined order. For example, after studying color terminology in more than 100 languages, Berlin and Kay (1991, 1999) discovered 10 basic color terms: *white, black, red, yellow, blue, green, brown, pink, orange,* and *purple* (they evolved in more or less that order). The number of terms varied with cultural complexity. Representing one extreme were Papua New Guinea cultivators and Australian hunters and gatherers, who used only two basic terms, which translate as *black* and *white* or *dark* and *light.* At the other end of the continuum were European and Asian languages with all the color terms. Color terminology was most developed in areas with a history of using dyes and artificial coloring.

Language, culture, and thought are interrelated. However, and in opposition to the Sapir-Whorf hypothesis, it might be more reasonable to say that changes in culture produce changes in language and thought than the reverse. Consider differences between female and male Americans in regard to the color terms they use (Lakoff 2004, 2017). Distinctions implied by such terms as *salmon, rust, peach, beige, teal, mauve, cranberry,* and *dusky orange* aren't in the vocabularies of most American men. However, many of them weren't even in American women's lexicons 70 years ago. Color terms and distinctions have increased with the growth of the fashion and cosmetic industries. A similar contrast (and growth) in Americans' lexicons shows up in football, baseball, basketball, and hockey vocabularies. Sports fans, more often males than females, use more terms in reference to—and make more elaborate distinctions involving—the games they watch. Cultural contrasts and changes affect lexical distinctions (for instance, *peach* versus *salmon*) within semantic domains (for instance, color terminology). **Semantics** refers to a language's meaning system.

Meaning

Speakers of particular languages use sets of terms to organize, or categorize, their experiences and perceptions. Linguistic terms and contrasts encode (embody) differences in meaning that people perceive. **Ethnosemantics** studies such classification systems in various languages. Well-studied ethnosemantic *domains* (sets of related things, perceptions, or concepts named in a language) include kinship terminology and color terminology. When we study such domains, we are examining how those people perceive and distinguish between kin relationships or colors. Other such domains include ethnomedicine—the terminology

SOCIOLINGUISTICS

No language is a uniform system in which everyone talks just like everyone else. The field of **sociolinguistics** investigates relationships between social and linguistic variation (Eckert 2018; Meyerhoff 2019; Simpson 2019). How do different speakers use a given language? How do linguistic features correlate with social diversity and stratification, including regional, class, ethnic, and gender differences (Coates 2016; Eckert and McConnell-Ginet 2013; Talbot 2019; Tannen 2017)? How is language used to gain, express, reinforce, or resist power (Lakoff 2017; McConnell-Ginet 2020; Mooney and Evans 2019; Simpson et al. 2018)? How does language vary in the context of new media (Danesi 2020)?

Linguistic Diversity within Nations

As an illustration of the linguistic variation that is encountered in all nations, consider the contemporary United States. Ethnic diversity is revealed by the fact that millions of Americans learn first languages other than English. Spanish is the most common. Most of those people eventually become bilinguals, adding English as a second language. In many multilingual (including colonized) nations, people use two or more languages on different occasions: one in the home, for example, and the other on the job or in public. In India, where some 22 languages are spoken, a person may need to use three different languages when talking, respectively, with a boss, a spouse, and a parent. Only about one-tenth of India's population speaks English, the colonial language. As they interact today with one of the key instruments of globalization—the Internet—even those English speakers appreciate being able to read, and to find Internet content in, their own regional languages.

sociolinguistics
The study of language in society.

semantics
A language's meaning system.

ethnosemantics
The study of lexical (vocabulary) categories and contrasts.

Whether bilingual or not, we all vary our speech depending on context; we engage in **style shifts.** In 2013, I traveled to India with a friend, an India-born American who speaks perfectly good American English. During the time we spent in India, it was fascinating to watch as he shifted back and forth between Hindi, English with a strong Indian accent (when speaking to Indians in English), and Standard American English (when speaking to his American fellow travelers). In certain parts of Europe, people regularly switch dialects. This phenomenon, known as **diglossia,** applies to "high" and "low" variants of the same language, for example, in German and Dutch. People employ the "high" variant at universities and in writing, professions, and the mass media. They use the "low" variant for ordinary conversation with family members and friends.

Regional Variation

We all have stereotypes about how people in other regions talk. Some stereotypes, spread by the media, are more generalized than others. Most Americans think they can imitate a "Southern accent." Americans also stereotype speech in Canada ("oot" for "out") and Boston ("I pahked the kah in Hahvahd Yahd"). The Boston accent is on full display in a 2020 Super Bowl Hyundai Sonata commercial showing that car's "Smaht Pahk" (Smart Park) capability. You can see that commercial, featuring Bostonians Rachel Dratch, Chris Evans, John Krasinski, and David "Big Papi" Ortiz. at the following website https://www.youtube.com/watch?v=85iRQdjCzj0.

Although many people assume, erroneously, that midwesterners don't have accents, people from that region do exhibit significant linguistic variation (see Eckert 1989, 2000). One of the best examples is pronunciation of the *e* vowel sound (called the /e/ phoneme), in such words as *ten, rent, section, lecture, effect, best,* and *test.* In southeastern

Michigan, there are four different ways of pronouncing this *e* sound. African Americans and immigrants from Appalachia often pronounce *ten* as "tin," just as Southerners habitually do. Some Michiganders say "ten," the correct pronunciation in Standard English. However, two other pronunciations also are common. Instead of "ten," many Michiganders say "tan" or "tun" (as though they were using the word *ton,* a unit of weight).

I remember, for example, how one of my Michigan-raised teaching assistants appeared deliriously happy one afternoon. When I asked why, she replied, "I've just had the best suction." "What?" I asked, and she replied more precisely. "I've just had the best saction." She considered this a clearer pronunciation of the word *section.* Another TA complimented me, "You luctured to great effuct today." After an exam, a student lamented that she had not done her "bust on the tust" (i.e., "best on the test"). The truth is, regional patterns affect the way we all speak.

Linguistic Diversity in California

Is there a "California accent"? Popular stereotypes about how Californians talk reflect exposure to media images of blond surfer boys who say things like "dude" and "gnarly" and white Valley girls who intone "Like, totally!" and "Gag me with a spoon!" Such stereotypes have some accuracy, as we'll see. Just as striking, however, is the linguistic diversity that also marks contemporary California.

To document this diversity, annually since 2009, Professor Penelope Eckert, a sociolinguist at Stanford University, and her graduate students are engaged in an ongoing research project called Voices of California (see http://www.stanford.edu/dept/linguistics/VoCal/). A team of 10–15 researchers visits a new site each fall, spending

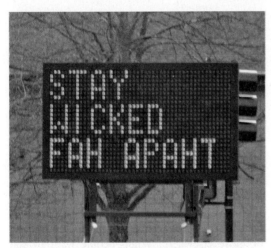

This traffic sign, posted in Maynard, Massachusetts, on April 23, 2020, uses the Boston accent to remind residents to practice social distancing.
Kenneth Martin/Alamy Stock Photo

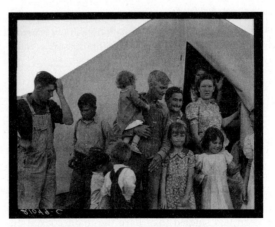

Members of this family from Oklahoma (father, mother, and eleven children), shown here in a migrant labor camp in Brawley, California, found seasonal work as pea harvesters. Such depression-era migrants from Oklahoma's Dust Bowl left their mark on California speech.
Library of Congress Prints & Photographs Division [LC-USF34-021049-C]

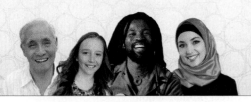

appreciating DIVERSITY

Words of the Year

Annual lists of "words of the year" provide an excellent illustration of how vocabulary shifts in response to cultural changes. Organizations in various countries routinely publish such lists, from which one increasingly common word or phrase is generally chosen as the winner—the "word of the year." Table 5.1 lists the word of the year chosen by the American Dialect Society (ADS) for every year between 2000 ("chad") and 2019 ((my) pronouns). The list tells us a lot about recent American history and culture, especially the concerns that have dominated the news and public discourse from year to year. For instance, we see how certain key words—often just one word or phrase—can sum up the presidential elections of 2000 (*chad*), 2004 (*red state, blue state, purple state*), and 2016 (*dumpster fire*). National crises of 2001, 2002, 2007, and 2008 are encapsulated respectively by *9-11, weapons of mass destruction, subprime,* and *bailout.* Years of protest show up in *occupy* (2011) and *#blacklivesmatter* (2014). *Tweet* (2009), *app* (2010), and *hashtag* (2012) summarize changes in technology and communication. Sometimes, the words are more playful, like *metrosexual* (2003), *truthiness* (2005), and plutoed (2006)—coined from the demotion of our former ninth planet. And finally, in less exciting years, the Dialect Society may single out a common word that is being used in a new way. For example, *because* (2013) no longer

TABLE 5.1 Words of the Year 2000–2019, as Chosen by the American Dialect Society

2000: chad (from the "hanging chads" on several ballots cast in Florida in the 2000 U.S. presidential election)

2001: 9-11 (for obvious reasons)

2002: weapons of mass destruction (used by the George W. Bush administration as a pretense for invading Iraq)

2003: metrosexual (a fashion-conscious heterosexual male)

2004: red state, blue state, purple state (from the 2004 U.S. presidential election)

2005: truthiness (from *The Colbert Report;* preferring concepts or facts one wishes to be true, rather than concepts or facts known to be true)

2006: plutoed (demoted or devalued, like the former planet Pluto)

2007: subprime (a risky loan, mortgage, or investment)

2008: bailout (government rescue of a company on the brink of failure)

2009: tweet (a message sent via Twitter)

2010: app (short for *application,* as on a smartphone, now extended to any computer program)

2011: occupy (as in Occupy Wall Street)

2012: hashtag (a word or phrase preceded by a hash symbol, as on Twitter)

2013: because (when used to introduce a noun, adjective, or other part of speech, as in "because awesome")

2014: #blacklivesmatter (hashtag used to protest killings of African Americans by police)

2015: singular they (as a gender-neutral pronoun; also word of the decade 2010-2019)

2016: dumpster fire (a disastrous or chaotic situation, representing the public discourse and preoccupations surrounding the 2016 U.S. presidential election)

2017: fake news (meaning either: [1] disinformation or falsehoods presented as real news or [2] actual news that is claimed to be untrue)

2018: tender-age shelter (also *tender-age facility* or *tender-age camp,* are terms used euphemistically to describe the government-run detention centers housing the children of asylum seekers at the U.S./Mexico border)

about 10 days interviewing about 100 residents who grew up in the area. Much of their research has been done in inland California, which has been less studied than have the main coastal cities. The researchers always test certain words that elicit specific pronunciations. These words include *wash,* sometimes pronounced "warsh," *greasy* ("greezy"), and *pin* and *pen,* which some people pronounce the same. Interviews in Merced and Shasta Counties have revealed ways that Depression-era migrants from Oklahoma's Dust Bowl left their mark on California speech, such as

their pronunciation of *wash* and *greasy* (see King 2012).

Another factor contributing to linguistic diversity is how people feel about their home community versus the outside world. In California's Central Valley, which is economically depressed, young people must choose whether to stay put or move elsewhere. When people want to stay involved in their home community, they tend to talk like locals. A desire *not* to be perceived as being from a particular place can motivate people to change their speech (King 2012).

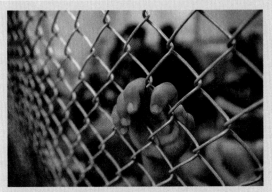

August 12, 2019: In McAllen, Texas, children are detained inside this U.S. Border Patrol Central Processing Center. According to Border Patrol officials, 1,267 people were being held and processed here on this day. Terms including "tender-age shelter," "tender-age facility," and "tender-age camp" were used euphemistically to describe such detention centers at the U.S./Mexico border.

Carolyn Van Houten/Getty Images

2019: (my) pronouns (referring to the sharing of one's set of personal pronouns, as in "Becky Smith--pronouns: she/her" or "Pat Roberts--pronouns they/ them")

SOURCE: Adapted from the Words of the Year website of the American Dialect Society. https://www.americandialect.org/woty.

has to be followed by *of* or a full clause. People now say "because science" or "because tired," rather than "because of science" or "because I'm tired." As one advocate put it, *because* deserved to be the 2013 Word of the Year "because useful"! (See https://www.americandialect.org/because-is-the-2013-word-of-the-year.)

In 2015, not just the ADS, but other organizations as well, chose the singular form of the common pronoun *they* as word of the year, and in 2019 the Society made *singular "they"* its Word of the Decade (2010-2019). *They* is a third-person pronoun that is gender neutral; it includes males, females, and nonbinary individuals. Although grammatically *they* is a plural pronoun, it also is employed (increasingly) as a singular pronoun. Someone can use *they* when they want to avoid having to use "he or she" in a sentence—as I just did. Historical documents show that *they* has been used as a singular pronoun for over 600 years (Baron 2015).

Although for centuries, *they* has been used as both a singular and a plural pronoun, singular *they* began to meet resistance around 1800. Grammarians discouraged its use because of lack of agreement between an apparently plural pronoun and a singular verb (e.g., "They eats dinner."). Those grammatical purists who still resist singular *they* might be reminded that the singular pronoun *you* in English began as a plural pronoun, which eventually replaced *thou* and *thee* as a singular pronoun. It appears that the time has come for a similar shift to using *they* instead of the more unwieldy "he or she." If someone wants to do that, they won't get any flak from me.

In its 30th annual words of the year vote, the ADS chose *"(my) pronouns"* as its Word of the Year (2019) and, as mentioned, *singular "they"* as its Word of the Decade (2010-2019). *"(My) pronouns"* was recognized for its use in sharing one's set of personal pronouns (as in "pronouns: she/her"). *Singular "they"* was recognized for its use to refer to someone whose gender identity is nonbinary. As noted, *singular "they"* had been previously selected by the Society as the Word of the Year for 2015. The selection of *"(my) pronouns"* recognizes how the personal expression of gender identity has become an increasing part of our shared discourse. That trend is also reflected in singular *they* for individuals whose gender identities don't conform to the binary of *he* and *she.*

In addition to regional diversity, the speech of Californians also reflects ethnic contrasts. The most recently available census figures show that Latinxs (Hispanics) outnumber non-Hispanic whites in California (39.3 percent to 36.8 percent). A large and diverse group of Asian Americans constitute 15 percent of the state's population, with African Americans at 6.5 percent. California's Mexican-derived (Chicano) populations have the longest continuous (nonindigenous) linguistic history in the state, having contributed its most important place names, including Los Angeles,

San Francisco, San Diego, and Sacramento. So strong is the Spanish heritage that Spanish-like vowels even influence the way English is spoken by Hispanics who learn English as their first, or native, language. For example, among Chicano speakers in northern California the vowel in the second syllable of *nothing* has come to resemble the Spanish "ee" sound (see Eckert and Mendoza-Denton 2002)

Despite the well-documented diversity in California speech, linguists have detected trends toward uniformity as well, particularly among coastal whites. Since the 1940s, a distinctive "California accent" has been developing, and some of its features were indeed highlighted in Moon Unit Zappa's 1982 recording of "Valley Girl." This accent is most evident in vowels. For example, the vowels in *hock* and *hawk,* or *cot* and *caught,* are pronounced the same, so that *awesome* rhymes with *possum*. Second, the vowel sound in *boot* and *dude* has shifted and now is pronounced as in *cute* or *pure* (thus, *boot* becomes "beaut," and *dude* becomes "dewed," rather than "dood") (see Eckert and Mendoza-Denton 2002). Third, the vowel sound in *but* and *cut* is shifting, so that those words sound more like "bet" and "ket" (see Eckert and Mendoza-Denton 2002).

Such coordinated phonological changes are known as chain shifts. The most extreme versions of these chain-shifted vowel sounds are found in the speech of young white Californians. Young people tend to be leaders in speech innovations, which is why linguists spend a lot of time studying them. California's communities bring together adolescents from varied backgrounds. Their linguistic styles, like their clothing and behavioral styles, influence one another. Hostility may cause people to differentiate and diversify their styles, while curiosity or admiration may cause people to copy, or adopt elements from, other styles.

Variation within a language at any given time is historic change in progress. The same forces that, working gradually, have produced large-scale linguistic change over the centuries are still at work today. Linguistic change occurs not in a vacuum but in society. When new ways of speaking are associated with social factors, they are imitated, and they spread. In this way, a language changes. Sociolinguists focus on features that vary systematically with social position and situation. To study variation, sociolinguists must observe, define, and measure variable use of language in real-world situations (see Tusting 2020) Let's consider some additional examples.

Study these menus from two restaurants, one more upscale than the other. Note the use of names of farms (food origin) in one menu and the use of adjectives such as *delicious, fresh,* and *premium* in the other. Which menu is from the more upscale restaurant?

Both: Mark Dierker/McGraw Hill Education

The Language of Food
In his book *The Language of Food,* linguist Dan Jurafsky (2014) describes some of his studies of sociolinguistic variation as it relates to restaurant food. Jurafsky and his colleagues analyzed the menus of 6,500 contemporary American restaurants. One of

their goals was to see how the food vocabularies of upscale restaurants differed from those of cheaper establishments. One key difference they found was that upscale restaurants were much more likely to include on their menus the sources of the foods they served. They named specific farms, gardens, ranches, pastures, woodlands, and farmers' markets. They were careful to mention, if the season was right, that their tomatoes or peas were heirloom varieties. Very expensive restaurants mentioned the origin of food more than 15 times as often as inexpensive restaurants.

Word length was another differentiator. Menu words averaged half a letter longer in upscale restaurants than in the cheaper establishments. Cheaper eateries, for instance, were more likely to use *decaf,* rather than *decaffeinated,* and *sides* rather than *accompaniments.* Diners had to pay higher prices for those longer words: Every increase of one letter in the average length of words describing a dish meant an average increase of $0.18 in the price of that dish.

Cheaper restaurants were more apt to use linguistic fillers. These included positive but vague words like *delicious, tasty, mouthwatering,* and *flavorful,* or other positive, but impossible to measure, adjectives such as *terrific, wonderful, delightful,* and *sublime.* Each positive vague word for a dish in a modest restaurant reduced its average price by 9 percent. Downscale restaurants also were more likely to assure their diners that their offerings were *fresh.* Expensive restaurants expect their patrons to assume that their offerings are fresh, without having to say it. Next time you eat out, pay attention to these findings about "the language of food" (see also Karrebæk et al. 2018)

Southwestern Spanglish
Linguist Jane Hill also examined restaurant menus as reflective of sociolinguistic differences. How is Spanish used on menus of restaurants serving Mexican-themed food in southern Arizona? Hill examined the online menus of every such restaurant south of the Gila River that had a web presence. In an article titled "A Linguist Walks into a Mexican Restaurant," Hill described and explained the mixtures of Spanish and English she encountered.

She noted that many English-speaking Arizonans pepper their speech with occasional Spanish words like "adiós" and "gracias." They also use mock Spanish expressions like "no problemo," "el cheapo," and "bad hombre." Such Spanishisms help them assert their regional identity. "Knowing a little Spanish" might also make them appear a little bit cosmopolitan (but not too much). Ironically, many of these same people view real Spanish as a threat to "America." Some get angry when they hear Spanish spoken in public, or see signs in Spanish, when "English is our national language."

To accommodate such attitudes, menus in Mexican-themed restaurants perform a delicate balancing act. They use just enough Spanish to make the restaurant seem authentic, but not so much as to threaten their nativist customers. They toss in a few small or familiar Spanish words, as in "Green Corn Tamale y Cheese Enchilada" or "deliciously grande." (All examples come from real menus.) It helps if bigger Spanish words look like English words, as in "Elegante style." "Mucho" is good, because it's just English with an o tacked on. Mock Spanish is okay, too, as in "Burrito Loco," "Macho Burrito," "Gordo Burrito," and the "Smoky Señorita" cocktail. Hill's study shows how restaurant menus manage a treacherous linguistic environment.

Gender Speech Contrasts

Comparing men and women, we find differences in phonology, grammar, and vocabulary as well as in the body stances and movements that accompany speech (Coates 2016; Eckert and McConnell-Ginet 2013; Talbot 2019; Tannen 2017). In public contexts, traditional Japanese women tend to adopt an artificially high voice, for the sake of politeness. In North America and Great Britain, women's speech tends to be more similar to the standard dialect than men's speech. Consider the data in Table 5.2, gathered in Detroit (Wolfram & Fasold 1974). In all four social classes, but particularly in the working class, men were more apt to use double negatives (e.g., "I don't want none"). Women tend to be more careful about "uneducated speech." Men may adopt working-class speech because they associate it with masculinity. Perhaps women pay more attention to the media, where standard dialects are employed.

According to Robin Lakoff (2004, 2017), the use of certain types of words and expressions has been associated with women's traditional lesser power in American society (see also Tannen 1990, 2017). For example, *Oh dear, Oh fudge,* and *Goodness!* are less forceful than *Hell* and *Damn.* Watch the lips of a disgruntled player in a football game. What's the likelihood he's saying "Phooey on you"? Women are more likely than men to use such adjectives as *adorable, charming, sweet, cute, lovely,* and *divine.* A man may be called out for "mansplaining" when he attempts to "enlighten" a woman about a domain in which he assumes he has superior knowledge. Is there any linguistic practice that might be called "womansplaining" (See Caldas-Coulthard, ed. 2020)?

Differences in the linguistic strategies and behavior of men and women are examined in several books by the well-known sociolinguist Deborah Tannen (1990, 2017). Tannen uses the terms *rapport* and *report* to contrast women's and men's overall linguistic styles. Women, says Tannen, typically use language and the body movements that accompany it to build rapport, social connections with others. Men, on the other hand, tend to make reports, reciting information to establish a place for themselves in a hierarchy, as they also attempt to determine the relative ranks of their conversation mates.

Language and Status Position

Honorifics are terms used with people, often by being added to their names, to "honor" them. Such terms may convey or imply a status difference between the speaker and the person being referred to ("the good doctor") or addressed ("Professor Dumbledore"). Although Americans tend to be less formal than other nationalities, American English still has its honorifics. They include such terms as *Mr., Mrs., Ms., Dr., Professor, Dean, Senator, Reverend, Honorable,* and *President.* Often these terms are attached to names, as in "Dr. Wilson," "President Lincoln," and "Senator Murray," but some of them can be used to address someone without using his or her name, such as "Dr.," "Mr. President," "Senator," and "Miss." The British have a more developed set of honorifics, corresponding to status distinctions based on class, nobility (e.g., "Lord and Lady Trumble"), and special recognition (e.g., knighthood—"Sir Elton" or "Dame Judi").

In Japanese, several honorifics convey different degrees of respect. The suffix *-sama* (added to a name), showing great respect, is used to address someone of higher social status, such as a lord or a respected teacher. Women can use it to demonstrate love or respect for their husbands. The most common Japanese honorific, *-san,* attached to the last name, is respectful, but it is less formal than *Mr., Mrs.,* or *Ms.* in American English. Attached to a first name, *-san* denotes more familiarity (*Free Dictionary* 2004; Heinrich and Ohara 2019; Loveday 1986, 2001).

Kin terms, too, can be associated with gradations in age, rank, and status. *Dad* is a more familiar, less formal kin term than *Father,* but it still shows more respect than would using the father's first name. Outranking their children, parents routinely use their kids' first names, nicknames, or baby names, rather than addressing them as *son* and *daughter.* Southerners up to (and sometimes

honorifics
Terms of respect; used to honor people.

TABLE 5.2 Multiple Negation ("I don't want none") According to Gender and Class (in Percentages)

	UPPER MIDDLE CLASS	LOWER MIDDLE CLASS	UPPER WORKING CLASS	LOWER WORKING CLASS
Male	10.4	22.3	68.2	81.3
Female	6.0	2.4	41.2	74.3

long past) a certain age routinely use *ma'am* and *sir* for older or higher-status women and men.

Stratification and Symbolic Domination

We use and evaluate speech in the context of *extralinguistic* forces—social, political, and economic. Many Americans evaluate the speech of lower-status groups negatively, calling it "uneducated." This is not because these ways of speaking are bad in themselves but because they have come to symbolize low status. Consider variation in the pronunciation of *r*. In some parts of the United States, *r* is regularly pronounced, and in other (*r*-less) areas, it is not. Originally, American *r*-less speech was modeled on the fashionable speech of England. Because of its prestige, *r*-lessness was adopted in many areas and continues as the norm around Boston and in the South.

New Yorkers sought prestige by dropping their *r*'s in the 19th century, after having pronounced them in the 18th. However, contemporary New Yorkers are going back to the 18th-century pattern of pronouncing *r*'s. What matters, and what governs linguistic change, is not the reverberation of a strong midwestern *r* but *social* evaluation, whether *r*'s happen to be "in" or "out."

Studies of *r* pronunciation in New York City have clarified the mechanisms of phonological change. William Labov (1972*b*) focused on whether *r* was pronounced after vowels in such words as *car, floor, card,* and *fourth.* To get data on how this linguistic variation correlated with social class, he used a series of rapid encounters with employees in three New York City department stores, each of whose prices and locations attracted a different socioeconomic group. Saks Fifth Avenue (68 encounters) catered to the upper middle class, Macy's (125) attracted middle-class shoppers, and S. Klein's (71) had predominantly lower-middle-class and working-class customers. The class origins of store personnel tended to reflect those of their customers.

Having already determined that a certain department was on the fourth floor, Labov approached ground-floor salespeople and asked where that department was. After the salesperson had answered, "Fourth floor," Labov repeated his "Where?" in order to get a second response. The second reply was more formal and emphatic, the salesperson presumably thinking that Labov hadn't heard or understood the first answer. For each salesperson, therefore, Labov had two samples of /r/ pronunciation in two words.

Labov calculated the percentages of workers who pronounced /r/ at least once during the interview. These were 62 percent at Saks, 51 percent at Macy's, but only 20 percent at S. Klein's. He also found that personnel on upper floors, where he asked "What floor is this?" (and where more expensive items were sold), pronounced /r/ more

TABLE 5.3 Pronunciation of *r* in New York City Department Stores

STORE	NUMBER OF ENCOUNTERS	% *r* PRONUNCIATION
Saks Fifth Avenue	68	62
Macy's	125	51
S. Klein's	71	20

often than ground-floor salespeople did (see also Labov 2006).

In Labov's study, summarized in Table 5.3, /r/ pronunciation was clearly associated with prestige. Certainly the job interviewers who had hired the salespeople never counted *r*'s before offering employment. However, they did use speech evaluations to make judgments about how effective certain people would be in selling particular kinds of merchandise. In other words, they practiced sociolinguistic discrimination, using linguistic features in deciding who got certain jobs.

Many dialects coexist in the United States with Standard American English (SAE), which itself is a dialect that differs, say, from "BBC English," the preferred dialect in Great Britain. According to the principle of *linguistic relativity,* all dialects are equally effective as systems of communication, which is the main job of language. Our tendency to think of particular dialects as cruder or more sophisticated than others is a social rather than a linguistic judgment. We rank certain speech patterns as better or worse because we recognize that they are used by groups that we also rank. People who say *dese, dem,* and *dere* instead of *these, them,* and *there* communicate perfectly well with anyone who recognizes that the *d* sound systematically replaces the *th* sound in their speech. However, this form of speech is stigmatized; it has become an indicator of low social rank. We call it, like the use of *ain't,* "uneducated speech." The use of *dem, dese,* and *dere* is one of many phonological differences that Americans recognize and look down on (see Labov 2012).

Our speech habits help determine how others evaluate us and thus our access to employment and other material resources. Because of this, "proper language" itself becomes a strategic resource—and a path to wealth, prestige, and power (Gal 1989; Mooney and Evans 2019). Illustrating this, many ethnographers have described the importance of verbal skill and oratory in politics (Beeman 1986; Simpson et al 2019; Wodak and Forchtner 2018). Ronald Reagan, known as a "great communicator," dominated American society in the 1980s as a two-term president. Another twice-elected president, Bill Clinton, despite his Arkansas accent, is known for his verbal skills, as is former president Barack Obama. Communications flaws may have helped doom the presidencies of Gerald Ford,

Jimmy Carter, and George Bush (the elder). How do you evaluate the linguistic style and skills of the current leader of your country?

The speech habits of the 45th U.S. president, Donald J. Trump, have attracted the attention of linguistics. George Lakoff and Gil Duran, in a 2018 article, analyze how "Trump Has Turned Words into Weapons. And He's Winning the Linguistic War." In another 2018 article titled "The Unmonitored President," linguist John McWhorter points out that Trump is the first U.S. president who consistently eschews traditional presidential formal speech and instead just gets up and talks.

The French anthropologist Pierre Bourdieu views linguistic practices as *symbolic capital* that people, if trained properly, can convert into economic and social capital. The value of a dialect—its standing in a "linguistic market"—depends on the extent to which it provides access to desired positions in society. In turn, this reflects its legitimation by formal institutions: educational institutions, state, church, and prestige media. Even people who don't use the prestige dialect accept its authority and correctness, its "symbolic domination" (Bourdieu 1982, 1984; Labov 2012). Thus, linguistic forms, which lack power in themselves, take on the power of the groups they symbolize (see Mooney and Evans 2015). The education system, however (defending its own worth), denies linguistic relativity, misrepresenting prestige speech as being inherently better. The linguistic insecurity often felt by lower-class and minority speakers is a result of this symbolic domination.

African American Vernacular English (AAVE)

No one pays much attention when someone says "saction" instead of "section." But some nonstandard speech carries more of a stigma. Sometimes stigmatized speech is linked to region, class, or educational background; sometimes it is associated with ethnicity or "race."

The sociolinguist William Labov (1972a) and several associates, both white and Black, have conducted detailed studies of what they call **African American Vernacular English (AAVE).** (*Vernacular* means ordinary, casual speech.) AAVE is actually a complex linguistic system with its own rules, which linguists have described. Consider some of the phonological and grammatical differences between AAVE and SAE. One phonological difference is that AAVE speakers are less likely to pronounce *r* than SAE speakers are. Actually, many SAE speakers don't pronounce *r*'s that come right before a consonant (ca*r*d) or at the end of a word (ca*r*). But SAE speakers usually do pronounce an *r* that comes right before a vowel, either at the end of a word (fou*r* o'clock) or within a word (Ca*r*ol). AAVE speakers, by contrast, are much more likely to omit such intervocalic (between vowels) *r*'s. The result is that speakers of the two dialects have different *homonyms* (words that sound the same but have different meanings). AAVE speakers who don't pronounce intervocalic *r*'s have the following homonyms: *Carol/Cal; Paris/pass.*

Phonological rules also may lead AAVE speakers to omit *-ed* as a past-tense marker and *-s* as a marker of plurality. However, other speech contexts demonstrate that AAVE speakers do understand the difference between past- and present-tense verbs, and between singular and plural nouns. Confirming this are irregular verbs (e.g., *tell, told*) and irregular plurals (e.g., *child, children*), in which AAVE works the same as SE.

Linguists disagree about exactly how AAVE originated (McWhorter 2017; Rickford 1997, 2019; Rickford and Rickford 2000). Smitherman (1986) notes certain structural similarities between West African languages and AAVE. African linguistic backgrounds no doubt influenced how early African Americans learned English. Did they restructure English to fit African linguistic patterns? Or, possibly, in acquiring English, did enslaved Africans fuse English with African languages to make a pidgin or creole, which influenced the subsequent development of AAVE? Creole speech may have been introduced to the American colonies by the many slaves who were brought in from the Caribbean during the 17th and 18th centuries (Rickford 1997).

African American Vernacular English (AAVE)
The rule-governed dialect spoken by some African Americans.

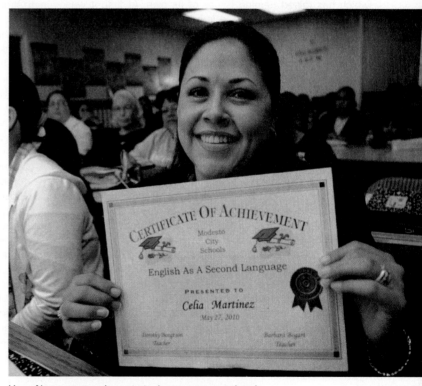

Use of language can be a strategic resource, correlated with wealth, prestige, and power. Shown here is a recent graduate of an ESL (English as a Second Language) class in Modesto, California. How necessary is it for Spanish speakers in the United States to learn English?
ZUMA Press Inc /Alamy Stock Photo

Naming a Pandemic: Do Geographic Names Stigmatize?

Naming is often relative, especially when geography is involved. In Charleston, South Carolina, I can drive down Savannah Highway, but in Savannah, that same road (more impartially, U. S. Highway 17) becomes Charleston Highway. What Americans recall as the Vietnam War is known as the American War in Vietnam. Anthropologist Hugh Gusterson (2020) points out similar relativity, but this time often tinged with prejudice, in disease names. Syphilis was known historically in England as "the French disease." In France, that same STI became "la maladie Anglaise" (the English illness). For the Russians, it was "the Polish disease."

The "Spanish flu" pandemic of 1918–19 did not originate in Spain. It got its name from the Spanish press, which reported more openly and truthfully about its extent and ravages than did media in Britain, France, Germany, and the United States, where that strain of influenza was killing more people. The *Times* of London christened it "the Spanish flu," and the name stuck (Gusterson 2020).

I am writing this during the 2020 coronavirus pandemic, which has raised naming issues of its own. At first, it was merely "coronavirus." As we learned that there are many coronaviruses, including the common cold, more precise naming became necessary. Avoiding its formal classificatory title, SARS-CoV-2, the media settled on COVID-19, short for a coronavirus that emerged in 2019. At a briefing on March 19, 2020, American President Donald Trump was seen to have crossed out "corona" in his prepared remarks and used a sharpie to insert "Chinese" instead. Thereafter, he repeatedly referred to "the Chinese virus," generating controversy (Gusterson 2020).

Was "Chinese virus" a racist or ethnic slur? Or was it merely a geographic name, as Trump contended, citing the fact that the virus first emerged in China. Trump's defenders brought up the "Spanish flu" and other diseases with geographic names—Lyme disease (Lyme, Connecticut), West Nile virus (West Nile district of Uganda), Ebola (the Ebola River in the Democratic Republic of Congo), and Middle East respiratory syndrome (MERS--Saudi Arabia). All those names refer to the place or region where that disease emerged or where it was first identified or discovered.

As Gusterson (2020) points out, however, those disease names refer to places on a map that are not also ethnic classifications. "Ebola" is not known as "the Congolese disease," nor has "Lyme disease" become "the American disease." As Congressman Ted Lieu of California has commented, there is

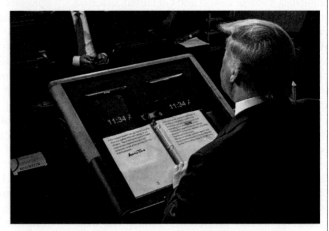

In President Donald Trump's notes for a COVID-19 briefing on March 19, 2020, the word "corona" in the term *coronavirus* was crossed out and replaced with the word "Chinese." On June 20, 2020, at a rally in Tulsa, Oklahoma, Trump would refer to the virus as "Kung Flu."
Jabin Botsford/Getty Images

a difference between saying the virus is from China and saying it is a Chinese virus (cited in Gusterson 2020). The World Health Organization (WHO) advises against geographic disease designations, precisely because they can cause stigmatization of the cities, countries, regions, or continents so named.

What might be better ways to name diseases? If we find names like SARS-CoV-2, or even COVID-19, too cumbersome, what are noncontroversial options? Many diseases or syndromes are named for their discoverers, including Parkinson, Huntington, Tourette, and Crohn. Salmonella gets its name not from the fish but from the veterinarian, Daniel Salmon, who discovered it. John Langdon Down authored the paper (written in the 1860s) that first described what is now known as Down syndrome (Gusterson 2020).

Gusterson (2020) suggests naming COVID-19 for one of the heroes of the pandemic, Yong-Zhen Zhang of the Shanghai Public Health Clinical Center & School of Public Health at Fudan University. On January 10, 2020, Zhang's team published the genome of the newly discovered coronavirus on an open platform. This globally circulated DNA sequence helped researchers develop tests for the virus and serves as a basis for an eventual vaccine.

A final alternative might be to name COVID-19 after the animal(s) from which it spread to humans. In this case, likely culprits are the bat plus some intermediate animals, perhaps the pangolin ("scaly anteater"). If we can name diseases "bird flu," "swine flu," and "mad cow disease," perhaps we should consider naming this one after the bat, a truly global mammal that has no respect for national boundaries.

SAE is not superior to AAVE as a linguistic system, but it does happen to be the prestige dialect—the one used in the mass media, in writing, and in most public and professional contexts.

SAE is the dialect that has the most "symbolic capital." In areas of Germany where there is diglossia, speakers of Plattdeusch (Low German) learn the High German dialect (originally spoken in the highlands of southern Germany) to communicate appropriately in the national context. High German is the standard literary and spoken form of German. Similarly, upwardly mobile AAVE-speaking students learn SAE.

HISTORICAL LINGUISTICS

Sociolinguists study contemporary variation in speech—language change in progress. **Historical linguistics** deals with longer-term change (see Burridge and Bergs 2017; Hock 2019). Language changes over time. It evolves—varies, spreads, divides into dialects and eventually into **subgroups** (languages within a taxonomy of related languages that are most closely related). Historical linguists can reconstruct many features of past languages by studying contemporary **daughter languages.** These are languages that descend

from the same parent language and that have been changing for hundreds or even thousands of years. We call the original language from which they diverge the **protolanguage.** Romance languages such as French and Spanish, for example, are daughter languages of Latin, their common protolanguage. German, English, Dutch, and the Scandinavian languages are daughter languages of proto-Germanic. Latin and proto-Germanic were both Indo-European (IE) languages (see Figure 5.2). Proto-Indo-European (PIE), spoken in the more distant past, was the common protolanguage of Latin, proto-Germanic, and many other ancient languages (see Kapovic 2017).

According to one theory, PIE was introduced by chariot-driving pastoralists who spread out from the Eurasian steppes above the Black Sea about 4,000 years ago and conquered Europe and Asia (see Wade 2012). The main line of evidence for this view is linguistic: PIE had a

historical linguistics
The study of languages over time.

subgroups
(Linguistic) closely related languages.

daughter languages
Languages sharing a common parent language, e.g., Latin.

protolanguage
A language ancestral to several daughter languages.

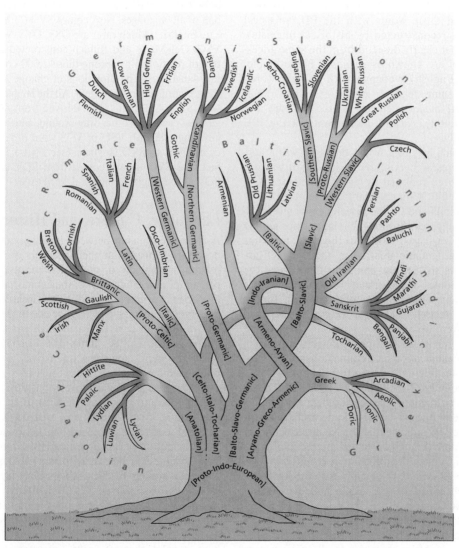

FIGURE 5.2 PIE Family Tree.

This is a family tree of the Indo-European languages. All can be traced back to a protolanguage, Proto-Indo-European (PIE). PIE split into dialects that eventually evolved into separate daughter languages, which, in turn, evolved into granddaughter languages such as Latin and proto-Germanic, which are ancestral to dozens of modern languages.

vocabulary for chariots and wagons that included words for "wheel," "axle," "harness-pole," and "to go or convey in a vehicle." These PIE words (as reconstructed by historical linguists) have recognizable descendant words in many IE languages. This suggests that wheeled vehicles must have been invented before PIE started diverging (Wade 2012). The earliest such vehicles date to 3500 B.C.E.

The main rival theory, first proposed by archaeologist Colin Renfrew (1987), is that PIE was spoken and spread by peaceful farmers who lived in Anatolia, now Turkey, about 9,000 years ago. More recent studies by the evolutionary biologist Quentin Atkinson and his colleagues in New Zealand support the Anatolian origin of PIE (see Bouckaert et al. 2012). Atkinson's team focused on a set of vocabulary items known to be resistant to linguistic change. These include pronouns, parts of the body, and family relations. For 103 IE languages, the researchers compared those words with the PIE ancestral word (as reconstructed by historical linguists). Words that clearly descend from the same ancestral word are known as *cognates*. For example, *mother* (English) is cognate with all these words for the same relative: *mutter* (German), *mat* (Russian), *madar* (Persian), *matka* (Polish), and *mater* (Latin). All are descendants of the PIE word *mehter*.

For each language, when the word was a cognate the researchers scored it 1; when it was not (having been replaced by an unrelated word), it was scored 0. With each language represented by a string of 1s and 0s, the researchers could establish a family tree showing the relationships among the 103 languages. Based on those relationships and the geographic areas where the daughter languages are spoken, the computer determined the likeliest routes of movement from an origin. The calculation pointed to Anatolia, southern Turkey. This is precisely the region originally proposed by Renfrew, because it was the area from which farming spread to Europe. Atkinson also ran a computer simulation on a grammar-based IE tree—once again finding Anatolia to be the most likely origin point for PIE (Wade 2012). Although many linguists still support the chariot/steppe origin theory, several lines of biological and archaeological evidence now indicate that the Neolithic economy spread more through the actual migration of farmers than through the diffusion of crops and ideas. This would seem to offer support to the Renfrew–Atkinson model of PIE origin and dispersal of Neolithic farmers.

Historically oriented linguists suspect that a very remote protolanguage, spoken perhaps 50,000 years ago in Africa, gave rise to all contemporary languages. Murray Gell-Mann and Merritt Ruhlen (2011), who co-direct the Program on the Evolution of Human Languages at the Sante Fe Institute, have reconstructed the syntax (word ordering) of

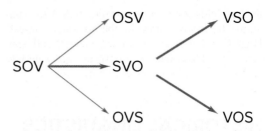

FIGURE 5.3 Evolution of Word Order from Original SOV (Subject, Object, Verb) in Ancient Ancestral Protolanguage.

this ancient protolanguage (see http://ehl.santafe.edu/intro1.htm). Their study focused on how subject (S), object (O), and verb (V) are arranged in phrases and sentences in some 2,000 contemporary languages. There are six possible word orders: SOV, SVO, OSV, OVS, VSO, and VOS. Most common is SOV ("I you like," e.g., Latin), present in more than half of all languages. Next comes SVO ("I like you," e.g., English). Much rarer are OSV, OVS, VOS, and VSO. Gell-Mann and Ruhlen constructed a family tree of relationships among those 2,000 contemporary languages. The directions of change involving the six word orders were clear. All the languages that were SVO, OVS, and OSV derived from SOV languages—never the other way around. Furthermore, any language with VSO or VOS word order always came from an SVO language (see Figure 5.3). The fact that SVO always comes from SOV confirms SOV as the original, ancestral word order.

Language, Culture, and History

A close relationship between languages does not necessarily mean that their speakers are closely related biologically or culturally, because people can adopt new languages. In the equatorial forests of Africa, "pygmy" hunters have discarded their ancestral languages and now speak those of the cultivators who have migrated to the area. Immigrants to the United States and Canada spoke many different languages on arrival, but their descendants now speak fluent English.

Knowledge of linguistic relationships is often valuable to anthropologists interested in history, particularly events during the past 5,000 years. Cultural features may (or may not) correlate with the distribution of language families. Groups that speak related languages may (or may not) be more culturally similar to each other than they are to groups whose speech derives from different linguistic ancestors. Of course, cultural similarities aren't limited to speakers of related languages. Even groups whose members speak unrelated languages have contact through trade, intermarriage, and warfare. Ideas and inventions diffuse widely among human groups. Many items of vocabulary in contemporary English come from French. Even without written documentation of France's influence after the Norman Conquest of England in 1066, linguistic evidence in contemporary English would reveal a long period of important firsthand contact with France. Similar linguistic evidence may confirm cultural contact and borrowing when written history is lacking. By considering which words have been borrowed, we also can make inferences about the nature of the contact.

Language Loss

One aspect of linguistic history is language loss. When languages disappear, cultural diversity is reduced as well. According to linguist K. David Harrison, "When we lose a language, we lose centuries of thinking about time, seasons, sea creatures, reindeer, edible flowers, mathematics, landscapes, myths, music, the unknown and the everyday" (quoted in Maugh 2007). Harrison's book *When Languages Die* (2007) notes that the world's linguistic diversity has been cut in half (measured by number of distinct languages) in the past 500 years, and half of the remaining languages are predicted to disappear during this century. Colonial languages (e.g., English, Spanish, Portuguese, French, Dutch, Russian) have expanded at the expense of indigenous ones. Of approximately 7,000 remaining languages, about 20 percent are endangered, compared with 18 percent of mammals, 8 percent of plants, and 5 percent of birds (Bradley and Bradley 2019; Harrison 2010; Maugh 2007).

The Endangered Languages Project (http://www.endangeredlanguages.com/) offers links to research and publications concerning the world's endangered languages, as well as a global map of those languages. The rate of endangerment is highest in northern Australia and adjacent New Guinea, where over 150 indigenous languages are endangered. However, if you consult that map, you

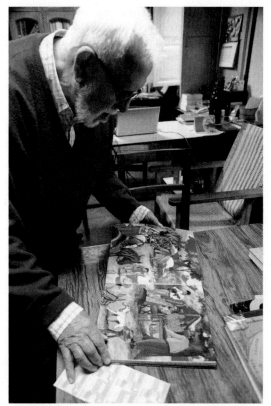

One way of preserving indigenous languages is through translation. In this photo, the Spanish anthropologist Bartomeu Melia displays his translation into Guarani (Paraguay's principal indigenous language) of Cervantes' *Don Quixote*. This translation is intended to reach young people in rural areas of Paraguay.
Noberto Duarte/AFP/Getty Images

will see that the endangerment threat is global in scope, as indigenous tongues have yielded, either voluntarily or through coercion, to a colonial language (see Harrison 2010).

for REVIEW

1. Wild primates use call systems to communicate. Environmental stimuli trigger calls, which cannot be combined when multiple stimuli are present. Contrasts between language and call systems include displacement, productivity, and cultural transmission. Over time, our ancestral call systems grew too complex for genetic transmission, and hominid communication began to rely on learning. Humans still use nonverbal communication, such as facial expressions, gestures, and body stances and movements. But language is the main system humans use to communicate. Chimps and gorillas can understand and manipulate nonverbal symbols based on language.

2. Phonology—the study of speech sounds—focuses on sound contrasts (phonemes) that distinguish meaning. Morphology studies how sounds combine to form morphemes—words and their meaningful parts. A language's lexicon is a dictionary containing all its morphemes and their meanings. Syntax refers to the arrangement and order of words in phrases and sentences. The grammar and lexicon of a language can influence how its speakers perceive and think about the world.

summary

Specialized sets of terms and distinctions that are particularly important to certain groups are known as focal vocabulary. Studies of ethnosemantic domains such as kinship, color terminologies, and pronouns show that speakers of different languages categorize their experiences differently.

3. Linguistic anthropologists share anthropology's general interest in diversity in time and space. Sociolinguistics investigates relationships between social and linguistic variation by focusing on the actual use of language. Only when features of speech acquire social meaning are they imitated. If they are valued, they will spread. People vary their speech, shifting styles, dialects, and languages. As linguistic systems, all languages and dialects are equally complex, rule-governed, and effective for communication. However, speech is used, is evaluated, and changes in the context of political, economic, and social forces. Often the linguistic traits of a low-status group are negatively evaluated. This devaluation is not because of *linguistic* features per se. Rather, it reflects the association of such features with low *social* status. One dialect, supported by the dominant institutions of the state, exercises symbolic domination over the others.

4. Historical linguistics is useful for anthropologists interested in historical relationships among populations. Cultural similarities and differences often correlate with linguistic ones. Linguistic clues can suggest past contacts between cultures. Related languages—members of the same language family—descend from an original protolanguage. Relationships between languages don't necessarily mean that there are biological ties between their speakers, because people can learn new languages.

5. One aspect of linguistic history is language loss. The world's linguistic diversity has been cut in half in the past 500 years, and half of the remaining 7,000 languages are predicted to disappear during this century.

key terms

African American Vernacular English (AAVE) 95

call systems 82

cultural transmission 83

daughter languages 97

diglossia 89

displacement 83

ethnosemantics 88

focal vocabulary 87

historical linguistics 97

honorifics 93

kinesics 85

language 81

lexicon 85

morphology 85

phoneme 85

phonemics 86

phonetics 86

phonology 85

productivity 83

protolanguage 97

Sapir-Whorf hypothesis 87

semantics 88

sociolinguistics 88

style shifts 89

subgroups 97

syntax 85

think like an anthropologist

1. What dialects and languages do you speak? Do you tend to use different dialects, languages, or speech styles in different contexts? Why or why not?

2. Culture always plays a role in shaping what we understand as "natural." What does this mean? Provide three examples of the relevance of this fact in the context of human language and communication.

3. Consider how changing technologies are altering the ways you communicate with family, friends, and even strangers. Suppose your best friend decides to study sociolinguistics in graduate school. What ideas about the relationship among changing technologies, language, and social relations could you suggest to him or her as worth studying?

4. List some stereotypes about how different people speak. Are those real differences, or just stereotypes? Are the stereotypes positive or negative? Why do you think those stereotypes exist?

5. What is language loss? Why are some researchers and communities worldwide so concerned by this growing phenomenon?

credits

Design Elements: Understanding Ourselves: muha/123RF (rock paintings); Focus on Globalization: janrysavy/Getty Images (globe); Appreciating Diversity (left to right): Floresco Productions/age footstock; Hero/Corbis/Glow Images, Hill Street Studios/Blend Images, Billion Photos/Shutterstock; Understanding Ourselves : Hemera Technologies/Alamy (Cymbal), LACMA - Los Angeles County Museum of Art (Trefoil Oinochoe), Ingram Publishing/SuperStock (Coin), ChuckSchugPhotography/Getty Images (Rug).

CHAPTER 6

Ethnicity and Race

▸ What is social status, and how does it relate to ethnicity?

▸ How are race and ethnicity socially constructed in various societies?

▸ What are the positive and negative aspects of ethnicity?

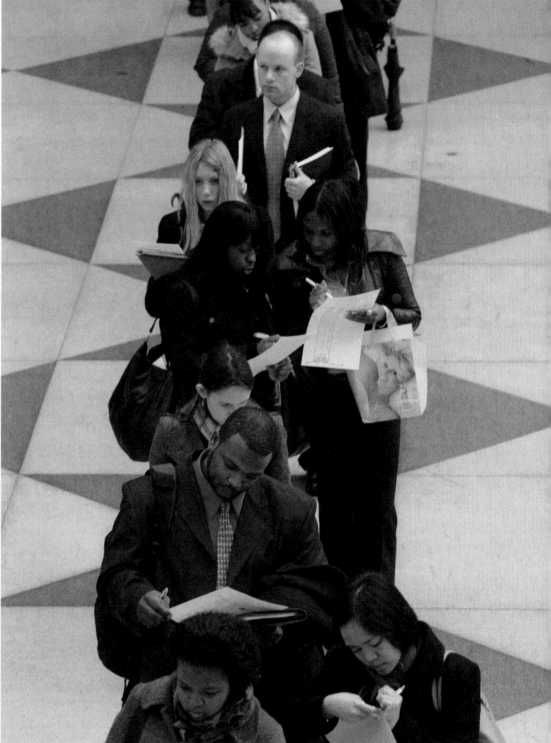

Don Emmert/Getty Images

Hundreds of job seekers line up at the City University of New York's Big Apple Job Fair on March 20, 2009. Around 6,000 students and alumni showed up to apply for jobs offered by 100 or so potential employers. Note the diversity in the crowd.

understanding **OURSELVES**

When asked "Who are you?" what first comes to mind? Think of the last person you met, or the person sitting nearest you. What labels pop into your head to describe that person? What kinds of identity cues and clues do people use to figure out the kinds of people they are dealing with, and how to act in various social situations? Part of human adaptive flexibility is our ability to shift self-presentation in response to context. Italians, for example, maintain separate sets of clothing to be worn inside and outside the home. They invest much more in their outside wardrobe (thus supporting a vibrant Italian fashion industry)—and what it says about their public persona—than in indoor garb, which is for family and intimates to see. Identities and behavior change with context: "I may be a Neandertal at the office, but I'm all *Homo sapiens* at home." Many of the social statuses we occupy, the "hats" we wear, depend on the situation. A person can be both Black and Hispanic, or both a father and a ballplayer. One identity is claimed or perceived in certain settings, another in different ones. Among African Americans a "Hispanic" baseball player might be Black; among Hispanics, Hispanic.

When our claimed or perceived identity varies depending on the context, this is called the *situational negotiation of social identity*. Depending on the situation, the same woman might declare: "I'm Jimmy's mother." "I'm your boss." "I'm an African-American woman." "I'm your professor." In face-to-face encounters, other people see who we are—actually, who they perceive us to be. They may expect us to think and act in certain (stereotypical) ways based on their perception of our identity (e.g., Latina woman, older white male golfer). Although we can't know which aspect of identity they'll focus on (e.g., ethnicity, gender, age, or political affiliation), face to face it's hard to be anonymous or to be someone else entirely. That's what masks, costumes, disguises, and hiding are for. Who's that little man behind the curtain?

Unlike our early ancestors, people today don't just interact face to face. We routinely give our money and our trust to individuals and institutions we've never laid eyes on. We phone, text, write, and—more than ever—use the Internet, where we must choose which aspects of ourselves to reveal. The Internet allows myriad forms of cybersocial interaction, and people can create new personas by using different "handles," including fictitious names and identities. In anonymous regions of cyberspace, people can manipulate ("lie about") their ages, genders, and physical attributes and create their own cyberfantasies. In psychology, multiple personalities are abnormal, but for anthropologists, multiple identities are more and more the norm.

ETHNIC GROUPS AND ETHNICITY

Ethnicity is based on cultural similarities (with members of the same ethnic group) and differences (between that group and others). Ethnic groups must deal with other such groups in the nation or region they inhabit. Interethnic relations are important in the study of any nation or region—especially so because of the ongoing transnational movement of migrants and refugees (see Marger 2015; Parrillo 2016, 2019).

Members of an **ethnic group** share certain beliefs, values, habits, customs, and norms because of their common background. They define themselves as different and special because of cultural features.

This distinction may arise from language, religion, historical experience, geographic placement, kinship, or "race" (see Spickard 2013; Tamai et al. 2019; Warne 2015). Markers of an ethnic group may include a collective name, belief in common descent, a sense of solidarity (belonging together), and an association with a specific territory, which the group may or may not hold (Ryan 1990, pp. xiii, xiv).

Ethnicity means identification with, and feeling part of, an ethnic group and exclusion from certain other groups because of this affiliation. Issues of ethnicity can be complex. Ethnic feelings and associated behavior vary in intensity within ethnic groups and countries and over time. A change in the degree of importance attached to an ethnic identity may reflect political changes (Soviet rule ends—ethnic feeling rises) or individual life-cycle changes (old people relinquish, or young people reclaim, an ethnic background).

Status and Identity

Ethnicity is only one basis for group identity. Cultural differences also are associated with class, region, religion, and other social variables (see Warne 2015). Individuals often have more than one group identity. In a complex society such as the United States or Canada, people negotiate their social identities continually. All of us "wear different hats," presenting ourselves sometimes as one thing, sometimes as another.

These different social identities are known as statuses. In daily conversation, we hear the term *status* used as a synonym for *prestige*. In this context, "She's got a lot of status" means she's got a lot of prestige; people look up to her. Among social scientists, that's not the primary meaning of *status*. Social scientists use **status** more neutrally—for any position, no matter what its prestige, that someone occupies in society. Parent is a social status. So are professor, student, factory worker, Republican, salesperson, homeless person, labor leader, ethnic-group member, and thousands of others. People always occupy multiple statuses (e.g., Hispanic, Catholic, preteen, brother). Among the statuses we occupy, particular ones dominate in particular settings, such as son or daughter at home and student in the classroom.

Some statuses are **ascribed:** People have limited choice about occupying them. Age is an ascribed status. We can't choose not to age, although many people, especially wealthy ones, use cultural means, such as plastic surgery, to try to disguise the biological aging process. Race and gender usually are ascribed; most people are born members of a given race or gender and remain so all their lives. **Achieved statuses,** by contrast, aren't automatic; they come through choices, actions, efforts, talents, or accomplishments and may be positive or negative. Examples of achieved statuses include physician, senator, convicted felon, salesperson, union member, father, and college student.

From the media, you will be familiar with cases in which gender and race have become achieved rather than ascribed statuses. Transgender individuals, including the widely reported media figure Caitlyn Jenner, modify the gender status they were assigned at birth or during childhood. People who were born members of one race have chosen to adopt another. In some cases, individuals who were born African American have passed as white, Hispanic, or Native American. In a case widely reported in 2015, a woman known as Rachel Dolezal, who was born white, changed her racial identity to Black or African American as an adult. In doing this, she modified her physical characteristics by changing her hairstyle to better fit her new identity. Given what culture can do to biology, few statuses are absolutely ascribed.

ethnic group
One among several culturally distinct groups in a society or region.

ethnicity
Identification with, and feeling part of, an ethnic group and exclusion from certain other groups because of this affiliation

ascribed status
Social status based on limited choice.

achieved status
Social status based on choices or accomplishments.

status
Any position, no matter what its prestige, that someone occupies in society.

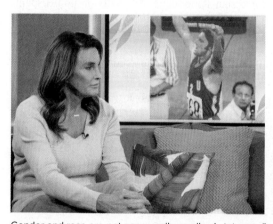
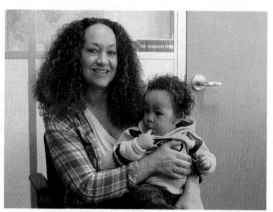

Gender and race are not necessarily ascribed statuses: (Left) Caitlyn Jenner (born Bruce, whose image also is shown in this photo) is interviewed on the "This Morning" TV show in London in May 2017. (Right) Rachel Dolezal poses for a 2017 photo with her son in Spokane, Washington. Dolezal, who was born white, rose to prominence as a Black civil rights leader and has legally changed her name to Nkechi Amare Diallo.

(left): Ken McKay/ITV/Shutterstock; (right): Nicholas K. Geranios/AP Images

American Ethnic Groups

Often status is contextual: One identity is used in certain settings, another in different ones. We call this the *situational negotiation of social identity* (Spickard 2013; Warne 2015). Members of an ethnic group may shift their ethnic identities. Hispanics, for example, may use different ethnic labels (e.g., *Cuban* or *Latino*) to describe themselves depending on context. In one study, about half (51 percent) of American Hispanics surveyed preferred to identify using their family's country of origin (as in *Mexican, Cuban,* or *Dominican*) rather than *Hispanic* or *Latino*. Just one-quarter (24 percent) chose one of those two pan-ethnic terms, while 21 percent said they use the term *American* most often (Taylor et al. 2012). (Because, in Spanish and Portuguese, *Latino* is a term that refers to males, and *Latina* to females, the term *Latinx* [plural *Latinxs*] has come into favor to designate someone of this ethnicity without regard to gender.)

Latinxs with different national roots may mobilize around issues of general interest to Hispanics, such as a path to citizenship for undocumented immigrants, while acting as separate interest groups in other contexts. Among Hispanics, Cuban Americans are older and richer on average than Mexican Americans and Puerto Ricans, and their class interests and voting patterns differ. Cuban Americans are more likely to vote Republican than are Puerto Ricans and Mexican Americans. Some Mexican Americans whose families have lived in the United States for generations have little in common with new Hispanic immigrants, such as those from Central America. (Table 6.1 lists American ethnic groups, based on 2019 figures.)

The Hispanic share of the U.S. population grew rapidly, by 71 percent, between 2000 and 2019, from 35.2 million to 60.1 million people. However, the annual Asian growth rate (about 3 percent) now exceeds that of Hispanics (about 2 percent). The Hispanic growth rate has slowed because immigration to the United States from Mexico has leveled off and the fertility rate among Hispanic women has declined (see Krogstad 2017). *Hispanic* is a category based mainly on language.

It includes whites, Blacks, and "racially" mixed Spanish speakers and their ethnically conscious descendants. (There also are Native American and even Asian Hispanics.) The label *Hispanic* lumps together people of diverse geographic origin—Mexico, Puerto Rico, El Salvador, Cuba, the Dominican Republic, Guatemala, and other Spanish-speaking countries of Central and South America and the Caribbean. *Latino* is a broader category, which also can include Brazilians (who speak Portuguese). Mexicans constitute about two-thirds of American Hispanics. Next come Puerto Ricans at around 9 percent. Salvadorans, Cubans, Dominicans, and Guatemalans living in the United States all number more than one million people per nationality.

Of the major racial and ethnic groups in the United States, Hispanics are by far the youngest. Non-Hispanic whites are the oldest of any racial or ethnic group, with a median age of 44, versus 31 years old for all minorities, 30 for Latinx, and 38 for the U.S. population overall (Schaeffer 2019, https://www.pewresearch.org/fact-tank/2019/07/30/most-common-age-among-us-racial-ethnic-groups/).

Minority Groups and Stratification

Minority groups are so called because, as a group, they occupy subordinate (lower) positions within a social hierarchy. Minority groups have less power and wealth than *majority groups* do. Minority groups are obvious features of stratification in the United States. The 2018 poverty rate was 8.1 percent for non-Hispanic whites, 10.1 percent for Asian Americans, 17.6 percent for Hispanics, and 20.8 percent for African Americans (Semega et al. 2019). Inequality shows up consistently in unemployment figures as well as in income and wealth. Median household incomes in 2018 were as follows: $87,194 for Asian Americans, $70,642 for non-Hispanic whites, $51,450 for Hispanics, and $41,361 for African Americans (Semega et al. 2019). As of 2016, the median African American family owned just 2 percent, and the median Hispanic family

TABLE 6.1   Racial/Ethnic Identification in the United States, 2019

CLAIMED IDENTITY	NUMBER (MILLIONS)	PERCENTAGE
White (non-Hispanic)	198.2	60.4%
Hispanic	60.1	18.3%
Black	44.0	13.4%
Asian	19.4	5.9%
Other	6.5	2.0%
Total population	328.2	100.0%

SOURCE: Quick Facts, United States Census, Population estimates July 1, 2019 (V2019). https://www.census.gov/quickfacts/fact/table/US/PST045219.

GROUP	POVERTY RATE	MEDIAN HOUSEHOLD INCOME
Non-Hispanic whites	8.1%	$70,642
Asian Americans	10.1%	$87,194
Hispanic Americans	17.6%	$51,450
African Americans	20.8%	$41,361
Overall	11.8%	$63,179

SOURCE: U.S. Census Bureau. *Income and Poverty in the United States: 2018,* September, 2019. https://www.census.gov/content/dam/Census/library/publications/2019/demo/p60-266.pdf

just 4 percent, of the wealth of the median non-Hispanic white family (see https://inequality.org/facts/wealth-inequality/#racial-wealth-divide).

(Some of these measures of stratification are summarized in Recap 6.1.)

HUMAN BIOLOGICAL DIVERSITY AND THE RACE CONCEPT

The photos in this book illustrate just a fraction of the world's human biological diversity. Additional illustration comes from your own experience. Look around you in your classroom, at the mall, or at a large public event. Inevitably, you'll see people whose ancestors lived in many lands. The first (Native) Americans had to cross a land bridge that once linked Siberia to North America. For later immigrants, perhaps including your own parents or grandparents, the voyage may have been across the sea, or overland from nations to the south. They came for many reasons; some came voluntarily, while others were brought in chains. The scale of migration in today's world is so vast that millions of people routinely cross national borders or live far from the homelands of their grandparents. Now meeting every day are diverse human beings whose biological features reflect adaptation to a wide range of environments other than the ones they now inhabit. Physical contrasts are evident to anyone. Anthropology's job is to explain them.

Historically, scientists have approached the study of human biological variation in two main ways: (1) racial classification (now largely abandoned) versus (2) the current explanatory approach, which focuses on understanding specific biological differences. The study of human biological variation is a key part of anthropology, but this variation is not packaged in discrete units called races (see Marks 2016). First, we'll consider problems with **racial classification** (the attempt to assign humans to discrete categories—races—based on common ancestry), to understand why it's been abandoned. Then we'll offer some explanations for specific aspects of human biological diversity.

Biological differences are real, important, and apparent to us all. Modern scientists find it most productive to seek explanations for this diversity, rather than trying to pigeonhole people into categories called races (see Tattersall and DeSalle 2018).

What is race anyway? In theory, a biological race would be a geographically isolated subdivision of a species. Such a *subspecies* would be capable of interbreeding with other subspecies of the same species, but it would not actually do so because of its geographic isolation. Some biologists also use *race* to refer to "breeds," as of dogs or roses. Thus, a pit bull and a Chihuahua would be different races of dogs. Such domesticated "races" have been bred by humans for generations. Humanity (*Homo sapiens*) lacks such races because human populations have not been isolated enough from one another to develop into such discrete groups. Nor have humans experienced controlled breeding like that which has created the various kinds of dogs and roses.

When an ethnic group is assumed to have a biological basis (distinctively shared "blood" or genes), it is called a **race** (see Mukhopadhyay et al. 2014; Wade 2015). Discrimination against such a group is called **racism**. Traditional racial classification has been guided by two erroneous assumptions: (1) that humans belong to distinct races and (2) that each race has a biological basis (shared "blood" or genes). Today, most anthropologists agree that race is unreal as a set of biological facts, but it is very real as a set of social, political, and experiential facts (Benedict 2019; Marks 2016). As anthropologist Angela Jenks (2016) puts it: "race is not a helpful way of understanding human biological variation, but . . . as a cultural system, it has powerful effects on our lives." Race is a *cultural* category rather than a biological reality. That is, "races" are based on contrasts perceived and perpetuated in particular societies, rather than on scientific classifications based on common genes (see Fairbanks 2015). Racial distinctions and racial discrimination vary from one society to another (see Desmond 2020; Lentin 2020; Prasad 2016).

Racism is discrimination against a group perceived to have a biological basis. Racism has not

race
An ethnic group assumed to have a biological basis.

racism
Discrimination against an ethnic group assumed to have a biological basis.

racial classification
Assigning humans to categories (purportedly) based on common ancestry.

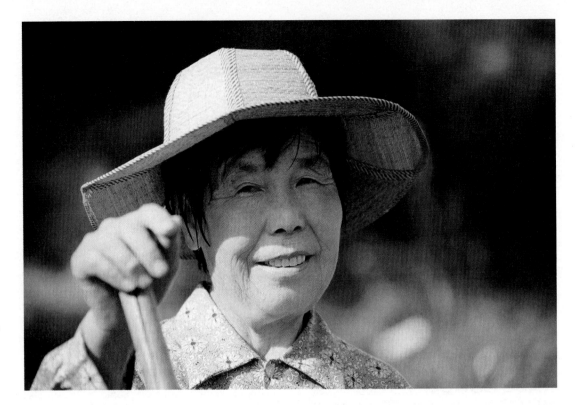

The photos in this chapter illustrate only a small part of the range of human biological diversity. This woman wearing a sun hat is from Emerald Valley, Huangshan, Anhui Province, China.

Rodrigo A Torres/Glow Images

always existed, nor is it intrinsic to humanity. Consider studies by the classics scholar Frank Snowden, Jr., of intergroup relations in the ancient world. Snowden (1970, 1995) draws on classical studies and ancient art to show that Europeans and Africans coexisted in the ancient world and that social relations and business transactions occurred free of discrimination based on skin color. Most Roman slaves were foreigners, and slavery was not based on race. The Romans enslaved prisoners of war and other people captured or bought outside Roman territory. Needy Roman citizens sometimes sold their own children into slavery. Slaves looked so similar to Roman citizens that the Senate once considered making them wear special clothing so that they could be easily identified. Although there were African slaves in the Roman Empire, other Africans were free and worked in varied professions, for example, as writers, philosophers, generals, and Roman officials.

A race is supposed to reflect shared genetic material (inherited from a common ancestor), but early scholars instead used phenotypical traits (such as skin color and facial features) for racial classification. **Phenotype** refers to an organism's evident traits, its "manifest biology"—anatomy and physiology. Humans display hundreds of evident (detectable) physical traits. They range from skin color, hair form, eye color, and facial features (which are visible) to blood groups, color blindness, and enzyme production (which become evident through testing).

Racial classification based on phenotype raises the problem of deciding which trait(s) should be primary. Should races be defined by height,

phenotype
The expressed or evident biological characteristics of an organism.

weight, body shape, facial features, teeth, skull form, or skin color? Like their fellow citizens, early European and American scientists gave priority to skin color. Many schoolbooks and encyclopedias still proclaim the existence of three great races: the white, the black, and the yellow. This overly simplistic classification was compatible with the political use of race during the colonial period of the late 19th and early 20th centuries (see Gravlee 2009). Such a tripartite scheme kept white Europeans neatly separate from their African and Asian subjects. Colonial empires began to break up, and scientists began to question established racial categories, after World War II (see Tattersall and DeSalle 2018).

Races Are Not Biologically Distinct

History and politics aside, one obvious problem with classifying people by skin color is that the terms *white, black,* and *yellow* do not accurately describe human skin colors. So-called "white" people are more pink, beige, or tan than white. "Black" people are various shades of brown, and "yellow" people are tan or beige. It does not make the tripartite division of human races any more accurate when we use the more scientific-*sounding* synonyms—*Caucasoid, Negroid,* and *Mongoloid*—rather than *white, black,* and *yellow.*

Another problem with classifying people by skin color is that many populations do not fit neatly into any one of the three "great races." For example, where would one put the Polynesians? *Polynesia* is a triangle of South Pacific islands formed by Hawaii to the north, Easter

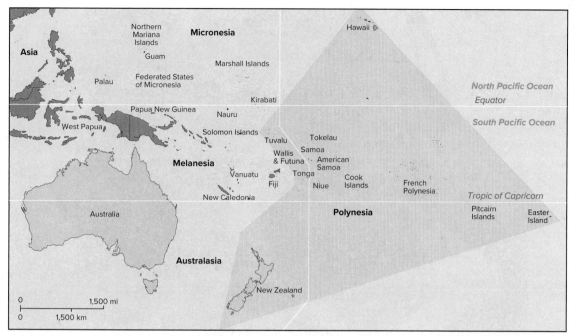

FIGURE 6.1 The Polynesian Triangle (right) in relation to other Pacific Islands and Australia.

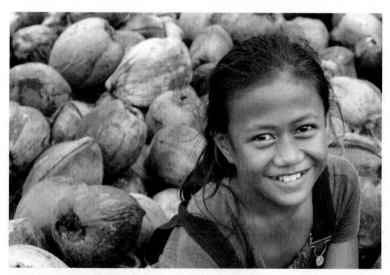

This girl is a coconut vendor in Apia, Samoa, Polynesia.

Thomas Cockrem/Alamy Stock Photo

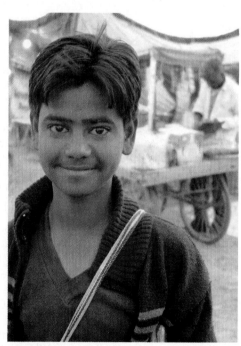

A boy at the Pushkar livestock fair, Rajasthan, India.

Conrad P. Kottak

Island to the east, and New Zealand to the southwest (see Figure 6.1). Does the "bronze" skin color of Polynesians connect them to the Caucasoids or to the Mongoloids? Some scientists, recognizing this problem, enlarged the original tripartite scheme to include the Polynesian race. Native Americans presented a similar problem. Were they red or yellow? Some scientists added a fifth race—the "red," or Amerindian—to the major racial groups.

Many people in southern India have dark skins, but scientists have been reluctant to classify them with "black" Africans because of their Caucasoid facial features and hair form. Some, therefore, have created a separate race for these people. What about the Australian Aborigines, hunters and gatherers indigenous to what has been, throughout human history, the most isolated continent? By skin color, one might place some indigenous Australians in the same race as tropical Africans. However, similarities to Europeans in hair color (light or reddish) and facial features have led some scientists to classify them as Caucasoids. But there is no evidence that Australians are closer genetically to either of these groups than they are to Asians. Recognizing this problem, scientists often regard indigenous Australians as a separate race.

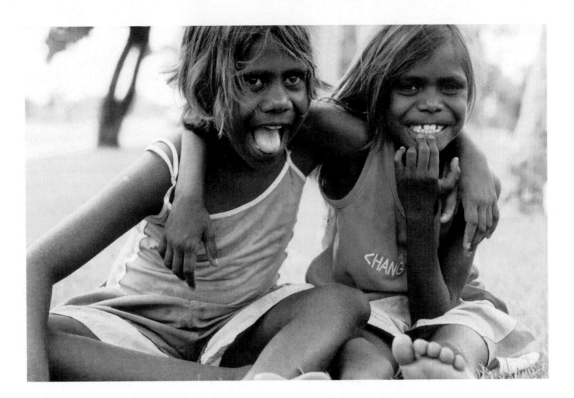

Indigenous Australian children from Australia's Northern Territory.

agefotostock/Alamy Stock Photo

Finally, consider the *San* ("Bushmen") of the Kalahari Desert in southern Africa. Scientists have perceived their skin color as varying from brown to yellow. Some who regard San skin as "yellow" have placed them in the same category as Asians. In theory, people of the same race share more recent common ancestry with each other than they do with anyone else. There is, however, no evidence for recent common ancestry between San and Asians. Somewhat more reasonably, some scholars assign the San to the Capoid race (from the Cape of Good Hope), which is seen as being different from other groups inhabiting tropical Africa.

Similar problems arise in using any phenotypical trait for racial classification. An attempt to use facial features, height, hair type, or any other phenotypical trait is fraught with difficulties. For example, consider the *Nilotes,* who live in the upper Nile region of Uganda and South Sudan. Nilotes tend to be tall and to have long, narrow noses. Certain Scandinavians also are tall, with similar noses. Given the distance between their homelands, however, there is no reason to assume that Nilotes and Scandinavians are more closely related to each other than either is to shorter and nearer populations with different kinds of noses.

Would racial classifications be better if we based them on a combination of physical traits rather than a single trait such as skin color, height, or nose form? To do so would avoid some of the problems raised using a single trait, but other problems would arise. The main problem is that physical features do not go together in a coherent and consistent bundle. Some tall people have dark skin; others are lighter. Some short people have

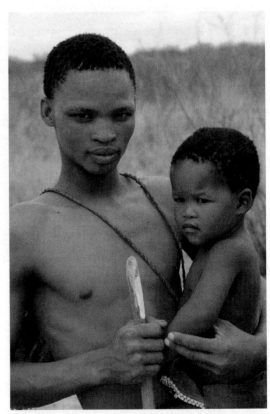

A Naro San ("Bushman") father and son, Central Kalahari, Botswana.

Ariadne Van Zandbergen/Alamy Stock Photo

curly hair; others have straight hair. Imagine the various possible combinations of skin color, stature, and skull form. Add to that facial features such as nose form, eye shape, and lip thickness.

People with dark skin may be tall or short and have hair ranging from straight to very curly. Dark-haired populations may have light or dark skin, along with various skull forms, facial features, and body sizes and shapes. The number of combinations is very large, and the amount that heredity (versus environment) contributes to such phenotypical traits is often unclear (see also Anemone 2011; Beall 2014; Goodman 2020). Using a combination of physical characteristics would not solve the problem of constructing an accurate racial classification scheme.

There is a final objection to racial classification based on phenotype. The characteristics on which races are based supposedly reflect genetic material that is shared and that has stayed the same for long periods of time. But phenotypical differences and similarities don't necessarily have a genetic basis. Because of changes in the environment that affect individuals during growth and development, the range of phenotypes characteristic of a population may change without any genetic change whatsoever. There are several examples. In the early 20th century, the anthropologist Franz Boas (1940/1966) described changes in skull form (e.g., toward rounder heads) among the children of Europeans who had migrated to North America. The reason for this was not a change in genes, for the European immigrants tended to marry among themselves. Also, some of their children had been born in Europe and merely raised in the United States. Something in the environment, probably in the diet, was producing this change. We know now that changes in average height and weight produced by dietary differences in a few generations are common and may have nothing to do with race or genetics.

Explaining Skin Color

Traditional racial classification assumed that biological characteristics such as skin color were determined by heredity and that they were stable (immutable) over many generations. We now know that a biological similarity does not necessarily indicate recent common ancestry. Tropical Africans and southern Indians, for example, can share dark skin color for reasons other than common ancestry. Scientists have made considerable progress in explaining variation in human skin color, along with many other features of human biological diversity. We shift now from racial classification to *explanation,* in which natural selection plays a key role.

Natural selection is the process by which the forms most fit to survive and reproduce in a given environment do so. Over the generations, the less fit organisms die out, and the favored types survive by producing more offspring. The role of natural selection in producing variation in skin color will illustrate the explanatory approach to human biological diversity. Comparable explanations have

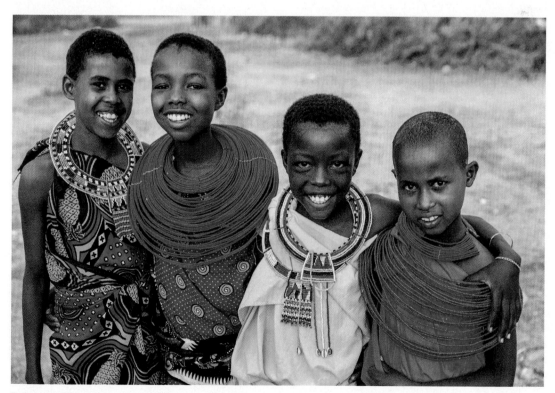

Before the 16th century, almost all the very dark-skinned populations of the world lived in the tropics, as do these Samburu girls from Kenya.

Bartosz Hadyniak/Getty Images

been provided for many other aspects of human biological variation.

How has natural selection affected human skin color? Skin color is a complex biological trait—influenced by several genes (see Jablonski 2006, 2012). **Melanin,** the primary determinant of human skin color, is a chemical substance manufactured in the epidermis, or outer skin layer. The melanin cells of darker skinned people produce more and larger granules of melanin than do those of lighter skinned people. By screening out ultraviolet (UV) radiation from the sun, melanin offers protection against a variety of maladies, including sunburn and skin cancer. It is advantageous to have lots of melanin if one lives in the tropics, where UV radiation is intense.

Before the 16th century, most of the world's very dark-skinned peoples did live in the **tropics,** a belt extending about 23 degrees north and south of the equator, between the Tropic of Cancer to the north and the Tropic of Capricorn to the south. The association between dark skin color and a tropical habitat existed throughout the Old World, where humans and their ancestors have lived for millions of years. The darkest populations of Africa evolved not in shady equatorial forests but in sunny open grassland, or savanna, country.

Outside the tropics, skin color gets lighter. Moving north in Africa, for example, there is a gradual transition from dark brown to medium brown. Average skin color continues to lighten as one moves through the Middle East, into southern Europe, through central Europe, and to the north. (Gradual shifts in gene frequencies between neighboring groups are called *clines.*) South of the Tropic of Capricorn, skin color also is lighter. In the Americas, however, tropical populations do not have very dark skin. This is true because the settlement of the New World by light-skinned Asian ancestors of Native Americans was relatively recent, probably dating back no more than 20,000 years.

How, aside from recent migrations, can we explain the geographic distribution of human skin color? Natural selection provides an answer. In the tropics, intense UV radiation poses a series of threats, including severe sunburn, which make light skin color an adaptive disadvantage (Recap 6.2 summarizes those threats). By damaging sweat glands, sunburn reduces the body's ability to perspire and thus to regulate its own temperature. Sunburn also can increase susceptibility to disease. Another disadvantage of having light skin color in the tropics is that exposure to UV radiation can cause skin cancer. Melanin, nature's own sunscreen, confers a selective advantage (i.e., a better chance to survive and reproduce) on darker skinned people living in the tropics. (Today, there are cultural alternatives that allow people with various skin colors to live wherever they choose. Thus, light-skinned people can survive in the tropics by staying indoors and by using cultural products,

Melanin
"Natural sunscreen" produced by skin cells responsible for pigmentation.

tropics
Zone between 23 degrees north (Tropic of Cancer) and 23 degrees south (Tropic of Capricorn) of the equator.

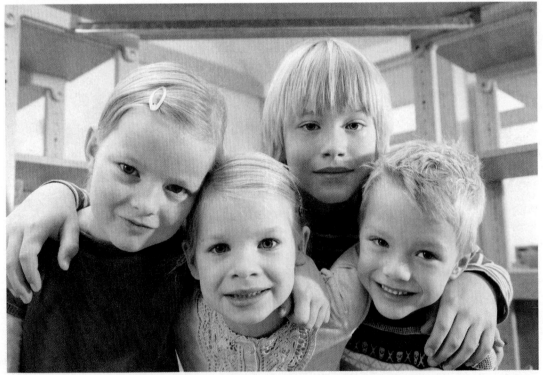

Very light skin color, illustrated by these German children, maximizes absorption of ultraviolet radiation by those few parts of the body exposed to direct sunlight during northern winters.
Robert Niedring/Getty Images

Also shown are cultural alternatives that can make up for biological disadvantages and examples of natural selection (NS) operating today in relation to skin color.

		CULTURAL ALTERNATIVES	NS IN ACTION TODAY
DARK SKIN COLOR	Melanin is natural sunscreen.		
Advantage	In tropics: screens out UV radiation		
	Reduces susceptibility to folate destruction and thus to neural tube defects (NTDs), including spina bifida		
	Prevents sunburn and thus enhances sweating and temperature regulation		
	Reduces disease susceptibility		
	Reduces risk of skin cancer		
Disadvantage	Outside tropics: reduces UV absorption	Foods, vitamin D supplements	East Asians in northern U.K.; Inuit with modern diets
	Increases susceptibility to rickets, osteoporosis		
LIGHT SKIN COLOR	No natural sunscreen		
Advantage	Outside tropics: admits UV		
	Body manufactures vitamin D and thus prevents rickets and osteoporosis		
Disadvantage	Increases susceptibility to folate destruction and thus to NTDs, including spina bifida	Folic acid/folate supplements	Whites still have more NTDs
	Impaired spermatogenesis		
	Increases susceptibility to sunburn and thus to impaired sweating and poor temperature regulation	Shelter, sunscreens, lotions, etc.	
	Increases disease susceptibility		
	Increases susceptibility to skin cancer		

such as umbrellas and lotions, to screen sunlight.) Outside the tropics, however, the fact that melanin screens out UV radiation can become a selective *dis*advantage.

Many years ago, W. F. Loomis (1967) focused on the role of UV radiation in stimulating the manufacture of vitamin D by the human body. The unclothed human body can produce its own vitamin D when exposed to sufficient sunlight. However, in a cloudy environment that also is so cold that people have to wear clothes much of the year (such as northern Europe, where very light skin color evolved), clothing interferes with the body's manufacture of vitamin D, as does having too much melanin in one's skin. The ensuing shortage of vitamin D diminishes the absorption of calcium in the intestines. A nutritional disease known as **rickets,** which softens and deforms the bones, may develop. In women, deformation of the pelvic bones from rickets can interfere with childbirth. In cold northern areas, light skin color maximizes the absorption of UV radiation and the manufacture of vitamin D by the few parts of the body that are exposed to direct sunlight during northern winters. *There has been selection against dark skin color in northern areas because melanin screens out UV radiation.*

This natural selection continues today: East Asians who have migrated recently from India and Pakistan to northern areas of the United Kingdom have a higher incidence of rickets and osteoporosis (also related to vitamin D and calcium deficiency) than the general British population. A related example involves Eskimos (Inuit) and other indigenous inhabitants of northern Alaska and northern Canada. According to Nina Jablonski (quoted in Iqbal 2002), "Looking at Alaska, one would think that the native people should be pale as ghosts" (to maximize their UV absorption and vitamin D). One reason they are not pale is that they haven't inhabited this region very long in terms of geological time. Even more important, their traditional diet, rich in fish oils, supplied sufficient vitamin D to make a reduction in pigmentation unnecessary. (This is another example of how a cultural alternative can help overcome a disadvantageous biological trait.) However, and again illustrating natural selection at work today, "when these people don't eat their aboriginal diets of fish and marine mammals, they suffer tremendously high rates of vitamin D-deficiency diseases such as rickets in children and osteoporosis in adults" (Jablonski quoted in Iqbal 2002). Far from being stable and unchanging,

rickets
Vitamin D deficiency marked by bone deformation.

skin color can become an evolutionary liability very quickly.

According to Jablonski and George Chaplin (2000; see also Jablonski 2006, 2012), another way in which natural selection has affected human skin color involves the destructive effects of UV radiation on folate, an essential nutrient that the human body manufactures from folic acid. Humans require folate for cell division and the production of new DNA. Pregnant women require particularly large amounts of folate to support rapid cell division in the embryo. Folate deficiency during pregnancy can cause neural tube defects (NTDs) in human embryos. NTDs are marked by the incomplete closure of the neural tube, so the spine and spinal cord fail to develop completely. One NTD, anencephaly (with the brain an exposed mass), results in stillbirth or death soon after delivery. With spina bifida, another NTD, survival rates are higher, but babies have severe disabilities, including paralysis. NTDs are the second most common human birth defect after cardiac abnormalities. Folate also plays a role in another process that is central to reproduction, spermatogenesis—the production of sperm. In mice and rats, folate deficiency can cause male sterility; it may well play a similar role in humans.

Dark skin color, as we have seen, is adaptive in the tropics because it protects against such UV hazards as sunburn and its consequences. We have seen that UV radiation destroys folate in the human body. By blocking UV radiation, and thus preventing this destruction, dark skin color helps conserve folate, thus protecting against NTDs (Jablonski and Chaplin 2000). Africans and African Americans rarely experience severe folate deficiency, which primarily affects light-skinned people. Today, pregnant women are routinely advised to take folic acid or folate supplements as a hedge against NTDs. Even so, light skin color still is correlated with a higher incidence of spina bifida.

Jablonski and Chaplin (2000) explain variation in human skin color as resulting from a balancing act between the evolutionary needs (1) to protect against all UV hazards (thus favoring dark skin in the tropics) and (2) to have an adequate supply of vitamin D (thus favoring lighter skin outside the tropics). This discussion of skin color shows that common ancestry, the presumed basis of race, is not the only reason for biological similarities. Natural selection, still at work today, makes a major contribution to variations in human skin color as well as to many other human biological differences and similarities.

The AAA RACE Project

To broaden public understanding of human diversity, the American Anthropological Association (AAA) offers its RACE Project, which includes an award-winning public education program titled RACE Are We So Different? This program, whose intended audience is middle-school-aged children through adults, includes an interactive website and a traveling museum exhibit www.understandingrace.org.

RACE Are We So Different? examines the race concept through the eyes of history, science, and lived experience (see Goodman 2020 for a collection of essays related to the project). It explains how human variation differs from race, when and why the idea of race was invented, and how race and racism affect our everyday lives. The program's three key messages are that (1) race is a recent human invention; (2) race is about culture, not biology; and (3) race and racism are embedded in institutions and everyday life (see also Gravlee 2009; Hartigan 2013).

In addition to its RACE project, the AAA has issued a statement on race (https://www.americananthro.org/ConnectWithAAA/Content.aspx?ItemNumber=2583). It discusses the social construction of race, for example, under colonialism. The AAA statement also stresses that inequalities among "racial" groups are not consequences of their biological inheritance but products of social, economic, educational, and political circumstances (see also Benedict 2019; Hartigan 2015).

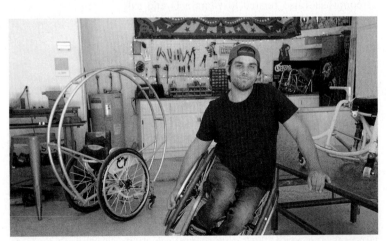

Although Aaron 'Wheelz' Fotheringham lacks control over his legs, he holds six sporting world records. Aaron, age 27 in this 2019 photo, was born with spina bifida, which often causes paralysis of the lower limbs. He got his first wheelchair at age three and eventually became a Wheelchair Motocross (WCMX) rider. His sport combines skateboard and BMX tricks, performed in a wheelchair.
Jessica Sherry/Getty Images

RACE AND ETHNICITY

In American culture, we hear the words *ethnicity* and *race* frequently, without clear distinctions made between them. For example, the term *race* often is used inappropriately to refer to Hispanics, who, in fact, can be of any race. The following example provides one illustration of confusion about ethnicity and race in American culture. Eight years prior to her appointment to the U.S. Supreme Court, Sonia Sotomayor, then an appeals court judge, gave a talk

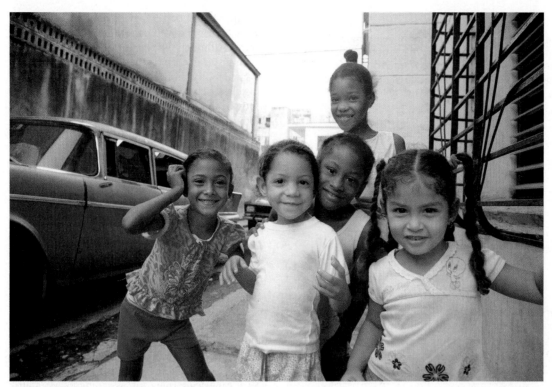

Hispanic and *Latino* are ethnic categories that crosscut "racial" contrasts such as that between *Black* and *white*. Note the physical diversity among these children in Old Havana, Cuba.

Kumar Sriskandan/Alamy Stock Photo

titled "A Latina Judge's Voice," at the University of California, Berkeley, School of Law. As part of a much longer speech, Sotomayor declared

> I would hope that a wise Latina woman with the richness of her experiences would more often than not reach a better conclusion than a white male who hasn't lived that life (Sotomayor 2001/2009).

On hearing about that speech, conservatives, including former House Speaker Newt Gingrich and radio talk show host Rush Limbaugh, seized on this declaration as evidence that Sotomayor was a "racist" or a "reverse racist." Her critics ignored the fact that "Latina" is an ethnic (and gendered-female) rather than a racial category. I suspect that Sotomayor also was using "white male" as an ethnic-gender category, to refer to nonminority men. Our popular culture does not consistently distinguish between ethnicity and race (see Ansell 2013; Banton 2015; Golash-Boza 2019). Can you think of any recent examples? Why might "Chinese virus" be considered both an ethnic and a racist slur?

THE SOCIAL CONSTRUCTION OF RACE

Most Americans believe (incorrectly) that their population includes *biologically based* races to which various labels are applied. Such racial

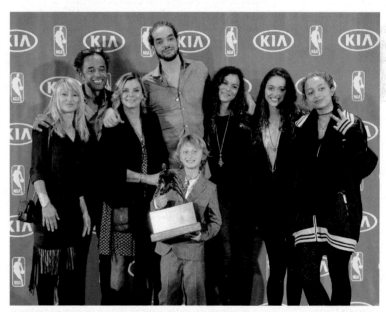

An international and multiethnic American family. Joakim Noah, center, is an All-Star professional basketball player, who played in college for the Florida Gators. Also shown are his mother, a former Miss Sweden, and father, a French singer and tennis player who won the French open in 1983. Joakim's grandfather, Zacharie Noah, was a professional soccer player from the African nation of Cameroon. What is Joakim Noah's race?

Matt Marton/AP Images

terms include "white," "Black," "yellow," "red," "Caucasoid," "Negroid," "Mongoloid," "Amer-indian," "Euro-American," "African American," "Asian American," and "Native American."

5. Please provide information for each person living here. If there is someone living here who pays the rent or owns this residence, start by listing him or her as Person 1. If the owner or the person who pays the rent does not live here, start by listing any adult living here as Person 1.

What is Person 1's name? *Print name below.*

First Name   MI

[ ][ ][ ][ ][ ][ ][ ][ ][ ][ ][ ][ ][ ][ ][ ]   [ ]

Last Name(s)

[ ][ ][ ][ ][ ][ ][ ][ ][ ][ ][ ][ ][ ][ ][ ][ ][ ]

6. What is person 1's sex? *Mark* [X] *ONE box.*

☐ Male   ☐ Female

7. What is Person 1's age and what is Person 1's date of birth? *For babies less than 1 year old, do not write the age in months. Write 0 as the age.*

Print numbers in boxes.

Age on April 1, 2020   Month   Day   Year of birth

[ ][ ][ ] Years   [ ][ ]   [ ][ ]   [ ][ ][ ][ ]

→ **NOTE: Please answer BOTH Question 8 about Hispanic origin and Question 9 about race. For this census, Hispanic origins are not races.**

8. Is Person 1 of Hispanic, Latino, or Spanish origin?

☐ No, not of Hispanic, Latino, or Spanish origin

☐ Yes, Mexican, Mexican Am., Chicano

☐ Yes, Puerto Rican

☐ Yes, Cuban

☐ Yes, another Hispanic, Latino, or Spanish origin – *Print, for example, Salvadoran, Dominican, Colombian, Guatemalan, Spaniard, Ecuadorian, etc.* ⤴

[ ][ ][ ][ ][ ][ ][ ][ ][ ][ ][ ][ ][ ][ ][ ][ ][ ]

FIGURE 6.2   Questions about Hispanic Origin in the 2020 Census.

SOURCE: U.S. Census Bureau, Census 2020 questionnaire.

descent
Social identity based on ancestry.

hypodescent
Children of mixed unions assigned to the same group as their minority parent.

We have seen that races, while assumed to have a biological basis, actually are socially constructed in particular societies. Let's consider now several examples of the social construction of race, beginning with the United States.

Hypodescent: Race in the United States

Most Americans acquire their racial identity at birth and stick with it throughout their lives, but race isn't based on biology or on simple ancestry. Consider a child with one Black and one white parent. Although 50 percent of that child's DNA comes from each parent, American culture overlooks heredity and classifies this child as Black. This classificatory rule is arbitrary. On the basis of genotype (genetic composition), it would be just as logical to classify the child as white. Operating here is a rule of **descent** (it assigns social identity on the basis of ancestry), but of a sort that is rare outside the contemporary United States. It is called **hypodescent** (Harris and Kottak 1963) because it automatically places children of mixed unions in the group of their minority parent (*hypo* means "lower"). Hypodescent divides American society into groups that have been unequal in their access to wealth, power, and prestige.

The hypodescent rule may be arbitrary, but it is very strong. How else can we explain the common assertion that Barack Obama was the first Black president, rather than the first biracial president, of the United States? (This chapter's "Appreciating Diversity" focuses on another successful biracial or multiracial American, Tiger Woods, in a discussion of the lack of racial diversity in golf.) American rules for assigning racial status can be even more arbitrary, as the following case illustrates.

Governments (federal or, in this case, the state of Louisiana) can play a decisive role in defining and assigning racial and ethnic identities (see Mullaney 2011). Susie Guillory Phipps, a light-skinned woman with straight black hair, discovered as an adult that she was Black. When Phipps ordered a copy of her birth certificate, she found her race listed as "colored." Since she had been "brought up white and married white twice," Phipps challenged a 1970 Louisiana law declaring anyone with at least one-thirty-second "Negro blood" to be legally Black. Although the state's lawyer admitted that Phipps "looks like a white person," the state of Louisiana insisted that her racial classification as colored was proper (Yetman 1991, pp. 3–4).

Race in the Census

The U.S. Census Bureau has gathered data by race since 1790. The most recent (2020) census asks for detailed information about Hispanic origin and race for each household member. Question 8 asks whether a person is "of Hispanic, Latino, or Spanish origin" (Figure 6.2). One can choose among several options, the first being "No"–not Hispanic, the rest asking about specific national origins: (1) Mexican, (2) Puerto Rican, (3) Cuban, and (4) another Hispanic origin (Salvadoran, etc.).

Question 9 (Figure 6.3) asks "What is a person's race?–Mark one or more boxes." The first three choices are: (1) white, (2) Black or African American, (3) American Indian or Alaska Native. Each category provides space for specifying a particular national origin, with examples of such origins. For whites, those examples are "German, Irish, English, Italian, Lebanese, Egyptian, etc." African Americans are offered these examples: "African American, Jamaican, Haitian, Nigerian, Ethiopian, Somali, etc." For Native Americans, the choices suggested are "Navajo Nation, Blackfeet Tribe, Mayan, Aztec, Native Village of Barrow Inupiat Traditional Government, Nome Eskimo Community, etc." Below those three categories come several individual boxes specifying Asian and Pacific Island origins: Chinese, Vietnamese, Native Hawaiian, Filipino, Korean, Samoan, Asian Indian, Japanese, Chamorro, Other Asian, and Other Pacific Islander. Finally, there is a box offered the respondent the chance to specify "Some other race."

For each question in the 2020 census, the bureau addresses "Why we ask this question?" The statistics about ethnicity provided by question 8 will help "federal agencies monitor compliance with anti-discrimination provisions, such as those in the Voting Rights Act and the Civil Rights Act." The census bureau offers the same rationale (compliance with anti-discrimination provisions) for question 9 on race. Note that the 2020 census questions on ethnicity and race solicit the most specific and detailed information ever in the United States census.

Census data, including ethnic and racial classification, has always been a political issue involving access to resources, including jobs, voting districts, and programs aimed at minorities. The hypodescent rule results in all the population growth being attributed to the minority category. Attempts to add a "multiracial" category to the U.S. Census have been opposed by the National Association for the Advancement of Colored People (NAACP) and the National Council of La Raza (a Hispanic advocacy group). Minorities fear their political clout will decline if their numbers go down.

But things have changed. Choice of "some other race" in the U.S. Census tripled from 6.8 to 19 million people between 1980 and 2010—suggesting imprecision in and dissatisfaction with the existing categories. (Results of the 2020 census are not yet available as of this writing.) In the 2000 census, 2.4 percent of Americans chose a first-ever option of identifying themselves as belonging to more than one race. That figure rose to 2.9 percent in the 2010 census. The 2020 census instruction to "mark one or more boxes" will show how many Americans today consider themselves to be multiracial. The number of interracial marriages and children has been increasing, with implications for the traditional system of American racial classification. "Interracial," "biracial," or "multiracial" children undoubtedly identify with qualities of both parents. It may be troubling for many

9. What is person 1's race?

Mark [X] *one or more boxes* **AND** *print origins.*

☐ White – *Print, for example, German, Irish, English, Italian, Lebanese, Egyptian, etc.* ↗

☐ Black or African Am. – *Print, for example, African American, Jamaican, Haitian, Nigerian, Ethiopian, Somali, etc.* ↗

☐ American Indian or Alaska Native – *Print name of enrolled or principal tribe(s), for example, Navaje Nation, Blackfeet Tribe, Mayan, Aztec, Native Village of Barrow Inupiat Traditional Government, Nome Eskimo Community, etc.* ↗

☐ Chinese   ☐ Vietnamese   ☐ Native Hawaiian

☐ Filipino   ☐ Korean   ☐ Samoan

☐ Asian Indian   ☐ Japanese   ☐ Chamorro

☐ Other Asian – *Print, for example, Pakistani, Cambodian, Hmong, etc.* ↗   ☐ Other pacific Islander – *Print, for example, Tongan, Filian, Marshallese, etc.* ↗

☐ Some other race – *Print, race or origin.* ↗

→ **If more people were counted in Question 1 on the front page, continue with Person 2 on the next page.**

FIGURE 6.3 Questions about Race in the 2020 Census.

SOURCE: U.S. Census Bureau, Census 2020 questionnaire.

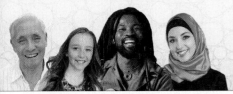
Why Are the Greens So White?

How do race and ethnicity figure in the world of golf, a sport whose popularity has been growing not only in the United States but also in Europe, Asia, and Australia? More than 20 million Americans play golf, an industry that also supports about 400,000 workers. For decades, golf has been the preferred sport of business tycoons and politicians—mainly white. President Dwight D. Eisenhower (1953–1960), whose love for golf was well known, etched a lasting (and accurate) image of golf as a Republican sport (despite the fact that former presidents Bill Clinton and Barack Obama also play the game). A recent survey found that only 2 of the top 125 PGA touring pros identified as Democrats. The most recent Republican president, Donald Trump, is both a business tycoon and an avid golfer.

A glance at golfers in any televised game reveals a remarkable lack of variation in skin color. American golf was the nation's last major sport to desegregate, and minorities traditionally have been relegated to supporting roles. Latinos maintain the game's greens and physical infrastructure. Until the motorized golf cart replaced them, African Americans had significant opportunities to observe and learn the game by caddying. Indeed, there once was a tradition of African American caddies becoming excellent golfers.

The best example of this trajectory is Dr. Charlie Sifford (1922–2015), who in 1961 broke the color barrier in American professional golf. Sifford began his golf career as a caddie for white golfers. He went on to dominate the all-Black United Golf Association, winning five straight national titles, but he wanted to play with the world's best golfers. At the age of 39, Sifford successfully challenged—and ended—the white-only policy of the Professional Golfers' Association of America (PGA), becoming its first African American member.

Sifford, who had to endure phone threats, racial slurs, and other indignities at the beginning of his PGA career, went on to win

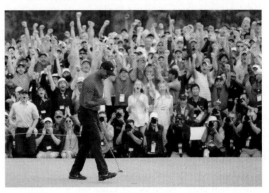

On April 14, 2019, in Augusta, Georgia, Tiger Woods celebrates as he wins his fifth Masters title, his first major championship in 11 years.
David Cannon/Getty Images

the Greater Hartford Open in 1967, the Los Angeles Open in 1969, and the 1975 Senior PGA Championship. In 2004, he became the first African American inducted into the World Golf Hall of Fame. His major regret was that he never got to play in a Masters Tournament. That event, held annually in Augusta, Georgia, did not invite its first Black player until Lee Elder in 1975. Sifford's bitterness about

of them to have so important an identity as race dictated by the arbitrary rule of hypodescent.

Rather than race, the Canadian census (conducted every 5 years) asks about "visible minorities." That country's Employment Equity Act defines such groups as "persons, other than Aboriginal [First Nations] peoples, who are non-Caucasian in race or non-white in colour." The visible minority population consists mainly of the following groups: South Asian, Chinese, Black, Filipino, Latin American, Arab, Southeast Asian, West Asian, Korean and Japanese (Statistics Canada 2016). "South Asian" and "Chinese" are Canada's largest visible minorities (see Figure 6.4). Canada's visible minority population of 22.4 percent in 2016 (up from 11.2 percent in 1996) contrasts with a figure of 39 percent for the United States (in 2017, up from 25 percent in 2000).

As is true of the minority population of the United States, Canada's visible minority population has been growing much faster than the country's overall population. In 1981, visible minorities accounted for just 4.7 percent of the Canadian population, versus 22.4 percent in 2016. Visible minorities accounted for 88 percent of Canada's total population growth between 2011 and 2016. If recent immigration trends continue, by 2031 visible minorities are projected to comprise almost one-third (31 percent) of the Canadian population (Statistics Canada 2010).

Not Us: Race in Japan

Japan presents itself and is commonly viewed as a nation that is homogeneous in race, ethnicity, language, and culture (see Toyosaki and Eguchi 2017). Although Japan's population is in fact less diverse than those of most nations, it does contain significant minority groups (see Graburn, Ertle, and Tierney 2008; Weiner 2009). Constituting

his own exclusion from the Masters was tempered somewhat by his pleasure when Tiger Woods, another African American golfer, won the first of his five green Masters jackets in 1997.

In terms of diversity, golf has actually regressed since the 1970s, when 11 African Americans played on the PGA Tour. As of this writing, there are only 2 African Americans (Tiger Woods and Harold Varner III) among the 125 top players on the PGA Tour. In Britain, only 2 percent of an estimated 850,000 regular golfers are non-white.

Economic factors continue to limit minority access to golf, compared with baseball, football, and especially basketball—all of which offer greater public access. As Harold Varner puts it, "golf is really expensive. Why would I spend $30 a day to play golf when I can spend 30 bucks a month and go to the 'Y' and play basketball" (quoted in Bianchi 2017). Prospective golfers need money for instruction, equipment, access to courses, and travel to tournaments. Asian Americans, who enjoy a relatively high socioeconomic status, are the only minority group in the United States with a growing representation in golf, for both men and women.

For years, Tiger Woods has been the standout non-white individual in this mainly white, affluent, Republican sport. Woods became one of America's most celebrated and popular athletes by combining golfing success with a carefully cultivated reputation as a family man. He presented himself as the hard-working and achievement-oriented son of an Asian mother and an African American father, and as the devoted husband and father of his Scandinavian wife and two photogenic children. Woods's fall from grace began late in 2009, as a flood of media reports converted his image from family man into serial philanderer. Although his marriage did not survive his transgressions, his golfing career did.

Woods gradually reintegrated into the world of golf, even receiving the 2013 PGA Tour Player of the Year Award. For several years thereafter, however, he struggled with back injuries, surgeries, and other woes. By July 2017, his ranking among the world's golfers had fallen to 1,005th.

Yet Tiger Woods was far from done. In September 2018, he claimed victory in the 2018 Tour Championship at Atlanta's East Lake Golf Club—his first win since the WGC-Bridgestone Invitational in 2013. He had played in 41 PGA Tour events between those two victories. His 2018 win (his 80th) placed him just two victories shy of Sam Snead's record of 82. On April 14, 2019, in Augusta, Georgia, Woods won his fifth Masters title and his 15th major tournament, his first major championship in 11 years.

A resurgent champion at age 43, a decade after his fall from grace, Tiger Woods seemed destined for additional victories. Whatever the future holds, he will be remembered historically as a pioneer among African American golfers, and one of that sport's all-time greats. What role, if any, do you think race, ethnicity, racism, and racial stereotyping have played in the rise, fall, resurgence, and overall career of Tiger Woods?

SOURCE: Ferguson, D., "First Black Player on PGA Tour Dies," *Associated Press,* Post and Courier, Charleston, SC, February 5, 2015; Riach, J., "Golf's Failure to Embrace Demographics across Society Is Hard to Stomach," *The Guardian,* May 22, 2013. http://www.theguardian.com/sport/blog/2013/may/22/uk-golf-clubs-race-issues.; Starn, O., *The Passion of Tiger Woods: An Anthropologist Reports on Golf, Race, and Celebrity Scandal.* Durham, NC: Duke University Press, 2011.

about 10 percent of Japan's total population, those groups include aboriginal Ainu, annexed Okinawans, outcast *burakumin,* children of mixed marriages, and immigrant nationalities, especially Koreans, who number more than 700,000 (Ryang and Lie 2009). The (majority) Japanese define themselves by opposition to others, whether minority groups in their own nation or outsiders—anyone who is "not us." Furthermore, assimilation is discouraged. Cultural mechanisms, including residential segregation and taboos on "interracial" marriage, work to keep minorities "in their place."

To describe racial attitudes in Japan, Jennifer Robertson (1992) used Kwame Anthony Appiah's (1990) term "intrinsic racism"—the belief that a (perceived) racial difference is a sufficient reason to value one person less than another. In Japan the valued group is majority ("pure") Japanese, who are believed to share "the same blood." Thus, the caption to a printed photo of a Japanese American model reads: "She was born in Japan but raised in Hawaii. Her nationality is American but no foreign blood flows in her veins" (Robertson 1992, p. 5). Something like hypodescent also operates in Japan, but less precisely than in the United States, where mixed offspring automatically become members of the minority group. The children of mixed marriages between majority Japanese and others (including Euro-Americans and African Americans) may not get the same "racial" label as their minority parent, but they are still stigmatized for their non-Japanese ancestry (see Yamashiro 2017).

Biracial Japanese
One exception to this stigma has been tennis's Naomi Osaka, who beat Serena Williams in the final of the 2018 U.S. Open. Osaka, who is the daughter of a Haitian American father and a Japanese mother, became the first Japanese-born

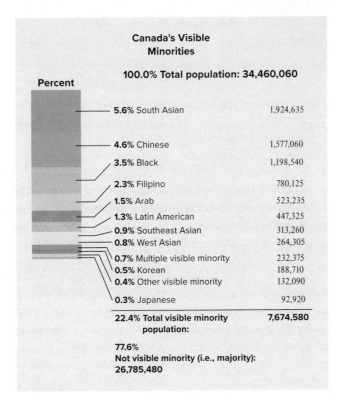

Canada's Visible Minorities

100.0% Total population: 34,460,060

Percent		
5.6%	South Asian	1,924,635
4.6%	Chinese	1,577,060
3.5%	Black	1,198,540
2.3%	Filipino	780,125
1.5%	Arab	523,235
1.3%	Latin American	447,325
0.9%	Southeast Asian	313,260
0.8%	West Asian	264,305
0.7%	Multiple visible minority	232,375
0.5%	Korean	188,710
0.4%	Other visible minority	132,090
0.3%	Japanese	92,920
22.4%	**Total visible minority population:**	**7,674,580**

77.6%
Not visible minority (i.e., majority):
26,785,480

FIGURE 6.4 Visible Minority Population of Canada, 2016, According to the Most Recent Canadian Census.

SOURCE: From Statistics Canada, Census Profile, 2016 Census.http://www12.statcan.gc.ca/census-recensement/2016/dp-pd/prof/details/page.cfm?Lang=E&Geo1=PR&Code1=01&Geo2=&Code2=&Data=Count&SearchText=Canada&SearchType=Begins&SearchPR=01&B1=All&TABID=1

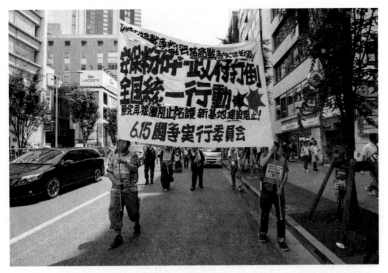

On June 12, 2016, in Tokyo, Japan, burakumin protesters seek greater respect and protection from the government and society. The term "burakumin" literally means "hamlet people," and originates from a now-defunct caste system that existed in the Edo Period (1603–1867).

Alessandro Di Ciommo/NurPhoto/Getty Images

appearance, parentage, or the fact that she had been raised in the United States and spoke halting Japanese. Like a proper Japanese, she did not display excessive joy when she won (in fact, she even apologized), and, despite her aggressive play, she is humble in interviews and bows appropriately (Rich 2018).

This warm reception by the press struck some as hypocritical while Japan's pure-blood definition of ethnicity persists. Many biracial people in Japan still feel undervalued. One term applied to them is *hafu*, derived from the English word "half"—a label that implies "not whole," incomplete, or "less than."

Could Osaka's reception be a sign that things are changing? Other evidence: In 2015 Ariana Miyamoto, a half-Black, half-Japanese woman, was chosen Miss Universe Japan. A year later, another mixed-race woman, Priyanka Yosikawa, won the same crown. In Brazil, it often is said that "Money whitens." In other words, someone who is wealthy will be perceived as having lighter skin color than a physically similar person who is less well off. Media treatment of Osaka, Miyamoto, and Yosikawa suggest that something comparable may be going on in Japan. Can we conclude that "celebrity Japanizes"?

Burakumin

In its construction of race, Japanese culture regards certain ethnic groups as having a biological basis, when there is no evidence that they do. The best example is the burakumin, a stigmatized group of some 3 million outcasts, sometimes compared to India's untouchables. The burakumin are physically and genetically indistinguishable from other Japanese. Many of them "pass" as (and marry) majority Japanese, but a deceptive marriage can end in divorce if burakumin identity is discovered (Amos 2011).

Based on their ancestry (and thus, it is assumed, their "blood," or genetics), burakumin are considered "not us." Majority Japanese try to keep their lineage pure by discouraging mixing. The burakumin are residentially segregated in neighborhoods (rural or urban) called *buraku,* from which the racial label is derived. Compared with majority Japanese, the burakumin are less likely to attend high school and college. When burakumin attend the same schools as majority Japanese, they face discrimination. Majority children and teachers may refuse to eat with them because burakumin are considered unclean.

In applying for university admission or a job and in dealing with the government, Japanese must list their address, which becomes part of a registry. This list makes residence in a buraku, and likely burakumin social status, evident. Schools and companies use this information to discriminate. (The best way to pass is to move so often that the buraku address eventually disappears from the registry.) Majority Japanese also limit "race"

tennis player to win a Grand Slam championship. Her victory was widely celebrated in Japan as one for that country. Japanese media focused on Osaka's cultural "Japaneseness" rather than her

mixture by hiring marriage mediators to check out the family histories of prospective spouses. They are especially careful to check for burakumin ancestry (Amos 2011).

The origin of the burakumin lies in a historical tiered system of stratification (from the Tokugawa period, 1603–1868). The top four ranked categories were warrior-administrators (*samurai*), farmers, artisans, and merchants. The ancestors of the burakumin were below this hierarchy. They did "unclean" jobs such as animal slaughter and disposal of the dead. Burakumin still do similar jobs, including work with leather and other animal products (see Hankins 2014). They are also more likely than majority Japanese to do manual labor (including farm work) and to belong to the national lower class. Burakumin and other Japanese minorities also are more likely to have careers in crime, prostitution, entertainment, and sports.

Like Blacks in the United States, the burakumin are internally **stratified.** In other words, there are class contrasts within the group. Because certain jobs are reserved for the burakumin, people who are successful in those occupations (e.g., shoe factory owners) can be wealthy. Burakumin also have found jobs as government bureaucrats. Financially successful burakumin can temporarily escape their stigmatized status by travel, including foreign travel.

Discrimination against the burakumin is strikingly like the discrimination that Blacks have experienced in the United States. The burakumin often live in communities with poor housing and sanitation. They have limited access to education, jobs, amenities, and health facilities. In response to burakumin political mobilization, Japan has dismantled the legal structure of discrimination against burakumin and has worked to improve conditions in the buraku. (The website http://www.blhrri.org/old/blhrri_e/blhrri/about.htm is sponsored by the Buraku Liberation and Human Rights Research Institute and includes the most recent information about the burakumin liberation movement.) However, discrimination against nonmajority Japanese is still the rule in companies. Some employers say that hiring burakumin would give their company an unclean image and thus create a disadvantage in competing with other businesses.

Phenotype and Fluidity: Race in Brazil

There are more flexible, less restrictive ways of socially constructing race than those used in the United States and Japan. Consider Brazil, which shares a history of slavery with the United States but lacks the hypodescent rule. Nor does Brazil have racial aversion of the sort found in Japan.

Brazilians use many more racial labels—over 500 were once reported (Harris 1970)—than Americans or Japanese do. In northeastern Brazil, I found 40 different racial terms in use in Arembepe, a village of only 750 people (Kottak 2018). Through their traditional classification system, Brazilians recognize and attempt to describe the physical variation that exists within their population. The American classification system, which recognizes only a few races, obscures an equivalent range of evident physical contrasts. Brazilian racial classification has other significant features. In the United States, one's race is assigned automatically by hypodescent and usually doesn't change. In Brazil, racial identity is more flexible, more of an achieved status.

Brazilian racial classification pays attention to phenotype. Scientists distinguish between *genotype*, or hereditary makeup, and *phenotype*—expressed physical characteristics. Genotype is what you are genetically; phenotype is what you appear as. Identical twins and clones have the same genotype, but their phenotypes vary if they have been raised in different environments. Phenotype describes an organism's evident traits, its "manifest biology"—physiology and anatomy, including skin color, hair form, facial features, and eye color. A Brazilian's phenotype and racial label may change because of environmental factors, such as the tanning rays of the sun or the effects of humidity on the hair.

A Brazilian also can change his or her "race" (say from "Indian" to "mixed") by altering his or her speech, clothing, location (e.g., rural to urban), and even attitude (e.g., by adopting urban behavior). Two racial/ethnic labels used in Brazil are *indio* (indigenous, Native American) and *cabôclo* (someone who "looks *indio*" but wears modern clothing and participates in Brazilian culture, rather than living in an indigenous community). Similar shifts in racial/ethnic classification occur in other parts of Latin America, for example,

stratified
Class structured, with differences in wealth, prestige, and power.

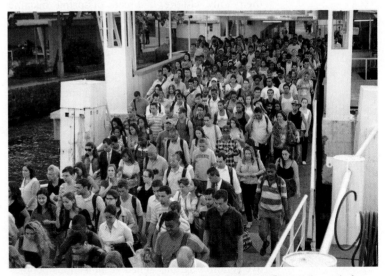

In Rio de Janeiro, Brazil, commuters make their way onto a ferry at the end of a work day. This heterogeneous crowd offers just a glimpse of the phenotypical diversity encountered among contemporary Brazilians.
Melanie Stetson Freeman/Getty Images

Guatemala (see Wade 2010, 2017). Racial perceptions are influenced not just by one's physical phenotype but also by how one dresses and behaves.

Furthermore, racial differences in Brazil may be so insignificant in structuring community life that people may forget the terms they have applied to others. Sometimes they even forget the ones they've used for themselves. In Arembepe, I made it a habit to ask the same person on different days to tell me the races of others in the village (and my own). In the United States, I am always "white" or "Euro-American," but in Arembepe I got lots of terms besides *branco* ("white"). I could be *claro* ("light"), *louro* ("blond"), *sarará* ("light-skinned redhead"), *mulato claro* ("light mulatto"), or *mulato* ("mulatto"). The racial term used to describe me or anyone else varied from person to person, week to week, even day to day. My best informant, a man with very dark skin color, changed the term he used for himself all the time—from *escuro* ("dark") to *preto* ("black") to *moreno escuro* ("dark brunet").

For centuries the United States and Brazil have had mixed populations, with ancestors from Native America, Europe, Africa, and Asia. Although races have mixed in both countries, Brazilian and American cultures have constructed the results differently. The historical reasons for this contrast lie mainly in the different characteristics of the settlers of the two countries. The mainly English early settlers of the United States came as women, men, and families, but Brazil's Portuguese colonizers were mainly men—merchants and adventurers. Many of these Portuguese men married indigenous women and recognized their racially mixed children as their heirs. Like their North American counterparts, Brazilian plantation owners had sexual relations with their slaves. But the Brazilian landlords more often freed the children that resulted. (Sometimes these were their only children.) Freed offspring became plantation overseers and foremen and filled many intermediate positions in the emerging Brazilian economy. They were not classed with the slaves but were allowed to join a new intermediate category. No hypodescent rule developed in Brazil to ensure that whites and blacks remained separate (see Degler 1970; Harris 1964).

In today's world system, Brazil's system of racial classification is changing in the context of international identity politics and rights movements. Just as more and more Brazilians claim indigenous identities, an increasing number now assert their blackness and self-conscious membership in the African diaspora. Particularly in such northeastern Brazilian states as Bahia, where African demographic and cultural influence is strong, public universities have instituted affirmative action programs aimed at indigenous peoples and especially at Afro-Brazilians. Racial identities firm up in the context of international (e.g., pan-African and pan–Native American) mobilization and access to strategic resources based on race.

nation
A society that shares a language, religion, history, territory, ancestry, and kinship.

state
A society with a central government, administrative specialization, and social classes.

nation-state
An autonomous political entity; a country.

ETHNIC GROUPS, NATIONS, AND NATIONALITIES

The term **nation** once was synonymous with *tribe* or *ethnic group*. All three of these terms have been used to refer to a single culture sharing a single language, religion, history, territory, ancestry, and kinship. Thus, one could speak interchangeably of the Seneca (Native American) nation, tribe, or ethnic group. Now *nation* has come to mean **state**—an independent, centrally organized political unit, or a government. *Nation* and *state* have become synonymous. Combined in **nation-state** they refer to an autonomous political entity, a country.

Because of migration, conquest, and colonialism, few nation-states are ethnically homogeneous. In a study of "Ethnic and Cultural Diversity by Country," James Fearon (2003) found that a single ethnic group formed an absolute majority of the population in about 70 percent of all countries. The average population share of that majority group was 65 percent. The average size of the *second* largest group, or largest ethnic minority, was 17 percent. (Notice that the United States today is similar to this distribution, with the majority group [non-Hispanic whites] at 60.4 percent and the largest minority [Hispanics] at 18.3 percent.) In Fearon's study, only 18 percent of all countries, including Brazil and Japan, had a single ethnic group representing 90 percent or more of its population.

Ethnic Diversity by Region

There is substantial regional variation in countries' ethnic structures. The German researcher Erkan Gören (2013) measured cultural diversity in more than 180 countries, based on each country's degree of diversity in ethnicity, race, and language (see Morin 2013). In Gören's study, the most culturally diverse countries were in Africa. Heading his list were Chad, Cameroon, Nigeria, Togo, and the Democratic Republic of the Congo. African countries tend to rank high on any diversity index because of their multiple ethnic groups and languages. The only Western country among the 20 most diverse was Canada. The United States ranked near the middle, a bit more diverse than Russia but slightly less so than Spain (Morin 2013).

The world's least diverse countries included Argentina and Uruguay. Although Argentina (like Brazil) has experienced significant German and Italian immigration, Spanish remains its almost universal language, and most Argentines are white and Roman Catholic. Gören also placed Brazil among the least diverse, because virtually all Brazilians speak Portuguese regardless of their racial characteristics or ethnic backgrounds.

Most Latin American and Caribbean countries contain a majority group (speaking a European language, such as Portuguese or Spanish) and a single minority group—indigenous peoples. The latter is a catch-all category encompassing several small Native American tribes or remnants. Exceptions are Guatemala and the Andean countries of Bolivia, Peru, and Ecuador, with large indigenous populations (see Gotkowitz 2011; Wade 2010, 2017).

Most countries in Asia and the Middle East/North Africa have ethnic majorities. The Asian countries of Myanmar, Laos, Vietnam, and Thailand contain a large lowland majority edged by more fragmented mountain folk. Several oil-producing countries in the Middle East, including Saudi Arabia, Bahrain, United Arab Emirates, Oman, and Kuwait, contain an ethnically homogeneous group of citizens who form either a plurality or a bare majority; the rest of the population consists of ethnically diverse noncitizen workers. Other countries in the Middle East/North Africa contain two principal ethnic or ethnoreligious groups: Arabs and Berbers in Morocco, Algeria, Libya, and Tunisia; Muslims and Copts in Egypt; Turks and Kurds in Turkey; Greeks and Turks in Cyprus; and Palestinians and Transjordan Arabs in Jordan (Fearon 2003).

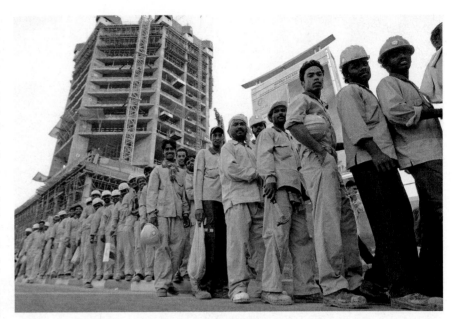

Foreign workers await transport by bus to their living quarters as their shift ends at a construction site in Dubai. Like other Arab Emirates, Dubai relies on a large population of workers from outside.

KARIM SAHIB/AFP/Getty Images

Nationalities without Nations

Strong central governments, particularly in Europe (e.g., France), have deliberately and actively worked to homogenize their diverse premodern populations to a common national identity and culture (see Beriss 2004). Benedict Anderson (1991/2006) traces Western European *nationalism* (the feeling of belonging to a nation), back to the 18th century. He stresses the crucial role of the printed word in the growth of national consciousness in England, France, and Spain. The novel and the newspaper were "two forms of imagining" communities (consisting of all the people who read the same sources and thus witnessed the same events) that flowered in the 18th century (Anderson 1991/2006, pp. 24–25).

Groups that have, once had, or wish to have or regain, autonomous political status (their own country) are called **nationalities.** As a result of political upheavals, wars, and migration, many nationalities have been split up and placed in separate nation-states. For example, the German and Korean homelands were artificially divided after wars, according to communist and capitalist ideologies. World War I dispersed the Kurds, who form a majority in no state, but exist as minority groups in Turkey, Iran, Iraq, and Syria.

Colonialism—the foreign domination of a territory—established a series of multitribal and multiethnic states. The new national boundaries that were created under colonialism often corresponded poorly with preexisting cultural divisions. However, colonial institutions also helped forge new identities that extended beyond nations and nationalities. A good example is the idea of *négritude* ("black identity") developed by African intellectuals in Francophone (French-speaking) West Africa. Négritude can be traced to the association and common experience in colonial times of youths from Guinea, Mali, the Ivory Coast, and Senegal at the William Ponty School in Dakar, Senegal (Anderson 1991/2006, pp. 123–124).

ETHNIC TOLERANCE AND ACCOMMODATION

Ethnic diversity may be associated with either positive group interaction and coexistence or with conflict (to be discussed shortly). There are nation-states in which multiple ethnic groups live together in reasonable harmony, including some less-developed countries.

Assimilation

Assimilation describes the process of change that ethnic groups may experience when they move to a country where another culture dominates. In assimilating, the immigrant group adopts the patterns and norms of its host culture. It is incorporated into the dominant culture to the point that it no longer exists as a separate cultural unit. Some countries, such as Brazil, are more assimilationist than others. Germans, Italians, Japanese, Middle Easterners, and Eastern Europeans started migrating to Brazil late in the

nationalities
Ethnic groups that have, once had, or want their own country.

assimilation
The absorption of minorities within a dominant culture.

colonialism
The political, social, economic, and cultural domination of a territory and its people by a foreign power for an extended time.

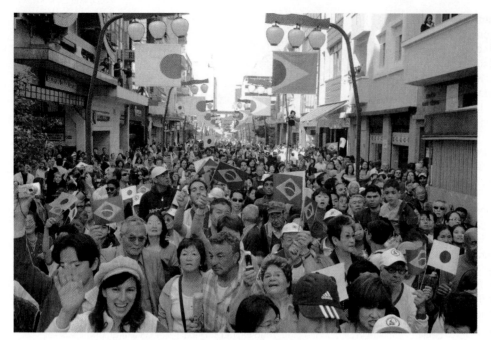

Brazil is home to the world's largest community of Japanese descendants outside Japan. Numbering about 1.5 million people, these Japanese Brazilians live mostly in and around the city of São Paulo. Shown here, well-wishers gather to welcome then Crown Prince, now Emperor of Japan, Naruhito to Liberdade, São Paulo's largest Japanese neighborhood, on June 20, 2008.

The Asahi Shimbun/Getty Images

multiculturalism
The view of cultural diversity as valuable and worth maintaining.

plural society
A society with economically interdependent ethnic groups.

and exchange with one another. When different ethnic groups exploit the *same* ecological niche, the militarily more powerful group usually will replace the weaker one. If they exploit more or less the same niche, but the weaker group is better able to use marginal environments, they also may coexist (Barth 1958/1968, p. 331). Given niche specialization, ethnic boundaries and interdependence can be maintained, although the specific cultural features of each group may change. By shifting the analytic focus from individual cultures or ethnic groups to *relationships* between cultures or ethnic groups, Barth (1958/1968, 1969) made important contributions to ethnic studies (see also Kamrava 2013).

Multiculturalism

The view of cultural diversity in a country as something good and desirable is called **multiculturalism** (see Kottak and Kozaitis 2012). The multicultural model is the opposite of the assimilationist model, in which minorities are expected to abandon their cultural traditions and values, replacing them with those of the majority population. The multicultural view encourages the practice of cultural–ethnic traditions. A multicultural society socializes individuals not only into the dominant (national) culture but also into an ethnic culture. Thus, in the United States millions of people speak both English and another language, eat both "American" foods (apple pie, steak, hamburgers) and "ethnic" dishes, and celebrate both national (July 4, Thanksgiving) and ethnic–religious holidays.

Multiculturalism seeks ways for people to understand and interact that depend not on sameness but rather on respect for differences. Multiculturalism assumes that each group has something to offer to and learn from the others. The United States and Canada have become increasingly multicultural, focusing on their internal diversity. Rather than as "melting pots," they are better described as ethnic "salads" (each ingredient remains distinct, although in the same bowl, with the same dressing).

Several forces have propelled North America away from the assimilationist model toward multiculturalism. First, multiculturalism reflects the fact of recent large-scale migration, particularly from the "less-developed" countries to the "developed" nations of North America, as well as Western Europe. The global scale of modern migration introduces unparalleled ethnic variety to host nations (see Marger 2015; Parrillo 2016). People

19th century. These immigrants have assimilated to a common Brazilian culture, which has Portuguese, African, and Native American roots. The descendants of these immigrants speak the national language (Portuguese) and participate in the national culture. (During World War II, Brazil, which was on the Allied side, forced assimilation by banning instruction in any language other than Portuguese—especially in German.) The United States was much more assimilationist during the early 20th century than it is today, as the multicultural model has become more prominent (see "Multiculturalism," later in this section).

The Plural Society

Assimilation isn't inevitable, and there can be ethnic harmony without it. Through a study of three ethnic groups in Swat, Pakistan, Fredrik Barth (1958/1968) showed that ethnic groups can be in contact for generations without assimilating and can live in peaceful coexistence.

Barth (1958/1968, p. 324) defines **plural society** (an idea he extended from Pakistan to the entire Middle East) as a society combining ethnic contrasts, ecological specialization (i.e., use of different environmental resources by each ethnic group), and the economic interdependence of those groups. In his view, ethnic boundaries are most stable and enduring when the groups occupy different ecological niches. That is, they make their living in different ways and don't compete. Ideally, they should depend on one another's activities

migrate to nations whose life-styles they learn about through the media and from tourists who increasingly visit their own countries. Much of the increasing ethnic diversity in Europe's former colonial powers, such as France and the United Kingdom, reflects migration from former colonies.

Migration also is fueled by rapid population growth, coupled with insufficient jobs (for both educated and uneducated people), in the less-developed countries. As traditional rural economies decline or mechanize, displaced farmers move to cities, where they and their children often are unable to find jobs. As people in the less-developed countries get better educations, they seek more skilled employment, often outside their country of origin. Urban migration and unemployment also fuel crime, including the growth of gangs in such countries as El Salvador in Central America. Fear of gangs then becomes a powerful push factor in migration.

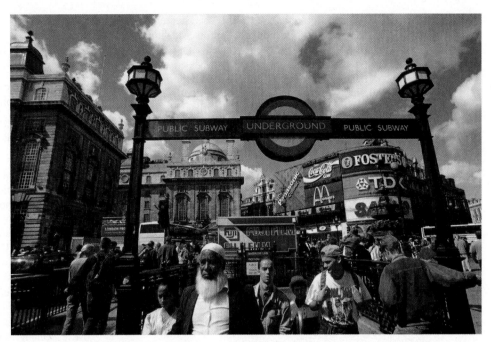

In the United States, Canada, and Western Europe, multiculturalism is of growing importance, as is suggested by this contemporary scene from London, England. Can you find evidence for both multiculturalism and globalization in this photo?
H. & D. Zielske/Alamy Stock Photo

The Backlash to Multiculturalism

When Barack Obama was first elected president of the United States in 2008, it seemed to many commentators that the United States had entered a postracial era. It was taken as a sign of progress in racial and ethnic relations that an African American man could be elected to the highest office in the land. The backlash began soon after Obama's election, culminating in Donald Trump's election as president in 2016. The period between 2008 and 2010 saw the growth of the Tea Party wing of the Republican Party and a dramatic reduction in the power of Democrats after the 2010 election. A similar coalition of young people, women, and minorities that backed Obama in 2008 and 2012 enabled Hillary Clinton to win the popular vote in 2016 but was insufficient to propel her to an Electoral College victory and the presidency.

One of the rallying cries of Tea Party voters was to "take our country back." A similar sentiment was prominent in the 2016 presidential campaign. Tycoon and reality TV star Donald Trump rose to prominence as a Republican presidential candidate by promising to "make America great again." Prominent in his campaign was open *ethno-nationalism,* the idea of an association between ethnicity—traditionally and predominantly European derived and Christian—and the right to rule the United States. Trump advocated deportation of undocumented immigrants,

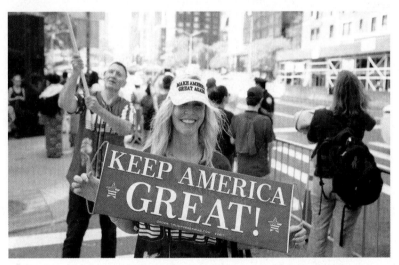

On September 23, 2019, a supporter of U.S. President Donald Trump awaits the motorcade bringing him to the United Nations building, where he would attend a gathering of world leaders. How might a sociocultural anthropologist cite features of language, ethnicity, race, and gender to explain Trump's rise to political prominence?
Kay Nietfeld/dpa/Alamy Live News

focusing on Mexicans. He envisioned a wall along the southern border of the United States to keep out Mexicans and other Latinos. He proposed various bans on Muslim entry into the United States. He blamed a global pandemic on a "Chinese virus" that he eventually referred to as "Kung Flu."

Trump and other Republican candidates also decried multiculturalism and "political correctness," which they saw as excessive caution about using language and labels that might offend particular groups. Trump, in particular, used the claim of hypersensitive political correctness to justify his stereotyping of Mexicans as "bad hombres" and of Muslims as terrorists. Anyone who complained about insults was "overreacting"—just being a hypersensitive snowflake. Trump's successful candidacy harnessed and expressed the backlash against the multicultural model of ethnic relations that has been gaining ground in the United States for the past few decades.

Rarely, if ever, does cultural change occur without opposition, and rarely does a backlash not produce a backlash of its own. Sure enough, in the 2018 midterm elections, an Obama-like voting coalition reassembled. Democrats won 24 of 35 open Senate seats, and picked up 41 seats in the House of Representatives, to take control of the latter.

CHANGING DEMOGRAPHICS IN THE UNITED STATES

In October 2006, the population of the United States reached 300 million people, just 39 years after reaching 200 million (in 1967) and 91 years after reaching the 100 million mark (in 1915). The country's ethnic composition has changed dramatically in the past 50 years. The 1970 census, the first to attempt an official count of Hispanics, found they represented no more than 4.7 percent of the American population. By 2019, this figure had risen to 18.3 percent—more than 60 million Hispanics. The percentage of African Americans grew from 11.1 percent in 1967 to 13.4 percent in 2019, while (non-Hispanic) whites ("Anglos") declined from 83 to 60.4 percent (Krogstad 2017; Quick Facts, United States Census Bureau 2019).

In 1973, 78 percent of students in American public schools were white, and 22 percent were minorities. By 2004, only 57 percent of public school students were white. In fall 2014, for the first time, the overall number of Latino, African American, and Asian students in public K–12 classrooms surpassed the number of non-Hispanic whites (Maxwell 2014).

The Gray and the Brown

In 2018, for the first time, the combined nonWhite U.S. population—Blacks, Hispanics, Asians, persons identifying as multiracial, and as some other race—constituted the dominant share (50.1 percent) of the under age *15* population (Frey 2019). Just two years later, the minority share of the American population under age *18* also passed 50 percent. The median age of non-Hispanic whites is 44 years, significantly higher than those of all other racial or ethnic groups. Latinos, in particular, are much younger, with a median age of 30 (Saenz 2020).

Drawing on a Brookings Institution (2010) report titled *State of Metropolitan America: On the Front Lines of Demographic Transformation,* Ronald Brownstein (2010) analyzes an intensifying confrontation between groups he describes as "the gray and the brown." Brownstein and demographer William Frey, an author of the Brookings report, focus on two key U.S. demographic trends (see also Frey 2019):

1. Ethnic/racial diversity is increasing, especially among the young.

2. The country is aging, and most of the senior population is white.

Frey sees these trends as creating a "cultural generation gap"—a sharp contrast in the attitudes, priorities, and political leanings of younger and older Americans (Brookings Institution 2010, pp. 26, 63; see also Vespa et al. 2020). Politically the two groups—the gray (older) and the brown (younger)—are poles apart. The aging white population appears increasingly resistant to taxes and public spending, while younger people and minorities value government support of education (e.g., free tuition at public colleges), health (e.g., Medicare for all), and social welfare. In recent presidential elections, young people, especially minorities, have strongly supported the Democratic candidates, Barack Obama (2008 and 2012) and Hillary Clinton (2016), while white seniors voted solidly for Republicans John McCain, Mitt Romney, and Donald Trump.

The history of U.S. national immigration policy helps us understand how the gap between the gray and the brown arose. Federal policies established in the 1920s had severely curtailed immigration from areas other than northern Europe. However, in 1965, Congress loosened restrictions—resulting in an eventual influx of immigrants from southern Europe, Asia, Africa, the Caribbean, and Latin America (see Vigil 2012).

Non-Hispanic whites comprised the overwhelming majority of Americans through the mid-20th century, including the post–World War II baby boom (1946–1964). Most baby boomers grew up and have lived much of their lives in white suburbs, residentially isolated from minorities (Brownstein 2010). As they age and retire, many older white Americans are reconstituting such communities in racially homogeneous enclaves in the Southeast and Southwest.

In such communities, except for their yard and construction workers and house cleaners, older white Americans live apart from the minorities who represent a growing share of the national population. Since 1965, expanded immigration and higher fertility rates among minorities have transformed American society. As recently as 1980, minorities made up only 20 percent of the total population (versus 40 percent today), and 25 percent of children under 18, versus 50 percent as of 2020. Similar trends are evident in western Europe and are everyday expressions of globalization.

The Gray Need the Brown

The gray and the brown are more interdependent economically than either usually realizes. Minority children may benefit disproportionately from public education today, but minority workers will pay a growing share of the payroll taxes needed to sustain Social Security and Medicare in the future. These are government programs that most directly benefit old white people.

The year 2030 will mark a demographic turning point for the United States (Vespa et al. 2018). By that year, all baby boomers will be older than 65 years. By 2035, for the first time in American history, old people will outnumber children. The older (65+) population of the United States is projected to nearly double in size, from 49 million today to 95 million in 2060. In percentage terms, older Americans will constitute 23 percent of the population in 2060 versus about 16 percent today. This demographic shift will affect the ratio of workers to nonworkers.

Furthermore, in coming decades, the youth dependency ratio—the number of children under 18 for every 100 working-age adults (aged 18 to 64)—is projected to shrink. By 2060 there will be only 35 children for every 100 working-age adults, versus 65 children in 1960, when the baby boom was nearing its end. As this youth ratio contracts, the aged ratio will expand. By 2060, the old-age dependency ratio will nearly double, rising from 21 today to 41. In other words, there will be 41 seniors for every 100 adults of working age. Unless working patterns change substantially, the overall dependency ratio among Americans (35 children + 41 seniors per 100 workers) will be significantly higher than it is today (Vespa et al. 2018).

Immigration will be needed to supply workers for this increasingly dependent population. The aging of America explains why immigration is projected to overtake (probably around 2030) natural increase (the number of births over deaths) as the main engine that drives U.S. population growth. And the "gray" will become increasingly "brown." As its deaths exceed its births, the non-Hispanic white population is projected to shrink from 199 million (60.7 percent) in 2020 to 179 million (44.3 percent) in 2060 (see Figure 6.5), even as the overall U.S. population grows (slowly) (Vespa et al. 2018). Can you speculate about if and how the political orientations of American minorities are likely to change as they, too, age during coming decades?

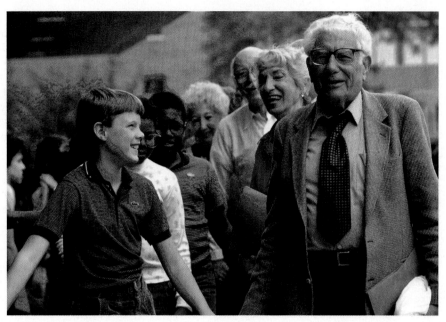

In this recent American photo, contrast the visible ethnic diversity in the line of children with the racially more uniform line of older people.

James Marshall/Corbis

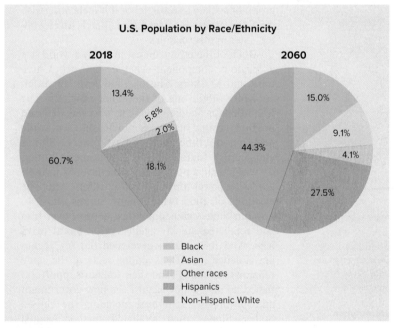

FIGURE 6.5 Ethnic Composition of the United States.
The proportion of the American population that is white and non-Hispanic is declining. The projection for 2060 shown here comes from a 2018 report. Note especially the dramatic rise in the Hispanic and Asian portions of the American population between 2018 and 2060.

2018 data from Population Estimates, Quick Facts, United States Census Bureau, July 1, 2018; 2060 projection from Vespa, J., D. M. Armstrong, and L. Medina. 2018. Demographic Turning Points for the United States: Population Projections for 2020 to 2060, U.S. Census Bureau, Current Population Reports P25-1144, March.

ETHNIC CONFLICT

Ethnic differences can exist harmoniously, for example, in plural societies or through multiculturalism. However, ethnic differences also can lead to interethnic confrontation and discrimination. The perception of cultural differences can have disastrous effects on social interaction. Why are ethnic differences often associated with conflict and violence? Ethnic groups may compete economically and/or politically. An ethnic group may react if it perceives prejudice or discrimination by another

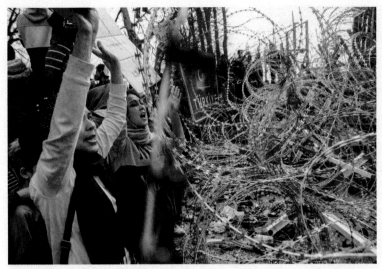

On March 6, 2020, refugees and would-be migrants protest at the Greek border fence in Edirne, Turkey. Thousands of refugees approached this border after Turkey announced that it would open border gates for 72 hours to allow refugees to continue their journey into Europe.

Burak Kara/Getty Images

group or society as a whole, or if it feels otherwise devalued or disadvantaged (see "Black Lives Matter" later in this section).

Much of the ethnic unrest in today's world has a religious component—whether between Christians and Muslims, Muslims and Jews, or different sects within one of the major religions. The Iraqi dictator Saddam Hussein, who was deposed in 2003, favored his own Sunni Muslim sect while fostering discrimination against others (Shiites and Kurds). Sunnis, although a numeric minority within Iraq's population, were favored in their access to power, prestige, and position. After the elections of 2005, which many Sunnis chose to boycott, Shiites gained political control over Iraq and retaliated quickly against prior Sunni privilege. A civil war soon developed out of "sectarian violence" (conflicts among sects of the same religion) as Sunnis (and their foreign supporters) fueled an insurgency against the new government and its foreign supporters, including the United States. Shiites then retaliated further against Sunni attacks and a history of Sunni favoritism. The Sunnis, lacking power in the new Iraqi government, eventually helped form the so-called Islamic state (IS), also known as ISIS, ISIL, and Daesh.

Iraq and Syria each contain substantial Muslim populations of Shiites, Sunnis, and Kurds (along with various ethno-religious minorities). Syria's president, Bashar al-Assad, like his father and predecessor in office, Hafez al-Assad (who ruled from 1971 to 2000), has favored his own minority Muslim group (Alawites—allied with the Shiites) over his country's Sunni majority. Syria has experienced devastating internal warfare since 2011, when, as in other parts of the Middle East, a series of uprisings known collectively as the Arab Spring

arose in opposition to authoritarian governments. The Assad regime fanned the flames of civil war by its violent suppression of the protesters and eventual rebels.

The parties to the conflict in Syria have included (1) the Assad government and its foreign allies, including Russia, Shiite Iran, and the Lebanese militia Hezbollah; (2) Sunni-led ISIS, whose influence (now substantially reduced) was strongest in parts of northern and eastern Syria, adjacent to and extending into Iraq; and (3) "moderate" rebels, presumably including Sunnis opposed to both Assad and ISIS. These rebels, whose numbers, commitment, and effectiveness are unclear, have been supported by the United States and other Sunni-majority countries in the Middle East. Finally, (4) the Kurds, who have been particularly effective in the fight against ISIS.

The Syrian conflict has displaced at least half of Syria's population of 23 million. Some 6.3 million people have been uprooted internally, while more than 5 million others have fled Syria as refugees. The latter have sought refuge primarily in other Middle Eastern countries, including Turkey, Lebanon, Jordan, Iraq, and Egypt. Other Syrian refugees have traveled by boat across the Aegean Sea to the Greek islands and mainland, and from there into Europe via the Balkans. Others have crossed the Mediterranean into Italy, and some have crossed from North Africa to Spain. Sweden and, particularly, Germany have been the most welcoming European countries. In Syria itself, if Assad eventually vacates the presidency, Sunni reprisals are likely against Alawites and other religious minorities, including Christians and Shiite Muslims.

Prejudice and Discrimination

Members of an ethnic group may be the targets of prejudice (negative attitudes and judgments) or discrimination (punitive action). **Prejudice** means devaluing (looking down on) a group because of its assumed behavior, values, capabilities, or attributes. People are prejudiced when they hold stereotypes about groups and apply them to individuals. (**Stereotypes** are fixed ideas—often unfavorable—about what the members of a group are like.) Prejudiced people assume that members of the group will act as they are "supposed to act" (according to the stereotype) and interpret a wide range of individual behaviors as evidence of the stereotype. They use this behavior to confirm their stereotype (and low opinion) of the group.

Discrimination refers to policies and practices that harm a group and its members. Discrimination may be legally sanctioned—*de jure* (part of the law), or it may be *de facto* (practiced, but not legally sanctioned). Segregation in the southern United States and *apartheid* in South Africa provide two historical examples of de jure discrimination. In both systems, by law, blacks and whites

prejudice
Devaluing a group because of its assumed attributes.

stereotypes
Fixed ideas—often unfavorable—about what members of a group are like.

discrimination
Policies and practices that harm a group and its members.

had different rights and privileges. Also, their social interaction ("mixing") was legally curtailed. An example of de facto discrimination is the harsher treatment that American minorities (compared with other Americans) tend to get from the police and the judicial system. This unequal treatment isn't legal, but it happens anyway, as the next section documents.

Black Lives Matter

Anyone who follows the news regularly will have heard of a series of cases in which African Americans, mostly young men, have been shot dead by (usually white) police officers. The "Black Lives Matter" movement arose in the United States in response to these and other incidents in which Black lives have not seemed to matter much to local officials. As described by Elizabeth Day (2015), the movement originated in July 2013, when an African American woman named Alicia Garza reacted to the acquittal of George Zimmerman, a neighborhood watch volunteer, in the shooting of Trayvon Martin, an unarmed Black teenager, in Sanford, Florida. Stunned by Zimmerman's acquittal on charges of second-degree murder and manslaughter, Garza posted the following message on Facebook: "Black people. I love you. I love us. Our lives matter."

Garza's friend Patrisse Cullors adopted Garza's words and began to post them online using the hashtag #blacklivesmatter. The two women wanted to raise public awareness about the apparent devaluation of Black lives in the American judicial and enforcement systems. Using Facebook, Tumblr, and Twitter, Garza and Cullors encouraged users to share stories of why #blacklivesmatter. In August 2014, another unarmed African American teenager, 18-year-old Michael Brown, was killed by 12 rounds of ammunition from the gun of a white police officer in Ferguson, Missouri. Garza helped organize a "Freedom Ride" to Ferguson that brought some 500 people to the St. Louis suburb. On arrival, she was astonished to see her own phrase being shouted by protesters and written on their banners. There were additional protests in Ferguson after a grand jury failed to indict the white police officer. Thereafter, with a series of additional cases in which unarmed Black men were shot by white police officers, the slogan "Black Lives Matter" rose to national prominence. The American Dialect Society even named #blacklivesmatter as their word of the year for 2014. By 2016, Black Lives Matter chapters had opened throughout the country (Day 2015).

The movement has grown not only in response to police shootings and brutality but also following the mass murder on June 17, 2015, of nine African American churchgoers in Charleston, South Carolina, by a white supremacist domestic terrorist. That tragic event prompted the governor to call for and achieve the removal of a contentious and

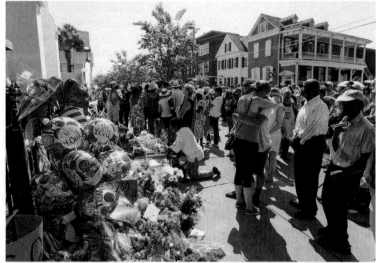

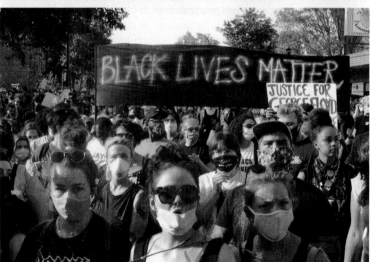

Top: People gather outside the Emanuel AME Church prior to the first service following the mass murder (on June 21, 2015) of nine unarmed African American congregants by an avowed white supremacist. *Bottom:* Demonstrators protest the death of George Floyd on June 5, 2020 in Minneapolis, Minnesota. Floyd died while in police custody on May 25, after former Minneapolis police officer Derek Chauvin kneeled on his neck for nearly nine minutes while detaining him. Floyd's death sparked weeks of demonstrations and protests nationally and internationally and gave new impetus to the Black Lives Matter (BLM) movement.

(top): Cem Ozdel/Anadolu Agency/Getty Images; (bottom): Scott Olson/Getty Images

racially charged symbol, the Confederate battle flag, from prominent display in the state capital, Columbia.

Social media continue to be prominent in linking and organizing the #blacklivesmatter movement. Activists have been able to respond quickly to an ongoing series of widely reported incidents (e.g., in Cleveland, Baltimore, North Charleston, and Chicago, and more recently in Baton Rouge, Louisiana; Falcon Heights, Minnesota; South Bend, Indiana; Minneapolis, Louisville, Atlanta, and Kenosha, Wisconsin—tragically, the list continues to grow) in which Black people have been killed by police or died in police custody. Most notably, the death of George Floyd on May 25, 2020 in Minneapolis, Minnesota while in police custody sparked weeks of demonstrations and protests nationally and internationally and gave new impetus to the Black Lives Matter (BLM) movement. Former Minneapolis police officer Derek Chauvin killed Floyd by kneeling on his neck for almost nine minutes while detaining him, while three other police officers watched. All four officers were fired one day after Floyd's murder. Subsequently, Derek Chauvin was charged with second-degree murder; and the three other former officers, with aiding and abetting murder.

Critics of the BLM movement contended that not only "Black lives" but "all lives" should matter, as indeed they should. However, this criticism ignores, and would diminish needed attention to, the disproportionate likelihood of arrest, incarceration, mistreatment, injury, and death by cop that African Americans, in particular, face. Americans have not heard in recent years a series of reports about unarmed white men being shot or choked to death by police officers. Even if discrimination against American minorities is no longer *de jure,* it certainly remains *de facto.*

Anti-ethnic Discrimination

This section considers some of the more extreme forms of anti-ethnic discrimination, including genocide, forced assimilation, ethnocide, ethnic expulsion, and cultural colonialism (see also Lange 2017). The most extreme form is **genocide,** the deliberate elimination of a group (such as Jews in Nazi Germany, Muslims in Bosnia, or Tutsi in Rwanda) through mass murder (see Bachman 2019; Hinton and O'Neill 2009; Jones 2017).

Most of us are familiar with the genocidal Holocaust carried out by the Nazis during World War II. The Bosnian and Rwandan genocides are less well-known. Until 1992, Bosnia was part of Yugoslavia, a nonaligned Socialist country outside the former Soviet Union (USSR). Like the USSR, Yugoslavia began to fall apart, mainly along ethnic and religious lines, in the early 1990s. Among Yugoslavia's ethnic groups were Roman Catholic Croats, Eastern Orthodox Serbs, Muslim Slavs (Bosniaks), and ethnic Albanians. Separating from Yugoslavia in 1991–92 were Slovenia, Croatia, and Bosnia-Herzegovina—all now independent countries. The Yugoslav Serbs reacted violently, with military intervention, after a 1992 vote for the independence of Muslim-led Bosnia, whose population is one-third Serbian, but with a Bosniak majority of over 40 percent. Bosnian Serbs initiated a policy of forced expulsion—"ethnic cleansing"—against Croats, but mainly against Bosniaks. Yugoslav Serbs, who controlled the national army, supported the Bosnian Serbs in their ethnic cleansing, which culminated in the massacre of some 7,000 Bosniak men and boys in the town of Srebrenica in July 1995. This was the worst wartime atrocity and genocide in Europe since World War II and the Holocaust. With Bosnia's capital, the multiethnic city of Sarajevo, under siege, the conflict was suspended after a December 1995 settlement was signed in Dayton, Ohio.

Over a period of about 100 days in Rwanda (East Africa) in 1994, extremist members of the Hutu ethnic majority hunted down and slaughtered an estimated 800,000 members of the Tutsi minority. Constituting just 15 percent of the Rwandan population, the Tutsi, like the Sunni Muslims in Iraq under Saddam Hussein, traditionally had enjoyed favored access to wealth and political power. Political disputes and ethnic resentment fueled the Rwandan genocide.

More recently, in the Darfur region of western Sudan, government-supported Arab militias, called the *Janjaweed,* have forced black Africans off their land. The militias are accused of genocide, of killing up to 30,000 darker-skinned Africans.

Ethnocide is the deliberate suppression or destruction of an ethnic culture by a dominant group. One way of implementing a policy of ethnocide is through *forced assimilation,* in which the dominant group forces an ethnic group to adopt the dominant culture. Many countries have penalized or banned the language and customs of an ethnic group (including its religious observances). One example of forced assimilation is the anti-Basque campaign that the dictator Francisco Franco (who ruled between 1939 and 1975) waged in Spain. Franco banned Basque books, journals, newspapers, signs, sermons, and tombstones and imposed fines for using the Basque language in schools. In reaction to his policies, nationalist sentiment strengthened in the Basque region, and a Basque terrorist group took shape.

A policy of *ethnic expulsion* aims at removing from a country groups that are culturally different. There are many examples, including Bosnia-Herzegovina in the 1990s. Uganda expelled 74,000 Asians in 1972. The neofascist parties of contemporary Western Europe advocate repatriation (expulsion) of immigrant workers, such as Algerians in France and Turks in Germany. As of this writing (2020), the United States contains approximately 11 million undocumented immigrants. They are here without documents because they overstayed their visas or work permits, entered unofficially, or were smuggled in. Millions of them work, pay taxes, and have children born in the United States, who are American citizens. What are their prospects? The future of undocumented immigrants became a particularly contentious political issue during the 2016 presidential election. More than one of the Republican candidates for president advocated their mass deportation. No one explained the logistics of deporting 11 million people. Such deportation would be a form of forced expulsion, although America's undocumented immigrants come from many countries and lack legal documents granting them the right to remain in the United States.

Ethnocide
The deliberate suppression or destruction of an ethnic culture by a dominant group.

genocide
The deliberate elimination of a group through mass murder.

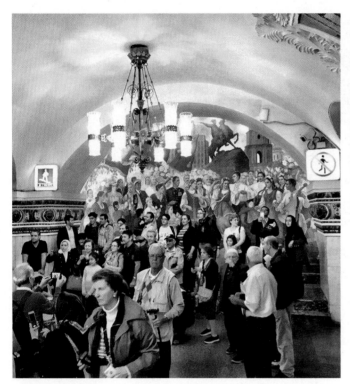

The author took the photo above in August 2017 in a Moscow metro station named for Kiev, the Ukrainian capital. A group of tourists from the former Soviet Union pose in front of a colorful mosaic depicting Ukrainian folk life and friendly Russian soldiers.

Conrad P. Kottak

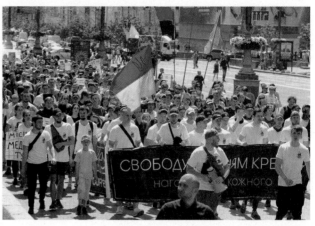

In the photo above, taken on June 1, 2019 in Kiev, Ukraine, activists and relatives of Ukrainians captured and jailed by Russia (in Russia, the Crimea, and Eastern Ukraine) carry placards with the prisoners' names and portraits. This "Freedom for the Kremlin Prisoners!" march urged the Ukrainian government to intensify its efforts to secure the release of those prisoners..

NurPhoto/Getty Images

When members of an ethnic group are expelled, they often become **refugees**—people who have been forced (involuntary refugees) or who have chosen (voluntary refugees) to flee a country, to escape persecution or war. A government policy of ethnic expulsion is only one source of refugees. The Syrian refugees discussed previously have been driven from their homes by civil war and reprisals by various factions and their foreign allies. They are not, by and large, voluntary refugees, but they were not forced out by a government policy of ethnic expulsion.

Cultural colonialism refers to the internal domination by one group and its culture or ideology over others. One example is how the Russian people, language, and culture and the communist ideology dominated the former Soviet empire. In cultural colonialism, the dominant culture makes itself the official culture. This is reflected in schools, the media, and public interaction. Under Soviet rule, ethnic minorities had very limited self-rule in republics and regions controlled by Moscow. All the republics and their peoples were to be united by the oneness of "socialist internationalism." A common technique in cultural colonialism is to flood ethnic areas with members of the dominant ethnic group. In the former Soviet Union, ethnic Russian colonists were sent to many areas, to diminish the cohesion and clout of the local people.

For example, when Ukraine belonged to the Soviet Union, Moscow promoted a policy of Russian in-migration and Ukrainian out-migration, so that ethnic Ukrainians' share of the population of Ukraine declined from 77 percent in 1959 to 73 percent in 1991. That trend reversed after Ukraine gained independence, so that, by the turn of the 21st century, ethnic Ukrainians made up more than three-fourths of their country's population. Russians still constitute Ukraine's largest minority, but they now represent less than one-fifth of the population. They are concentrated in eastern Ukraine, where ethnic Russians have rebelled against Ukraine's pro-Western government. Eastern Ukraine, especially those provinces dominated by the Russian language and ethnicity, is considered a potential target of Russian annexation. In 2014, Russia did annex Crimea, where ethnic Russians (constituting more than 60 percent of the Crimean population) and the Russian language dominate. Recap 6.3 summarizes the various types of ethnic interaction—positive and negative—that have been discussed.

The fall of the Soviet Union in 1991 was accompanied by a resurgence of ethnic feeling among formally dominated groups. The ethnic groups and nationalities once controlled by Moscow have sought, and continue to seek, to forge their own separate and viable nation-states. This celebration of ethnic autonomy is part of an ethnic florescence that—as surely as globalization and transnationalism—is a trend of the late 20th and early 21st centuries. The new assertiveness of long-resident ethnic groups extends to the Welsh and Scots in the United Kingdom, Bretons and Corsicans in France, and Basques and Catalans in Spain.

refugees
People who flee a country to escape persecution or war.

cultural colonialism
The internal domination by one group and its culture or ideology over others.

TYPE	NATURE OF INTERACTION	EXAMPLES
POSITIVE		
Assimilation	Ethnic groups absorbed within dominant culture	Brazil; United States in early, mid-20th century
Plural society	Society or region contains economically interdependent ethnic groups	Areas of Middle East with farmers/herders; Swat, Pakistan
Multiculturalism	Cultural diversity valued; ethnic cultures coexist with dominant culture	Canada; United States in 21st century
NEGATIVE		
Prejudice	Devaluing a group based on assumed attributes	Worldwide
Discrimination de jure	Legal policies and practices harm ethnic group	South African apartheid; former segregation in southern United States.
Discrimination de facto	Not legally sanctioned but practiced	Worldwide
Genocide	Deliberate elimination of ethnic group through mass murder	Nazi Germany; Bosnia; Rwanda; Cambodia; Darfur
Ethnocide	Cultural practices attacked by dominant culture or colonial power	Spanish Basques under Franco
Ethnic expulsion	Forcing ethnic group(s) out of a country or region	Ugandan Asians; Serbia; Bosnia; Kosovo

for REVIEW

summary

1. *Ethnic group* refers to members of a particular culture in a nation or region that contains others. Ethnicity is based on cultural similarities (among members of the same ethnic group) and differences (between that group and others). A race is an ethnic group assumed to have a biological basis.

2. Because of a range of problems involved in classifying humans into racial categories, contemporary biologists focus on specific differences and try to explain them. Because of extensive gene flow and interbreeding, *Homo sapiens* has not evolved subspecies or distinct races.

3. Biological similarities between groups may reflect—rather than common ancestry—similar but independent adaptations to similar natural selective forces, such as degrees of ultraviolet radiation from the sun in the case of skin color.

4. Human races are cultural (rather than biological) categories that derive from contrasts perceived in particular societies. Racial labels such as *white* and *Black* designate socially constructed races—categories defined by American culture. In American racial classification, governed by the rule of hypodescent, children of mixed unions, no matter what their appearance, are classified with the minority group parent.

5. Racial attitudes in Japan illustrate intrinsic racism—the belief that a perceived racial difference is a sufficient reason to value one person less than another. The valued group is majority (pure) Japanese, who define themselves in opposition to others, anyone who is "not us." In Brazil, racial identity is more of an achieved status, which can change during someone's lifetime, reflecting phenotypical changes.

6. The term *nation,* which once was synonymous with *ethnic group,* now means a state—a centrally organized political unit. Most nation-states are not ethnically homogeneous. Ethnic groups that seek autonomous political status are nationalities.

7. An ethnic group may undergo assimilation when it moves to a country where another culture dominates. It adopts the patterns and norms of its host culture. A plural society combines ethnic contrasts and economic interdependence between ethnic groups. Multiculturalism socializes individuals not only into the dominant (national) culture but also into an ethnic one.

8. Ethnic conflict often arises in reaction to prejudice (attitudes and judgments) or discrimination (action). The most extreme form of ethnic discrimination is genocide, the deliberate elimination of a group through mass murder. A dominant group may try to destroy certain ethnic practices (ethnocide), or to force ethnic group members to adopt the dominant culture (forced assimilation). *Cultural colonialism* refers to internal domination by one group and its culture or ideology over others.

key terms

1. What's the difference between a culture and an ethnic group? In what culture(s) do you participate? To what ethnic group(s) do you belong? What is the basis of your primary cultural identity? Do others readily recognize this basis and identity? Why or why not?
2. Describe three problems with human racial classification.
3. What explains skin color in humans? Are the processes that determined skin color in humans still continuing today? If so, what are some examples of this?
4. Would "All Lives Matter" be a useful slogan for a civil rights movement? How might social media function in organizing social and political movements?
5. This chapter describes different types of ethnic interaction. What are they? Are they positive or negative? Anthropologists have made and continue to make important contributions to understanding past and ongoing cases of ethnic conflict. What are some examples of this?

think like an anthropologist

Design Elements: Understanding Ourselves: muha/123RF (rock paintings); Focus on Globalization: janrysavy/ Getty Images (globe); Appreciating Diversity (left to right): Floresco Productions/age footstock; Hero/Corbis/ Glow Images, Hill Street Studios/Blend Images, Billion Photos/Shutterstock; Understanding Ourselves : Hemera Technologies/Alamy (Cymbal), LACMA - Los Angeles County Museum of Art (Trefoil Oinochoe), Ingram Publishing/SuperStock (Coin), ChuckSchugPhotography/Getty Images (Rug).

credits

Making a Living

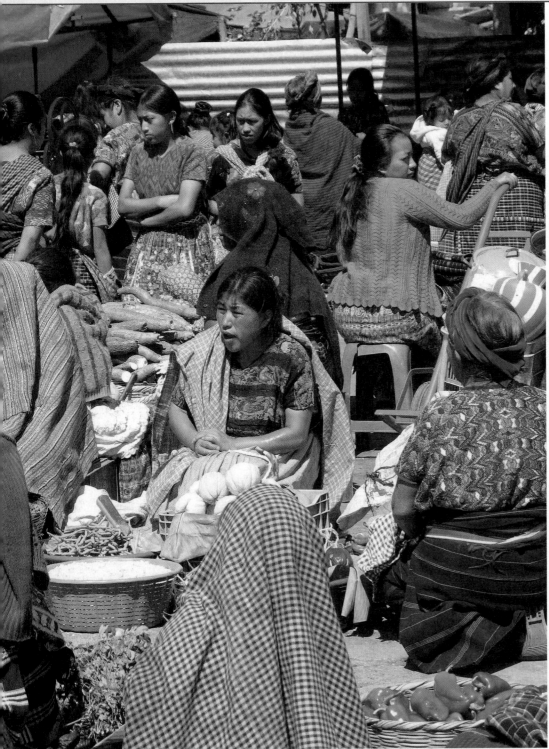

▶ How do people make a living in different types of society?

▶ What is an economy, and what is economizing behavior?

▶ What principles regulate the exchange of goods and services in various societies?

Lissa Harrison

A Guatemalan outdoor vegetable market with vendors and shoppers buying and selling produce.

understanding OURSELVES

The necessities of work, marriage, and raising children are fundamental. However, in the non-Western societies where the study of anthropology originated, the need to balance work (economy) and family (society) wasn't as stark as it is for us. In traditional societies, one's workmates usually were also one's kin. There was no need for a "take your child to work" day, because most women did that every day. People didn't work with strangers. Home and office, society and economy, were intertwined.

The fact that subsistence and sociality are both basic human needs creates conflicts in modern society. People have to make choices about allocating their time and energy between work and family. Parents in dual-earner and single-parent households always have faced a work–family time bind, and the number of Americans living in such households has doubled in recent decades. Fewer than one-third of American wives worked outside the home in 1960, compared with almost twice that fraction today. That same year, only one-fifth of married women with children under age 6 were in the workforce, versus three-fifths today.

Think about the choices your parents have made in terms of economic versus social goals. Have their decisions maximized their incomes, their lifestyles, their individual happiness, family benefits, or what? What about you? What factors motivated you when you chose to apply to and attend college? Did you want to stay close to home, to attend college with friends, or to maintain a romantic attachment (all social reasons)? Did you seek the lowest tuition and college costs—or get a generous scholarship (economic decisions)? Did you choose prestige, or perhaps the likelihood that one day you would earn more money because of the reputation of your alma mater (maximizing prestige and future wealth)? Economists tend to assume that the profit motive rules in contemporary society. However, different individuals, like different cultures, may choose to pursue goals other than monetary gain.

Studies show that most American women now expect to join the paid labor force, just as men do. But the family remains attractive. Many young women also plan to stay home with small children and return to the workforce once their children enter school. How about you? If you have definite career plans, how do you imagine your work will fit in with your future family life—if you have one planned? What do your parents want most for you—a successful career or a happy family life with children? Probably both. Will it be easy to fulfill such expectations?

Communities and societies throughout the world are being incorporated, at an accelerating rate, into larger systems (Caldararo 2014). The first major acceleration in the growth of human social systems can be traced back to around 12,000–10,000 years ago, when humans started intervening in the reproductive cycles of plants and animals. Food production refers to human control over the reproduction of plants and animals, and it contrasts with the foraging economies that preceded it and that still persist in some parts of the world today.

To make their living, foragers hunt, gather, and collect what nature has to offer. Foragers may harvest, but they don't plant. They may hunt animals, but (except for the dog) they don't domesticate them. Only food producers systematically select and breed for desirable traits in the plants they cultivate and the animals they keep and herd. The origin and spread of

food production (plant cultivation and animal domestication) accelerated human population growth and led to the formation of larger and more powerful social and political systems. The pace of cultural transformation increased enormously. This chapter provides a framework for understanding a variety of human adaptive strategies and economic systems.

ADAPTIVE STRATEGIES

The anthropologist Yehudi Cohen (1974) used the term *adaptive strategy* to describe a society's main system of economic production. He argued that the most important reason for social and cultural similarities among unrelated societies is their possession of a similar adaptive strategy. In other words, similar economies have similar sociocultural characteristics. For example, there are clear similarities among societies that have a foraging (hunting and gathering) strategy. Cohen developed a classification or *typology* of societies based on correlations between their economies and their social features. His typology includes these five adaptive strategies: foraging, horticulture, agriculture, pastoralism, and industrialism. Industrialism is the focus of the last two chapters of this book. The present chapter focuses on the first four adaptive strategies, which are characteristic of nonindustrial societies.

FORAGING

Foraging—an economy and way of life based on hunting and gathering—was humans' only way of making a living until about 12,000 years ago, when people began experimenting with food production. To be sure, environmental differences created substantial contrasts among foragers living in different parts of the world (see Kelly 2013). Some, like the people who lived in Europe during the ice ages, were big-game hunters (see Lemke 2018). Today, foragers in the Arctic still focus on large animals. They also fish, but their diets are much less varied, with fewer plant foods, than those of tropical foragers.

Animal domestication (initially of sheep and goats) and plant cultivation (of wheat and barley) began 12,000 to 10,000 years ago in the Middle East. Cultivation based on different crops, such as corn (maize), manioc (cassava), and potatoes, arose independently in the Americas. In both hemispheres, most societies eventually turned from foraging to food production. Today most foragers have at least some dependence on food production or on food producers (Codding and Kramer 2016; Kent 1996).

Foraging economies survived into modern times in certain forests, deserts, islands, and very cold areas—places where cultivation was not practicable with simple technology (see Ikeya and Hitchcock 2016; Lee and Daly 1999). Figure 7.1 presents a partial distribution of recent foragers. Their habitats tend to have one thing in common—their *marginality*. Posing major obstacles to food production, these environments did not attract farmers or herders. The difficulties of cultivating at the North Pole are obvious. In southern Africa, the Dobe Ju/'hoansi San area studied by Richard Lee and others is surrounded by a huge waterless belt (Solway and Lee 1990). Farming could not exist in much of California without irrigation, which is why its native populations were foragers.

We should not assume that foragers will inevitably turn to food production once they learn of its existence. In fact, foragers in many areas have been—and still are—in contact with farmers or herders, but they have chosen to maintain their foraging lifestyle. Their traditional economy supported them well enough, lacked the greater labor requirements associated with farming and herding, and provided an adequate and nutritious diet. In some places, people tried food production, only to abandon it eventually and return to foraging.

Today, all foragers live in nation-states. Typically, they are in contact with food-producing neighbors as well as with missionaries and other outsiders. We should not view contemporary foragers as isolated or pristine survivors of the Stone Age. Modern foragers are influenced by national and international policies and political and economic events in the world system.

Geographic Distribution of Foragers

It will be helpful to refer to Figure 7.1 throughout this section. Africa contains two broad belts of contemporary or recent foraging. One is the Kalahari Desert of southern Africa. This is the home of the San ("Bushmen"), who include the Ju/'hoansi (see Barnard 2019; Kent 1996; Lee 2012, 2013). The other main African foraging area is the equatorial forest of central and eastern Africa, home of the Mbuti, Efe, and other "pygmies" (Bailey et al. 1989; Turnbull 1965).

People still do, or until recently did, subsistence foraging in certain remote forests in Madagascar, South and Southeast Asia, Malaysia, and the Philippines, and on certain islands off the Indian coast. In addition, some of the best-known recent foragers are the Aborigines of Australia. Those Native Australians lived on their island continent for 65,000 years without developing food production.

The Western Hemisphere also had recent foragers. The Eskimos, or Inuit, of Alaska and Canada are well-known hunters. These (and other) northern foragers now use modern technology, including rifles and snowmobiles, in their subsistence activities. The native populations of the North Pacific Coast of North America (northern California, Oregon, Washington, British Columbia, and

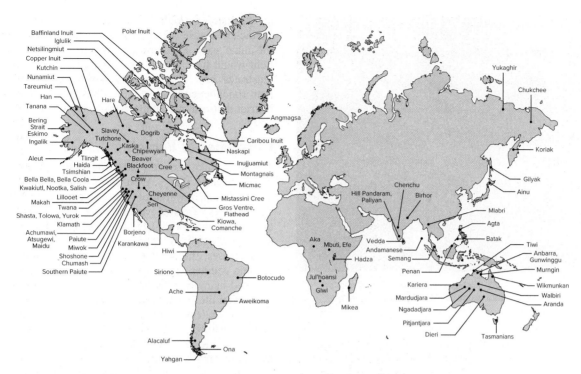

FIGURE 7.1 Worldwide Distribution of Selected Hunter-Gatherers.

southern Alaska) all were foragers, as were those of inland subarctic Canada and the Great Lakes. For many Native Americans, fishing, hunting, and gathering remain important subsistence (and sometimes commercial) activities. Considering South America, there were coastal foragers along that continent's southern tip, in Patagonia. Additional foragers inhabited the grassy plains of Argentina, southern Brazil, Uruguay, and Paraguay.

Jana Fortier (2009) summarizes key attributes of foragers in South Asia, which today is home to more full- and part-time hunter-gatherers than any other world area. In India, Nepal, and Sri Lanka, about 40 societies and an estimated 150,000 people continue to derive their subsistence from full- or part-time foraging. Hill Kharias and Yanadis are the largest contemporary South Asian foraging populations, with about 20,000 members each. Several other ethnic groups are highly endangered, with fewer than 350 members still doing subsistence foraging.

Surviving South Asian foraging societies are those whose members, despite having lost many of their natural resources to deforestation and spreading farming populations, have been unwilling to adopt food cultivation and its cultural correlates. These hunter-gatherers share features with other foragers worldwide: small social groups, mobile settlement patterns, sharing of resources, immediate food consumption, egalitarianism, and decision making by mutual consent (Fortier 2009; Widlock 2017).

As is true elsewhere, specific foraging techniques reflect variations in environment and resource distribution. Foragers living in the hills and mountains of South Asia focus their hunting on medium-sized prey (langur monkey, macaque,

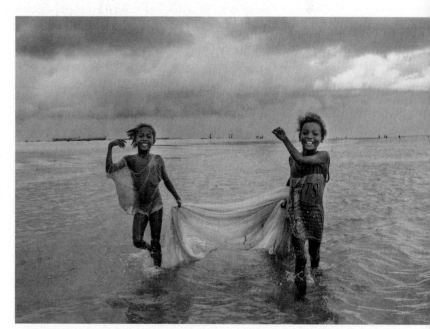

In southwestern Madagascar, two young Vezo girls (members of a maritime ethnic group) fish in the coastal waters of the Mozambique Channel, which separates Madagascar from Africa.

Cristina Mittermeier/National Geographic Creative

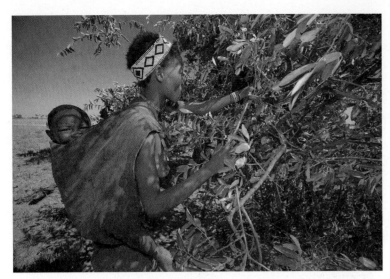

Gathering: This photo, taken in April, 2012, shows a Ju/'hoansi (San) woman picking berries from a bush on the open plains of the Kalahari, Botswana.

Neil Aldridge/Alamy Stock Photo

correlation
An association; when one variable changes, another does, too.

band
The basic social unit among foragers; fewer than a hundred people; may split up seasonally.

porcupine). Other groups pursue smaller species or practice broad-spectrum hunting of bats, porcupines, and deer. Larger groups use communal hunting techniques, such as spreading nets over large fig trees to entangle sleeping bats. Some South Indian foragers focus on such wild plant resources as yams, palms, and taro, in addition to more than 100 locally available plants. Harvesting honey and beeswax has been prominent in many South Asian foraging societies (Fortier 2009).

Their members cherish their identities as people who forage for a living in biologically rich and diverse environments. They stress their need for ongoing access to rich forest resources to continue their lifestyles, yet many have been evicted from their traditional habitats. Their best chances for cultural survival depend on national governments that maintain healthy forests, allow foragers access to their traditional natural resources, and foster cultural survival rather than assimilation (Fortier 2009).

Some governments have done quite the opposite. For example, between 1997 and 2002, the government of Botswana (in southern Africa) carried out a relocation scheme affecting about 3,000 Basarwa San Bushmen (Motseta 2006). The government forced these people to leave their ancestral territory, which became a wildlife reserve. After some of them sued, Botswana's High Court eventually ruled that the Basarwa had been wrongly evicted, and issued a court order allowing them to return, but under very restrictive conditions. Although 3,000 people had been moved out, only the 189 people who actually filed the lawsuit were granted an automatic right of return with their children. The many other Basarwa San who wanted to return to their ancestral territory would need to apply for special permits. Even the 189 favored people would be allowed to build only temporary structures and to use just enough water

for subsistence needs. Water would be a major obstacle, because the government had shut down the main well. Furthermore, anyone wishing to hunt would have to apply for a permit. This case illustrates how contemporary governments can limit the independence of indigenous peoples and restrict their traditional lifestyle.

Correlates of Foraging

Typologies like Cohen's adaptive strategies are useful because they suggest **correlations**—that is, association or covariation between two or more variables. (Correlated variables are factors that are linked and interrelated, such as food intake and body weight, such that when one increases or decreases, the other changes as well.) Ethnographic studies in hundreds of societies have revealed many correlations between the economy and social life. Associated (correlated) with each adaptive strategy is a bundle of particular sociocultural features. Correlations, however, rarely are perfect. Some foragers lack cultural features usually associated with foraging, and some of those features are found in groups with other adaptive strategies.

What are some correlates of foraging? Foragers often, but not always, lived in band-organized societies. Their basic social unit, the **band,** was a small group of fewer than a hundred people, all related by kinship or marriage. Among some foragers, band size stayed about the same year-round. In others, the band split up for part of the year. Families left to gather resources that were better exploited by just a few people. Later, they regrouped for cooperative work and ceremonies.

Typical characteristics of the foraging life are flexibility and mobility. In many San groups, as among the Mbuti of Congo, people shifted band membership several times in a lifetime. One might be born, for example, in a band in which one's mother had kin. Later, one's family might move to a band in which the father had relatives. Because bands were exogamous (people married outside their own band), one's parents came from two different bands, and one's grandparents might have come from four. People could join any band to which they had kin or marital links. A couple could live in, or shift between, the husband's band and the wife's band.

Foraging societies tend to be *egalitarian.* That is, they make few status distinctions, and the ones they make are based mainly on age, gender, and personal qualities or achievements. For example, old people—elders—may receive respect as guardians of myths, legends, stories, and traditions. Younger people may value the elders' special knowledge of ritual and practical matters. A good hunter, an especially productive gatherer, or a skilled midwife or shaman may be recognized as such. But foragers are known for sharing rather than bragging. Their status distinctions are not associated with differences in wealth and power, nor are they inherited. When considering issues of "human nature," we should remember that the egalitarian society associated with foraging was a basic form of human social life for most of our history. Food production has existed less than 1 percent of the time *Homo* has spent on Earth. However, it has produced huge social differences. We now consider the main economic features of food-producing strategies.

ADAPTIVE STRATEGIES BASED ON FOOD PRODUCTION

The three adaptive strategies based on food production in nonindustrial societies are horticulture, agriculture, and pastoralism. With horticulture and agriculture, plant cultivation is the mainstay of the economy, whereas with pastoralism, herding is key. All three strategies originated in nonindustrial societies, although they may persist as ways of making a living even after some degree of industrialization reaches the nation-states that include them. In fully industrial societies, such as the United States and Canada, most cultivation has become large-scale, commercial, mechanized, agrochemical-dependent farming. Rather than simple pastoralism, industrial societies use technologically sophisticated systems of ranch and livestock management.

A society's adaptive strategy (e.g., pastoralism) refers to its *primary* way of making a living, even though its people may also engage in other economic activities. Pastoralists (herders), for example, consume milk, blood, and meat from their animals as mainstays of their diet. However, they also add plant food to their diet by doing some cultivating or by trading with neighbors.

Horticulture

The two types of plant cultivation found in nonindustrial societies are **horticulture** (nonintensive, shifting cultivation) and **agriculture** (intensive, continuous cultivation). Both differ from the commercially oriented farming systems of industrial nations, which use large land areas and rely on machinery and petrochemicals.

Horticulture is cultivation that does *not* make intensive use of land, labor, or machinery. When food production arose, both in the Middle East and in the Americas, the earliest cultivators were rainfall-dependent horticulturalists. More recently, horticulture has been—and in many cases still is—the primary form of cultivation in parts of Africa, Southeast Asia, the Pacific islands, Mexico, Central America, and the South American tropical forest.

Horticulturalists use simple tools such as hoes and digging sticks to grow their crops.

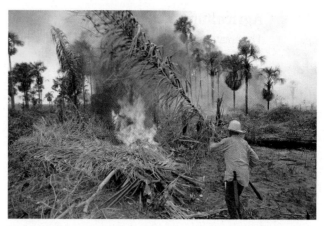

In slash-and-burn cultivation, the land is cleared by cutting down (slashing) and burning trees and brush, using simple technology, as we see here in Brazil's Amazon region.

Nigel Dickinson/Alamy Stock Photo

They preserve their ecosystems by allowing their fields to lie fallow for varying lengths of time. Horticulturalists typically rely on *slash-and-burn* techniques. Farmers clear land by cutting down (slashing) trees, saplings, and brush. Then they burn that vegetation. They also may set fire directly to grasses and weeds on their farm plots before planting. Slashing and burning not only gets rid of unwanted vegetation, but it also kills pests and provides ashes that help fertilize the soil. The farmers then sow, tend, and harvest their crops on the cleared plot. They do not use that plot continuously; often they farm it for only a year or two.

Horticulture also is known as *shifting cultivation,* because farmers shift back and forth between plots, rather than using any one of those plots continuously. With shifting cultivation, horticulturalists farm a plot for a year or two, then abandon it, clear another plot, cultivate it for a year or two, then abandon it, and so on. After the original plot lies fallow for several years (the duration varies in different societies), it can be farmed again.

Shifting cultivation doesn't mean that whole villages must move when plots are abandoned. Horticulture can support large, permanent villages. Among the Kuikuru of the South American tropical forest, for example, one village of 150 people remained in the same place for 90 years (Carneiro 1956). Kuikuru houses are large and well made. Because the work involved in building them is great, the Kuikuru preferred to walk farther to their fields, rather than construct a new village. They chose to shift their plots rather than their villages. By contrast, other horticulturalists in the montaña (Andean foothills) of Peru maintained small villages of about thirty people (Carneiro 1961/1968). Their houses were small, simple, and easy to rebuild, so that they would stay a few years in one place, then move on to a different site near their fields where they would build new homes. They preferred rebuilding to walking even a half-mile to their fields.

horticulture
Nonintensive, shifting cultivation with fallowing.

agriculture
Cultivation using land and labor continuously and intensively.

Agriculture

The greater labor demands associated with agriculture, as compared with horticulture, reflect its use of domesticated animals, irrigation, or terracing.

Domesticated Animals

Many agriculturalists use animals as means of production—for transport, as cultivating machines, and for their manure. Asian farmers typically incorporate cattle and/or water buffalo into agricultural economies based on rice production. Rice farmers may use cattle to trample pretilled flooded fields, thus mixing soil and water, prior to transplanting. Many agriculturalists attach animals to plows and harrows for field preparation before planting or transplanting. Also, agriculturalists typically collect manure from their animals, using it to fertilize their plots, thus increasing yields. Animals are attached to carts for transport as well as to implements of cultivation.

Irrigation

cultivation continuum

A continuum of land and labor use running from horticulture (noncontinuous, nonintensive) to agriculture (continuous, intensive).

While horticulturalists must await the rainy season, agriculturalists can schedule their planting in advance, because they control water—they irrigate their fields. Like other irrigation experts in the Philippines, the Ifugao (Figure 7.2) irrigate their fields with canals that divert water from rivers, streams, springs, and ponds. Irrigation makes it possible to cultivate a plot year after year. Irrigation enriches the soil, because the irrigated field is a unique ecosystem with several species of plants and animals, many of them minute organisms, whose wastes fertilize the land.

An irrigated field is a capital investment that usually increases in value. It takes time for a field to start yielding; it reaches full productivity only after several years of cultivation. The Ifugao, like other irrigators, have farmed the same fields for generations. In some agricultural areas, including the Middle East, however, salts carried in the irrigation water can make fields unusable after 50 or 60 years.

Terracing

Terracing is another agricultural technique the Ifugao have mastered. Their homeland has small valleys separated by steep hillsides. Because the population is dense, people need to farm the hills. However, if they simply planted on the steep hillsides, fertile soil and crops would be washed away during the rainy season. To prevent this, the Ifugao cut into the hillside and build stage after stage of terraced fields rising above the valley floor. Springs located above the terraces supply their irrigation water. Building and maintaining a system of terraces requires a lot of work. Terrace walls crumble and must be repaired or rebuilt. The canals that bring water down through the terraces also need maintenance.

Costs and Benefits of Agriculture

Agriculture requires considerable labor to build and maintain irrigation systems, terraces, and other works. People must feed, water, and care for their animals. Given sufficient labor input and proper management, agricultural land can yield one or two crops annually for years or even generations. An agricultural field does not necessarily produce a higher single-year yield than does a horticultural plot. The first crop grown by horticulturalists on long-idle land may be larger than that from an agricultural plot of the same size. Furthermore, because agriculturalists have to work more hours than horticulturalists do, agriculture's yield relative to the labor time invested also is lower. Agriculture's main advantage is that the long-term yield per area is far greater and more dependable. Because a single field sustains its owners year after year, there is no need to maintain a reserve of uncultivated land as horticulturalists do. This is why agricultural societies tend to be more densely populated than are horticultural ones.

The Cultivation Continuum

Because nonindustrial economies can have features of both horticulture and agriculture, it is useful to discuss cultivators as being arranged along a **cultivation continuum**. Horticultural systems stand at one end—the "low-labor, shifting-plot" end. Agriculturalists are at the other—the "labor-intensive, permanent-plot" end.

We speak of a continuum because there are intermediate economies, which combine horticultural and agricultural features. In such economies, cultivation is more intensive than with annually shifting horticulture, but less so than

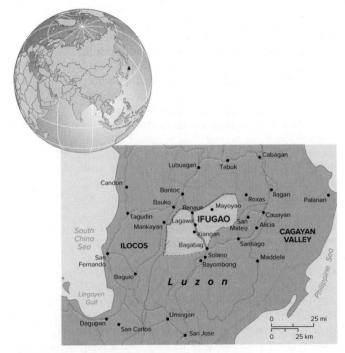

FIGURE 7.2 Location of the Ifugao.

with permanent agriculture. The South American Kuikuru, for example, grow two or three crops of *manioc,* or cassava—an edible tuber—before abandoning their plots. Cultivation is even more intensive in certain densely populated areas of Papua New Guinea, where plots are planted for two or three years, allowed to rest for three to five, and then recultivated. After several of these cycles, the plots are abandoned for a longer fallow period. Such intermediate economies, which support denser populations than does simple horticulture, also are found in parts of West Africa, and in the highlands of Mexico, Peru, and Bolivia.

The one key difference between horticulture and agriculture is that *horticulture always has a fallow period,* whereas agriculture does not.

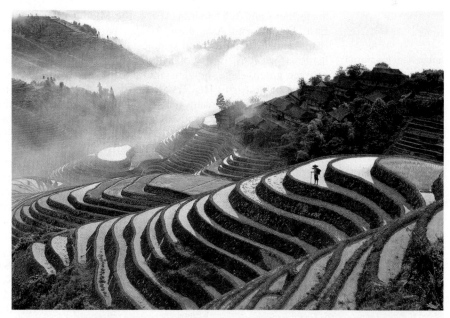

Agriculture requires longer hours than horticulture does and uses land intensively and continuously. Labor demands associated with agriculture reflect its use of domesticated animals, irrigation, and terracing. Shown here, irrigated rice terraces surround a farming village in Longsheng, Guangxi province, China.

KingWu/iStockphoto.com

Intensification: People and the Environment

The range of environments available for cultivation has widened as people have increased their control over nature. Agriculturalists have been able to colonize many areas that are too arid for nonirrigators or too hilly for nonterracers. Agriculture's increased labor intensity and permanent land use have major demographic, social, political, and environmental consequences.

How, specifically, does agriculture affect society and environment? Because of their permanent fields, agriculturalists tend to be sedentary. People live in larger and more permanent communities located closer to other settlements. Growth in population size and density increases contact between individuals and groups. There is more need to regulate interpersonal relations, including conflicts of interest. Economies that support more people usually require more coordination in the use of land, labor, and other resources.

Intensive agriculture has significant environmental effects. Irrigation ditches and paddies (fields with irrigated rice) become repositories for organic wastes, chemicals (such as salts), and disease microorganisms. Intensive agriculture typically spreads at the expense of trees and forests, which are cut down to be replaced by fields. Accompanying such deforestation is a loss of environmental diversity (see Srivastava, Smith, and Forno 1999). Compared with horticulture, agricultural economies are specialized. They focus on one or a few caloric staples, such as rice, and on the animals that are raised and tended to aid the agricultural economy. Because tropical horticulturalists typically cultivate dozens of plant species simultaneously, a horticultural plot tends to mirror the botanical diversity found in a tropical

forest. Agricultural plots, by contrast, reduce ecological diversity by cutting down trees and concentrating on just a few staple foods.

Agriculturalists attempt to reduce risk in production by counting on a reliable annual harvest and long-term production. Tropical foragers and horticulturalists, by contrast, attempt to reduce risk by relying on multiple species and benefiting from ecological diversity. The agricultural strategy is to put all one's eggs in one big and dependable basket. Of course, even with agriculture, there is a possibility that the single staple crop may fail, and famine may result. The strategy of horticulturalists is to have several, smaller baskets, a few of which may fail without endangering subsistence. The agricultural strategy makes sense when there are lots of children to raise and adults to be fed. Horticulture, like foraging, is associated with smaller, sparser, and more mobile populations.

Many indigenous groups, especially foragers and horticulturalists, have done a reasonable job of managing their resources and preserving their ecosystems (see also Menzies 2006). Such societies had traditional ways of categorizing resources and regulating their use. Increasingly, however, these traditional management systems have been challenged by national and international incentives to exploit and degrade the environment (see Dove, Sajise, and Doolittle 2011).

Pastoralism

Herders, or **pastoralists,** are people whose activities focus on such domesticated animals as cattle, sheep, goats, camels, yak, and reindeer. They live

pastoralists
Herders of domesticated animals.

in northern and sub-Saharan Africa, the Middle East, Europe, and Asia. East African pastoralists, like many others, live in symbiosis with their herds. (*Symbiosis* is an obligatory interaction between groups—here, humans and animals—that is beneficial to each.) Herders attempt to protect their animals and to ensure their reproduction in return for food (dairy products and meat) and other products, such as leather.

People use livestock in various ways. Natives of North America's Great Plains, for example, didn't eat, but only rode, their horses. (They got those horses after Europeans reintroduced them to the Western Hemisphere; the native American horse had become extinct thousands of years earlier.) For Plains Indians, horses served as "tools of the trade," means of production used to hunt buffalo, the main target of their economies. So the Plains Indians were not true pastoralists but hunters who used horses—as many agriculturalists use animals—as means of production.

Pastoralists, by contrast, typically use their herds for food. They consume the animals' meat, blood, and milk, from which they make yogurt, butter, and cheese. Although some pastoralists rely on their herds more completely than others do, it is impossible to base subsistence solely on animals. Most pastoralists therefore supplement their diet by hunting, gathering, fishing, cultivating, or trading.

The Samis (also known as Lapps or Laplanders) of Norway, Sweden, and Finland domesticated the reindeer, which their ancestors once hunted, in the 16th century. Like other herders, they follow their animals as they make an annual trek, in this case from coast to interior. Today's Samis use modern technology, such as snowmobiles and four-wheel-drive vehicles, to accompany their herds on their annual nomadic trek, and they market reindeer products to outsiders, including tourists. Some of them probably use reindeer management software on their laptops, tablets, personal digital assistants (PDAs), or smartphones. Although their environment is harsher, the Samis, like other herders, live in nation-states and must deal with outsiders, including government officials, as they follow their herds and make their living through animal husbandry, trade, and sales (Paine 2009).

Unlike foraging and plant cultivation, which existed throughout the world before the Industrial Revolution, herding was confined almost totally to the Old World. Before European conquest, the only herders in the Americas lived in the Andean region of South America. They used their llamas and alpacas for food and wool and in agriculture and transport. Much more recently, the Navajo of the southwestern United States developed a pastoral economy based on sheep, which were brought to North America by Europeans. The populous Navajo became the major pastoral population in the Western Hemisphere.

Two patterns of movement occur with pastoralism: nomadism and transhumance. Both are based on the fact that herds must move to use pasture available in particular places in different seasons. In **pastoral nomadism,** the entire group—women, men, and children—moves with the animals throughout the year. The Middle East and North Africa provide numerous examples of pastoral nomads (see Salzman 2008). In Iran, for example, the Basseri and the Qashqai ethnic groups traditionally followed a nomadic route more than 300 miles (480 kilometers) long (see Salzman 2004).

With **transhumance,** part of the group moves with the herds, but most people stay in the home

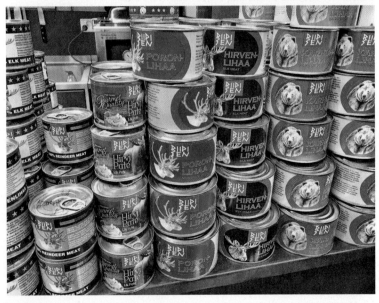

Reindeer (and bear) products on display at a tourist-oriented market in Helsinki, Finland.

Conrad P. Kottak

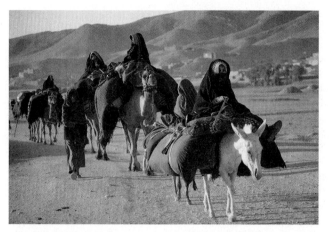
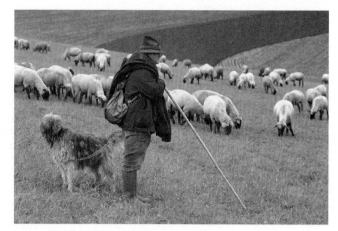

Pastoralists may be nomadic or transhumant, but they don't typically live off their herds alone. They either trade or cultivate. On the left we see a caravan of Kuchi nomads on the move in Ghor province, central Afghanistan, on August 11, 2011. Around 10-15,000 nomads pass through this mountainous province every summer, to graze their cattle in high pastures. The photo on the right shows a transhumant shepherd with his herd in Eifel, Rheinland Pfalz, Germany.

(left): Jerome Starkey/Getty Images; (right): tbkmedia.de/Alamy Stock Photo

RECAP 7.1	Yehudi Cohen's Adaptive Strategies (Economic Typology) Summarized	
ADAPTIVE STRATEGY	**ALSO KNOWN AS**	**KEY FEATURES/VARIETIES**
Foraging	Hunting-gathering	Mobility, use of nature's resources
Horticulture	Slash-and-burn, shifting cultivation, dry farming	Fallow period
Agriculture	Intensive farming	Continuous use of land, intensive use of labor
Pastoralism	Herding	Nomadism and transhumance
Industrialism	Industrial production	Factory production, capitalism, socialist production

village. There are examples from Europe and Africa. In Europe's Alps, it is just the shepherds and goatherds—not the whole hamlet, village, or town—who accompany the flocks to highland meadows in summer. Among the Turkana of Uganda, men and boys take the herds to distant pastures, while much of the village stays put and does some horticultural farming. During their annual trek, pastoral nomads trade for crops and other products with more sedentary people. Transhumants don't have to trade for crops. Because only part of the population accompanies the herds, transhumants can maintain year-round villages and grow their own crops. (Recap 7.1 summarizes the major adaptive strategies.)

MODES OF PRODUCTION

An **economy** is a system of production, distribution, and consumption of resources; *economics* is the study of such systems. Economists, however, focus on modern nations and capitalist systems. Anthropologists have broadened understanding of economic principles by gathering data on nonindustrial economies. *Economic anthropology* brings a comparative, cross-cultural perspective to the study of economics (see Carrier 2012; Chibnik 2011; Gudeman 2016; Hann and Hart 2011; Sahlins 1972/2017).

A **mode of production** is a way of organizing production—"a set of social relations through which labor is deployed to wrest energy from nature by means of tools, skills, organization, and knowledge" (Wolf 1982, p. 75). In the *capitalist* mode of production, money buys labor power, and there is a social gap between the people (bosses and workers) involved in the production process. By contrast, in nonindustrial societies, labor is not usually bought but is given as a social obligation. In such a *kin-based* mode of production, mutual aid in production is one among many expressions of a larger web of social relations (see Graca and Zingarelli 2015).

Societies representing each of the adaptive strategies just discussed (e.g., foraging) tend to have roughly similar modes of production. Variation in the mode of production within a given strategy can reflect differences in the resources they target. Thus, a foraging mode of production may be based on individual hunters or teams, depending on whether the game is solitary, or a herd or flocking animal. Gathering is usually more individualistic than hunting, although collecting teams may assemble when abundant resources ripen and must be harvested quickly. Fishing may be done alone (as in ice fishing or spearfishing) or in crews (as with open-sea fishing and hunting of sea mammals).

mode of production
A specific set of social relations that organizes labor.

economy
A system of resource production, distribution, and consumption.

Production in Nonindustrial Societies

Although some kind of division of economic labor based on age and gender is a cultural universal, the specific tasks assigned to females, males, and people of different ages vary (see Malefyt and McCabe 2020). Many horticultural societies assign a major productive role to women, but some make men's work primary. Similarly, among pastoralists, men generally tend large animals, but in some cultures women do the milking. Tasks that depend on teamwork in some cultivating societies may be carried out by smaller groups or individuals in other societies.

The Betsileo of Madagascar have two stages of teamwork in rice cultivation: transplanting and harvesting. Team size varies with the size of the field. Both transplanting and harvesting feature a traditional division of labor by age and gender that is well known to all Betsileo and is repeated across the generations. The first job in the transplanting process is the trampling of a previously tilled and flooded field by young men driving cattle, in order to mix earth and water. The young men yell at and beat the cattle, striving to drive them into a frenzy, so that they will trample the fields properly. Trampling breaks up clumps of earth and mixes irrigation water with soil to form a smooth mud, into which women will soon transplant seedlings. Once the tramplers leave the field, older men arrive. With their spades, they break up the clumps that the cattle missed. Meanwhile, the owner and other adults uproot rice seedlings and take them to the field, where women will transplant them.

At harvest time, four or five months later, young men cut the rice off the stalks. Young women carry it to a clearing above the field, where older women arrange and stack it. The oldest men and women then stand on the stack, stomping and compacting it. Three days later, young men thresh the rice, beating the stalks against a rock to remove the grain. Older men then attack the stalks with sticks to make sure all the grains have fallen off.

Most of the other tasks in Betsileo rice cultivation are done by individual owners and their immediate families. All household members help weed the rice field. It is a man's job to till the fields with a spade or a plow. Individual men repair the irrigation and drainage systems and the earth walls that separate one plot from the next. Among other agriculturalists, however, repairing the irrigation system can be a task involving teamwork and communal labor.

Means of Production

The relationship between the worker and the means of production is more intimate in nonindustrial societies than it is in industrial nations. **Means,** or **factors, of production** include land (territory), labor, technology, and capital.

Land

Ties between people and land are less permanent among foragers than among food producers. The borders between foraging territories are neither precisely demarcated nor enforced. A hunter's stake in pursuit of an animal is more important than where that animal finally dies. One acquires the right to use a band's territory by being born in that band or by joining it through a tie of kinship or marriage. On changing bands, one immediately acquires rights to hunt or gather in the new band's territory.

Among food producers, rights to the means of production also come through kinship and marriage. Descent groups (groups whose members claim common ancestry) are common among nonindustrial food producers, and those who descend from the founder share the group's territory and resources. If the adaptive strategy is horticulture, the estate includes garden and fallow land for shifting cultivation. With pastoralism, descent group members have access to animals to start their own herds, to grazing land, to garden land, and to other means of production.

means (factors) of production

Major productive resources, e.g., land, labor, technology, capital.

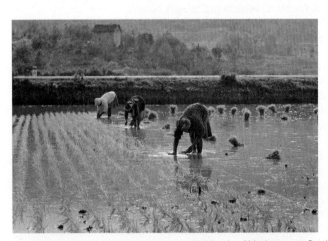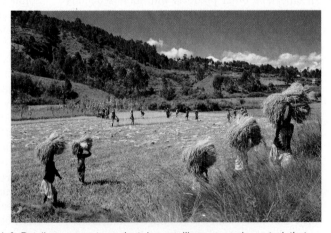

Transplanting and harvesting rice in the highlands of Madagascar. On the left, Betsileo women transplant rice seedlings—an arduous task that places considerable strain on the back. On the right, Betsileo women carry sheaves of rice to an open area for threshing.

(Left): RGB Ventures/SuperStock/Alamy Stock Photo; (Right): Michele Burgess/Alamy Stock Photo

Labor, Tools, and Specialization

Like land, labor is a means of production. In nonindustrial societies, access to both land and labor comes through social links such as kinship, marriage, and descent. The labor that is mutually given in production is merely one aspect of ongoing social relations that are expressed on many other occasions.

Nonindustrial societies contrast with industrial nations in regard to another means of production: technology. Manufacturing often is linked to age and gender. Women may weave, and men may make pottery, or vice versa. Most people of a particular age and gender share the technical knowledge associated with that age and gender. If married women customarily make baskets, all or most married women know how to make baskets. Neither technology nor technical knowledge is as specialized as it is in states.

However, some tribal societies do promote specialization. Among the Yanomami of Venezuela and Brazil (Figure 7.3), for instance, certain villages manufacture clay pots and others make hammocks. They don't specialize, as one might suppose, because certain raw materials happen to be available near particular villages. Clay suitable for pots is widely available. Everyone knows how to make pots, but not everybody does so. Craft specialization reflects the social and political environment rather than the natural environment. Such specialization promotes trade, which is the first step in creating an alliance with enemy villages (Chagnon 2013a, 2013b). Specialization contributes to keeping the peace, although it has not prevented intervillage warfare.

Alienation in Industrial Economies

There are significant contrasts between nonindustrial economies and industrial ones. In the former, economic relations are just one part of a larger, multidimensional social matrix. People don't just work for and with others; they live with those same people, and they pray with, feast with, and care about them. One works for and with people with whom one has long-term personal and social bonds (e.g., kin and in-laws).

In industrial societies, by contrast, workers sell their labor to bosses who can fire them. Work and the workplace are separated—*alienated*—from one's social essence. The term *alienation* is used to describe a situation in which a worker has produced something but sees that product as belonging to someone else, rather than to the man or woman whose labor actually produced it. Rather than expressing an ongoing, mutual social relationship, labor becomes a thing (commodity) to be paid for, bought, and sold—and from which the boss can generate an individual profit. Furthermore, industrial workers usually don't work with their relatives and neighbors. If coworkers are friends, the personal relationship often develops out of their common employment rather than a previous social tie. (This chapter's "Focus on Globalization" describes the increasingly impersonal nature of today's global economy.)

In nonindustrial societies, the individual who has made an item can use or dispose of it as he or she sees fit. That maker may feel pride in his or her own product and, if it is given away, a renewed commitment to the social relationship that is reinforced by the gift. On the other hand, when factory workers produce for someone else's profit, their products, as well as their labor, are alienated. Human labor and its products belong to someone other than the individual producer. Unlike

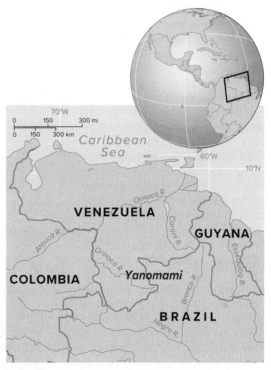

FIGURE 7.3 Location of the Yanomami.

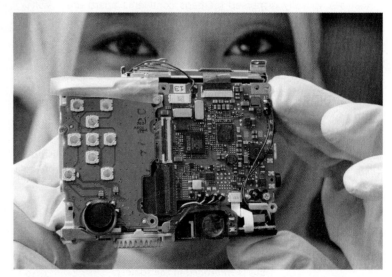

A technician displays the circuit board for a compact digital camera at a Canon factory in Petaling Jaya, Malaysia. Throughout Southeast Asia, hundreds of thousands of young women from peasant families now work in factories. Chances are good that you own one of their products.

Goh Seng Chong/Bloomberg via Getty Images

focus on GLOBALIZATION

Our Global Economy

Economic systems are based on production, distribution, and consumption. All these processes now have global, and increasingly impersonal, dimensions. The products, images, and information we consume each day can come from anywhere. How likely is it that the item you last bought from a website, an outlet, or a retail store was made in the United States, rather than Canada, Mexico, Peru, or China?

The national has become international. Consider a few familiar "American" brands: Good Humor, French's mustard, Frigidaire, Adidas, Caribou Coffee, Church's Chicken, Trader Joe's, Holiday Inn, Dial soap, T-Mobile, and Toll House Cookies. All of them have foreign ownership. As well, the following iconic brands have been bought by foreign companies: Budweiser, Burger King, Alka-Selzer, Hellmann's, Ben and Jerry's, 7-Eleven, Popsicle, *Woman's Day,* Purina, Gerber, Vaseline, Firestone, and *Car and Driver* magazine. Also foreign owned are such American architectural icons as New York's Plaza Hotel, Flatiron Building, and Chrysler Building, along with the Indiana Toll Road and the Chicago Skyway.

Much of America, including 39 percent of the U.S. national debt, is held by foreigners, versus merely 5 percent in the 1970s. Foreign countries have invested heavily in U.S. Treasury securities because of their liquidity and safety. As of February, 2020, Japan owned $1.15 trillion of U.S. national debt, with China close behind at $1.07 trillion. Next were the UK at $333 billion and Brazil at $282 billion (see https://www.thebalance.com/who-owns-the-u-s-national-debt-3306124).

The Internet is a vital organ of our 21st-century global economy. All kinds of products—music, movies, clothing, appliances, this book, you name it—are produced, distributed, and consumed via the Internet. Economic functions that are spatially dispersed (perhaps continents apart) are coordinated online in real time. Activities that once involved face-to-face contact are now conducted impersonally, often across vast distances. When you order something via the Internet, the only human being you might speak to is the delivery driver. However, even that human contact is in danger of being replaced by a drone. The computers that take and process your order from Amazon can be on different continents. The products you order can come from a warehouse anywhere in the world. Transnational finance has shifted the economic control of local life to outsiders. Greeks, for example, blamed Germans for austerity measures imposed on their country.

How different is today's global economy from British poet Henry Wadsworth Longfellow's vision of production—noble, local, and autonomous:

Under a spreading chestnut-tree

The village smithy stands. . . .

Toiling—rejoicing—sorrowing,

Onward through life he goes;

Each morning sees some task begin,

Each evening sees it close.

(Longfellow, "The Village Blacksmith," 1839)

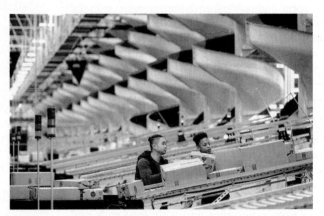

This photo, taken on February 5, 2019, shows workers at a distribution station in an Amazon fulfillment center in Staten Island, New York. Inside this huge warehouse, thousands of robots distribute items sold by Amazon.
Johannes Eisele/Getty Images

assembly-line workers, producers in nonindustrial societies typically see their work through from start to finish and feel a sense of accomplishment.

In nonindustrial societies, the economic relation between coworkers is just one aspect of a more general social relation. They aren't just coworkers but kin, in-laws, or celebrants in the same ritual. In such settings, the relations of production, distribution, and consumption are *social relations with economic aspects.* Economy is not a separate entity but is *embedded* in the society.

A Case of Industrial Alienation

For decades, the government of Malaysia has promoted export-oriented industry, allowing transnational companies to install labor-intensive manufacturing operations in rural Malaysia. The industrialization of Malaysia is part of a global strategy. In search of cheaper labor, corporations headquartered in Japan, Western Europe, and the United States have been moving labor-intensive factories to developing countries. Malaysia has hundreds of Japanese and American subsidiaries, which produce mainly garments, foodstuffs, and electronics components. In electronics plants in rural Malaysia, thousands of young women from peasant families now assemble microchips and microcomponents for transistors and capacitors. Aihwa Ong (1987, 2010) did a study of electronics assembly workers in an area where 85 percent of the workers were young, unmarried females from nearby villages.

Ong found that, unlike village women, female factory workers had to cope with a rigid work routine and constant supervision by men. The discipline that factories enforce was being taught in local schools, where uniforms helped prepare girls for the factory dress code. Village women wore loose, flowing tunics, sarongs, and sandals, but factory workers had to don tight overalls and heavy rubber gloves, in which they felt constrained. Labor in these factories illustrates the alienation that Karl Marx considered the defining feature of industrial work. One woman said about her bosses, "They exhaust us very much, as if they do not think that we too are human beings" (Ong 1987, p. 202). Nor does factory work bring women a substantial financial reward, given low wages, job uncertainty, and family claims on wages. Young women typically work just a few years. Production quotas, three daily shifts, overtime, and surveillance take their toll in mental and physical exhaustion.

One response to factory relations of production has been spirit possession (factory women are possessed by spirits). Ong interprets this phenomenon as the women's unconscious protest against labor discipline and male control of the industrial setting. Sometimes possession takes the form of mass hysteria. Spirits have simultaneously invaded as many as 120 factory workers. Weretigers (the Malay equivalent of the werewolf) arrive to avenge the construction of a factory on aboriginal burial grounds. Disturbed earth and grave spirits swarm on the shop floor. First the women see the spirits; then their bodies are invaded. The women become violent and scream abuses. The weretigers send the women into sobbing, laughing, and shrieking fits. To deal with possession, factories employ local medicine men, who sacrifice chickens and goats to fend off the spirits. This solution works only some of the time; possession still goes on. Factory women continue to act as vehicles to express their own frustrations and the anger of avenging ghosts.

Ong argues that spirit possession expresses anguish at, and resistance to, capitalist relations of production. By engaging in this form of rebellion, however, factory women avoid a direct confrontation with the source of their distress. Ong concludes that spirit possession, while expressing repressed resentment, doesn't do much to modify factory conditions. (Other tactics, such as unionization, would do more.) Spirit possession may even help maintain the current system by operating as a safety valve for accumulated tensions. (Chapter 14's "Appreciating Anthropology" describes a different kind of alienation—that which follows the job *loss* associated with deindustrialization.)

ECONOMIZING AND MAXIMIZATION

Economic anthropologists have been concerned with two main questions:

1. How are production, distribution, and consumption organized in different societies? This question focuses on *systems* of human behavior and their organization.

2. What *motivates* people in different cultures to produce, distribute or exchange, and consume? Here the focus is not on systems of behavior but on the motives of the *individuals* who participate in those systems.

Anthropologists view both economic systems and motivations in a cross-cultural perspective. Motivation is a concern of psychologists, but it also has been, implicitly or explicitly, a concern of economists and anthropologists. Economists assume that our decisions are guided by the *profit motive*—the desire to make a monetary profit. Although anthropologists know that the profit motive is not universal, the assumption that individuals try to maximize profits is basic to the capitalist world economy and to much of Western economic theory. In fact, the subject matter of economics often is defined as **economizing,** or the rational (profit-oriented) allocation of scarce means (resources) to alternative ends (uses) (see Chibnik 2011).

What does that mean? Classical economic theory assumes that our wants are infinite and that our means are limited. Since means are limited, people must make choices about how to use their scarce resources: their time, labor, money, and capital. (This chapter's "Appreciating Diversity" disputes the idea that people always make economic choices based on scarcity.) Economists assume that when confronted with choices and decisions, people tend to make the one that maximizes profit. This is assumed to be the most rational (reasonable) choice.

The idea that individuals choose to maximize profit was a basic assumption of the classical economists of the 19th century and is one that is still held by many contemporary economists. However, certain economists now recognize that individuals in Western cultures, as in others, may be motivated by many other goals. Depending on the society and the situation, people may try to maximize profit, wealth, prestige, pleasure, comfort, or social harmony. Individuals may want to realize their personal or family ambitions or those of another group to which they belong (see Chibnik 2011; Sahlins 1972/2017).

economizing

The allocation of scarce means (resources) among alternative ends.

Alternative Ends

To what uses do people in various societies put their scarce resources? Throughout the world,

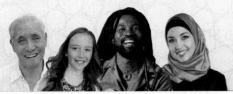

Scarcity and the Betsileo

The Betsileo of Madagascar have two stages of teamwork in rice cultivation: transplanting and harvesting. Team size varies with the size of the field. Both transplanting and harvesting feature a traditional division of labor by age and gender that is well known to all Betsileo and is repeated across the generations. The first job in the transplanting process is the trampling of a previously tilled and flooded field by young men driving cattle, in order to mix earth and water. The young men yell at and beat the cattle, striving to drive them into a frenzy, so that they will trample the fields properly. Trampling breaks up clumps of earth and mixes irrigation water with soil to form a smooth mud, into which women will soon transplant seedlings. Once the tramplers leave the field, older men arrive. With their spades, they break up the clumps that the cattle missed. Meanwhile, the owner and other adults uproot rice seedlings and take them to the field, where women will transplant them.

In the realm of cultural diversity, perceptions and motivations can change substantially over time. Consider some changes I've observed among the Betsileo of Madagascar during the decades I've been studying them. Initially, compared with modern consumers, the Betsileo had little perception of scarcity. Now, with population increase and the spread of a cash-oriented economy, their perceived wants and needs have increased relative to their means. Their motivations have changed, too, as people increasingly seek profits, even if it means stealing from their neighbors or destroying ancestral farms.

During the 1960s, my wife and I lived among the Betsileo people of Madagascar, studying their economy and social life (Kottak 1980, 2004). Soon after our arrival we met two well-educated schoolteachers (first cousins) who were interested in our research. The woman's father was a congressional representative who became a cabinet minister during our stay. Their family came from a historically important Betsileo village called Ivato, which they invited us to visit with them.

We had traveled to many other Betsileo villages, where often we were unhappy with our reception. As we drove up, children would run away screaming. Women would hurry inside. Men would retreat to doorways, where they lurked bashfully. This behavior expressed the Betsileo's great fear of the *mpakafo*. Believed to cut out and devour his victim's heart and liver, the mpakafo is the Malagasy vampire. These cannibals are said to have fair skin and to be very tall. Because I have light skin and stand well over 6 feet tall, I was a natural suspect. The fact that such creatures were not known to travel with their wives offered a bit of assurance that I wasn't really a mpakafo.

When we visited Ivato, its people were different—friendly and hospitable. Our very first day there we did a brief census and found out who lived in which households. We learned people's names and their relationships to our schoolteacher friends and to each other. We met an excellent informant who knew all about the local history. In a few afternoons I learned much more than I had in the other villages in several sessions.

Ivatans were so willing to talk because we had powerful sponsors, village natives who had succeeded in the outside world, people the Ivatans knew would protect them. The schoolteachers vouched for us, but even more significant was the cabinet minister, who was like a grandfather and benefactor to everyone in town. The Ivatans had no reason to fear us because their influential native son had asked them to answer our questions.

Once we moved to Ivato, the elders established a pattern of visiting us every evening. They came to talk, attracted by the inquisitive foreigners but also by the food and wine we offered. I asked questions about their customs and beliefs. I eventually developed interview schedules about various subjects, including rice production. I used these forms in Ivato and in two other villages I was studying less intensively. Never have I interviewed as easily as I did in Ivato.

As our stay neared its end, our Ivatan friends lamented, saying, "We'll miss you. When you leave, there won't be any more cigarettes (I smoked then), any more wine, or any more questions." They wondered what it would be like for us back in the United States. They knew we had an automobile and that we could afford to buy products they never would have. They commented, "When you go back to your country, you'll need a lot of money for things like cars, clothes, and food. We don't need to buy those things. We make almost everything we use. We don't need as much money as you, because we produce for ourselves."

The Betsileo weren't unusual for nonindustrial people. Strange as it may seem to an American

people devote some of their time and energy to building up a *subsistence fund* (Wolf 1966). In other words, people must work to subsist, to feed themselves, to go on living. People also have to invest in a *replacement fund*. They must maintain their technology and other items essential to production. If a hoe or plow breaks, they must repair or replace it. They also must obtain and replace items that are essential not to production but to everyday life, such as clothing and shelter.

People also have to invest in a *social fund*. They have to help their friends, relatives, in-laws, and neighbors. It is useful to distinguish between a social fund and a *ceremonial fund*. The latter term refers to expenditures on ceremonies or rituals. To prepare a festival honoring one's

consumer, those rice farmers actually believed they had all they needed. The lesson from the Betsileo of the 1960s is that scarcity, which economists view as universal, is variable. Although shortages do arise in nonindustrial societies, the concept of scarcity (insufficient means) is much less developed in stable subsistence-oriented societies than in industrial societies, particularly as the reliance on consumer goods increases.

But with globalization over the past few decades, significant changes have affected the Betsileo—and most nonindustrial peoples. On my last visit to Ivato, the effects of cash and of rapid population increase were evident there—and throughout Madagascar—where the national growth rate has been about 3 percent per year. Madagascar's population doubled between 1966 and 1991—from 6 to 12 million people. Today it exceeds 28 million—more than four times as many people to feed as when I first did fieldwork there. One result of population pressure has been agricultural intensification. In Ivato, farmers who formerly had grown only rice in their rice fields now were using the same land for cash crops, such as carrots, after the annual rice harvest. Another change affecting Ivato in recent years has been the breakdown of social and political order, fueled by increasing demand for cash.

Cattle rustling has become a growing threat. Cattle thieves (sometimes from neighboring villages) have terrorized peasants who previously felt secure in their villages. Some of the rustled cattle are driven to the coasts for commercial export. Prominent among the rustlers are relatively well-educated young men, who have studied enough

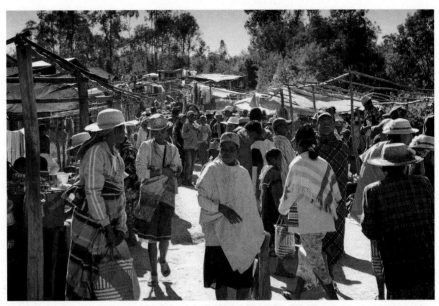

A market in Betsileo country, southcentral Madagascar. The Betsileo increasingly participate in a cash economy—buying and selling at markets and interacting impersonally with outsiders.
Neil McAllister/Alamy Stock Photo

to be comfortable negotiating with outsiders, but who are unable to find formal work and are unwilling to toil in the rice fields. The formal education system has familiarized them with external institutions and norms, including the need for cash. The concepts of scarcity, commerce, and negative reciprocity now thrive among the Betsileo.

I've witnessed other striking evidence of the new addiction to cash during my most recent visits to Betsileo country. Near Ivato's county seat, people now sell semiprecious stones—tourmalines, which originally were found by chance in local rice fields. We saw an amazing sight: dozens of villagers destroying an ancestral resource, digging up a large rice field, seeking tourmalines—clear evidence of the

encroachment of cash on the local subsistence economy. You can't eat gemstones.

Throughout the Betsileo homeland, population growth and density are propelling emigration. Locally, land, jobs, and money are all scarce. One woman with ancestors from Ivato, herself now a resident of the national capital (Antananarivo), remarked that half the children of Ivato now lived in that city. Although she was exaggerating, a census of all the descendants of Ivato reveals a substantial emigrant and urban population.

Ivato's recent history is one of increasing participation in a cash economy. That history, combined with the pressure of a growing population on local resources, has made scarcity not just a concept but a reality for Ivatans and their neighbors.

ancestors, for example, requires time and the outlay of wealth.

Citizens of nation-states also must allocate scarce resources to a *rent fund.* We think of rent as payment for the use of property. However, the term has a wider meaning. It refers to resources that people must render to an individual or agency that is superior politically or economically. Tenant

farmers and sharecroppers, for example, either pay rent or give some of their produce to their landlords, as peasants did under feudalism.

Peasants are small-scale agriculturalists who live in state-organized societies and have rent fund obligations. They produce to feed themselves, to sell their produce, and to pay rent. All peasants have two things in common:

peasant
A small-scale farmer with rent fund obligations.

1. They live in state-organized societies.

2. They produce food without the elaborate technology—chemical fertilizers, tractors, airplanes to spray crops, and so on—of modern farming or agribusiness.

In addition to paying rent to landlords, peasants must satisfy government obligations, paying taxes in the form of money, produce, or labor. The rent fund is not simply an *additional* obligation for peasants. Often it becomes their foremost and unavoidable duty. Sometimes, to meet the obligation to pay rent, their own diets suffer. The demands of paying rent may divert resources from subsistence, replacement, social, and ceremonial funds.

Motivations vary from society to society, and people often lack freedom of choice in allocating their resources. Because of obligations to pay rent, peasants may allocate their scarce means toward ends that are not their own but those of landlords or government officials. Thus, even in societies where there is a profit motive, people are often prevented from rationally maximizing self-interest by factors beyond their control.

DISTRIBUTION AND EXCHANGE

The economist Karl Polanyi (1968) was a key early contributor to the comparative study of exchanges (e.g., gift giving, trade), and several anthropologists followed his lead. Polanyi defined three principles that guide exchanges: the market principle, redistribution, and reciprocity. All three principles can be present in the same society, but in that case they govern different kinds of transactions. In any society, one of them usually dominates. The principle that dominates in a given society is the one that determines how the means of production are exchanged (see Chibnik 2011; Hann and Hart 2011).

The Market Principle

In today's world capitalist economy, the **market principle** dominates. It governs the distribution of the means of production—land, labor, natural resources, technology, knowledge, and capital. With market exchange, items are bought and sold, using money, with an eye to maximizing profit, and value is determined by the *law of supply and demand* (things cost more the scarcer they are and the more people want them). Bargaining is characteristic of market principle exchanges. The buyer and the seller strive to maximize—to get their "money's worth." The bargainers don't need to meet personally, but their offers and counteroffers usually take place within a fairly short time period.

Redistribution

Redistribution operates when products, such as a portion of the annual harvest, move from the local level to a center from which they eventually flow back out. That center may be a capital, a regional collection point, or a storehouse near a chief's residence. Redistribution typically occurs in societies that have chiefs. To reach the center, where they will be stored, products often move through a hierarchy of officials. Along the way, those officials and their dependents may consume some, but never all, of the products. After reaching the center, the flow of goods eventually will reverse direction—out from the center, down through the hierarchy, and back to the common people. Redistribution is a way of moving a variety of goods from different areas to a central point, where they are stored and eventually redistributed to the public. The custom of tithing encouraged by many religions is a form of redistribution, because what the church receives can be used (redistributed) to benefit the needy.

One ethnographic example of redistribution comes from the Cherokee, Native Americans who were the original owners of the Tennessee Valley. The Cherokee were productive cultivators of maize, beans, and squash, which they supplemented by hunting and fishing. They also had chiefs. Each of their main villages had a central plaza, where meetings of the chief's council took place, and where redistributive feasts were held. According to Cherokee custom, each family farm had an area where the family set aside a portion of its annual harvest for the chief. This supply of corn was used to feed the needy, as well as travelers journeying through Cherokee territory. This store of food was available to all who needed it, with the understanding that it "belonged" to the chief and was dispersed through his generosity. The chief also hosted redistributive feasts held in the main settlements. On those occasions, ordinary people were able to consume some of the produce they had previously given in the chief's name (Harris 1978).

Reciprocity

Reciprocity is the act of reciprocating—giving back, returning a favor, repaying a debt. More specifically, economic anthropologists use the term **reciprocity** to refer to exchanges between social equals, people who are related by some kind of personal tie, such as kinship or marriage. Because it occurs between social equals, reciprocity is the dominant exchange principle in the more egalitarian societies—among foragers, cultivators, and pastoralists.

There are three forms of reciprocity: generalized, balanced, and negative (Sahlins 1968, 2017; Service 1966). These may be imagined as areas along a continuum defined by these questions:

1. How closely related are the parties to the exchange?

2. How quickly and unselfishly are gifts reciprocated?

The exchanges that occur between the most closely related people illustrate *generalized reciprocity.* There is no expectation of immediate return of a gift or favor. With *balanced reciprocity,* social distance increases, as does the need to reciprocate. In *negative reciprocity,* social distance is greatest and reciprocation is most calculated. This range, from generalized through balanced to negative, is called the **reciprocity continuum.**

With **generalized reciprocity,** someone gives to another person and expects nothing concrete or immediate in return. Such exchanges (including parental gift giving in contemporary North America) are not primarily economic transactions but expressions of personal relationships. Most parents don't keep accounts of all the time, money, and energy they expend on their children. They merely hope that the children will respect their culture's customs involving love, honor, loyalty, and other obligations to parents.

Among foragers, generalized reciprocity—unselfish giving with no immediate expectation of return—is the norm. People routinely share with other band members. A study of the Ju/'hoansi San (Figure 7.4) found that 40 percent of the population contributed little to the food supply (Lee 1968/1974). Children, teenagers, and people over 60 depended on other people for their food. Despite the high proportion of dependents, the average worker spent less than half as much time hunting or gathering (12 to 19 hours a week) as the average American works. Nonetheless, there was always food, because different people worked on different days.

So strong is the ethic of reciprocal sharing that most foragers lack an expression for "thank you." To offer thanks would imply that a particular act of sharing, which is the keystone of egalitarian society, was unusual. Among the Semai, foragers of central Malaysia (Dentan 1979, 2008), to express gratitude would suggest surprise at a hunter's generosity or success (see also Widlok 2017; Zhang 2016).

Balanced reciprocity characterizes exchanges between people who are more distantly related than are members of the same band or household. In a horticultural society, for example, a man presents a gift to someone in another village. The recipient may be a cousin, a trading partner, or a brother's fictive kinsman. The giver expects something in return. This may not come immediately, but the social relationship will be strained if there is no eventual and more or less equivalent return gift.

Exchanges in nonindustrial societies also may illustrate **negative reciprocity,** mainly in dealing with people outside or on the fringes of their social systems. To people who live in a world of close personal relations, exchanges with outsiders are full of ambiguity and distrust. Exchange is one way of establishing friendly relations with outsiders, but especially when trade begins, the relationship still is tentative. Often, the initial exchange is close to

being purely economic; people want to get something back immediately. Just as in market economies, but without using money, they try to get the best possible immediate return for their investment (see Clark 2010; Hann and Hart 2009).

Generalized and balanced reciprocity are based on trust and a social tie (see this chapter's "Appreciating Anthropology"). With negative reciprocity, the goal is to get something immediately and as cheaply as possible, even if it means being cagey or deceitful or even cheating. Among the most extreme and "negative" examples of negative reciprocity was 19th-century horse thievery by North American Plains Indians. Men would sneak into camps and villages of neighboring tribes to steal horses. Such thefts were likely to be reciprocated. A similar pattern of cattle raiding continues today in East Africa, among tribes such as the Kuria (Fleisher 2000). In these cases, the party that starts the raiding can expect reciprocity—a raid on their own village—or worse. The Kuria hunt down cattle thieves and kill them. It's still reciprocity, governed by "Do unto others as they have done unto you."

reciprocity continuum
A continuum running from generalized reciprocity (closely related/deferred return) to negative reciprocity (strangers/immediate return).

generalized reciprocity
Exchanges among closely related individuals.

balanced reciprocity
The midpoint on the reciprocity continuum, between generalized and negative reciprocity.

negative reciprocity
Potentially hostile exchanges among strangers.

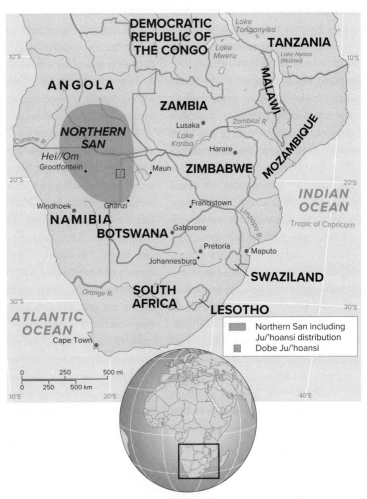

FIGURE 7.4 Location of the San, Including Ju/'hoansi.

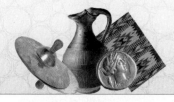

To Give Is Good: Reciprocity and Human Survival

In an article titled "Is a More Generous Society Possible," Leah Shaffer (2019), describes problem-oriented fieldwork by anthropologist Cathryn Townsend in Uganda. In 2016, Townsend began a restudy of the Ik, a group of about 11,600 people who subsist by foraging and subsistence farming. They live in an inhospitable area of Uganda, in arid mountain terrain. Townsend chose this group based on a previous study by anthropologist Colin Turnbull, who had described them most unsympathetically. In his book *The Mountain People* (1972), Turnbull, who studied the Ik in the mid-1960s, characterized them as "loveless," "inhospitable," and "generally mean." To support this negative portrayal, he cited cases of children abandoned to starvation and food being snatched from the mouths of elderly people. We know now, however that Turnbull studied this group during a period of extreme famine, and that his ethnographic account was an inaccurate portrayal of the Ik as they normally live.

Townsend was a participant in The Human Generosity Project (HGP), a multidisciplinary endeavor that examines patterns of cooperation and generosity in different cultures (see http://www.humangenerosity.org/). The Project was initiated in 2014 and is now co-directed by Lee Cronk, a Rutgers University anthropologist, and Athena Aktipis, a psychologist at Arizona State University. The project's goal is to investigate the determinants of human generosity. The HGP now includes more than 20 researchers, who employ a variety of methods to understand the nature and evolution of human generosity, including fieldwork (at nine field sites), laboratory experiments, and computer modeling. Townsend chose to restudy the Ik, based on Turnbull's account, as a likely counterexample to generous cultures–a truly selfish society. The Project wanted to see how an allegedly "selfish" society operated. Townsend's fieldwork would reveal, however, that the Ik were far from the loveless and ungenerous group that Turnbull described (Shaffer 2019).

The findings of the HGP are confirming that patterns of generalized reciprocity (as described in the text) are common in many cultures. That is, people regularly give to others, especially those in need, with no expectation of immediate return. Project researchers are concluding that generosity is a widespread and long-standing human tradition that helps communities survive when times get tough.

In other words, human altruism has adaptive value. In subsistence-oriented societies, generosity plays the role that commercial insurance fulfills in our own. It helps people cope with risk and unforeseen circumstances. When disaster strikes, people readily help one another—they assume the community would do the same for them under similar circumstances. HGP researchers call this form of reciprocity "need-based transfer." On the reciprocity scale mentioned in the text, it stands a bit closer to generalized than to balanced reciprocity. There is no expectation of immediate return, although there is an expectation that mutual community support will be available when need arises.

As an American example of need-based transfer, Shaffer (2019) cites "the Cajun Navy," a group of boat owners that formed originally to perform rescues during the flooding that accompanied Hurricane Katrina in 2005. Twelve years later, the Cajun Navy voyaged to Texas to assist in rescue efforts during flooding caused by hurricane Harvey. They also assisted when Hurricane Florence hit North Carolina in 2018.

Volunteerism illustrates both need-based transfer and generalized reciprocity. The Cajun Navy expects neither payment nor an immediate return. Of course, victims of Hurricanes Katrina, Harvey, and Florence relied even more heavily on insurance policies they had paid for, although many found to their surprise that ordinary homeowners' insurance does not cover floods. A separate policy—flood insurance—is needed. The Cajun Navy example does indicate, however, that generalized reciprocity persists in market-oriented societies and even extends to nonrelatives.

HGP researchers have used a computer-based simulation to compare outcomes in three kinds of community.

1. The first community uses need-based transfer (comparable to generalized reciprocity).

2. In the second community, sharing occurs, but people expect repayment. The Project calls this practice "account keeping," and it seems analogous to balanced reciprocity.

3. The third community does not share (negative reciprocity).

The researchers based their simulation of outcomes on pastoralists like the East African Maasai, who routinely share cattle and other resources. As droughts and disease threats were simulated randomly, the researchers observed how the herds fared in each community. It turned out that both forms of sharing (equivalent to generalized and balanced reciprocity) had better outcomes in terms of herd survival than in the community in which no sharing occurred (a form of negative reciprocity). Sharing, it seems, is good for human survival (Shaffer 2019).

The HGP may have to abandon its search for a truly selfish society. Cathryn Townsend found no evidence for the kind of selfishness that Turnbull described. Rather than snatching food from the mouths of the aged, she watched community members take food to an old man who lived alone. The Ik are no strangers to sharing.

How much should we trust Turnbull's account? Maybe more than we would like. Maybe the Ik did display the selfish behavior that he described. Maybe for that year, and perhaps that year only, they truly became "the selfish people." Famine brings true scarcity, capable of leading a community to abandon its normal altruistic behavior. Having survived the famine, although still far from prosperous, the Ik, as observed by Townsend, now maintain a culture of community sharing.

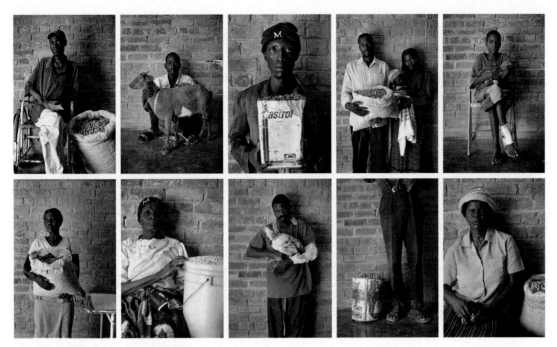

At Zimbabwe's Chidamoyo Hospital, patients often barter farm products for medical treatment. How does barter fit with the exchange principles discussed here?

Robin Hammond/*The New York Times*/Redux Pictures

One way of reducing the tension in situations of potential negative reciprocity is to engage in "silent trade." One example is the silent trade of the Mbuti "pygmy" foragers of the African equatorial forest and their neighboring horticultural villagers. There is no personal contact during their exchanges. A Mbuti hunter leaves game, honey, or another forest product at a customary site. Villagers collect it and leave crops in exchange. The parties can bargain silently. If one feels the return is insufficient, he or she simply leaves it at the trading site. If the other party wants to continue trade, it will be increased.

Coexistence of Exchange Principles

In contemporary North America, the market principle governs most exchanges, from the sale of property to the sale of consumer goods. We also have redistribution. Some of our tax money goes to support the government, but some also comes back to us in the form of social services, education, health care, and infrastructure. We also have reciprocity. Generalized reciprocity characterizes the relationship between parents and children. However, even here the dominant market mentality surfaces in comments about the high cost of raising children and in the stereotypical statement of the disappointed parent: "We gave you everything money could buy."

Exchanges of gifts, cards, and invitations exemplify reciprocity, usually balanced. Everyone has heard remarks like "They invited us to their daughter's wedding, so when ours gets married,

we'll have to invite them" and "They've been here for dinner three times and haven't invited us yet. I don't think we should ask them back until they do." Such precise balancing of reciprocity would be out of place in a foraging band, where resources are communal (common to all) and sharing is normal and essential to social life and survival (see Widlok 2017).

Generalized reciprocity is the most widespread form of exchange, because it exists in every kind of society, from foraging bands to industrial nations. The larger social and economic networks typically found among food producers (compared with foragers) allow for wider and more distant exchanges characterized by balanced and even negative reciprocity. Societies with chiefs have redistribution. The market principle tends to dominate exchanges in state-organized societies, to be examined further in Chapter 8, on political systems.

POTLATCHING

The **potlatch** is a festive event among tribes of the North Pacific Coast of North America, including the Salish and Kwakiutl of Washington and British Columbia and the Tsimshian of Alaska (Figure 7.5). Potlatching is a form of competitive feasting among villages that participate in a regional exchange network. Historically, at a potlatch, the sponsoring community gave away food and wealth items, such as blankets and pieces of copper, to visitors from other villages. The sponsoring community received prestige in return. That prestige

potlatch
A competitive feast on the North Pacific Coast of North America.

increased with the lavishness of the potlatch. Some North Pacific tribes still practice the potlatch, sometimes as a memorial to the dead (Kan 1986, 2016).

The potlatching tribes were foragers, but very atypical ones. Rather than living in nomadic bands, they were sedentary and had chiefs. They enjoyed access to a wide variety of land and sea resources. Among their most important foods were salmon, herring, candlefish, berries, mountain goats, seals, and porpoises (Piddocke 1969).

The economist Thorstein Veblen (1934) criticized potlatching, which he saw as an out-of-control form of conspicuous consumption. He emphasized the lavishness and supposed wastefulness, especially of Kwakiutl potlatches, to support his contention that in some societies people strive to maximize prestige at the expense of their material well-being. Anthropologists have challenged his interpretation.

Ecological anthropology, also known as *cultural ecology,* is a theoretical school in anthropology that attempts to interpret cultural practices, such as the potlatch, in terms of their possible long-term role in helping humans adapt to their environments (see Haenn, Wilk, and Harnish 2016). The ecological anthropologists Wayne Suttles (1960) and Andrew Vayda (1961/1968) viewed potlatching not in terms of its apparent wastefulness but in terms of its long-term role as a cultural adaptive mechanism (see also Trosper 2009). This view not only helps us understand potlatching; it also helps explain similar patterns of lavish feasting in many other parts of the world. Here is the ecological interpretation: *Customs like the potlatch are cultural adaptations to alternating periods of local abundance and shortage.*

How did this work? The overall natural environment of the North Pacific Coast is favorable, but resources fluctuate from year to year. Salmon and herring aren't equally abundant every year in a given locality. One village can have a good year while another is experiencing a bad one. Later their fortunes reverse. In this context, the potlatch cycle had adaptive value. It was not just a competitive display; it also brought material benefits.

A village enjoying an especially good year had a surplus of subsistence items, which it could trade for more durable wealth items, such as blankets, canoes, or pieces of copper. Such wealth, in turn, could be given away and thereby converted into prestige. Members of several villages were invited to any potlatch and got to take home the resources that were distributed. In this way, potlatching linked villages together in a regional economy—an exchange system that distributed food and wealth from wealthy to needy communities.

The long-term adaptive value of potlatching becomes clear when we consider what happened when a formerly prosperous village had a run of bad luck. Its people started accepting invitations to potlatches in villages that were doing better. The tables were turned as the temporarily rich became temporarily poor and vice versa. The newly needy accepted food and wealth items. They were willing to receive rather than bestow gifts and thus to relinquish some of their stored-up prestige. They hoped their luck would eventually improve, so that resources could be recouped and prestige regained.

The potlatch linked local groups along the North Pacific Coast into a regional alliance and exchange network. Potlatching and intervillage exchange had adaptive functions, regardless of the motivations of the individual participants. The anthropologists who stressed rivalry for prestige were not wrong. They were merely emphasizing *motivations* at the expense of an analysis of economic and ecological *systems.*

The use of feasts to enhance individual and community reputations and to redistribute wealth

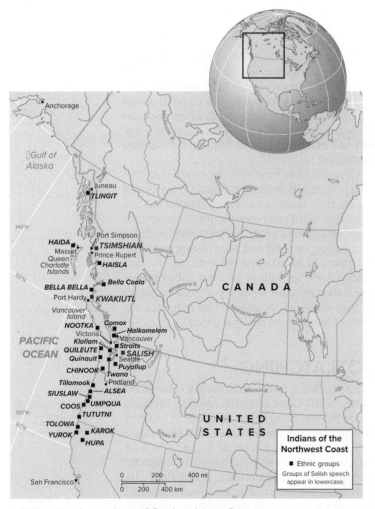

FIGURE 7.5 Location of Potlatching Groups.

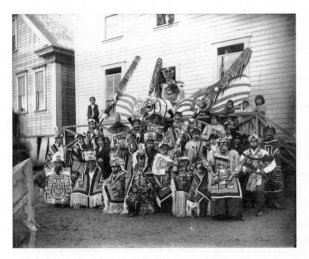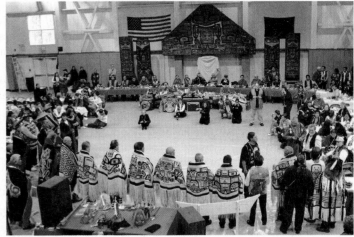

The potlatch then and now. The historic (1904) photo shows guests at a potlatch in Sitka, Alaska. In the photo on the right, taken in 2004, Tlingit clan members in Sitka celebrate the 100th anniversary of that potlatch.

(left): Source: Sitka National Historical Park/National Park Service/U.S. Department of the Interior; (right): *Daily Sitka Sentinel*, James Poulson/AP Images

is not unique to populations of the North Pacific Coast. Competitive feasting is widely characteristic of nonindustrial food producers. But among most foragers, who live, remember, in marginal areas, resources are too meager to support feasting on such a level. Among foragers living in marginal areas, sharing rather than competition prevails.

for REVIEW

summary

1. Cohen's adaptive strategies include foraging (hunting and gathering), horticulture, agriculture, pastoralism, and industrialism. Foraging was the only human adaptive strategy until the advent of food production (farming and herding) 12,000–10,000 years ago. Food production eventually replaced foraging in most places. Almost all modern foragers have at least some dependence on food production or food producers.

2. Horticulture and agriculture stand at opposite ends of a continuum based on labor intensity and continuity of land use. Horticulture doesn't use land or labor intensively. Horticulturalists cultivate a plot for one or two years and then abandon it. Farther along the continuum, horticulture becomes more intensive, but there is always a fallow period. Agriculturalists farm the same plot of land continuously and use labor intensively. They use one or more of the following: irrigation, terracing, and domesticated animals as means of production and manuring.

3. The pastoral strategy is mixed. Nomadic pastoralists trade with cultivators. Part of a transhumant pastoral population cultivates while another part takes the herds to pasture. Except for some Peruvians and the Navajo, who are recent herders, the New World lacks native pastoralists.

4. Economic anthropology is the cross-cultural study of systems of production, distribution, and consumption. In nonindustrial societies, a kin-based mode of production prevails. One acquires rights to resources and labor through membership in social groups, not impersonally through purchase and sale. Work is just one aspect of social relations expressed in varied contexts.

5. Economics has been defined as the science of allocating scarce means to alternative ends. Western economists assume that the notion of scarcity is universal—which it isn't—and that in making choices, people strive to maximize personal profit. In nonindustrial societies, indeed as in our own, people often maximize values other than individual profit.

6. In nonindustrial societies, people invest in subsistence, replacement, social, and ceremonial funds. States add a rent fund: People must share their output with social superiors. In states, the obligation to pay rent often becomes primary.

7. In addition to studying production, economic anthropologists study and compare exchange systems. The three principles of exchange are the market principle, redistribution, and reciprocity.

The market principle, based on supply and demand and the profit motive, dominates in states. With redistribution, goods are collected at a central place, but some of them are eventually given back, or redistributed, to the people. Reciprocity governs exchanges between social equals. It is the characteristic mode of exchange among foragers and horticulturalists. Reciprocity, redistribution, and the market principle may coexist in a society, but the primary exchange mode is the one that allocates the means of production.

8. Patterns of feasting and exchanges of wealth among villages are common among nonindustrial food producers, as well as among the potlatching cultures of North America's North Pacific Coast. Such systems help even out the availability of resources over time.

key terms

agriculture 137

balanced reciprocity 149

band 136

correlation 136

cultivation continuum 138

economizing 145

economy 141

food production 134

foraging 134

generalized reciprocity 149

horticulture 137

market principle 148

means (factors) of production 142

mode of production 141

negative reciprocity 149

nomadism (pastoral) 140

pastoralists 139

peasant 147

potlatch 151

reciprocity 148

reciprocity continuum 149

redistribution 148

transhumance 140

think like an anthropologist

1. When considering issues of "human nature," why should we remember that the egalitarian band was a basic form of human social life for most of our history?

2. Intensive agriculture has significant effects on social and environmental relations. What are some of these effects? Are they good or bad?

3. What does it mean when anthropologists describe nonindustrial economic systems as "embedded" in society?

4. What are your scarce means? How do you make decisions about allocating them?

5. Give examples from your own exchanges of different degrees of reciprocity. Why are anthropologists interested in studying exchange across cultures?

credits

Design Elements: Understanding Ourselves: muha/123RF (rock paintings); Focus on Globalization: janrysavy/Getty Images (globe); Appreciating Diversity (left to right): Floresco Productions/age footstock; Hero/Corbis/Glow Images, Hill Street Studios/Blend Images, Billion Photos/Shutterstock; Understanding Ourselves : Hemera Technologies/Alamy (Cymbal), LACMA - Los Angeles County Museum of Art (Trefoil Oinochoe), Ingram Publishing/SuperStock (Coin), ChuckSchugPhotography/Getty Images (Rug).

Political Systems

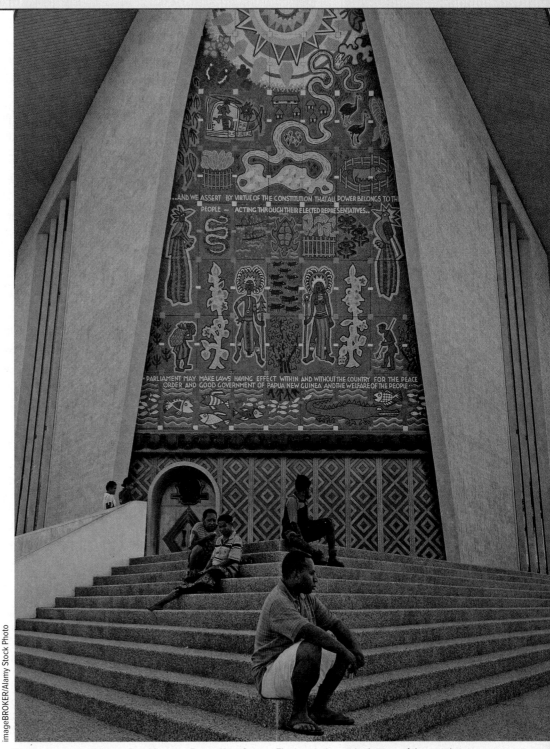

▶ What kinds of
political systems
have existed
worldwide,
and what are
their social
and economic
correlates?

▶ How does the
state differ from
other forms
of political
organization?

▶ What is social
control, and how
is it established
and maintained in
various societies?

imageBROKER/Alamy Stock Photo

The Parliament building in Port Moresby, Papua New Guinea. The inscription at the bottom of the mural states,
"Parliament may make laws having effect within and without the country for the peace, order, and good government
of Papua New Guinea and the welfare of the people."

understanding **OURSELVES**

You've probably heard the expression "big man on campus" (BMOC) used to describe a collegian who is very well known and/or popular. BMOC status might be the result of having a large network of friends, a trendy car or way of dressing, good looks, a nice smile, a sports connection, and a sense of humor. "Big man" has a different but related meaning in anthropology. Many indigenous cultures of the South Pacific had a kind of political figure that anthropologists call the "big man." Such a leader achieved his status through hard work, amassing wealth in the form of pigs and other native riches. Characteristics that distinguished the big man from his fellows, enabling him to attract loyal supporters (a large network of friends), included wealth, generosity, eloquence, physical fitness, bravery, and supernatural powers. Those who became big men did so because of their personalities rather than by inheriting their wealth or position.

Do any of the factors that make for a successful big man (or BMOC, for that matter) contribute to political success in a modern nation such as the United States? Although American politicians often use their own wealth, inherited or created, to finance campaigns, they also solicit labor and monetary contributions (rather than pigs) from supporters. And like big men, successful American politicians try to be generous with their supporters. Payback may take the form of a night in the Lincoln bedroom, an invitation to a strategic dinner, an ambassadorship, largesse to a particular area of the country, or favored access to federal stimulus funds. Tribal big men amass wealth and then give away pigs. Successful American politicians also dish out "pork."

As with the big man, communication skills contribute to political success (e.g., Ronald Reagan, Bill Clinton, Barack Obama, Donald Trump), although lack of such skills isn't necessarily fatal (e.g., either President Bush). What about physical fitness? Hair, height, health (and even a nice smile) are certainly political advantages. Bravery, as demonstrated through distinguished military service, may help political careers, but it certainly isn't required. Nor does it guarantee success. Just ask John McCain or John Kerry. Supernatural powers? Candidates who proclaim themselves atheists are as rare as self-identified witches or warlocks. Almost all political candidates claim to belong to a mainstream religion. Some even present their candidacies or policies as promoting God's will. However, contemporary politics isn't just about personality, as big man systems are. We live in a state-organized, stratified society with inherited wealth, power, and privilege, all of which have political implications. As is typical of states, kin connections play a role in—but once again can't guarantee—political success. Think of Kennedys, Bushes, and Clintons.

Anthropologists share with political scientists an interest in political systems, power, and politics. Here again, however, the anthropological approach is global and comparative and includes nonstates, whereas political scientists tend to focus on contemporary and recent nation-states (O'Neil 2018; Samuels 2021). Anthropological studies have revealed substantial variation in authority and in legal systems in different societies (see Goodale 2017; Pirie 2013; Walton and Suarez 2016). (**Power** is the ability to exercise one's will over others; *authority* is the formal, socially approved use of power, e.g., by government officials.) (See Plessner 2018; Schwartz, Turner, and Tuden 2011; Qian and Huo 2018.)

WHAT IS "THE POLITICAL"?

Morton Fried offered the following definition of political organization:

> Political organization comprises those portions of social organization that specifically relate to the individuals or groups that manage the affairs of public policy or seek to control the appointment or activities of those individuals or groups. (Fried 1967, pp. 20–21)

This definition certainly fits contemporary North America. Under "individuals or groups that manage the affairs of public policy" come various agencies and levels of government. Those who seek to influence public policy include political parties, unions, corporations, lobbyists, activists, political action committees (including super PACs), religious groups, and nongovernmental organizations (NGOs).

In nonstates, by contrast, it's often difficult to detect any "public policy." For this reason, I prefer to speak of *socio*political organization in discussing the exercise of power and the regulation of relations among groups and their representatives. *Political regulation* includes such processes as decision making, dispute management, and conflict resolution. The study of political regulation draws our attention to those who make decisions and resolve conflicts. Are there formal leaders? If not, who leads and how? (See Rhodes and Hart 2014; Stryker and Gonzalez 2014; Wolf with Silverman 2001.)

TYPES AND TRENDS

Ethnographic and archaeological studies in hundreds of places have revealed many correlations between the economy and social and political organization. Decades ago, the anthropologist Elman Service (1962) listed four types, or levels, of political organization: band, tribe, chiefdom, and state. Today, none of the first three types can be studied as a self-contained form of political organization, because all now exist within nation-states. There is archaeological evidence for early bands, tribes, and chiefdoms that existed before the first states appeared. However, because anthropology originated long after states did, anthropologists rarely if ever have observed "in the flesh" a band, tribe, or chiefdom outside the influence of some state. There still may be local political leaders (e.g., village heads) and regional figures (e.g., chiefs) of the sort discussed in this chapter, but all now exist and function within the context of state organization.

A *band* is a small, kin-based group (all its members are related by kinship or marriage) found among hunter-gatherers, such as the San ("Bushmen") of southern Africa or indigenous Australians. **Tribes** have economies based on horticulture and pastoralism. Living in villages and organized into kin groups based on common descent (clans and lineages), tribes have no formal government and no reliable means of enforcing political decisions. *Chiefdom* refers to a form of sociopolitical organization intermediate between the tribe and the state. In chiefdoms, social relations are based mainly on kinship, marriage, descent, age, generation, and gender—just as in bands and tribes. However, although chiefdoms are kin based, they feature **differential access** to resources (some people have more wealth, prestige, and power than others do) and a permanent political structure. The *state* is a form of sociopolitical organization based on a formal government structure and socioeconomic stratification.

The four labels in Service's typology are much too simple to account for the full range of political diversity and complexity known to archaeology and ethnography. We'll see, for instance, that tribes have varied widely in their political systems and institutions. Nevertheless, Service's typology does highlight some significant contrasts in political organization, especially those between states and nonstates. For example, in bands and tribes—unlike states, which have clearly visible governments—political organization does not stand out as separate and distinct from the total social order. In bands and tribes, it is difficult to characterize an act or event as political rather than merely social.

Service's labels *band, tribe, chiefdom,* and *state* are categories or types within a *sociopolitical typology.* These types are associated with particular adaptive strategies or economic systems.

power
The ability to exercise one's will over others.

tribe
A food-producing society with a rudimentary political structure.

differential access
Favored access to resources by superordinates over subordinates.

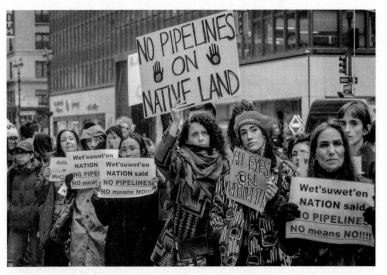

February 2, 2020: A rally organized in New York by a coalition of indigenous Peoples and indigenous-led organizations and held outside the Canadian Consulate and Permanent Mission to the United Nations. Demonstrators gather to support the Wet'suwet'en Nation of British Columbia, Canada, in their opposition to a Coastal GasLink pipeline scheduled to enter their traditional territory. As anthropologist Margaret Mead once observed about political mobilization, small groups of committed citizens have the capacity to change the world.
Erik McGregor/Getty Images

Thus, foragers (an economic type) tend to have band organization (a sociopolitical type). Similarly, many horticulturalists and pastoralists live in tribes. Although most chiefdoms have farming economies, herding has been important in some Middle Eastern chiefdoms. Nonindustrial states usually have an agricultural base.

Food production led to larger, denser populations and more complex economies than existed among foragers. New forms of sociopolitical organization emerged in response to the increased regulatory demands associated with cultivation, herding, and population increase. Archaeologists have studied these developments through time, and ethnographers have documented a range of sociopolitical forms among recent and contemporary societies (see Shore, Wright, and Però 2011).

BANDS AND TRIBES

This chapter will discuss, as case studies, a series of societies with different political systems. A common set of questions will be addressed for each one. What kinds of social groups does the society have? How do those groups deal with one another? How are their internal and external relations regulated? To answer these questions, we begin with bands and tribes and then consider chiefdoms and states.

Foraging Bands

Modern foragers are very different from their Stone Age predecessors (see Lee 2018). They live within nation-states, and in an interlinked world. All foragers now trade with food producers. The pygmies of Congo, for example, for generations have shared a social world and economic exchanges with neighbors who are cultivators. Furthermore, most contemporary hunter-gatherers rely on governments, missionaries, and other outsiders for at least part of what they consume.

The San

Chapter 7 described how the Basarwa San of Botswana have been affected by government policies that relocated them after converting their ancestral lands into a wildlife reserve (Motseta 2006). More generally, San speakers ("Bushmen") of southern Africa have been influenced by Bantu speakers (farmers and herders) for 2,000 years and by Europeans for centuries. Edwin Wilmsen (1989) contends that many San descend from herders who were pushed into the desert by poverty or oppression. He sees the San today as a rural underclass in a larger political and economic system dominated by Europeans and Bantu food producers. Within this system, many San now tend cattle for wealthier Bantu rather than foraging independently. San also have their own domesticated animals, further illustrating their movement away from a foraging lifestyle.

The nature of San life has changed considerably since the 1950s and 1960s, when a series of anthropologists from Harvard University, including Richard B. Lee, embarked on a systematic study of their lives. Studying the San over time, Lee and others have documented many changes (see Lee 2012, 2013, 2018; Tanaka 2014). Such longitudinal research monitors variation in time, while fieldwork in many San areas has revealed variation in space. One of the most important contrasts is between settled (sedentary) and nomadic groups (Kent and Vierich 1989). Although sedentism has increased substantially in recent years, some San groups (along rivers) have been sedentary for generations. Others, including the Dobe Ju/'hoansi San studied by Lee (2012, 2013) and the Kutse San whom Susan Kent (2002) studied, have retained more of the hunter-gatherer lifestyle.

To the extent that foraging continues to be their subsistence base, groups like the San can illustrate links between a foraging economy and other aspects of life in bands. For example, San groups that still are mobile, or that were so until recently, emphasize social, political, and gender equality, which are traditional band characteristics. A social system based on kinship, reciprocity, and sharing is appropriate for an economy with few people and limited resources. People have to share meat when they get it; otherwise, it rots. The nomadic pursuit of wild plants and animals tends to discourage permanent settlement, wealth accumulation, and status distinctions.

Marriage and kinship create ties between members of different bands. Trade and visiting also link them. Band leaders are leaders in name only. Bands are *egalitarian* societies. That is, they make only a few social distinctions, based mainly on age, gender, and individual talents or achievements. In

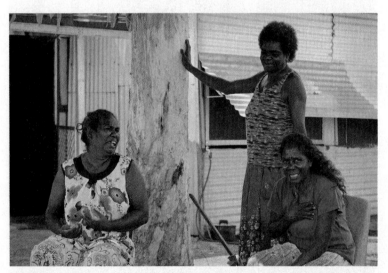

Like these indigenous women living in the Nyinyikay Homeland, East Arnhem Land, Northern Territory, Australia. most recent and contemporary foragers and their descendants participate in the modern world system.

Lynn Gail /Getty Images

these egalitarian societies, the "leaders" are merely first among equals. If they give advice or make decisions, they have no sure way to enforce those decisions.

The Inuit

The aboriginal Inuit (Hoebel 1954, 1954/1968), another group of foragers, provide a classic example of methods of settling disputes—**conflict resolution**—in stateless societies. All societies have ways of settling disputes (of variable effectiveness) along with cultural rules or norms about proper and improper behavior. *Norms* are cultural standards or guidelines that enable individuals to distinguish between appropriate and inappropriate behavior in a given society (N. Kottak 2002). Although rules and norms are cultural universals, only state societies, those with established governments, have laws that are formulated, proclaimed, and enforced (see Donovan 2007; Goodale 2017; Pirie 2013).

Foragers lacked formal **law** in the sense of a legal code with trial and enforcement, but they did have methods of social control and dispute settlement. The absence of law did not mean total anarchy. As described by E. A. Hoebel (1954) in a classic ethnographic study of conflict resolution, a sparse population of some 20,000 Inuit spanned 6,000 miles (9,500 kilometers) of the Arctic region (Figure 8.1). The most significant social groups were the nuclear family and the band. Personal relationships linked the families and bands. Some bands had headmen. There also were shamans (part-time religious specialists). However, these positions conferred little power on those who occupied them. Each Inuit had access to the resources he or she needed to sustain life. Every man could hunt, fish, and make the tools necessary for subsistence. Every woman could obtain the materials needed to make clothing, prepare food, and do domestic work. Inuit men could even hunt and fish in the territories of other local groups. There was no notion of private ownership of territory or animals.

Hunting and fishing by men were the primary Inuit subsistence activities. The diverse and

conflict resolution
Means of settling disputes.

law
A legal code of a state-organized society, with trial and enforcement.

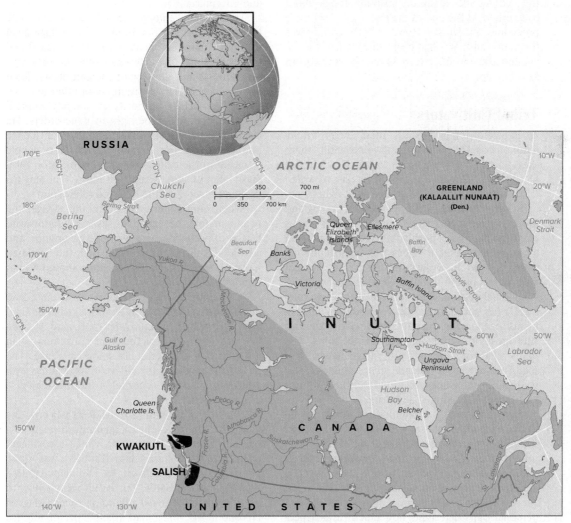

FIGURE 8.1 Location of the Inuit.

abundant plant foods available in warmer world areas, where female labor in gathering is important, were absent in the Arctic. Traveling on land and sea in a bitter environment, Inuit men faced more dangers than women did. The traditional male role took its toll in lives, so that adult women outnumbered men. This permitted some men to have two or three wives. The ability to support more than one wife conferred a certain amount of prestige, but it also encouraged envy. (*Prestige* is social esteem, respect, or approval.) If a man seemed to be taking additional wives just to enhance his reputation, a rival was likely to steal one of them. Most Inuit disputes were between men and originated over women, caused by wife stealing or adultery.

A jilted husband had several options. He could try to kill the wife stealer. However, if he succeeded, one of that man's relatives surely would try to kill him in retaliation. One dispute might escalate into several deaths as kinsmen avenged a succession of murders. No government existed to intervene and stop such a *blood feud* (a murderous feud between families). However, one also could challenge a rival to a song battle. In a public setting, contestants made up insulting songs about each other. At the end of the match, the audience proclaimed the winner. However, if the winner was the man whose wife had been stolen, there was no guarantee she would return. Often she stayed with her abductor.

Tribal Cultivators

As is true of foraging bands, there are no totally autonomous tribes in today's world. Still, there are societies, for example, in Papua New Guinea and in South America's tropical forests, in which tribal principles continue to operate. Tribes typically have a horticultural or pastoral economy and are organized into villages and/or *descent groups* (kin groups whose members trace descent from a common ancestor). Tribes lack socioeconomic stratification (i.e., a class structure) and a formal government of their own. A few tribes still conduct small-scale warfare, in the form of intervillage raiding. Tribes have more effective regulatory mechanisms than foragers do, but tribal societies have no sure means of enforcing political decisions. The main regulatory officials are village heads, "big men," descent-group leaders, village councils, and leaders of pantribal associations. All these figures and groups have limited authority.

Like foragers, horticulturalists tend to be egalitarian, although some have marked *gender stratification:* an unequal distribution of resources, power, prestige, and personal freedom between men and women. Horticultural villages usually are small, with low population density and open access to strategic resources. Age, gender, and personal traits determine how much respect people receive and how much support they get from others. Egalitarianism diminishes, however, as village size and population density increase. Horticultural villages usually have headmen—rarely, if ever, headwomen.

The Village Head

The Yanomami (Chagnon 2013*a;* Ferguson 1995; Ramos 1995) are Native Americans who live in southern Venezuela and an adjacent portion of Brazil. When anthropologists first studied them, they numbered about 26,000 people, living in 200 to 250 widely scattered villages, each with a population between 40 and 250. The Yanomami are horticulturalists who also hunt and gather. Their staple crops are bananas and plantains (a banana-like crop). There are more significant social groups among the Yanomami than exist in a foraging society. The Yanomami have families, villages, and descent groups. Their descent groups, which span more than one village, are patrilineal (ancestry is traced back through males only) and exogamous (people must marry outside their own descent group). However, branches of two different descent groups may live in the same village and intermarry.

Traditionally among the Yanomami the only leadership position has been that of **village head** (always a man). A village head is chosen based on his personal characteristics (e.g., bravery, persuasiveness) and the support he can muster from fellow villagers. The position is not inherited, and the village head's authority is severely limited. The headman lacks the right to issue orders. He can only persuade, harangue, and try to influence public opinion. For example, if he wants people to clean up the central plaza in preparation for a feast, he must start sweeping it himself, hoping his covillagers will take the hint and relieve him.

When conflict erupts within the village, the headman may be called on as a mediator who listens to both sides. He will give an opinion and advice. If a disputant is unsatisfied, the headman has no power to back his decisions and no way to impose punishments.

A Yanomami village headman also must lead in generosity. Expected to be more generous than any other villager, he cultivates more land. His garden provides much of the food consumed when his village hosts a feast for another village. The headman represents the village in its dealings with outsiders, including Venezuelan and Brazilian government agents.

Napoleon Chagnon (2013*a*) describes how one village headman, Kaobawa, guaranteed safety to a delegation from a village with which a covillager of his wanted to start a war. Kaobawa was a particularly effective headman. He had demonstrated his fierceness in battle, but he also knew how to use diplomacy to avoid offending other villagers. No one in his village had a better personality for the headship. Nor (because Kaobawa had many brothers) did anyone have more supporters. Among the Yanomami, when a village is dissatisfied with its headman, its members can leave and found a new village. This happens from time to time and is called *village fissioning.*

With its many villages and descent groups, Yanomami sociopolitical organization is more complicated than that of a band-organized society. The Yanomami face more problems in regulating relations between groups and individuals. Although a headman sometimes can prevent a specific violent act, intervillage raiding has been a feature of some areas of Yanomami territory, particularly those studied by Chagnon (2013a, 2013b).

The Yanomami are not isolated from outside events. They live in two nation-states, Venezuela and Brazil, and attacks by outsiders, especially Brazilian ranchers and miners, have plagued them (Chagnon 2013a; *Cultural Survival Quarterly* 1989; Ferguson 1995). During a Brazilian gold rush between 1987 and 1991, one Yanomami died each day, on average, from such attacks. By 1991, some 40,000 miners had reached the Brazilian Yanomami homeland. They introduced new diseases, and the swollen population ensured that old diseases became epidemic. Brazilian Yanomami were dying at a rate of 10 percent annually, and their fertility rate had dropped to zero. Since then, one Brazilian president has declared a huge Yanomami territory off limits to outsiders. Unfortunately, local politicians, miners, and ranchers have managed to evade the ban. The future of the Yanomami remains uncertain, especially with the election in 2018 of a Brazilian president, Jair Bolsonaro, who has shown little interest in preserving indigenous peoples and their territories.

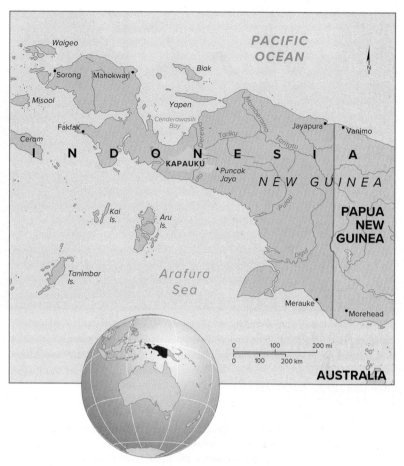

FIGURE 8.2 Location of the Kapauku.

The "Big Man"

Many societies of the South Pacific, particularly on the Melanesian Islands and in Papua New Guinea, had a kind of political leader that we call the big man. The **big man** (almost always a male) was an elaborate version of the village head, but with one significant difference. Unlike the village head, whose leadership was limited to one village, the big man had supporters in several villages. The big man thus was a regulator of regional political organization (Lederman 2015).

Consider the Kapauku Papuans, inhabitants of Irian Jaya, Indonesia (located on the island of New Guinea) (see Figure 8.2). Anthropologist Leopold Pospisil (1978) studied the Kapauku (then 45,000 people), who grew crops (with the sweet potato as their staple) and raised pigs. Their economy was too labor intensive to be described as simple horticulture. It required mutual aid in turning the soil before planting. The digging of long drainage ditches, which a big man often helped organize, was an even more complex endeavor. Kapauku cultivation supported a larger and denser population than does the simpler horticulture of the Yanomami. The Kapauku economy required collective cultivation and political regulation of the more complex tasks.

The key political figure among the Kapauku was the big man. Known as a *tonowi,* he achieved that status through hard work, amassing wealth in the form of pigs and other native riches. Big men were marked by certain characteristics that distinguished them from their fellows. Key attributes included wealth, generosity, eloquence, physical fitness, bravery, supernatural powers, and the ability to gain the support and loyalty of others. Big man was not an inherited position; men achieved that status through hard work and good judgment. They created wealth by breeding, raising, and trading pigs. As a man's pig herd and prestige grew, he attracted supporters. He sponsored pig feasts in which pork (provided by the big man and his supporters) was distributed to guests, bringing him more prestige and widening his network of support (see also O'Connor 2015).

The *tonowi*'s supporters, acknowledging past favors and anticipating future rewards, recognized him as a leader and accepted his decisions as binding. The *tonowi* was an important regulator of regional events in Kapauku life. He helped determine the dates for feasts and markets. He initiated

big man
A generous tribal entrepreneur with multivillage support.

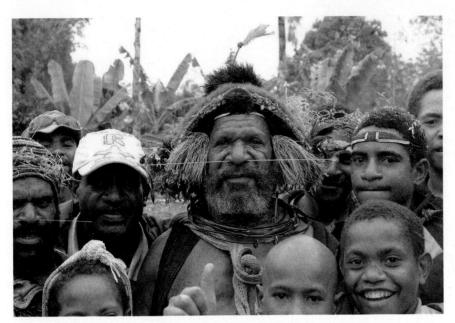

The "big man," like this one from highland Papua New Guinea, persuades people to organize feasts, which distribute pork and wealth. Big men owe their status to their individual personalities rather than to inherited wealth or position. Does our society have equivalents of big men?

Edward Reeves/Alamy Stock Photo

economic projects requiring the cooperation of a regional community.

The Kapauku big man again exemplifies a generalization about leadership in tribal societies: If someone achieves wealth and widespread respect and support, he or she must be generous. The big man worked hard not to hoard wealth but to be able to give away the fruits of his labor, to convert wealth into prestige and gratitude. A stingy big man would lose his support. Selfish and greedy big men sometimes were killed by their fellows (Zimmer-Tamakoshi 1997).

Pantribal Sodalities

Big men could forge regional political organization, albeit temporarily, by mobilizing supporters from several villages. Other principles in tribal societies—such as a belief in common ancestry, kinship, or descent—could be used to link local groups within a region. The same descent group, for example, might span several villages, and its dispersed members might recognize the same leader.

Principles other than kinship also can link local groups, especially in modern societies. People who live in different parts of the same nation may belong to the same labor union, sorority or fraternity, political party, or religious denomination. In tribes, nonkin groups called *associations* or *sodalities* may serve a similar linking function. Often, sodalities are based on common age or gender, with all-male sodalities more common than all-female ones.

pantribal sodalities
Non–kin-based groups with regional political significance.

Pantribal sodalities are groups that extend across the whole tribe, spanning several villages.

Such sodalities were especially likely to develop in situations of warfare with a neighboring tribe. Mobilizing their members from multiple villages within the same tribe, pantribal sodalities could assemble a force to attack or retaliate against another tribe.

The best examples of pantribal sodalities come from the Central Plains of North America and from tropical Africa. During the 18th and 19th centuries, Native American populations of the Great Plains of the United States and Canada experienced a rapid growth of pantribal sodalities. This development reflected an economic change that followed the spread of horses, which had been reintroduced to the Americas by the Spanish, to the area between the Rocky Mountains and the Mississippi River. Many Plains Indian societies changed their adaptive strategies because of the horse. At first they had been foragers who hunted bison (buffalo) on foot. Later they adopted a mixed economy based on hunting, gathering, and horticulture. Finally, they changed to a much more specialized economy based on horseback hunting of bison (eventually with rifles).

As the Plains tribes were undergoing these changes, other tribes also adopted horseback hunting and moved into the Plains. Attempting to occupy the same area, groups came into conflict. A pattern of warfare developed in which members of one tribe raided another, usually for horses. The economy demanded that people follow the movement of the bison herds. During the winter, when the bison dispersed, a tribe fragmented into small bands and families. In the summer, when huge herds assembled on the Plains, the tribe reunited. They camped together for social, political, and religious activities, but mainly for communal bison hunting.

Two activities demanded strong leadership: organizing and carrying out raids on enemy camps (to capture horses) and managing the summer bison hunt. All the Plains societies developed pantribal sodalities, and leadership roles within them, to police the summer hunt. Leaders coordinated hunting efforts, making sure that people did not cause a stampede with an early shot or an ill-advised action. Leaders imposed severe penalties, including seizure of a culprit's wealth, for disobedience.

Many of these tribes had once been foragers for whom hunting and gathering had been individual or small-group affairs. They never had come together previously as a single social unit. Age and gender were available as social principles that could quickly and efficiently forge unrelated people into pantribal sodalities.

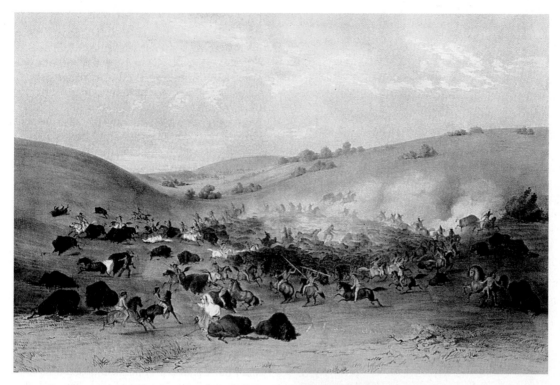

Natives of the Great Plains of North America originally hunted bison (buffalo) on foot, using the bow and arrow. The introduction of horses and rifles fueled a pattern of horse raiding and warfare. How far had the change gone, as depicted in this painting?

Popular Graphic Arts collection, Prints & Photographs Division, Library of Congress, LC-USZC2-3231

Raiding of one tribe by another, this time for cattle rather than horses, was common in eastern and southeastern Africa, where pantribal sodalities also developed. Among the pastoral Masai of Kenya, men born during the same four-year period were circumcised together and belonged to the same named group, an *age set,* throughout their lives. The sets moved through *age grades,* the most important of which was the warrior grade. Members of a set felt a strong allegiance to one another. Masai women lacked comparable set organization, but they also passed through culturally recognized age grades: the initiate, the married woman, and the female elder.

In certain parts of western and central Africa, pantribal sodalities are secret societies, made up exclusively of men or women. Like our college fraternities and sororities, these associations have secret initiation ceremonies. Among the Mende of Sierra Leone, men's and women's secret societies were very influential. The men's group, the Poro, trained boys in social conduct, ethics, and religion, and it supervised political and economic activities. Leadership roles in the Poro often overshadowed village headship and played an important part in social control, dispute management, and tribal political regulation. Age, gender, and ritual can link members of different local groups into a single social collectivity in a tribe and thus create a sense of ethnic identity, of belonging to the same cultural tradition.

Nomadic Politics

The political systems associated with pastoralism varied considerably, ranging from tribal societies

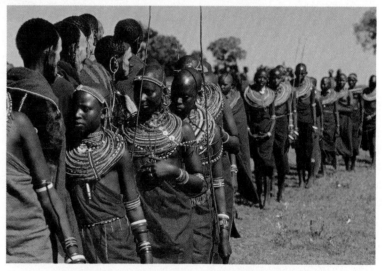

Among the Masai of Kenya and Tanzania, men born during the same four-year period belonged to the same named group, an age set, throughout their lives. The sets moved through grades, of which the most important was the warrior grade. Shown here is the *eunoto* ceremony in which young men become senior warriors and are allowed to choose wives.

imageBROKER/Alamy Stock Photo

to chiefdoms. The Masai (just discussed) live in a tribal society with no central leaders. Other pastoralists, however, have chiefs or similar leaders. (To *Game of Thrones* fans I offer Khal Drogo and Khaleesi Daenerys, successive leaders of the Dothraki people, as examples of such leaders in a nomadic society).

As ethnographic examples, consider two Iranian pastoral nomadic tribes—the Basseri and the Qashqai (Salzman 1974). Starting each year

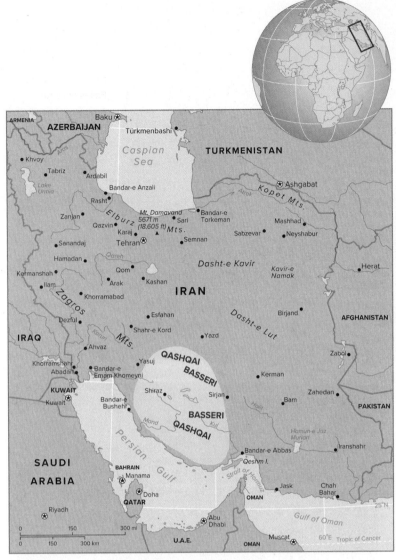

FIGURE 8.3 Location of the Basseri and Qashqai.

from a plateau near the coast, these groups took their animals to grazing land 17,000 feet (5,400 meters) above sea level (see Figure 8.3). The Basseri and the Qashqai shared this route with one another and with several other ethnic groups.

Use of the same pasture land at different times of year was carefully scheduled. Ethnic-group movements were tightly coordinated. Expressing this schedule is *il-rah,* a concept common to all Iranian nomads. A group's il-rah is its customary path in time and space. It is the schedule, different for each group, of when specific areas can be used in the annual trek.

Each tribe had its own leader, known not as the *khal,* but as the *khan* or *il-khan.* The Basseri khan, because he dealt with a smaller population, faced fewer problems in coordinating its movements than did the leaders of the Qashqai. Correspondingly, his rights, privileges, duties, and authority were weaker. Nevertheless, his authority exceeded that of any political figure discussed so far. The khan's authority still came from his personal traits rather than from his office. That is, the Basseri followed a particular khan not because of a political position he happened to fill but because of their personal allegiance and loyalty to him as a man. The khan relied on the support of the heads of the descent groups into which Basseri society was divided.

Among the Qashqai, however, allegiance shifted from the person to the office. The Qashqai had multiple levels of authority and more powerful chiefs or khans. Managing 400,000 people required a complex hierarchy. Heading it was the il-khan, helped by a deputy, under whom were the heads of constituent tribes (khans themselves), under each of whom were clan heads.

A case illustrates just how developed the Qashqai authority structure was. A hailstorm prevented some nomads from joining the annual migration at the appointed time. Although

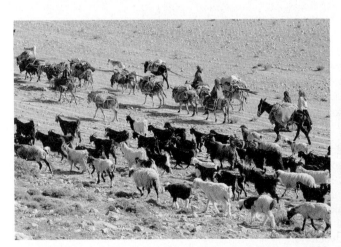

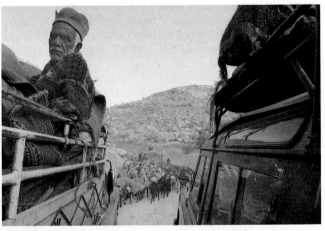

The Qashqai are pastoral nomads who traditionally trekked about 300 miles (480 kilometers) from highland summer pastures to lowland winter pastures near the Persian Gulf. The traditional migration is shown on the left; the modern trek, incorporating motor vehicles, on the right.

Left: Philippe Michel/age fotostock; right: Kaveh Kazemi/Getty Images News/Getty Images

everyone recognized that the latecomers were not to blame for their delay, the il-khan still assigned them less favorable grazing land, for that year only, in place of their usual pasture. The tardy herders and other Qashqai considered the judgment fair and didn't question it. This is one example of how Qashqai authorities regulated the annual migration. They also adjudicated disputes between people, tribes, and descent groups.

These Iranian cases can also illustrate the fact that pastoralism often is just one among many specialized economic activities within a nation-state. As part of a larger whole, pastoral tribes are constantly pitted against other ethnic groups. Within the context of the modern nation-state, that government becomes a final authority, a higher-level regulator that attempts to limit conflict among ethnic groups. State organization arose not just to manage agricultural economies but also to regulate the activities of multiple ethnic groups within expanding social and economic systems (see Das and Poole 2004).

CHIEFDOMS

A **chiefdom** is a polity with hereditary leaders and a permanent political structure. Some of its people and some of its settlements are ranked above others, and people with higher rank are favored in their access to resources. Often in chiefdoms, individuals are ranked in terms of their genealogical distance from the chief. The closer one is to the chief, the greater one's social importance, but the status distinctions are of degree rather than of kind. Chiefdoms are not divided into clearly defined social classes. Such social *stratification* is, however, a key feature of the state.

Geographic areas where chiefdoms once existed include the circum-Caribbean (e.g., Caribbean islands, Panama, Colombia), lowland Amazonia, the southeastern United States, and Polynesia. Chiefdoms created the megalithic cultures of Europe, including the one that built Stonehenge. Bear in mind that chiefdoms and states can fall (disintegrate) as well as rise. Before Rome's expansion, much of Europe was organized at the chiefdom level, to which it reverted for centuries after the fall of Rome in the fifth century C.E.

A **state** is a polity that has a formal, central government and *social stratification*—a division of society into classes. The first states developed about 5,500 years ago; and the first chiefdoms, a thousand or so years earlier. Today, in a world full of nation-states, there are few, if any, surviving chiefdoms. In many parts of the world, the chiefdom was a transitional form of political organization that emerged during the evolution of tribes into states. State formation began in Mesopotamia (currently Iran and Iraq). It next occurred in Egypt, the Indus Valley of Pakistan

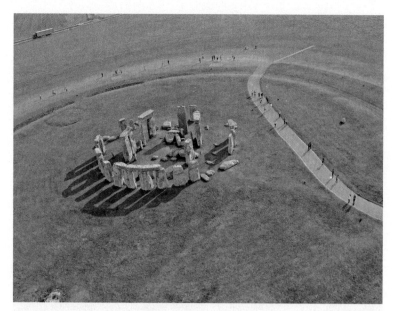

Chiefdoms as widespread as Mexico's Olmecs, Polynesia's Easter Island (Rapanui), and England's Stonehenge (shown here) are famed for their major works in stone. Stonehenge, built around 5,000 years ago, is comprised of standing stones arranged in a ring. Each stone is about 13 feet (4.0 m) high and 7 feet (2.1 m) wide and weighs about 25 tons.

Image Hans Elbers/Moment/Getty Images

and India, and northern China. A few thousand years later, states arose in two parts of the Western Hemisphere—Mesoamerica (Mexico, Guatemala, Belize) and the central Andes (Peru and Bolivia) (see Carneiro et al. 2017). Early states are known as archaic, or nonindustrial, states, in contrast to modern industrial nation-states. Robert Carneiro defines the state as "an autonomous political unit encompassing many communities within its territory, having a centralized government with the power to collect taxes, draft men for work or war, and decree and enforce laws" (1970, p. 733).

The *chiefdom* and the *state*, like many categories used by social scientists, are ideal types. That is, they are labels that make social contrasts seem sharper than they really are. In reality there is a continuum from tribe to chiefdom to state. Some societies had many attributes of chiefdoms but retained tribal features. Some advanced chiefdoms had many attributes of archaic states and thus are difficult to assign to either category. Recognizing this "continuous change" (Johnson and Earle 2000), some anthropologists speak of "complex chiefdoms" (Earle 1987, 1997), which are almost states.

Political and Economic Systems

Much of our ethnographic knowledge about chiefdoms comes from Polynesia (Kirch 2010, 2015, 2017), where they were common at the time of European exploration. In chiefdoms, social relations are mainly based on kinship, marriage,

chiefdom
A society with a permanent political structure, hereditary leaders, and social ranking but lacking class divisions.

state
A society with a central government, administrative specialization, and social classes.

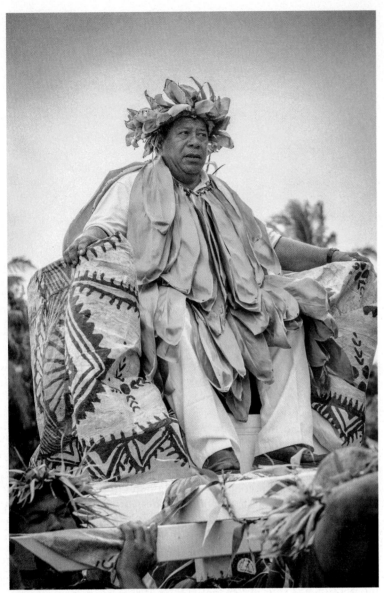

Citizens of Aitutaki, one of the Cook Islands in Polynesia, celebrate the investiture of Makirau Haurua as one of Aitutaki's four paramount chiefs. Dressed in traditional garb, Makirau Haurua is carried on a makeshift throne as part of his elevation to chiefly status.

Marco Pompeo Photography/Alamy Stock Photo

Polynesian chiefs were full-time specialists whose duties included managing the economy. They regulated production by commanding or prohibiting (often using religious taboos) the cultivation of certain lands and crops. Chiefs also regulated distribution and consumption. At certain seasons—often on a ritual occasion, such as a first-fruit ceremony—people would offer part of their harvest to the chief through his or her representatives. Products moved up the hierarchy, eventually reaching the chief. Conversely, illustrating obligatory sharing with kin, chiefs sponsored feasts at which they gave back some of what they had received (see O'Connor 2015). Unlike big men, chiefs were exempt from ordinary work and had special rights and privileges. Like big men, however, they still returned a portion of the wealth they took in.

Such a flow of resources to and then from a central place is known as *chiefly redistribution,* which offers economic advantages. If different parts of the chiefdom specialized in particular products, chiefly redistribution made those products available to the entire society. Chiefly redistribution also helped stimulate production beyond the basic subsistence level and provided a central storehouse for goods that might become scarce in times of famine (Earle 1987, 1997).

Status Systems

Social status in chiefdoms was based on seniority of descent. Polynesian chiefs kept extremely long genealogies. Some chiefs (without writing) managed to trace their ancestry back dozens of generations. Everyone in a chiefdom was related to everyone else. Presumably, all were descended from the same founding ancestors.

The chief would be the oldest child (usually son) of the oldest child of the oldest child, and so on. Degrees of seniority were calculated so intricately on some islands that there were as many ranks as people. For example, the third son would rank below the second, who in turn would rank below the first. The children of an eldest brother, however, would rank above the children of the next brother, whose children in turn would outrank those of younger brothers. However, even the lowest-ranking man or woman in a chiefdom was still the chief's relative, and everyone, including the chief, had to share with their relatives. It was difficult to draw a line between elites and common people.

Nevertheless, in chiefdoms as in states, some men, women, and even children had more prestige, wealth, and power than others did. These elites controlled resources such as land and water. Earle (1987) characterizes chiefs as "an incipient aristocracy with advantages in wealth and lifestyle" (p. 290).

Compared with chiefdoms, archaic states drew a much firmer line between elites and

descent, age, generation, and gender—as they are in bands and tribes. This is a basic difference between chiefdoms and states. States bring *nonrelatives* together and oblige them to pledge allegiance to a government.

Unlike bands and tribes, however, chiefdoms administer a regional political system that is permanent. Chiefdoms may include thousands of people living in many settlements. Regulation is carried out by the chief and his or her assistants, who occupy political offices. An **office** is a permanent position in a political structure; it must be refilled when it is vacated. The political system that is the chiefdom endures across the generations, thus ensuring permanent political regulation.

office
A permanent political position.

masses, distinguishing at least between nobles and commoners. Kinship ties did not extend from the nobles to the commoners because of *stratum endogamy*—marriage within one's own group. Commoners married commoners; elites married elites.

The Emergence of Stratification

We see that a key difference between chiefdom and state was the chiefdom's kinship basis. However, we know of historical instances in which ambitious chiefs and their closest relatives have launched an attack on their society's kinship basis. In Madagascar they would do this by demoting their more distant relatives to commoner status and banning marriage between nobles and commoners (Kottak 1980). Such moves, if accepted by the society, created separate social strata—unrelated groups that differ in their access to wealth, prestige, and power. (A *stratum* is one of two or more groups that contrast in social status and access to resources. Each stratum includes people of both genders and all ages.) The creation of separate social strata is called *stratification,* and its emergence signified the transition from chiefdom to state. The presence of stratification is one of the key distinguishing features of a state.

The influential sociologist Max Weber (1922/1968) defined three related dimensions of social stratification: (1) Economic status, or **wealth,** encompasses all a person's material assets, including income, land, and other types of property. (2) *Power,* the ability to exercise one's will over others—to get what one wants—is the basis of political status. (3) **Prestige**—the basis of social status—refers to esteem, respect, or approval for acts, deeds, or qualities considered exemplary. Prestige, or "cultural capital" (Bourdieu 1984), gives people a sense of worth and respect, which they may often convert into economic advantage (Table 8.1).

In archaic states—for the first time in human history—there were contrasts in wealth, power, and prestige between entire groups (social strata) of men and women. The **superordinate** (higher or elite) stratum had privileged access to valued resources. Access to those resources by members of the **subordinate** (lower or underprivileged) stratum was limited by the privileged group.

TABLE 8.1 Max Weber's Three Dimensions of Stratification

Wealth	→	Economic status
Power	→	Political status
Prestige	→	Social status

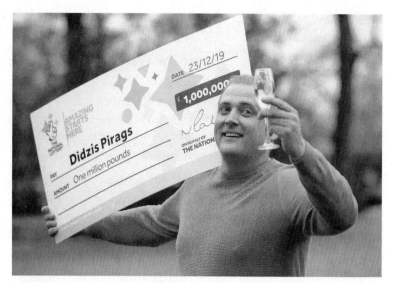

In Preston, Lancashire, United Kingdom, lottery winner Didzis Pirags, a single dad and chef, celebrates his £1 million win in the National Lottery Merry Millions game. Do lottery winners usually gain prestige, or merely money, as a result of their luck?
Danny Lawson/Newscom

STATE SYSTEMS

Recap 8.1 summarizes the information presented so far on bands, tribes, chiefdoms, and states. States, remember, are autonomous political units with social stratification and a formal government. States tend to be large and populous, and certain systems and subsystems with specialized functions are found in all states (see Sharma and Gupta 2006). They include the following:

1. Population control: fixing of boundaries, border control, establishment of citizenship categories, and censusing

2. Judiciary: laws, legal procedure, and judges

3. Enforcement: permanent military and police forces

4. Fiscal support: taxation

In archaic states, these subsystems were integrated by a ruling system or government composed of civil, military, and religious officials (Fried 1960). Let's look at the four subsystems one by one.

Population Control

To keep track of whom they govern, states enumerate—they conduct censuses. States also demarcate boundaries—borders—that separate that state from others. (See this chapter's "Appreciating Anthropology" for a discussion of border control issues in today's world.) Population displacements, within and between states, have increased with globalization and as war, famine, crime, and job seeking churn up migratory currents. Customs agents, immigration officers, navies, and coast guards

wealth
All a person's material assets; basis of economic status.

prestige
Esteem, respect, or approval.

superordinate
The upper, privileged group in a stratified society.

subordinate
The lower, underprivileged group in a stratified society.

SOCIOPOLITICAL TYPE	ECONOMIC TYPE	EXAMPLES	TYPE OF REGULATION
Band	Foraging	Inuit, San	Local
Tribe	Horticulture, pastoralism	Yanomami, Kapauku, Masai	Local, temporary regional
Chiefdom	Productive horticulture, pastoral nomadism, agriculture	Qashqai, Polynesia, Cherokee	Permanent regional
State	Agriculture, industrialism	Ancient Mesopotamia, contemporary United States and Canada	Permanent regional

patrol the frontiers. States also regulate population through administrative subdivision: provinces, districts, "states," counties, and parishes. Lower-level officials manage the subdivisions.

States often promote geographic mobility and resettlement, severing long-standing ties among people, land, and kin. Depending on the state, its citizens can identify by region, ethnicity, occupation, political party, religion, and team or club affiliation—rather than only as members of a descent group or an extended family.

States grant different rights to citizens and non-citizens. Status distinctions among citizens also are common. Archaic states granted different rights to nobles, commoners, and slaves. In American history prior to the Emancipation Proclamation, there were different laws for enslaved and free people. In European colonies, separate courts judged cases involving only natives and cases involving Europeans. In contemporary America, a military judiciary coexists alongside the civil system.

Judiciary

All states have laws based on precedent and legislative proclamations (see Dresch and Skoda 2012; Fikentscher 2016). Without writing, laws may be preserved in oral tradition. Crimes are violations of the legal code ("breaking the law"), with specified types of punishment. To handle crimes and disputes, all states have courts and judges (see Donovan 2007; Goodale 2017; Pirie 2013).

A striking contrast between states and non-states is intervention in internal and domestic disputes, such as violence within and between families. Governments step in to halt blood feuds and regulate previously private disputes. However, states aren't always successful in curbing internal conflict. Most of the world's armed conflicts since 1945 have begun within states—in efforts to overthrow a ruling regime or as disputes over ethnic, religious, or human rights issues.

Enforcement

How do states enforce laws and judicial decisions? All states have enforcement agents—some kind of police force, whose duties may include apprehending and imprisoning law-breakers. Confinement requires prisons and jailers. If there is a death penalty, executioners are needed. Government officials have the power to collect fines and confiscate property. The government uses its enforcement agents to maintain internal order, suppress disorder, and guard against external threats (with the military and border officials—see Maguire, Frois, and Zurawski 2014). As described in this chapter's "Focus on Globalization," censorship is another tool that governments employ to secure their authority.

Armies help states subdue and conquer neighboring nonstates, but conquest isn't the only reason state organization has spread. Although states impose hardships, they also offer advantages. States have formal agencies (e.g., military and police) designed to protect against external threats and to preserve internal order.

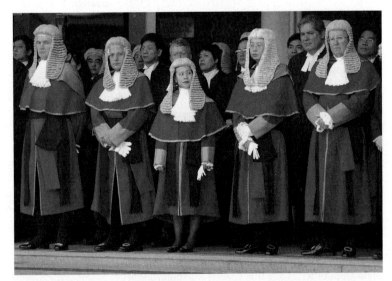

To handle disputes and crimes, all states have courts and judges. Shown here in a 2005 photo, judges in Hong Kong attend the annual ceremonial opening of the Legal Year at Hong Kong city hall. Does this photo say anything about cultural diffusion and/or colonialism?

Philippe Lopez/AFP/Getty Images

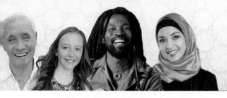

The Illegality Industry: A Failed System of Border Control

"Secure the border!" has become a familiar refrain in political discussion about undocumented immigrants to the United States. But what exactly does this mean? How can a border be truly secure in a world in which tens of millions of people, as well as migratory birds and mammals and the viruses they carry, are routinely on the move? What can anthropologists contribute to the discussion?

Ruben Andersson is a Swedish anthropologist who teaches in the Department of International Development at the University of Oxford. His 2014 book *Illegality, Inc.* is based on his ethnographic study of actual and would-be migrants to Europe, along with the people and agencies—some supportive, the majority just the opposite—they encounter along the way. The book's title reflects Andersson's contention that the European Union's migration policies have created an "illegality industry," which is fueling, rather than curbing, illegal activity.

According to the International Organization for Migration (IOM), at least 110,669 migrants and refugees reached Europe by sea in 2019. This was the sixth consecutive year with at least 100,000 people crossing via three Mediterranean Sea routes. The 2019 total was slightly below the 116,273 men, women and children who crossed in 2018.

Europe's migratory crisis year was 2015, when a million migrants and refugees sought asylum. The journey remains treacherous. The Mediterranean has claimed the lives of at least 19,164 migrants since 2014, mostly through drowning, as boats capsized. According to the IOM's Missing Migrants Project (MMP), at least 1,283 would-be migrants perished at sea in 2019, down from 2,299 in 2018. Most migrants are from West Africa, the Middle East, and Afghanistan. Political instability and war have been pushing refugees from the Middle East (especially Syria and Iraq) and Afghanistan toward Europe. Lack of job opportunities at home has been the main driver sending young West Africans toward Europe.

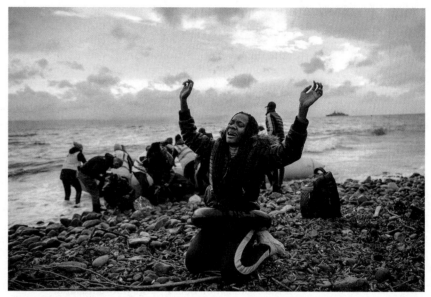

Alleluia! On February 29, 2020, a migrant from sub-Saharan Africa celebrates landing on the Greek island of Lesbos—having crossed from Turkey in a rubber dinghy.

Angelos Tzortzinis/Getty Images

Andersson did his fieldwork for his book between 2005 and 2014 and initially focused on would-be migrants from West Africa (mainly Senegal and Mali). Although his study took place before the recent refugee crisis in the Middle East, the lessons he derived can easily be applied to today's refugees.

Andersson began his research by focusing on a small sample of people with whom he established close personal relationships. He wanted to understand how border controls affect individual migrants. He was particularly struck by his informants' accounts of the various people and organizations they encountered (or tried to avoid) as they moved, and he extended his study to those intermediaries. He discovered an entire "illegality industry" deployed around, and benefiting financially from, migrants and their misfortunes. This industry supports border guards and police; defense, monitoring, and construction companies; nongovernmental aid organizations; journalists; and even academics building their careers on the study of migrants.

Among the greatest beneficiaries are human smugglers and traffickers, who increase their prices whenever and wherever border control tightens.

One of Andersson's main conclusions is that the current system of deterrence, although complex and expensive, is not working as intended. The European Union's border-control system includes razor-wire fences, naval blockades, drones, and command centers. In the nations through which migrants typically move (e.g., Turkey, Ukraine, Mauritania, Morocco, Libya), the EU subsidizes police officers to seek out and stop would-be migrants. Despite these barriers, migrants and refugees keep coming.

A more effective policy, Andersson argues, would be to normalize migration and provide people with legal, safe, and efficient ways of moving across national and continental borders (see also Andersson 2019). Can you apply lessons from Andersson's study to border control issues in contemporary North America? Is building walls likely to be an effective way to secure the border?

When they are successful in promoting internal peace, states enhance production. Their economies can support massive, dense populations, which supply armies and colonists to promote expansion.

Fiscal Support

States rely on financial, or **fiscal,** mechanisms (e.g., taxation) to support the government apparatus and agents just discussed. As in the chiefdom, the state intervenes in production, distribution, and consumption. The state may require a certain area to produce specific things, or ban certain activities in particular places. Like chiefdoms, states have redistribution ("spreading the wealth around"), but less of what comes in from the people actually goes directly back to the people.

In nonstates, people customarily share with their relatives, but people who live in states also have to turn over a significant portion of what they produce to the state. Officials standardize weights and measures and collect taxes on goods passing into or through the state. Of the revenues the state collects, it reallocates part for the general good and keeps another part (often larger) for itself—its agents and agencies.

State organization doesn't bring more freedom or leisure to the common people, who may be conscripted to build monumental public works. Some projects, such as dams and irrigation systems, may be economically necessary, but residents of archaic states also had to build temples, palaces, and tombs for the elites. Those elites reveled in the consumption of sumptuary goods—jewelry, exotic food and drink, and stylish clothing reserved for, or affordable only by, the rich. Peasants' diets suffered as they struggled to meet government demands for produce, currency, or labor (see Scott 2017). Commoners perished in territorial wars that had little relevance to their own needs. To what extent are these observations true of contemporary states?

Although it offers certain advantages, we should not think of the state as "better" than other forms of sociopolitical organization. Stratification and the state are antithetical to the egalitarian and free-ranging way of life practiced by our foraging ancestors. We have just considered some of the demands that states place on ordinary people. It should not be surprising, then, that certain groups have managed to resist or escape state organization by adopting lifestyles that are difficult for states to supervise. For example, James C. Scott (2009) discusses how a belt of Southeast Asian highland societies with economies based on shifting cultivation have survived for generations outside the control of states based in the lowlands of the same countries.

social control
Maintaining social norms and regulating conflict.

fiscal
Pertaining to finances and taxation.

hegemony
A stratified social order in which subordinates accept hierarchy as "natural."

SOCIAL CONTROL

In studying political systems, anthropologists pay attention not only to formal, governmental institutions but to other forms of social control as well. The concept of social control is broader than "the political." **Social control** refers to "those fields of the social system (beliefs, practices, and institutions) that are most actively involved in the maintenance of any norms and the regulation of any conflict" (N. Kottak 2002, p. 290). Norms are cultural standards or guidelines that enable individuals to distinguish between appropriate and inappropriate behavior.

Previous sections of this chapter have focused more on formal political organization than on sociopolitical process. We've seen how the scale of political organization has expanded through time and in relation to economic changes. We've examined means of conflict resolution, or their absence, in various types of society. We've looked at political decision making, including leaders and their limits. We've also recognized that all contemporary humans have been affected by states, colonialism, and the spread of the world system (see Kaplan 2014; Shore et al. 2011).

Sociopolitical was introduced as a key concept at the beginning of this chapter. So far, we've focused mainly on the political part of sociopolitical; now we focus on the social part. In this section we'll see that political systems have their informal, social, and subtle aspects along with their formal, governmental, and public dimensions.

Hegemony and Resistance

In addition to the formal mechanisms discussed in the "State Systems" section, what techniques do states employ to maintain social order? Antonio Gramsci (1971) developed the concept of **hegemony** for a stratified social order in which subordinates comply with domination by internalizing their rulers' values and accepting the "naturalness" of domination (this is the way things were meant to be). According to Pierre Bourdieu (1977, p. 164), every social order tries to make its own arbitrariness (including its mechanisms of control and domination) seem natural and in everyone's interest—even when that is not the case. Often promises are made (e.g., things will get better if you're patient).

Both Bourdieu (1977) and Michel Foucault (1979) argued that it is easier and more effective to dominate people in their minds than to try to control their bodies. Besides, and often replacing, physical coercion are more insidious forms of social control. These include various techniques of persuading and managing people and of monitoring and recording their beliefs, activities, and contacts.

Hegemony, the internalization of a dominant ideology, is one way in which elites curb resistance

The Political Role of New Media

Although the Internet makes possible the instantaneous global transmission of information, many countries restrict access to the Internet and other mass media for moral or political reasons. Many countries limit access to porn sites. In Cuba, Internet service is controlled by a state-owned telecom company. Availability is limited to crowded government-approved Wi-Fi hotspots in urban areas. Internet access is so limited and costly for most Cubans that formal censorship is unnecessary. China has a sophisticated censorship system—sometimes called the "Great Firewall of China." Off limits are social media websites, including Facebook, Twitter, and YouTube, that offer free interaction among people. The local search engine, Baidu, which observes the nation's censorship rules, drove Google out of China in 2010. Despite these roadblocks, China has more than twice as many Internet users (about half its population) as the United States (where about 90 percent have access).

Censorship can be a barrier to international business. The World Trade Organization (WTO) favors freedom of access to the Internet for commercial reasons: to allow free trade. WTO rules allow member nations to restrict trade to protect public morals or ensure public order, but with the understanding that such restrictions will disrupt trade as little as possible.

If the Internet and other media are used to promote free trade, how about free thought? The media have the capacity to enlighten by providing users with unfamiliar information and viewpoints and by offering a forum for dissident voices. Even when censorship is most stringent, people find ingenious ways of accessing forbidden information. North Korea's state-sanctioned television programming and screening, for example, has been penetrated by popular culture offerings from South Korean TV, and Western movies and cartoons smuggled in on DVDs.

More negatively, the media also spread and reinforce misinformation and stereotypes. In doing so, they blur the distinction between facts, evidence, and complexity, on the one hand, and propaganda, mere assertion, and oversimplification on the other. The media also promote fear, which often is manipulated for political reasons. Constant and instantaneous reporting has blurred the distinction between the international, the national, and the local. Geographic distance is obscured, and risk perception is magnified, by the barrage of "bad news" received daily from so many places. Many people have no idea how far away the disasters and threats really are. Was that suspicious package found in Paris or Pasadena? Did that subway bomb go off in New York or New Delhi? Votes in Athens, Greece, or Rome, Italy, can affect the American stock market more than votes in Athens or Rome, Georgia.

The political manipulation of media is not new. (Think of book banning and burning, for example. See http://www.ala.org/advocacy/bbooks/frequentlychallengedbooks for a list of books that have been challenged or banned in the United States between 2004 and 2018.) Would-be guardians of morality and authoritarian regimes always have sought to silence dissident voices. What is new is the potentially instantaneous and global reach of the voices that question both authority and democracy. New media, including cell phones, Facebook, Twitter, YouTube, and WhatsAp, have been used to muster public opinion and organize protests in places as distant as Rio de Janeiro, Brazil; Kiev, Ukraine; and Ferguson, Missouri. Can you think of examples of how new media have been used to question, and/or to reinforce, authority?

to their power and privileged position. Another way to discourage resistance is to make subordinates believe they eventually will gain power—as young people usually foresee when they let their elders dominate them. Yet another way to curb resistance is to separate or isolate people while supervising them closely, as is done in prisons (Foucault 1979).

Some contexts enable or encourage public resistance, particularly when people are allowed to assemble. The setting of a crowd offers anonymity, while also reinforcing and encouraging the common sentiments that have brought those people together. The elites, sensing the threat of surging crowds and public rebellion, often discourage such gatherings. They try to limit and control holidays, funerals, dances, festivals, and other occasions that might unite the oppressed. For example, in the American South before the Civil War, gatherings of five or more slaves were prohibited unless a white person was present.

Also working to discourage resistance are factors that interfere with community formation—such as geographic, linguistic, and ethnic separation. Elites want to isolate the oppressed rather than bringing them together in a group. Consequently, southern U.S. plantation owners sought slaves with diverse cultural and linguistic backgrounds, and limited their rights to assemble. Despite the measures used to divide them, the slaves did resist, developing their own popular culture, linguistic codes, and religious vision. The masters stressed portions of the Bible that emphasized compliance (e.g., the book of Job). The slaves, however, preferred the story of Moses and deliverance. The cornerstone of slave religion became the idea of a reversal in the conditions of whites and blacks. Slaves also resisted directly, through sabotage and flight. In many New World areas, slaves managed to establish free communities in the hills and other isolated areas (Price 1973).

Weapons of the Weak

The study of sociopolitical systems also should consider the sentiments and activity that may be hiding beneath the surface of evident, public behavior. In public, the oppressed may seem to accept their own domination, even when they are questioning it in private. James Scott (1990) uses the term "public transcript" to describe the open, public interactions between oppressed people and their oppressors. Scott uses "hidden transcript" to describe the critique of the power structure that goes on out of sight of those who hold power. In public, the elites and the oppressed may observe the etiquette of power relations. The dominants act like masters while their subordinates show humility and defer. But resistance often is seething beneath the surface (see Alexandrakis 2016).

Sometimes, the hidden transcript may include active resistance, but it is individual and disguised rather than collective and defiant. Scott (1985) uses Malay peasants, among whom he did field-work, to illustrate small-scale acts of resistance—which he calls "weapons of the weak." The Malay peasants used an indirect strategy to resist an Islamic tithe (religious tax). Peasants were expected to pay the tithe, usually in the form of rice, which was sent to the provincial capital. In theory, the tithe would come back as charity, but

it never did. Peasants didn't resist the tithe by rioting, demonstrating, or protesting. Instead, they used a "nibbling" strategy, based on small acts of resistance. For example, they failed to declare their land or lied about the amount they farmed. They underpaid, or they delivered rice contaminated with water, rocks, or mud to add weight. Because of this resistance, only 15 percent of what was due actually was paid (Scott 1990, p. 89).

Hidden transcripts tend to be expressed publicly at certain times (festivals and Carnavals) and in certain places (e.g., markets). Because of its costumed anonymity, Carnaval (Mardi Gras in New Orleans) is an excellent arena for expressing normally suppressed feelings. Carnavals celebrate freedom through immodesty, dancing, gluttony, and sexuality (DaMatta 1991). Carnaval may begin as a playful outlet for frustrations built up during the year. Over time, it may evolve into a powerful annual critique of stratification and domination and thus a threat to the established order (Gilmore 1987). (Recognizing this threat, the Spanish dictator Francisco Franco outlawed Carnaval.)

Shame and Gossip

Many anthropologists have noted the importance of "informal" processes of social control, such as fear, stigma, shame, and gossip, especially in small-scale societies. Gossip and shame, for example, can function as effective means of social control when a direct or formal sanction is risky or impossible. Gossip can be used to shame someone who has violated a social norm. Margaret Mead (1937) and Ruth Benedict (1946) distinguished between shame as an external sanction (i.e., forces set in motion by others, for example, through gossip) and guilt as an internal sanction, psychologically generated by the individual. They regarded shame as a more prominent form of social control in non-Western societies and guilt as a more dominant emotional sanction in Western societies. Of course, to be effective as a sanction, the prospect of being shamed or of shaming oneself must be internalized by the individual. In small-scale societies, in a social environment where everyone knows everyone else, most people try to avoid behavior that might harm their reputations and alienate them from their social network.

Nicholas Kottak (2002) studied political systems, and social control more generally, among the rural Makua of northern Mozambique (Figure 8.4). Social control mechanisms among the Makua extended well beyond the formal political system, as revealed in conversations about social norms and crimes. The Makua talk easily about norm

"Schwellkoepp," or "Swollen Heads," caricature local characters during a Carnaval parade in Mainz, Germany. Because of its costumed anonymity, Carnaval is an excellent arena for expressing typically suppressed speech. Is there anything like Carnaval in your society?

Daniel Roland/AP Images

violations, conflicts, and the sanctions that can follow them. Jail, sorcery, and shame are the main sanctions anticipated by the rural Makua.

Makua ideas about social control emerged most clearly in discussions about what would happen to someone who stole his or her neighbor's chicken. Most Makua villagers have a makeshift chicken coop in a corner of their home. Chickens leave the coop before sunrise each day and wander around, looking for scraps. Villagers may be tempted to steal a chicken when its owner seems oblivious to its whereabouts. The Makua have few material possessions and a meat-poor diet, making free-ranging chickens a real temptation. Their discussions about unsupervised chickens and the occasional chicken theft as community problems clarified their ideas about social control—about why people did *not* steal their neighbor's chickens.

The Makua perceived three main disincentives or sanctions: jail (*cadeia*), sorcery attack (*enretthe*), and shame (*ehaya*). (As used here, a *sanction* refers to a kind of punishment that follows a norm violation.) The main sanctions—sorcery and, above all, shame—came from society rather than from the formal political system. First, sorcery: Once someone discovered his chicken had been stolen, he would, the Makua thought, ask a traditional healer to launch a sorcery attack on his behalf. This would either kill the thief or make him very ill.

According to Nicholas Kottak (2002), the Makua repeatedly mention the existence of sorcerers and sorcery, although they aren't explicit about who the sorcerers are. They see sorcery as based on malice, which everyone feels at some point. Having felt malice themselves, individual Makua probably experience moments of self-doubt about their own potential status as a sorcerer. They recognize that others have similar feelings. Local theories see sickness, social misfortune, and death as caused by malicious sorcery. Life expectancy is short and infant mortality high in a Makua village. Health, life, and existence are far more problematic than they are for most Westerners. Such uncertainty heightens fears relating to sorcery. Any conflict or norm violation is dangerous because it might trigger a sorcery attack. The Makua see the chicken thief as the inevitable target of such an attack.

Makua fear sorcery, but they overwhelmingly mentioned shame as the main reason not to steal a neighbor's chicken. The chicken thief, having been discovered, would have to attend a formal, publicly organized village meeting, which would determine the appropriate punishment and compensation. The Makua were concerned not so much with a potential fine as with the intense and enduring shame or embarrassment they would feel as a confirmed chicken thief.

Rural Makua tend to live in one community for their entire lives. Such communities typically

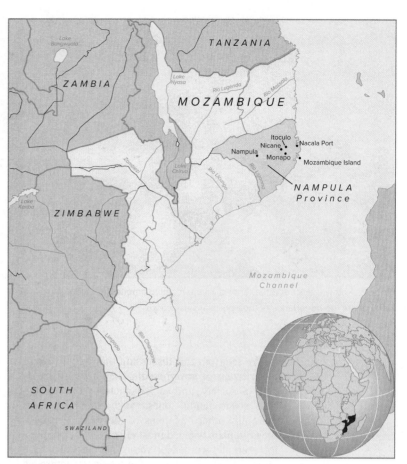

FIGURE 8.4 Location of the Makua and the Village of Nicane in the Province of Nampula in Northern Mozambique.

The Province of Nampula shown here is Makua territory.

have fewer than a thousand people, so that residents can easily keep track of one another's identities and reputations. Tight clustering of homes, markets, and schools facilitates the monitoring process. In this social environment, people try to avoid behavior that might spoil their reputations and alienate them from society.

Shame can be a very powerful sanction. Bronislaw Malinowski (1927) described how Trobriand Islanders might climb to the top of a palm tree and dive to their deaths because they couldn't tolerate the shame associated with public knowledge of some stigmatizing action. Makua villagers tell the story of a man rumored to have fathered a child with his stepdaughter. The political authorities imposed no formal sanctions (e.g., a fine or jail time) on this man, but gossip about the affair circulated widely. The gossip crystallized in the lyrics of a song that groups of young women would perform. After the man heard his name and behavior mentioned in that song, he hanged himself by the neck from a tree (N. Kottak 2002). (Previously we saw the role of song in the social control system of the Inuit. We'll see it again in the case of the Igbo Women's War, discussed in the next section.)

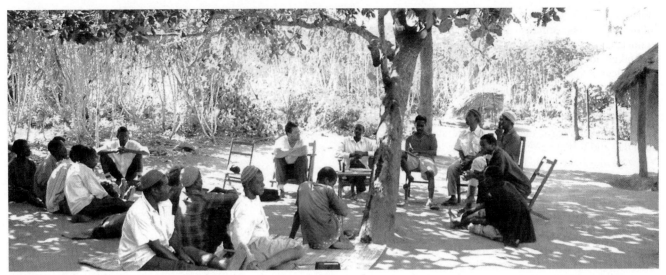

Nicholas Kottak (back center) attends a village meeting among the Makua of northern Mozambique. Two chiefs have called the meeting to renegotiate the boundaries of their political jurisdictions.

Nicholas C. Kottak

We see from this discussion that people aren't just citizens of governments; they are also members of society, and social sanctions exist alongside governmental ones. Such sanctions also exemplify other "weapons of the weak," because they often are wielded most effectively by people—for example, women or young people—who have limited access to the formal authority structure, as in the Igbo case, to which we now turn.

The Igbo Women's War

Shame and ridicule, used by women against men, played a decisive role in a protest movement in southeastern Nigeria in 1929. This is remembered

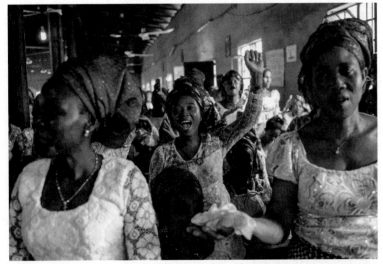

Igbo women dance and sing at a Catholic Church service in Aba, Nigeria on May 28, 2017. Political action by organized groups of Igbo women posed the first major challenge to British authority in Nigeria, and in West Africa more generally, during the colonial period.

Stefan Heunis/AFP/Getty Images

as the "Aba Women's Riots of 1929" in British colonial history and as the "Women's War" in Igbo history (see Dorward 1983; Martin 1988; Mba 1982; Oriji 2000; Van Allen 1971). During this two-month "war," at least 25,000 Igbo women joined protests against British officials, their agents, and their colonial policies. This massive revolt touched off the most serious challenge to British rule in the history of what was then the British colony of Nigeria.

In 1914, the British had implemented a policy of indirect rule by appointing local Nigerian men as their agents—known as "warrant chiefs." These chiefs became increasingly oppressive, seizing property, imposing arbitrary regulations, and imprisoning people who criticized them. Colonial administrators further stoked local outrage when they announced plans to impose taxes on Igbo market women. These women were key suppliers of food for Nigeria's growing urban population; they feared being forced out of business by the new tax. Market women were key organizers of the protests.

After hearing about the tax, thousands of Igbo women assembled in various towns to protest both the warrant chiefs and the taxes on market women. They used a traditional practice of censoring and shaming men through all-night song-and-dance ridicule (called "sitting on a man"). This process entailed constant singing and dancing around the houses and offices of the warrant chiefs. The women also followed the chiefs' every move, forcing the men to pay attention by invading their space (see also Walton and Suarez 2016). Wives of the warrant chiefs also urged their husbands to listen to the protesters' demands.

The protests were remarkably effective. The tax was abandoned, and many of the warrant chiefs resigned, some to be replaced by women. Other women were appointed to the Native courts as judges. The position of women improved in Nigeria, where market women especially remain a powerful political force to this day. Many Nigerian political events in the 1930s, 1940s, and 1950s were inspired by the Women's War, including additional tax protests. This Women's War inspired many other protests in regions all over Africa. The Igbo uprising is seen as the first major challenge to British authority in Nigeria and West Africa during the colonial period.

At the beginning of this chapter, *power* was defined as the ability to exercise one's will over others. It was contrasted with *authority*—the formal, socially approved use of power by government officials and others. The case of the Igbo Women's War shows how women effectively used their social power (through song, dance, noise, and "in-your-face" behavior) to subvert the formal authority structure and, in so doing, gained greater influence within that structure. Can you think of other, perhaps recent examples? We see how gossip, ridicule, and shaming can be effective processes of social control, which can even result in governmental change. The Igbo case also shows the importance of community organizing and political mobilization in effective resistance.

for REVIEW

summary

1. Although no ethnographer has been able to observe a sociopolitical system uninfluenced by some state, many anthropologists use a typology that classifies societies as bands, tribes, chiefdoms, or states. Foragers tended to live in egalitarian, band-organized societies. Personal networks linked individuals, families, and bands. Band leaders were first among equals, with no sure way to enforce decisions. Disputes rarely arose over strategic resources, which were open to all.

2. Political authority increased with growth in population size and density and in the scale of regulatory problems. More people means more relations among individuals and groups to regulate. Increasingly complex economies pose further regulatory problems.

3. Heads of horticultural villages are local leaders with limited authority. They lead by example and persuasion. Big men have support and authority beyond a single village. They are regional regulators, but temporary ones. In organizing a feast, they mobilize labor from several villages. Sponsoring such events leaves them with little wealth but with prestige and a reputation for generosity.

4. Age and gender also can be used for regional political integration. Among North America's Plains Indians, men's associations (pantribal sodalities) organized raiding and buffalo hunting. Such sodalities provide offense and defense when there is intertribal raiding for animals. Among pastoralists, the degree of authority and political organization reflects population size and density, interethnic relations, and pressure on resources.

5. The state is an autonomous political unit that encompasses many communities. Its government collects taxes, drafts people for work and war, and decrees and enforces laws. The state is a form of sociopolitical organization based on central government and social stratification. Early states are known as archaic, or nonindustrial, states, in contrast to modern industrial nation-states.

6. Unlike tribes, but like states, chiefdoms had permanent regional regulation and differential access to resources. But chiefdoms lacked stratification. Unlike states, but like bands and tribes, chiefdoms were organized by kinship, descent, and marriage. Chiefdoms emerged in several areas, including the circum-Caribbean, lowland Amazonia, the southeastern United States, and Polynesia.

7. Weber's three dimensions of stratification are wealth, power, and prestige. In early states—for the first time in human history—contrasts in wealth, power, and prestige between entire groups of men and women came into being. A socioeconomic stratum includes people of both genders and all ages. The superordinate—higher or elite—stratum enjoys privileged access to resources.

8. Certain systems are found in all states: population control, judiciary, enforcement, and fiscal. These are integrated by a ruling system or government composed of civil, military, and religious officials. States conduct censuses and demarcate boundaries. Laws are based on precedent and legislative proclamations. Courts and judges handle disputes and crimes. A police force maintains internal order, as a military defends against external threats. A financial, or fiscal, system supports rulers, officials, judges, and other specialists and government agencies.

9. *Hegemony* describes a stratified social order in which subordinates comply with domination by internalizing its values and accepting its "naturalness." Situations that appear hegemonic may have resistance that is individual and disguised rather than collective and defiant. "Public transcript" refers to the open, public interactions between the dominators and the oppressed. "Hidden transcript" describes the critique of power that goes on where the powerholders can't see it. Discontent also may be expressed in public rituals such as Carnaval.

10. Broader than the political is the concept of social control—those fields of the social system most actively involved in the maintenance of norms and the regulation of conflict. Sanctions are social as well as governmental. Shame, gossip, and fear of sorcery (among the Makua) can be effective social sanctions. The Makua and Igbo cases demonstrate how gossip, ridicule, and shaming can be effective processes of social control. In the Igbo Women's War, women effectively used their social power to subvert the formal authority structure and, in so doing, gained greater influence within that structure.

key terms

think like an anthropologist

1. This chapter notes that the labels *band, tribe, chiefdom,* and *state* are too simple to account for the full range of political diversity and complexity known to archaeologists and ethnographers. Why not get rid of this typology altogether if it does not accurately describe reality? What is the value, if any, of researchers retaining the use of ideal types to study society?

2. Why shouldn't modern hunter-gatherers be seen as representative of Stone Age peoples? What are some of the stereotypes associated with foragers?

3. What are sodalities? Does your society have them? Are they pantribal or pan-national? Do you belong to any? Why or why not?

4. What conclusions do you draw from this chapter about the relationship between population density and political hierarchy?

5. This chapter describes population control as one of the specialized functions found in all states. What are examples of population control? Have you had direct experiences with these controls? (Think of the last time you traveled abroad, registered to vote, paid taxes, or applied for a driver's license.) Do you think these controls are good or bad for society?

credits

Design Elements: Understanding Ourselves: muha/123RF (rock paintings); Focus on Globalization: janrysavy/ Getty Images (globe); Appreciating Diversity (left to right): Floresco Productions/age footstock; Hero/Corbis/ Glow Images, Hill Street Studios/Blend Images, Billion Photos/Shutterstock; Understanding Ourselves: Hemera Technologies/Alamy (Cymbal), LACMA - Los Angeles County Museum of Art (Trefoil Oinochoe), Ingram Publishing/SuperStock (Coin), ChuckSchugPhotography/Getty Images (Rug).

Gender

- ▶ How are biology and culture expressed in human sex/gender systems?

- ▶ How do gender, gender roles, and gender stratification correlate with other social, economic, and political variables?

- ▶ What is sexual orientation, and how do sexual practices vary cross-culturally?

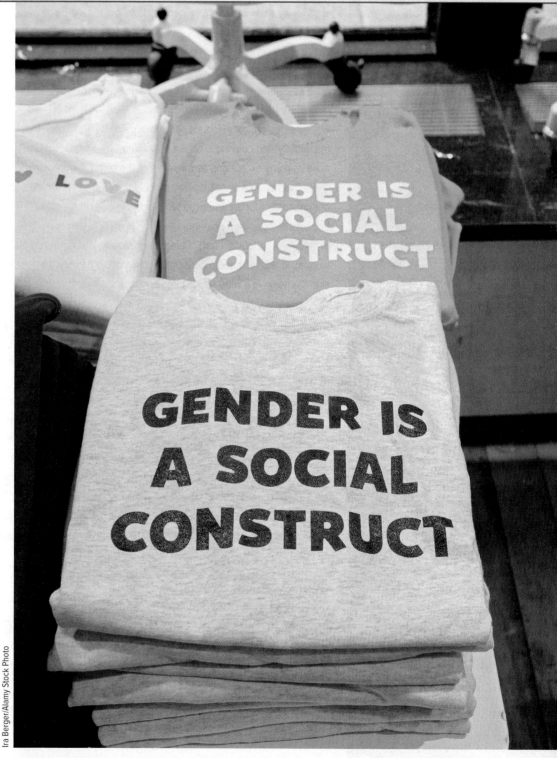

Ira Berger/Alamy Stock Photo

GENDER IS A SOCIAL CONSTRUCT

GENDER IS A SOCIAL CONSTRUCT

Unisex T-shirts for sale at PHLUID, which claims to be the world's first gender-free store, located on Broadway in Greenwich Village, Manhattan, New York.

understanding OURSELVES

A table (9.1) in this chapter lists activities that are generally done by the men in a society, generally done by the women in a society, or done by either men or women (swing). In this table, you will see some "male" activities familiar to our own culture, such as building houses, hunting, and butchering, along with activities that we consider typically female, such as doing the laundry and cooking. This list may bring to mind as many exceptions as followers of these "rules." Although it is not typical, it certainly is not unheard of for an American woman to hunt large game or an American man to cook (think of any male celebrity chef). Celebrities aside, women in our culture increasingly work outside the home in a wide variety of jobs—doctor, lawyer, accountant, professor—traditionally considered men's work. It is not true, however, that women have achieved equity in all types of employment. As of this writing, only 26 out of 100 U.S. senators are women. Only four women have ever served on the U.S. Supreme Court.

Ideas about proper gender behavior are changing just as inconsistently as are the employment patterns of men and women. Today's TV shows may feature characters who display nontraditional gender behavior and sexual behavior, while old beliefs, cultural expectations, and gender stereotypes linger.

The American expectation that proper female behavior should be polite, restrained, or unassuming poses a challenge for women, because American culture also values decisiveness and "standing up for what you believe in." When American men and women display similar behavior—speaking their minds, for example—they are judged differently. A man's assertive behavior may be admired and rewarded, but similar behavior by a woman may be labeled "aggressive," "nasty,"—or worse.

Both men and women are constrained by their cultural training, stereotypes, and expectations. For example, American culture has stigmatized male crying. It's okay for little boys to cry, but becoming a man often means giving up this natural expression of joy and sadness. Why shouldn't men be able to cry when they feel emotions? American men are trained as well to make decisions and stick to them. In our stereotypes, changing one's mind is more associated with women than with men and may be perceived as a sign of weakness. Politicians often criticize their opponents for being indecisive, for waffling or "flip-flopping" on issues. What a strange idea—that people shouldn't change their positions if they've discovered there's a better way. Males, females, and humanity may be equally victimized by aspects of cultural training.

Because anthropologists study biology, society, and culture, they are in a unique position to comment on nature (biological predispositions) and nurture (environment) as determinants of human behavior. Human attitudes, values, and behavior are limited not only by our genetic predispositions—which often are difficult to identify—but also by our experiences during enculturation. Our attributes as adults are determined both by our genes and by our environment during growth and development.

SEX AND GENDER

Questions about nature and nurture arise in the discussion of human sex-gender roles and sexuality. Men and women differ genetically. Women have two X chromosomes, and men have an X and a Y. The father determines a baby's sex because only he has the Y chromosome to transmit. The mother always provides an X chromosome.

The chromosomal difference is expressed in hormonal and physiological contrasts. Humans are sexually dimorphic, more so than some primates, such as gibbons (small, tree-living Asiatic apes), and less so than others, such as gorillas and orangutans. **Sexual dimorphism** refers to differences in male and female biology besides the contrasts in breasts and genitals. Women and men differ not just in primary (genitalia and reproductive organs) and secondary (breasts, voice, hair distribution) sexual characteristics but also in average weight, height, strength, and longevity. Women tend to live longer than men and have excellent endurance capabilities. In a given population, men tend to be taller and to weigh more than women do. Of course, there is a considerable overlap between the sexes in terms of height, weight, and physical strength, and there has been a pronounced reduction in sexual dimorphism during human evolution.

Just how far do these biological differences go, and what effects do they have on the way men and women act and are treated in different societies? Anthropologists have discovered both similarities and differences in the roles of men and women in different cultures. The predominant anthropological position on sex-gender roles and biology may be stated as follows:

> The biological nature of men and women [should be seen] not as a narrow enclosure limiting the human organism, but rather as a broad base upon which a variety of structures can be built. (Friedl 1975, p. 6)

Sex differences are biological, but gender encompasses all the traits that a culture assigns to and inculcates in males, females, and in some cases additional genders. **Gender,** in other words, refers to the cultural construction of whether one is female, male, or something else. Susan Bourque and Kay Warren (1987) emphasize the rich and varied constructions of gender among the world's cultures (see also Cornwall and Lindisfarne 2017). Margaret Mead did an early ethnographic study of variation in gender roles. Her book *Sex and Temperament in Three Primitive Societies* (1935/1950) was based on fieldwork in three societies in Papua New Guinea: the Arapesh, Mundugumor, and Tchambuli. The extent of personality variation in men and women among those three societies on the same island amazed Mead. She found that Arapesh men and women both acted as Americans traditionally have expected women to act: in a mild, parental, responsive way. Mundugumor men and women both, in contrast, acted as she believed we expect men to act: fiercely and aggressively. Finally, Tchambuli men were "catty," wore curls, and went shopping, but Tchambuli women were energetic and managerial and placed less

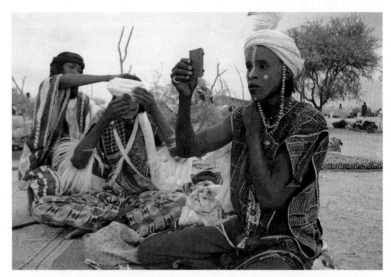

The realm of cultural diversity contains richly different social constructions and expressions of gender roles, as is illustrated by this Wodaabe man at the annual Gerewol male beauty contest in Niger.
Robert Harding World Imagery/Alamy Stock Photo

emphasis on personal adornment than did the men. (Drawing on their case study of the Tchambuli, whom they call the Chambri, Errington and Gewertz [1987], while recognizing gender malleability, have disputed the specifics of Mead's account.)

There is a well-established field of feminist scholarship within anthropology (Di Leonardo 1991; Lewin and Silverstein 2016; Rosaldo 1980b). Anthropologists have gathered systematic ethnographic data about similarities and differences involving gender in many cultural settings (Bonvillain 2021; Brettell and Sargent 2017; Burn 2019; Stimpson and Herdt 2014; Ward and Edelstein 2014). Anthropologists can detect recurrent themes and patterns involving gender differences. They also can observe that gender roles vary with environment, economy, adaptive strategy, and type of political system. Before we examine the cross-cultural data, some definitions are in order.

Gender roles are the tasks and activities a culture assigns by gender. Related to gender roles are **gender stereotypes,** which are oversimplified but strongly held ideas about the traits associated with different genders. **Gender stratification** describes inequality based on a gender hierarchy. There is differential access to socially valued resources, such as power, prestige, human rights, and personal freedom, based on gender.

In stateless societies, gender stratification often is more obvious in regard to prestige than it is in regard to wealth. In her study of the Ilongots of northern Luzon in the Philippines (Figure 9.1), Michelle Rosaldo (1980a) described gender differences related to the positive cultural value placed on adventure, travel, and knowledge of the external world. More often than women, Ilongot

sexual dimorphism
Marked differences in male and female biology besides the contrasts in breasts and genitalia.

gender
The cultural construction of whether one is female, male, or something else.

gender roles
The tasks and activities that a culture assigns to each sex.

gender stereotypes
Oversimplified, strongly held views about the characteristics of males and females.

gender stratification
The unequal distribution of social resources between men and women.

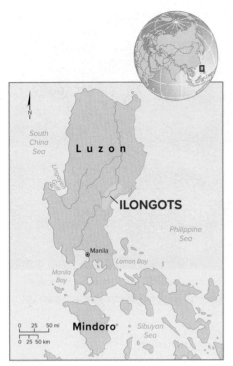

FIGURE 9.1 Location of Ilongots in the Philippines.

men, as headhunters, visited distant places. They acquired knowledge of the world outside, amassed experiences there, and returned to display their knowledge, adventures, and feelings in public oratory. They received acclaim as a result. Ilongot women had inferior prestige because they lacked external experiences on which to base knowledge and dramatic expression. We must distinguish between prestige systems and actual power in a given society (Ong 1989; see also Hodgson 2016). High male prestige does not necessarily mean that men wield economic or political power. (For more on Rosaldo's contributions to gender studies, see Lugo and Maurer 2000.)

RECURRENT GENDER PATTERNS

You probably had chores when you were growing up. If you had siblings, was there any gender bias in what you were asked to do, compared with a brother or sister? If you were raised by two parents, did any tension arise over your parents' division of labor? Based on cross-cultural data from 185 societies worldwide, Table 9.1 lists activities that are generally male, generally female, or swing

(either male or female). Before you look at that table, see if you can assign the following to one gender or the other (M or F): hunting large animals ( ), gathering wild plant foods ( ), tending crops ( ), fishing ( ), cooking ( ), fetching water ( ), making baskets ( ), making drinks ( ). Now consult the table and see how you did. Reflect on your results. Is what's true cross-culturally still true of the division of labor by gender in today's world, including the United States?

The data in the table illustrate cultural generalities rather than universals. For example, the table reports a general tendency for men to build boats, but there are societies that contradict the rule. One was the Hidatsa, a Native American group in which the women made the boats used to cross the Missouri River. (Traditionally, the Hidatsa were village farmers and bison hunters on the North American Plains; they now live in North Dakota.) Another exception is that Pawnee women worked wood; this is the only Native American group that assigned this activity to women. (The Pawnee, also traditionally Plains farmers and bison hunters, originally lived in what is now central Nebraska and central Kansas; they now live on a reservation in north central Oklahoma.)

Exceptions to cross-cultural generalizations may involve societies or individuals. That is, a society like the Hidatsa can contradict the cross-cultural generalization that men build boats by assigning that task to women. Or, in a society where men usually build boats, a particular woman or women can contradict that expectation by doing the male activity. Table 9.1 shows that in its sample of 185 societies, certain activities ("swing activities") are assigned to either or both men and women. Among the most important of these swing activities are planting, tending, and harvesting crops. Some societies customarily assign more farming chores to women, whereas others make men the primary farmers. Among the tasks almost always assigned to men, some (e.g., hunting large animals on land and sea) seem clearly related to the greater average size and strength of males. Others, such as working wood and making musical instruments, seem more arbitrary. Women, of course, are not exempt from arduous and time-consuming physical labor, such as gathering firewood and fetching water. In Arembepe, Bahia, Brazil, for example, women used to transport water in 5-gallon tins, balanced on their heads, from wells and lagoons located at long distances from their homes.

The original coding of the data in the table probably illustrates a male bias in that extradomestic activities received much more prominence than domestic activities did. Think about how female domestic activities could have been specified in greater detail. One wonders whether collecting wild honey is more necessary or time-consuming than nursing a baby (absent from the table). Also, notice that the table does not mention trade and

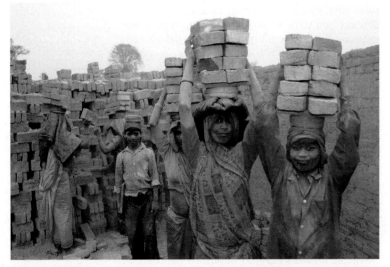

In many societies women (and children) routinely do hard physical labor, as is illustrated by these stone factory workers in Kathmandu, Nepal.

Horizons WWP/Alamy Stock Photo

TABLE 9.1 Generalities in the Division of Labor by Gender, Based on Data from 185 Societies

GENERALLY MALE ACTIVITIES	SWING (MALE OR FEMALE) ACTIVITIES	GENERALLY FEMALE ACTIVITIES
Hunting large aquatic animals (e.g., whales, walrus)	Making fire	Gathering fuel (e.g., firewood)
Smelting ores	Body mutilation	Making drinks
Metalworking	Preparing skins	Gathering wild plant foods
Lumbering	Gathering small land animals	Dairy production (e.g., churning)
Hunting large land animals	Planting crops	Spinning
Working wood	Making leather products	Doing the laundry
Hunting fowl	Harvesting	Fetching water
Making musical instruments	Tending crops	Cooking
Trapping	Milking	Preparing food (e.g., processing cereal grains)
Building boats	Making baskets	
Working stone	Caring for small animals	
Working bone, horn, and shell	Preserving meat and fish	
Mining and quarrying	Loom weaving	
Setting bones	Gathering small aquatic animals	
Butchering*	Clothing manufacture	
Collecting wild honey	Making pottery	
Clearing land		
Fishing		
Tending large herd animals		
Building houses		
Preparing the soil		
Making nets		
Carrying burdens		
Making mats		
Making rope		

*All the activities above "butchering" are almost always done by men; those from "butchering" through "making rope" usually are done by men.

SOURCE: Adapted from Murdock, G. P., and Provost, C., "Factors in the Division of Labor by Sex: A Cross-Cultural Analysis," Ethnology, vol. 12, no. 2, 1973, 202–225.

market activity, in which either or both men and women are active.

Both women and men have to fit their activities into 24-hour days. Turn now to Table 9.2, which shows that the time and effort spent in subsistence activities by men and women tend to be about equal. If anything, women do slightly more subsistence work than men do. In domestic activities and child care, however, female labor predominates. In about half the societies studied, men did virtually no domestic work. Even in societies where men did domestic chores, the bulk of domestic work was done by women. Adding together their subsistence activities and their domestic work, women tend to work more hours than men do. Furthermore, women had primary responsibility for young children in two-thirds of the societies studied.

What about access to mates? Table 9.3 shows that polygyny (multiple wives) is much more common than polyandry (multiple husbands). Furthermore, concerning premarital and extramarital sex, men tend to be less restricted than women are, although the restrictions were equal in about half the societies studied (Whyte 1978). Double standards that limit women more than men are one illustration of gender stratification, which we now examine more systematically.

GENDER ROLES AND GENDER STRATIFICATION

Economic roles influence gender stratification (the *unequal* distribution of social value by gender). In one cross-cultural study, Sanday (1974)

TABLE 9.2 Time and Effort Expended on Subsistence Activities by Men and Women*

More by men	16
Roughly equal	61
More by women	23

*Percentage of 88 randomly selected societies for which information was available on this variable.

SOURCE: Whyte, M. F., "Cross-Cultural Codes Dealing with the Relative Status of Women," *Ethnology,* vol. 17, no. 2, 1978, 211–239.

TABLE 9.3 Does the Society Allow Multiple Spouses?*

Only for males	77
For both, but more commonly for males	4
For neither	16
For both, but more commonly for females	2

*Percentage of 92 randomly selected societies for which information was available on this variable.

SOURCE: Whyte, M. F., "Cross-Cultural Codes Dealing with the Relative Status of Women," *Ethnology*, vol. 17, no. 2, 1978, 211–239.

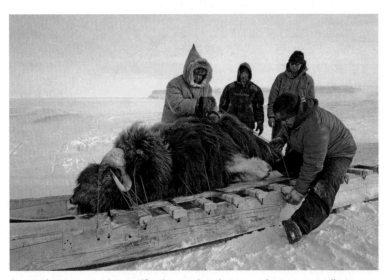

Among foragers, gender stratification tends to increase when men contribute much more to the diet than women do—as has been true among the Inuit and other northern hunters and fishers. Shown here, hunters transport a shot Muskox on a sledge, in Nunavut territory, Canada.

SeaTops/Alamy Stock Photo

domestic–public dichotomy
Work at home versus more valued work outside the home.

matrilineal descent
Descent traced through women only.

northern hunters and fishers. Among tropical and semitropical foragers, by contrast, gathering usually supplies more food than hunting and fishing do. Gathering is generally women's work. Men are the usual hunters and fishers, but women may do some fishing and hunt small animals, as is true among the Agta of the Philippines (Griffin and Estioko-Griffin 1985). Gender status tends to be more equal when gathering is prominent than it is when hunting and fishing are the main subsistence activities.

Gender status also is more equal when the domestic and public spheres are not sharply separated. (*Domestic* means within or pertaining to the home.) Strong differentiation between the home and the outside world is called the **domestic-public dichotomy** or the *private-public contrast.* The outside world can include politics, trade, warfare, or work. Often when domestic and public spheres are sharply separated, public activities have greater prestige than domestic ones do. This can promote gender stratification, because men are more likely to be active in the public domain than women are. Cross-culturally, women's activities tend to be closer to home than men's are. Another reason hunter-gatherers have less gender stratification than farmers and herders do is that the domestic–public dichotomy is less developed among foragers.

We've seen that certain gender roles are more sex-linked than others. Men are the usual hunters and warriors. Given such tools and weapons as spears, knives, and bows, men make better hunters and fighters because they are bigger and stronger on the average than are women in the same population (Divale and Harris 1976). The male hunter-fighter role also reflects a tendency toward greater male mobility.

Pregnancy, childbirth, lactation (nursing), and carrying infants interfere with female mobility, including her food gathering. However, among the Agta of the Philippines (Griffin and Estioko-Griffin 1985), women not only gather; they also hunt with dogs while carrying their babies. Still, given the effects of pregnancy and breast-feeding on mobility, it would be problematic for women to be the primary hunters (Friedl 1975). Warfare, which also requires mobility, is not typical of foraging societies, nor is interregional trade well developed. Warfare and trade are two public arenas that can contribute to status inequality of males and females among food producers.

Reduced Gender Stratification— Matrilineal–Matrilocal Societies

Cross-cultural variation in gender stratification is also related to rules of descent and postmarital residence (see Stone and King 2019). Many horticultural societies have **matrilineal descent** (descent traced through females only) and

found that gender stratification was least in societies in which men and women made roughly equal contributions to subsistence. Among foragers, gender stratification was most marked when men contributed much *more* to the diet than women did. This was true among the Inuit and other

matrilocality (residence after marriage with the wife's relatives). In such societies, female status tends to be high. Matriliny and matrilocality disperse related males, rather than consolidating them. By contrast, patriliny and patrilocality keep related males together, which is advantageous when warfare is present. Matrilineal–matrilocal systems tend to occur in societies where population pressure on strategic resources is minimal and warfare is infrequent.

Women tend to have high status in matrilineal-matrilocal societies for several reasons. Descent-group membership, succession to political positions, allocation of land, and overall social identity all come through female links. In Negeri Sembilan, Malaysia (Peletz 1988), matriliny gave women sole inheritance of ancestral rice fields. Matrilocality created solidary clusters of female kin. Women had considerable influence beyond the household. In such matrilineal contexts, women are the basis of the entire social structure. Although public authority may be (or may appear to be) assigned to the men, much of the power and decision making may actually belong to the senior women.

Matriarchy

If a *patriarchy* is a political system ruled by men, is a matriarchy necessarily a political system ruled by women? Or might we apply the term *matriarchy,* as anthropologist Peggy Reeves Sanday (2002) does, to a political system in which women play a much more prominent role than men do in social and political organization? One example would be the Minangkabau of West Sumatra, Indonesia, whom Sanday has studied for decades.

Sanday considers the Minangkabau a matriarchy because women are the center, origin, and foundation of the social order. The oldest village in a cluster of villages is called the "mother village." In ceremonies, women are addressed by the term used for their mythical Queen Mother. Women control land inheritance, and couples reside matrilocally. In the wedding ceremony, the wife collects her husband from his household and, with her female kin, escorts him to hers. If there is a divorce, the husband simply takes his things and leaves. Yet despite the special position of women, the Minangkabau matriarchy is not the equivalent of female rule, given the Minangkabau belief that all decision making should be by consensus.

Increased Gender Stratification– Patrilineal-Patrilocal Societies

Kay Martin and Barbara Voorhies (1975) link the decline of matriliny and the spread of the **patrilineal–patrilocal complex** (consisting of patrilineality, patrilocality, warfare, and male supremacy) to pressure on resources. (Societies

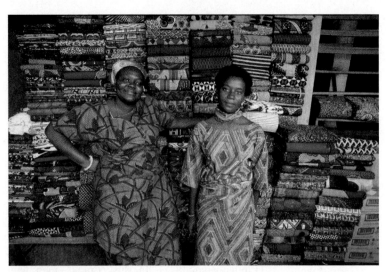

Many jobs that men do in some societies are done by women in others, and vice versa. In West Africa, women play a prominent role in trade and marketing. In Togo, shown here, women dominate textile sales. Is there a textile shop near you? Who runs it?

Pascal Deloche/GODONG/picture-alliance/Newscom

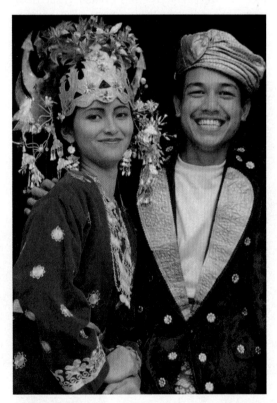

A Minangkabau bride and groom in West Sumatra, Indonesia, where anthropologist Peggy Reeves Sanday has conducted several years of ethnographic fieldwork.

Lindsay Hebberd/Corbis

with **patrilineal descent** trace descent through males only. In *patrilocal* societies a woman moves to her husband's village after marriage.) Faced with scarce resources, patrilineal-patrilocal cultivators such as the Yanomami often raid other villages. This favors patrilocality and

patrilineal-patrilocal complex

Male supremacy based on patrilineality, patrilocality, and warfare.

patrilineal descent

Descent traced through men only.

patriliny, customs that keep related men together in the same village, where they make strong allies in battle.

The patrilineal-patrilocal complex characterizes many societies in highland Papua New Guinea. Women work hard growing and processing subsistence crops, raising and tending pigs (the main domesticated animal and a favorite food), and doing domestic cooking, but they are isolated from the public domain, which men control. Men grow and distribute prestige crops, prepare food for feasts, and arrange marriages. The men even get to trade the pigs and control their use in ritual.

In densely populated areas of the Papua New Guinea highlands, male-female avoidance has been associated with strong pressure on resources (Lindenbaum 1972). In this context, men fear all contact with females, including sexual acts. They think that sexual contact with women will weaken them. Indeed, men see everything female as dangerous and polluting. They segregate themselves in men's houses and hide their precious ritual objects from women. They delay marriage, and some never marry. By contrast, the sparsely populated areas of Papua New Guinea, such as recently settled areas, lack such taboos on male-female contacts. The image of woman as polluter fades, male-female intercourse is valued, men and women live together, and reproductive rates are high.

Patriarchy and Violence

Patriarchy describes a political system ruled by men in which women have inferior social and political status, including basic human rights. Barbara Miller (1997), in a study of systematic neglect of females, describes women in rural northern India as "the endangered sex." Societies that feature a full-fledged patrilineal-patrilocal complex, replete with warfare and intervillage raiding, also typify patriarchy. Such practices as dowry murders, female infanticide, and clitoridectomy (removal of the clitoris) exemplify patriarchy, which extends from tribal societies such as the Yanomami to state societies such as India and Pakistan.

The gender inequality spawned by patriarchy and violence, which continues into the 21st century, can be deadly. Anyone who follows current events will have heard of recent cases of blatant abuse of women and girls, particularly in the context of warfare and terrorism, for example, in Bosnia, Syria, and Nigeria. In all of these places, rape has been used as a weapon of war or as punishment for transgressions committed by the victim's male relatives. In Afghanistan, Pakistan, and elsewhere, girls have been prevented from, or punished for, attending school. In 2014, Boko Haram, a jihadist rebel group in northern Nigeria, which also opposes female education, kidnapped nearly 300 schoolgirls, whom they subjected to abuse and forced marriages.

Sometimes, thankfully, such abuse fails in its attempt to silence female voices. Consider Malala Yousafzai (born in 1997 in northern Pakistan), who at the early age of 9 years embarked on her ongoing career as a forceful and persuasive advocate for female education.

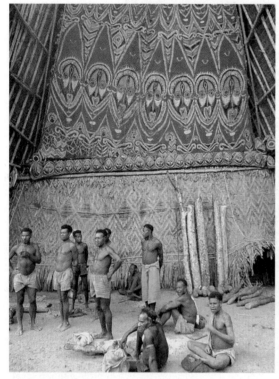

In some parts of Papua New Guinea, the patrilineal-patrilocal complex has extreme social repercussions. Regarding females as dangerous and polluting, men may segregate themselves in men's houses (such as this one, located near the Sepik River), where they hide their precious ritual objects from women. Are there places like this in your society?

George Holton/Science Source

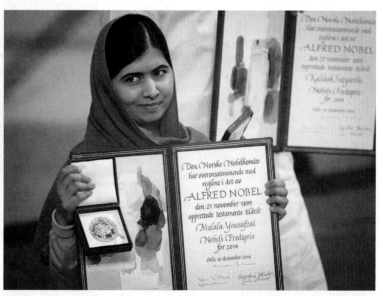

Education rights activist and Nobel Peace Prize winner Malala Yousafzai displays her medal and diploma during the Nobel awards ceremony in Oslo, Norway, on December 10, 2014.

Odd Andersen/AFP/Getty Images

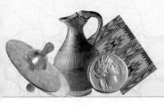

Patriarchy Today: Case Studies in Fundamentalist Communities

Patriarchy describes a society ruled by men in which women have inferior social and political status. Men systematically deprive women of basic human rights, including choices about their own bodies. In her recent (2020) book *Women in Fundamentalism,* anthropologist Maxine Margolis compares the status and treatment of women in three patriarchal religious communities. Each is an extreme fundamentalist offshoot of a major world religion, Christianity (Mormon polygamists), Judaism (Satmar Hasidim), and Islam (Afghan Pashtuns). Margolis describes how men, in each of these societies, exert patriarchal control over female bodies, activities, and associations.

Specifically, the three groups are: (1) Mormon polygamists known as the Fundamentalist Church of Jesus Christ of Latter-Day Saints (FLDS) of the American Southwest, (2) the Satmar Hasidim, mainly of New York state, and (3) the Pashtun ethnic group of Afghanistan and neighboring Pakistan. The FLDS Mormon polygamists live in Utah, Arizona, and Texas, with isolated enclaves in Canada and Mexico. The Satmar Hasidim live mainly in Williamsburg, Brooklyn, and in Kiryas Joel, a rapidly-growing town in Orange County, NY.

Each group values women principally as prolific child bearers. Particularly in the FLDS and Satmar communities, women are expected to give birth to as many children as possible. The FLDS community combines a preference for polygamy (multiple wives) with the expectation that each "sister wife" give birth to many children. Margolis quotes one FLDS boy who reported having about 55 aunts and uncles on his father's side and 22 on his mother's, with over a thousand cousins. In such families, he commented, it's hard to keep track of your own siblings, and impossible to remember all your cousins, aunts, and uncles.

Although the Satmar Hasidim do not practice polygamy, their birthrate–9 or 10 children per woman–is one of the highest in the United States. The village of Kiryas Joel is growing so rapidly that it has the youngest median age–a little over 13 years–of any municipality in the United States.

A Pashtun woman's prestige and influence within the extended family are determined by her number of sons. The birth of a baby boy is considered a success, but that of a baby daughter brings shame. Pity the poor woman who has no sons.

To ensure male control over female reproduction, each community requires modesty in female dress and behavior; restricts women's contact with outsiders—especially unrelated males; limits female educational opportunities; and maintains a sharp domestic–public dichotomy. Women interact mainly with family members and play no active role in political and religious institutions.

Women must do all they can to avoid attracting male attention. They should avoid form-fitting and flamboyant clothing, especially the color red. Satmar women should speak quietly and avoid laughing loudly or expressing enjoyment publicly, lest they excite some man's libido. Pashtun men protect their honor by closely supervising their female charges, whom they view as irrational and prone to seduction.

Pashtun women must cover their entire bodies in blue burqas, which have been likened to isolation chambers. Satmar women must shave their heads and wear wigs, often with an additional head covering; women's hair is considered enticing to men. Much of the body is clothed, including arms and legs (the latter with opaque stockings). FLDS women wear prairie-style dresses in pastel colors. Unlike the Satmar women, who must shave their heads, FLDS

women can never cut their hair. They wear it in a towering, sculpted hairstyle that requires hairspray to stay in place.

In all three groups, marriages are usually arranged, often between an older man and a younger, sometimes young teen, wife. If polygamy is practiced, as in the FLDS and Pashtun communities, the husband may be sexually experienced from a prior marriage, but the first-time wife almost never is. Among the Satmar, bride and groom are likely to be closer in age. Neither will know much, if anything, about sex, because of the rigid separation between boys and girls growing up and taboos on naming body parts involved in sex.

For the Pashtun, a woman's body belongs to a man, initially her father, eventually her husband. A Satmar woman moves at marriage from supervision and control by her father and male relatives to the same by her husband and in-laws. FLDS women make a similar transition from paternal to husbandly control.

How are these groups faring today? Despite efforts, mainly Western inspired, to enhance women's status in Afghanistan, there has been little progress, particularly among the rural Pashtun. FLDS membership has been declining as adherents have gained greater exposure to the outside world, including via the Internet. The Satmar, by contrast, are thriving, at least in terms of population growth and expansion within New York state.

Margolis's study reminds us that cultural anthropology is both ethnographic and comparative. The three patriarchal communities she describes, although offshoots of different religions, have developed remarkable similarities. All enforce male control over women, including over basic human rights such as marriage, reproduction, and presentation of self. To what extent do patriarchal institutions survive in the society in which you live?

Her courageous early work, including public speaking and a blog for the BBC (started when she was 11), criticized the Taliban for its efforts to block girls' education and prompted the Taliban to issue a death threat against her. In October 2012, a gunman shot Malala (then age 14) three times on a school bus as she was traveling home from school. She survived and has continued to speak out about the importance of education for girls. In 2014 she became the youngest person ever to receive the Nobel Peace Prize.

Family violence and domestic abuse of women are also widespread problems. Domestic violence certainly occurs in nuclear family settings, such as Canada and the United States, as well as in more blatantly patriarchal contexts. Cities, with their impersonality and isolation from extended kin networks, are breeding grounds for domestic violence, as also may be rural areas in which women lead isolated lives.

When a woman lives in her own birth village, she has kin nearby to protect her interests. Even in patrilocal polygynous (multiple wives) settings, women often count on the support of their cowives and sons in disputes with potentially abusive husbands. Unfortunately, settings in which women have a readily available social support network are disappearing from today's world. Patrilineal social forms and isolated families have spread at the expense of matriliny. Many nations have declared polygyny illegal. More and more women, and men, find themselves cut off from their families and extended kin.

With the spread of the women's rights and human rights movements, attention to abuse of women has increased. Laws have been passed, and mediating institutions established. Brazil's female-run police stations for battered women provide an example, as do shelters for victims of domestic abuse in the United States and Canada. A series of "Ladies Only" facilities, including trains and entry lines, can be found throughout India. But patriarchal institutions do persist in what should be a more enlightened world. (See this chapter's Appreciating Anthropology" for some examples.)

GENDER IN INDUSTRIAL SOCIETIES

The economic roles of men and women have changed and changed again over the course of American history. Nineteenth-century pioneer women worked productively in farming and home industry. As production shifted from home to factory, some women, particularly those who were poor or unmarried, turned to factory employment. Young white women typically worked outside the home only for a time, until they married and had children. The experience was different for African American women, many of whom, after abolition, continued working as field hands and domestic workers.

Changes in Gendered Work

Changing attitudes about women's work have reflected economic conditions and world events. In the United States, for example, the "traditional" idea that "a woman's place is in the home" developed as industrialism spread after 1900. One reason for this change was an influx of European immigrants, providing a male workforce willing to accept low wages for jobs, including factory work, that women previously might have done. Eventually, machine tools and mass production further reduced the need for female labor.

Anthropologist Maxine Margolis (2000) describes how gendered work, attitudes, and beliefs have varied in response to American economic needs. For example, when men are off fighting wars, work outside the home has been presented as women's patriotic duty, and the notion that women are biologically unfit for hard physical labor has faded.

The rapid population growth and business expansion that followed World War II created a demand for women to fill jobs in clerical work, public school teaching, and nursing (traditionally defined as female occupations). Inflation and the culture of consumption also have spurred female employment. When demand and/or prices rise, multiple paychecks help maintain family living standards.

Economic changes following World War II also set the stage for a women's movement, marked by the publication of Betty Friedan's influential book

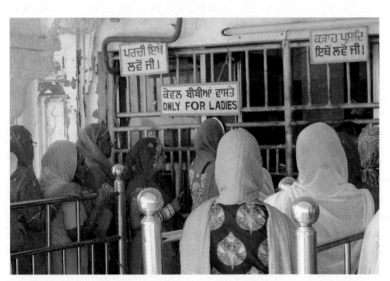

In many societies, especially patriarchal ones, women experience, and fear, intimidation as they increasingly enter the public sphere, especially in impersonal, urban settings. "Ladies Only" lines like this one at the Golden Temple in Amritsar, Punjab, India, are designed to help women move unmolested through public space.
Conrad P. Kottak

The Feminine Mystique in 1963 and the founding of NOW, the National Organization for Women, in 1966. Among other things, the movement promoted expanded work opportunities for women, including the goal (as yet unrealized) of equal pay for equal work.

As we see in Recap 9.1, in 1950 the 18.4 million American women who worked outside the home comprised less than one-third of all employed Americans. By 2000, that number had more than quadrupled—to 71.8 million—47 percent of the labor force. This percentage has stayed fairly constant since then, although the female-to-male earnings ratio has increased, from 60 cents on the dollar between 1950 and 1980 to 82 cents today. In 2018, there were 79.4 million employed American women—still 47 percent of the labor force (Semega et al. 2019). For one month (December) in 2019, women held slightly over half of all U. S. jobs on payrolls—those working full- or part-time for companies and other establishments. However, if we consider all jobs, including farm work and self-employment, the female share of the workforce remains about 47 percent.

Among the baby boomers (born between 1946 and 1964) who entered the American labor force in large numbers during the 1960s was a large influx of women. Female labor-force participation kept growing during the 1970s, 1980s, and 1990s, even during economic downturns. The rate of female participation peaked at 60 percent (of working-age American women) in 1999. Thereafter, it has declined, particularly during the severe recession of 2007–2009. Since 2008, the rate has declined further—to 57 percent in 2018 (U.S. Bureau of Labor Statistics 2018).

Although the female labor participation rate has fallen since 1999, the male rate has been falling, too. More women than men enter the workforce each year, and this has been true for several decades. Most dramatically, between 1964 and 1974, the number of employed American women grew by 43 percent, compared with 17 percent for men. Although the employment growth rate for both men and women slowed after the early 1980s, the female growth rate continued to exceed the male rate, and it still does. Women will continue to comprise a growing share of the American workforce.

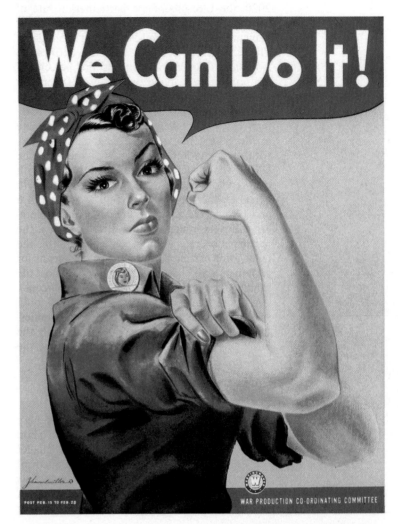

During the world wars, the notion that women were biologically unfit for hard physical labor faded. World War II's Rosie the Riveter—a strong, competent woman dressed in overalls and a bandana—was introduced as a symbol of patriotic womanhood. Is there a comparable poster woman today? What does her image say about modern gender roles?

National Archives and Records Administration (NWDNS-179-WP-1563)

RECAP 9.1	Female and Male Workforce Participation, Female–Male Employment Ratio, and Female-Male Earnings Ratio (Selected Years) 1950–2018

YEAR	MILLIONS OF WOMEN IN THE WORKFORCE	MILLIONS OF MEN IN THE WORKFORCE	FEMALE–MALE EMPLOYMENT RATIO	FEMALE-MALE EARNINGS RATIO
2018	79.4	88.1	.47	.82
2010	72.8	80.9	.47	.77
2000	71.8	80.6	.47	.74
1980	52.0	64.9	.44	.60
1960	30.6	50.0	.4	.61
1950	18.4	43.8	.3	.6

SOURCE: Semega, Jessica L., Kollar, Melissa A., Creamer, John, and Abinash Mohanty Table A-7. Number and Real Median Earnings of Total Workers and Full-Time, Year-Round Workers by Sex and Female-to-Male Earnings Ratio: 1960 to 2018. U.S. Census Bureau, *Current Population Reports*, P60–266. Washington, DC: U.S. Government Printing Office. https://www.census.gov/content/dam/Census/library/publications/2019/demo/p60-266.pdf

It's not mainly single women working today, as was the case in the 1950s. Prior to the massive unemployment caused by COVID-19 in 2020, the U.S. labor-force participation rate of parents with children under age 18 was about 70 percent for mothers and 93 percent for fathers. The U.S. Bureau of Labor Statistics defines the *labor force participation* rate as the percent of the population working or looking for work. In 2018 that rate was 72 percent for *all* American mothers with children under age 18. Currently *married* mothers were less likely to participate in the labor force, at 69 percent, than mothers with other marital statuses, at 77 percent. The labor force participation rate of *all* mothers with children under age 6 was 65 percent, rising to 76 percent when the youngest child was between 6 and 17 years old. Considering just *married* mothers with very young children (under age 3), the participation rate was 60 percent. In 2018, the labor force participation rate was 93 percent for *all* fathers with children under age 18, almost the same as the rate for married fathers (94 percent). Among married-couple families in 2018, both spouses were employed in 49 percent of families. In just 19 percent of those families was only the husband employed, while in 7 percent, only the wife worked outside the home.

Gender and Jobs

Thanks to automation and robotics, jobs have become less demanding in terms of physical labor. With machines to do the heavy work, the smaller average body size and lesser average strength of women are no longer significant impediments to blue-collar employment. But the main reason we don't see more modern-day Rosies working

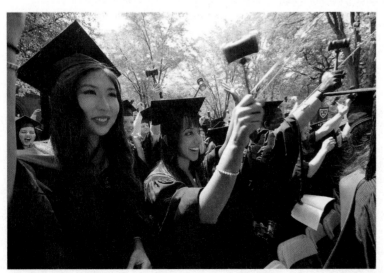

Harvard law school graduates wield their gavels in this 2015 commencement ceremony. Women are increasingly prominent among graduates of medical, law, and business schools.

Pat Greenhouse/Getty Images

alongside male riveters is that the U.S. workforce itself has been abandoning heavy-goods manufacture. In the 1950s, two-thirds of American jobs were blue-collar, compared with around 14 percent in 2019. The location of those jobs has shifted within the world capitalist economy. Developing countries, with their cheaper labor costs, produce steel, automobiles, and other heavy goods less expensively than the United States can, but the United States excels at services. The American mass education system has many deficiencies, but it does train millions of people for service and information-oriented jobs.

Another important change since the 1960s is the increasing levels of education and professional employment among women. For decades, more American women than men have attended and graduated from college. By 2019, women, ages 25 and older, had inched above 50 percent (50.2 actually) of the U.S. college-educated workforce—an 11 percent increase since 2000 (Matias 2019). Back in 1968, women made up less than 10 percent of the entering classes of MD (medicine), JD (law), and MBA (business) programs. The proportion of female students in those programs has risen to about 50 percent. Nowadays, female college graduates aged 30 to 34 are just as likely to be doctors, dentists, lawyers, professors, managers, and scientists as they are to be working in traditionally female professions, as teachers, nurses, librarians, secretaries, or social workers. In the 1960s, women were seven times more likely to be in the latter than in the former series of professions. Women now occupy more than half of professional and managerial positions. Almost 40 percent of all lawyers in the United States today are woman, compared with fewer than 10 percent in 1974.

In 1970, more than 60 percent of occupations were so male-dominated that 80 percent or more of their workers were male. Today that kind of occupational segregation has been reduced substantially. Only about a third of occupations have that degree of overrepresentation by males. At the same time, the share of occupations in which women make up 80 percent or more of workers has remained relatively constant at 10 percent.

Despite the many gains, female employment continues to lag noticeably in certain highly paid professions, such as computer science and engineering. In those fields, the percentage of female graduates has actually declined, to about 20 percent from 37 percent in 1980. By mid-career, twice the number of women as men leave their jobs in computer science, often because they perceive an uncomfortable and unsupportive workplace environment. Nearly 40 percent of women who left science, engineering, and technology jobs cited a "hostile macho culture" as their primary reason for doing so, versus only 27 percent who cited compensation (Council of Economic Advisers Report, 2014).

Work and Family: Reality and Stereotypes

As the workforce has changed, so, too, have ideas and attitudes about gender roles. Compare your grandparents and your parents. Chances are you have an employed mother, but your grandmother (and especially your great grandmother) was more likely to have been a stay-at-home mom. Your grandfather (and especially your great grandfather) is more likely than your father to have worked in manufacturing and to have belonged to a union. Your father is more likely than any of his male forebears to have participated significantly in child care and housework.

People everywhere have work and family obligations, but ideas about how to balance those responsibilities have changed considerably in recent years. As employment rose steadily after the 2008 recession and through 2019, Americans increasingly complained that work interferes with family—not the other way around. Some 46 percent of working men and women reported that job demands sometimes or often interfere with their family lives, up from 41 percent 15 years earlier (Parker and Livingston 2017).

Both men and women increasingly are questioning the notion that the man should be the breadwinner while the woman assumes domestic and child-care responsibilities. As of 2019, more than 40 percent of American mothers were the primary or sole source of income in their homes. This figure includes both single mothers and married mothers. Add to the rising percentage of female breadwinners the fact that fathers increasingly are taking on caregiving activities traditionally done by mothers. Seven percent of American families with children are father-only families. In general, American fathers spend significantly more time on child care and housework today than they did in the past. American fathers now do 4.6 more hours of child care, and 4.4 more hours of housework, per week than they did in 1965.

However, just as there are lingering barriers to women's progress in the workplace, obstacles remain to men's success at home. The reasons for this are both material and cultural. Material factors include the facts that women still do much more domestic work than men do, and the average man still works longer hours outside the home and earns more money than the average woman does, even in dual-earner households. There is a cultural lag as well. A stereotype that lingers is that of the incompetent male homemaker. For decades, clueless husbands and inept fathers have been a staple of television sitcoms—especially those produced after large numbers of women began to enter the workforce. Women still tend to think they are better homemakers than their husbands. Former Princeton professor Anne-Marie Slaughter (2013, 2015) cites examples of American women who maintain deeply entrenched stereotypes about

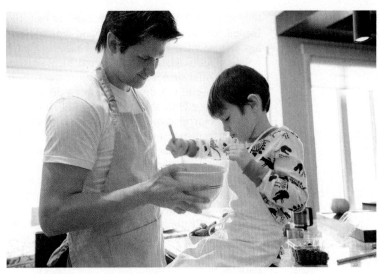

A father and son cooking in the kitchen. In married-couple households, American men have assumed a greater share of domestic and child-care responsibilities, and more single fathers are raising their children than was the case in the past.
Hero/Corbis/Glow Images

their own homemaking superiority and men's (lack of) domestic capabilities—from kids to kitchens (Slaughter 2013).

Slaughter discusses how, even when men seek, or are willing to play, a prominent domestic role, women may resist. The same woman who says she wants her husband to do more at home may then criticize him for not "doing things right" when he does pitch in. As Slaughter points out, "Doing things right" means doing things the woman's way. Practice, of course, does make perfect, and women still do a disproportionate share of housework and child care in 21st-century America. If the woman is the one who usually does the domestic work, and if she assumes she can do it better and faster than her husband, she probably will do so. A stereotype can become a self-fulfilling prophecy, often reinforced by material reality.

When women ask their husbands for "help" around the house or with the kids, they are affirming the feminine role as primary homemaker and child-care provider. The husband is viewed as merely a helper, rather than as an equal partner. Slaughter (2013, 2015) argues that Americans need to conceive and implement a whole new domestic order. Full gender equality would mean equality both at work and at home. There is still work to be done on both fronts. Men and women need to commit to and value a larger male domestic role, and employers need to make it easier for their employees to balance work and family responsibilities.

Both fathers and mothers increasingly have been seeking jobs that offer flexibility, require less travel, and include paid parental leave (including paternity leave). The United States lags behind other developed nations in providing such benefits, which help workers build long-term careers, as they also fulfill family responsibilities. In fact, the United States is the only developed country that has not adopted mandatory paid parental leave policies. Although a few states and local governments do offer such leave to their employees, most workers have to rely on an employer's decision to offer benefits. Only about 11 percent of American private-sector employers offer paid leave specifically for family reasons.

More than a quarter of American workers have encountered actual or threatened job loss because of an illness- or family-related absence. The work-family balancing act is particularly challenging for low-wage workers. They tend to have the least workplace flexibility, the most uncertain work hours, and the fewest benefits, and they can least afford to take unpaid leave. The toll is especially hard on single mothers.

The Feminization of Poverty

Alongside the economic gains of many American women, especially the college-educated, stands an opposite extreme: the feminization of poverty. This refers to the increasing representation of women (and their children) among America's poorest people. Table 9.4 shows the average income of married-couple families as more than twice that of families maintained by a single woman. The median female-headed one-earner family had an annual income of $48,098 in 2019 compared with $102,308 for a married-couple household.

The feminization of poverty isn't just a North American phenomenon. The percentage of single-parent (usually female-headed) households has been increasing worldwide. The figure ranges from about 10 percent in Japan, to between 10 and 20 percent in certain south Asian and southeast Asian countries, to almost 50 percent in certain African countries and the Caribbean. Among the developed Western nations, the United States maintains the largest percentage of single-parent households (around 30 percent), followed by the United Kingdom, Canada, Ireland, and Denmark (over 20 percent in each). Globally, households headed by women tend to be poorer than those headed by men. In the United States in 2018, the poverty rate for families maintained by just a woman was 27 percent, versus 5 percent for married-couple families (Semega et al. 2019, Figure 9).

Work and Happiness

Table 9.5 compares the rate of female labor-force participation by country with that country's rank on the most recent list of the world's happiest countries (Helliwell, Layard, and Sachs 2019). The highest rate of labor participation, 84 percent, was in Iceland. Of the countries listed in the table, the United States had the lowest female labor participation rate and also ranked lowest (among those countries) on the happiness index. Among countries not shown in Table 9.5, Turkey, which ranked lowest among all countries surveyed by female workforce participation (at 38 percent) also ranked 79th on the happiness index. You may wish to play around with the interactive table on age, gender, labor force participation, and unemployment by country at this site: https://stats.oecd.org/Index.aspx?DataSetCode=LFS_SEXAGE_I_R#.

There appears to be a relationship between a country's rate of female labor-force participation and its citizens' feelings of well-being. The *World Happiness Report,* which has been published annually since 2012, is an attempt to measure well-being and happiness in 156 countries. Its measurements are based on a set of six key variables, and a series of lesser ones. The six variables that are related

TABLE 9.4 Median Annual Income of U.S. Households, by Household Type, 2019

	NUMBER OF HOUSEHOLDS (1,000S)	MEDIAN ANNUAL INCOME (DOLLARS)	PERCENTAGE OF MEDIAN EARNINGS COMPARED WITH MARRIED-COUPLE HOUSEHOLDS
All households	128,451	68,703	67
Family households	83,677	88,149	86
Married-couple households	62,342	102,308	100
Male earner, no wife	6,503	69,244	68
Female earner, no husband	14,892	48,098	47
Nonfamily households	44,774	41,232	40
Single male	21,304	48,496	47
Single female	23,470	34,612	34

SOURCE: Semega, Jessica L.; Kollar, Melissa A.; Creamer, John; and Abinash Mohanty, Table A-1. Income Summary Measures by Selected Characteristics: 2017 and 2018.. Income and Poverty in the United States. U.S. Census Bureau, *Current Population Reports,* P60-266. Washington, DC: U.S. Government Printing Office. https://www.census.gov/content/dam/Census/library/publications/2019/demo/p60-266.pdf

TABLE 9.5 Female Labor-Force Participation Rate by Country, 2019

COUNTRY	ADULT FEMALE LABOR FORCE PARTICIPATION (2019)	RANK AMONG WORLD'S "HAPPIEST COUNTRIES" (2019)
Iceland	84	4
Sweden	82	7
Switzerland	81	6
Finland	77	1
Netherlands	77	5
New Zealand	77	8
Denmark	76	2
Norway	76	3
Canada	76	9
Germany	75	17
Australia	74	11
United Kingdom	74	15
United States	69	19

The labor-force participation rate is calculated as the labor force divided by the total working-age population. The working-age population refers to people aged 15 to 64.

SOURCE: Organisation for Economic Co-operation and Development,. Labor Force Participation by Age and Sex, Interactive Tables. https://stats.oecd.org/Index.aspx?DataSetCode=LFS_SEXAGE_I_R#.

John F, Helliwell, Richard Layard, and Jeffrey D. Sachs. *World Happiness Report 2019.* https://worldhappiness.report/ed/2019/.

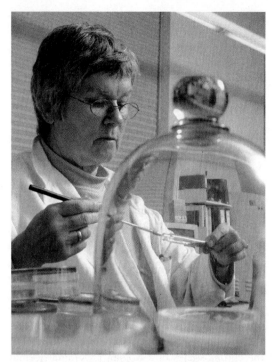

A scientist conducting laboratory research in Reykjavík, Iceland. What do you imagine this woman does when she gets home? Is it common for women to work outside the home in Iceland?

ARCTIC IMAGES/Alamy Stock Photo

most strongly to a country's sense of well-being are its per-capita gross domestic product (GDP, an indicator of its economic strength), social support, healthy life expectancy, freedom to make life choices, generosity in giving, and perceptions of corruption. The first five are positive variables: As they increase, so does the sense of well-being. The last one, perceptions of corruption, is a negative variable. That is, the less people perceive corruption, the happier they are. The 2019 *World Happiness Report,* issued by the Sustainable Development Solutions Network, can be found at https://worldhappiness.report/ed/2019/.

The top five countries in 2018 were Finland, Denmark, Norway, Iceland, and the Netherlands. Those countries rank highly on the main factors found to support happiness: caring, freedom, generosity, honesty, health, income, and good governance. Their averages are so close that small changes easily reorder the rankings from year to year.

Most of the countries with high female labor-force participation also ranked among the world's happiest. One wonders exactly why, as more women work outside the home, citizens might feel a greater sense of well-being. The greater financial security associated with dual-earner households may be part of the explanation. The world's happiest

countries not only have more employed women, but they also have a higher living standard and a more secure government safety net. Can you think of other factors that might explain a relationship between happiness and work outside the home?

BEYOND MALE AND FEMALE

Gender is socially constructed, and societies can recognize more than two genders (see Nanda 2014). In the contemporary United States, gender classification is in flux, with a proliferation of new options beyond male and female. A growing number of Americans self-identify as *transgender, nonbinary, gender-fluid,* or *gender-nonconforming.* These terms and identities complement and enlarge the traditional binary male-female contrast by recognizing that a person's gender can (1) transition from female to male, (2) transition from male to female, (3) be part male and part female, or (4) be neither male nor female. Someone who is gender-fluid or nonbinary may prefer to be referred to as *they,* rather than *he* or *she* (see the discussion of "[my] pronouns" and "they" as words of the year in the Appreciating Diversity box in Chapter 5.)

Cisgender refers to someone who still identifies with the gender assigned to them at birth (usually male or female). The terms *transgender* and *nonbinary* can be used to refer to individuals who do

cisgender
Individuals who identify with the gender assigned to them at birth.

not (see Risman 2018; Wortham 2018). Individuals may become **transgender** when their gender identity differs from their biological sex at birth and the gender identity that society assigned to them in infancy. Feeling that their previous gender assignment was incorrect, they assert, or seek to achieve, a new one.

The distinction between *intersex* and *transgender* is like the distinction between sex and gender. Sex, we have seen, refers to biology—chromosomes and their phenotypical manifestations—whereas gender is constructed socially (see Butler 1988, 1990, 2015). The term *intersex* is used to describe individuals who (usually) contrast biologically with biological males and females. *Both sex and gender, however, go beyond male and female.*

The term **intersex** describes a range of conditions resulting from an unusual combination of the X and Y chromosomes, or discrepancies involving the external genitals (penis, vagina, etc.) and the internal genitals (testes, ovaries, etc.). The causes of intersex are varied and complex (Kaneshiro 2009): (1) An XX intersex person has the chromosomes of a woman (XX) and normal ovaries, uterus, and fallopian tubes, but the external genitals appear male. Usually this results from a female fetus having been exposed to an excess of male hormones before birth. (2) An XY intersex person has the chromosomes of a man (XY), but the external genitals are incompletely formed, ambiguous, or female. The testes may be normal, malformed, or absent. (3) A true gonadal intersex person has both ovarian and testicular tissue. The external genitals may be ambiguous or may appear to be female or male. (4) Intersex also can result from an unusual chromosome combination, such as X0 (only one X chromosome, and no Y chromosome), XXY, XYY, and XXX. In the last three

cases there is an extra sex chromosome, either an X or a Y.

These chromosomal combinations don't typically produce a discrepancy between internal and external genitalia, but there may be issues involving sex hormone levels and overall sexual development. The XXY configuration, known as *Klinefelter's syndrome,* is the most common of these chromosomal combinations and the second most common condition (after Down syndrome) caused by the presence of extra chromosomes in humans. Klinefelter's syndrome occurs in about 1 of every 1,000 male births, but only about half of them have symptoms, such as small testicles and reduced fertility. With XXX, also known as *triple X syndrome,* there is an extra X chromosome in each cell of a human female. Triple X occurs in about 1 of every 1,000 female births. There usually is no physically distinguishable difference between triple X women and other women. The same is true of XYY compared with other males. Finally, *Turner syndrome* encompasses several conditions, of which 0X (absence of one sex chromosome) is most common. In this case, all or part of one of the sex chromosomes is absent. Girls with Turner syndrome typically are sterile because of nonworking ovaries and amenorrhea (absence of a menstrual cycle).

Many individuals affected by one of the biological conditions just described see themselves simply as male or female. Others identify as nonbinary, transgender, or even intersex (which then becomes a social as well as a biological term).

The anthropological record confirms that gender diversity beyond male and female exists in many societies and has taken many forms (see Nanda 2014; Peletz 2009). Consider, for example, the eunuch, or "perfect servant" (a castrated man who served as a safe attendant to harems in Byzantium [Tougher 2008]). Hijras, who live mainly in northern India, are culturally defined as "neither men nor women," or as men who become women by undergoing castration and adopting women's dress and behavior. Hijras identify with the Indian mother goddess and are believed to channel her power. They are known for their ritualized performances at births and marriages, where they dance and sing, conferring the mother goddess's blessing on the child or the married couple. Although culturally defined as celibate, some hijras now engage in prostitution (Nanda 1996, 1998). Hijra social movements have campaigned for recognition as a third gender, and in 2005, Indian passport application forms were updated with three gender options: M, F, and E (for male, female, and eunuch [i.e, hijra], respectively) (*Telegraph* 2005). Similarly, in the United States, California and Washington, among other states, now allow people to select "x" as their gender, instead of "male" or "female," on identity documents (Wortham 2018).

Several Native American tribes, including the Zuni of the American Southwest, included

On June 28, 2019, advocates for non-binary rights gather in Washington Square, Greenwich Village, New York, for the 15th Annual Trans Day of Action.
Erik McGregor/Getty Images

gender-variant individuals, described by the term "Two-Spirit." Depending on the society, as many as four genders might be recognized: feminine women, masculine women, feminine men, and masculine men. The Zuni Two-Spirit was a male who adopted social roles traditionally assigned to women and, through performance of a third gender, contributed to the social and spiritual well-being of the community (Roscoe 1991, 1998). Some Balkan societies included "sworn virgins," born females who assumed male gender roles and activities to meet societal needs when there was a shortage of men (Gremaux 1993).

Among the Gheg tribes of North Albania, "virginal transvestites" were biologically female, but locals consider them "honorary men" (Shryock 1988). Some Albanian adolescent girls have chosen to become men, remain celibate, and live among men, with the support of their families and villagers (Young 2000). And consider Polynesia. In Tonga the term *fakaleitis* describes males who behave as women do, thereby contrasting with mainstream Tongan men. Similar to Tonga's *fakaleitis,* Samoan *fa'afafine* and Hawaiian *mahu* are men who adopt feminine attributes, behaviors, and visual markers.

In the contemporary United States, the terms *transgender* and *nonbinary* encompass varied individuals whose gender performance and identity enlarge an otherwise binary gender structure. Transgender individuals are increasingly visible in the media and our everyday lives. The Amazon television series *Transparent,* whose principal character is a transgender woman, received several awards. The emergence of Caitlyn (formerly Bruce) Jenner as a transgender woman received considerable media attention in 2015. In November 2017, 33-year-old Danica Roem became the first transgender person to be elected to Virginia's House of Delegates. She defeated a 13-term

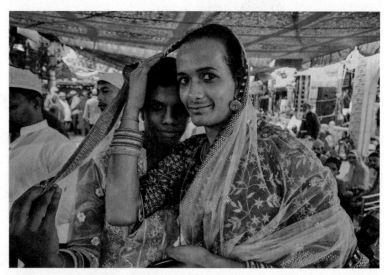

Neither men nor women, hijras constitute India's third gender. Many hijras get their income from performing at ceremonies, begging, or prostitution. Shown here, a group of hijras at a shrine in Rajasthan, India.

Tuul and Bruno Morandi/Alamy Stock Photo

Republican who had introduced a bill to bar transgender students from using the bathrooms of their choice.

In 2014, Facebook added a range of nonbinary gender identities and pronouns, offering more than 50 options for users who don't identify as male or female, including *agender, gender-questioning,* and *intersex* (Wortham 2018). Social media, especially Instagram and Facebook, provide a vital context for information on, and discussions of, gender identity and nonconformity. Especially for young people who are questioning, exploring, or developing their gender identities, social media sites offer advice, reassurance, and emotional support (see Darwin 2017; Wortham 2018).

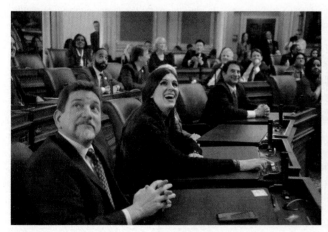

Delegate Danica Roem (center, smiling) casts a vote on her first day in office during the opening session of Virginia's House of Delegates on January 10, 2017, in Richmond. Roem is the first openly transgender person to be elected to the Virginia General Assembly.

Jahi Chikwendiu/*The Washington Post* via Getty Images

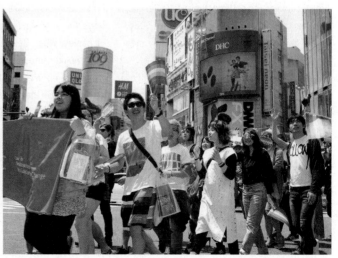

Some 5,000 participants joined this "Tokyo Rainbow Pride Parade," celebrating LGBT pride on May 8, 2016 in Tokyo, Japan.

The Asahi Shimbun via Getty Images

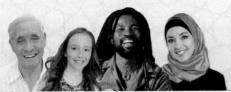
Gender, Ethnicity, and a Gold Medal for Fiji

On August 11, 2016, in Rio de Janeiro, Brazil, the island nation of Fiji won its first-ever Olympic medal. That gold medal, in men's rugby sevens, was awarded after Fiji trounced Great Britain, its former colonial master, by a score of 43 to 7. In Fiji, a Southwest Pacific nation of some 900,000 people, rugby is immensely popular. Specifically, Fijians excel at rugby sevens, a rapid game played by seven participants per side in just 14 minutes.

The addition of rugby to the roster of Olympic sports for the Rio summer games offered Fijians an opportunity to excel in a venue where previously Fiji had been woefully unrepresented. Only two Fijian athletes had qualified to participate in the games between 1956, when Fiji officially entered the Olympics, and 2016, when it won its gold medal.

Rugby is the national sport of Fiji, where its fans include men, women, and Fijians of all ethnic backgrounds. There are, however, dramatic differences in rugby participation between men and women, and between Fiji's two main ethnic groups: indigenous Fijians and Indo-Fijians. The latter are the descendants of immigrants from India who came to the island as indentured servants or free migrants during the 19th and 20th centuries, when both Fiji and India were British colonies. As anthropologist Niko Besnier, who has conducted fieldwork in Fiji since 1980, notes, participation in rugby is mainly by men who are indigenous Fijians.

In contrast to the success of the men's rugby team, the Fijian women's team—the Fijiana—managed only an eighth place finish out of 11 teams participating. This less-than-stellar result is not surprising given Fijian attitudes toward female players. Besnier and Brownell (2016) report that many Fijians view female rugby players as "tomboys"—women who act too

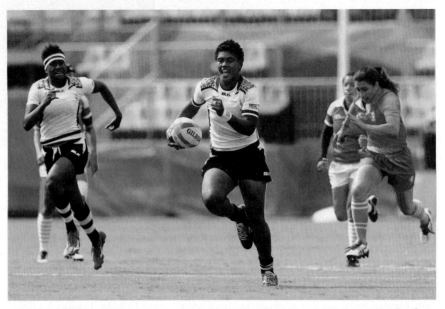

Fijiana player Rusila Nagasau rushes to score against Colombia during a women's rugby match on Day 2 (August 7) of the 2016 summer Olympic Games in Rio de Janeiro, Brazil.

David Rogers/Getty Images Sport/Getty Images

masculine by being independent, aggressive, and loud, and who often are assumed to be lesbians. Besnier heard stories of female players who had been beaten by their fathers or expelled from their family homes—an especially unhappy fate in a kin-based society. The Fijiana also receive little official support, with few corporate sponsors, unlike the men's team, which enjoys the sponsorship of the country's major companies. When Besnier visited the Fijiana at their training camp in March 2016, he found the women put up in a Christian camp, five people to a room, while the men's team was lodged at a luxury resort. Prior to the Olympic Games, there was even an attempt to replace some of the actual Fijiana national team with women from netball, who were more "feminine acting" even though they knew little about rugby (Besnier and Brownell 2016).

Women aren't the only Fijians who are discouraged from rugby. Indo-Fijians also face multiple barriers to participation in the sport. Indigenous Fijians contend that Indo-Fijians have slight physiques that make them unsuitable for rugby's roughness. Even Indo-Fijian parents discourage their sons from playing, fearing injury by the larger and rougher indigenous Fijians. In this ostensibly multicultural society, it is not uncommon for indigenous Fijians (57 percent of the population) to resent the Indian-derived minority (38 percent) because of its business success. Indo-Fijians fear physical expressions of this resentment on the playing field. Can you think of comparable barriers to sports participation and success based on gender and ethnic differences in other societies, including your own? Are these barriers physical, cultural, or a combination of the two?

As a gateway to a wider world, the Internet has become a place where almost anyone can find others like themselves, even if such others are absent or hidden in one's own hometown (Wortham 2018). This chapter's "Appreciating Diversity" illustrates how women who depart from cultural stereotypes involving "proper" behavior associated with gender identity can suffer domestic abuse, including expulsion from their family homes.

In recent years, the lesbian and gay rights movement has expanded to include bisexual, transgender, and "gender-Queer" (including nonbinary) individuals. The resulting LGBTQ community works to promote government policies and social practices that protect its members' civil and human rights. In recent years, this movement and its supporters have achieved many successes, including the repeal of the Defense of Marriage Act and of the "Don't Ask Don't Tell" policy of the U.S. armed services. The most notable achievement has been the legalization of same-sex marriage throughout the United States as of 2015. With reference specifically to transgender rights, more than 20 U.S. states, along with the District of Columbia, Guam, and Puerto Rico, offer legal protection against employment discrimination based either on sexual orientation or gender identity. On June 15, 2020, the U.S. Supreme Court ruled that the Civil Rights Act of 1964, which prohibits sex discrimination, applies to discrimination based on sexual orientation and gender identity, thus protecting gay and transgender workers from workplace discrimination. As of this writing, one unresolved issue affecting the rights of transgender and nonbinary Americans is whether public restroom and locker room access should be based on gender at birth or current gender identification (see Davis 2020) What do you think?

SEXUAL ORIENTATION

Gender identity refers to whether a person feels, acts, and is regarded as male, female, or something else. One's gender identity does not dictate one's sexual orientation. Men who have no doubt about their masculinity can be sexually attracted to women or to other men. Ditto women with regard to female gender identity and variable sexual attraction. **Sexual orientation** refers to a person's habitual sexual attraction to, and sexual activities with, persons of another sex, *heterosexuality;* the same sex, *homosexuality;* or both sexes, *bisexuality. Asexuality,* indifference toward or lack of attraction to either sex, also is a sexual orientation. All four of these forms are found throughout the world. But each type of desire and experience holds different meanings for individuals and groups (see Herdt 2021). For example, male–male sexual activity may be a private affair in Mexico, rather than public, socially sanctioned, and encouraged as it was among the Etoro of Papua New Guinea (see below).

In any society, individuals will differ in the nature, range, and intensity of their sexual interests and urges (see Blackwood 2010; Herdt and Polen-Petit 2021; Hyde and DeLamater 2019; Lyons and Lyons 2011; Nanda 2014; Naples 2020). No one knows for sure why such individual sexual differences exist. Part of the answer appears to be biological, reflecting genes or hormones. Another part may have to do with experiences during growth and development. But whatever the reasons for individual variation, culture always plays a role in molding individual sexual urges toward a collective norm. And such sexual norms vary from culture to culture.

What do we know about variation in sexual norms from society to society, and over time? A classic cross-cultural study (Ford and Beach 1951) found wide variation in attitudes about forms of sexual activity. Even in a single society, such as the United States, attitudes about sex vary over time and with socioeconomic status, region, and rural versus urban residence. However, even in the 1950s, prior to the "age of sexual permissiveness" (the pre-HIV period from the mid-1960s through the 1970s), research showed that almost all American men (92 percent) and more than half of American women (54 percent) admitted to masturbation. In the famous Kinsey report (Kinsey, Pomeroy, and Martin 1948), 37 percent of the men surveyed admitted having had at least one sexual experience leading to orgasm with another male. In a later study of 1,200 unmarried women, 26 percent reported same-sex sexual activities. (Because Kinsey's research relied on nonrandom samples, it should be considered merely illustrative, rather than a statistically accurate representation, of sexual behavior at the time.)

In almost two-thirds (63 percent) of the 76 societies in the Ford and Beach study, various forms of same-sex sexual activity were acceptable. Occasionally sexual relations between people of the same sex involved transvestism on the part of one of the partners (see Kulick 1998). Transvestism did not characterize male–male sex among the Sudanese Azande, who valued the warrior role (Evans-Pritchard 1970). Prospective warriors—young men aged 12 to 20—left their families and shared quarters with adult fighting men, who had sex with them. The younger men were considered temporary brides of the older men and did the domestic duties of women. Upon reaching warrior status, these young men took their own younger male brides. Later, retiring from the warrior role, Azande men married women. Flexible in their sexual expression, Azande males had no difficulty shifting from sex with older men (as male brides), to sex with younger men (as warriors), to sex with women (as husbands) (see Murray and Roscoe 1998).

An extreme example of tension involving male–female sexual relations in Papua New Guinea is provided by the Etoro (Kelly 1976), a group of 400

gender identity
A person's identification by self and others as male, female, or something else.

sexual orientation
Sexual attraction to persons of the opposite sex, same sex, or both sexes.

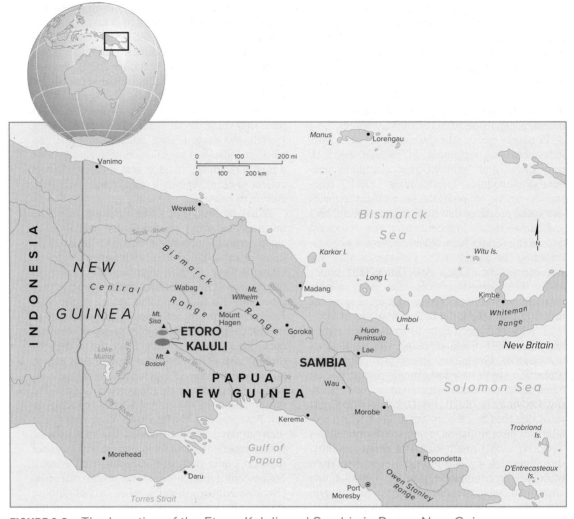

FIGURE 9.2 The Location of the Etoro, Kaluli, and Sambia in Papua New Guinea.
The western part of the island of New Guinea is part of Indonesia. The eastern part of the island is the independent nation of Papua New Guinea, home of the Etoro, Kaluli, and Sambia.

people who subsisted by hunting and horticulture in the Trans-Fly region (Figure 9.2). The Etoro illustrate the power of culture in molding human sexuality. The following account, based on ethnographic fieldwork by Raymond C. Kelly in the late 1960s, applies only to Etoro males and their beliefs. Etoro cultural norms prevented the male anthropologist who studied them from gathering comparable information about female attitudes and behavior. Note, also, that the activities described have been discouraged by missionaries. Since there has been no restudy of the Etoro specifically focusing on these activities, the extent to which these practices continue today is unknown. For this reason, I'll use the past tense in describing them.

Etoro opinions about sexuality were linked to their beliefs about the cycle of birth, physical growth, maturity, old age, and death. Etoro culture promoted the idea that semen was necessary to give life force to a fetus, which, they believed, was implanted in a woman by an ancestral spirit. A man was required to have sexual intercourse with his wife during her pregnancy in order to nourish the growing fetus with his semen. The Etoro believed, however, that men had a limited lifetime supply of semen. Any sex act leading to ejaculation was seen as draining that supply, and as sapping a man's virility and vitality. The birth of children, nurtured by semen, symbolized a necessary sacrifice that would lead to the husband's eventual death. Male-female intercourse, required for reproduction, was otherwise discouraged. Women who wanted too much sex were viewed as witches, hazardous to their husbands' health. Furthermore, Etoro culture allowed male-female intercourse only about 100 days a year. The rest of the time it was tabooed. Seasonal birth clustering shows the taboo was respected.

So objectionable was male-female sex that it was removed from community life. It could occur neither in sleeping quarters nor in the fields. Coitus could happen only in the woods, where it was risky because poisonous snakes, the Etoro believed, were attracted by the sounds and smells of male-female sex.

Although coitus was discouraged, sex acts between males were viewed as essential. Etoro believed that boys would not produce semen on their own. To grow into men and eventually give life force to their children, boys had to acquire semen orally from older men. No taboos were attached to this. This oral insemination could proceed in the sleeping area or garden. Every three years, young men around the age of 20 were formally initiated into manhood. They went to a secluded mountain lodge, where they were visited and inseminated by several older men.

A code of propriety governed male–male sexual activity among the Etoro. Although sexual relations between older and younger males were considered culturally essential, those between boys of the same age were discouraged. A boy who took semen from other youths was believed to be sapping their life force and stunting their growth. A boy's rapid physical development might suggest that he was getting semen from other boys. Like a sex-hungry wife, he might be shunned as a witch.

The sexual practices described in this section rested not on hormones or genes but on cultural beliefs and traditions. The Etoro shared a cultural pattern, which Gilbert Herdt (ed. 1984, 2006) calls "ritualized homosexuality," with some 50 other tribes in one area of Papua New Guinea. These societies illustrate one extreme of a male–female avoidance pattern that has been widespread in Papua New Guinea, and in patrilineal-patrilocal societies more generally.

Flexibility in sexual expression seems to be an aspect of our primate heritage. Both masturbation and same-sex sexual activity exist among chimpanzees and other primates. Male bonobos (pygmy chimps) regularly engage in a form of mutual masturbation that has been called "penis fencing." Female bonobos get sexual pleasure from rubbing their genitals against those of other females (de Waal 1997). Our primate sexual potential is molded by culture, the environment, and reproductive necessity. Male–female coitus is practiced in all human societies—which, after all, must reproduce themselves—but alternatives also are widespread (Rathus, Nevid, and Fichner-Rathus 2018). Like our gender roles, the sexual component of human identity—the ways in which we express our "natural," or biological, sexual urges—is a matter that culture and environment influence and limit.

for REVIEW

summary

1. *Gender roles* are the tasks and activities that a culture assigns to each sex. *Gender stereotypes* are oversimplified ideas about attributes of males and females. *Gender stratification* describes an unequal distribution of rewards by gender, reflecting different positions in a social hierarchy. Cross-cultural comparison reveals some recurrent patterns involving the division of labor by gender. Gender roles and gender stratification also vary with environment, economy, adaptive strategy, level of social complexity, and degree of participation in the world economy.

2. When gathering is prominent, gender status is more equal than it is when hunting or fishing dominates the foraging economy. Gender status is more equal when the domestic and public spheres aren't sharply separated. Foragers lack two public arenas that contribute to higher male status among food producers: warfare and organized interregional trade.

3. Gender stratification also is linked to descent and residence. Women's status in matrilineal societies tends to be high because overall social identity comes through female links. Women in many societies, especially matrilineal ones, wield power and make decisions. Scarcity of resources promotes intervillage warfare, patriliny, and patrilocality. The localization of related males is adaptive for military solidarity. Men may use their warrior role to symbolize and reinforce the social devaluation and oppression of women. *Patriarchy* describes a political system ruled by men in which women have inferior social and political status, including basic human rights.

4. Americans' attitudes toward gender vary with class and region. When the need for female labor declines, the idea that women are unfit for many jobs increases, and vice versa. The need for flexible employment, permitting a proper balance of work and family responsibilities, is increasingly important to both male and female workers. Despite the increased participation by women in the labor force and higher education, and by men in the domestic realm, including child care, barriers to full equality remain. Countering the economic gains of many American women is the feminization of poverty. This has become a global phenomenon, as impoverished female-headed households have increased worldwide.

5. Societies may recognize more than two genders. The term *intersex* describes a group of conditions, including chromosomal configurations, that may produce a discrepancy between external and internal genitals. In the contemporary United States, gender classification is in flux, with a proliferation of new options beyond male and female. A growing number of Americans self-identify as *transgender, nonbinary, gender-fluid,* or *gender-nonconforming.* These terms are used by individuals whose gender identity contradicts their biological sex at birth and the gender identity that society assigned to them in infancy. Self-identified transgender individuals may or may not contrast biologically with ordinary males and females.

6. *Gender identity* refers to whether a person feels, and is regarded as, male, female, or something else. One's gender identity does not dictate one's sexual orientation. *Sexual orientation* stands for a person's habitual sexual attraction to, and activities with, persons of the opposite sex (heterosexuality), the same sex (homosexuality), or both sexes (bisexuality). Sexual norms and practices vary widely from culture to culture.

key terms

cisgender 191

domestic–public dichotomy 182

gender 179

gender identity 195

gender roles 179

gender stereotypes 179

gender stratification 179

intersex 192

matrilineal descent 182

patriarchy 184

patrilineal descent 183

patrilineal-patrilocal complex 183

sexual dimorphism 179

sexual orientation 195

transgender 192

think like an anthropologist

1. How are sexuality, sex, and gender related to one another? What are the differences between these three concepts? Provide an argument about why anthropologists are uniquely positioned to study the relationships among sexuality, sex, and gender in society.

2. Using your own society, give an example of a gender role, a gender stereotype, and gender stratification.

3. What is the feminization of poverty? Where is this trend occurring, and what are some of its causes?

4. Is intersex the same as transgender? If not, how do they differ? How might biological, cultural, and personal factors influence gender identity?

5. This chapter describes Raymond Kelly's research among the Etoro of Papua New Guinea. What were his findings regarding Etoro male–female sexual relations? How did Kelly's own gender affect some of the content and extent of his study? Can you think of other research projects where the ethnographer's gender would have an impact?

credits

Design Elements: Understanding Ourselves: muha/123RF (rock paintings); Focus on Globalization: janrysavy/Getty Images (globe); Appreciating Diversity (left to right): Floresco Productions/age footstock; Hero/Corbis/Glow Images, Hill Street Studios/Blend Images, Billion Photos/Shutterstock; Understanding Ourselves : Hemera Technologies/Alamy (Cymbal), LACMA - Los Angeles County Museum of Art (Trefoil Oinochoe), Ingram Publishing/SuperStock (Coin), ChuckSchugPhotography/Getty Images (Rug).

Families, Kinship, and Descent

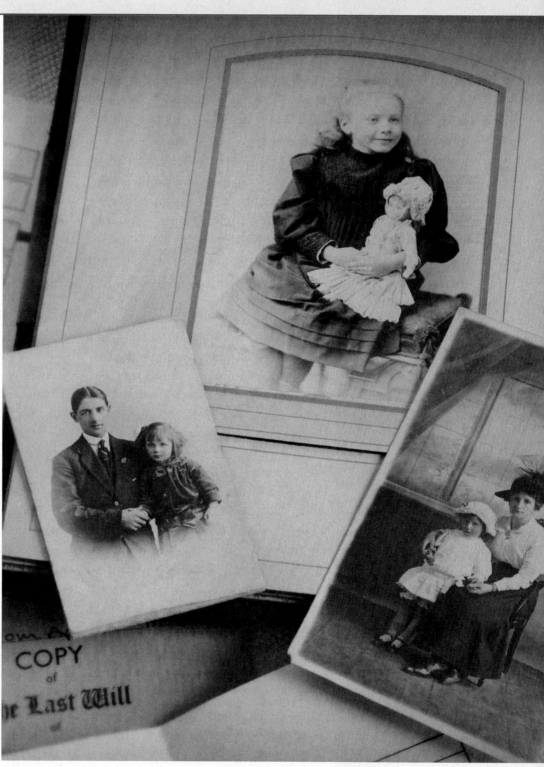

▶ Why and how do anthropologists study kinship?

▶ How do families and descent groups differ, and what are their social correlates?

▶ How is kinship calculated, and how are relatives classified, in various societies?

Andrew Bret Wallis/Getty Images

A vintage family photo album and documents from Harrogate in the United Kingdom.

understanding **OURSELVES**

Although it still is something of an ideal in our culture, the nuclear family (children living with their parents) now accounts for just 18 percent of all American households. What kind of family raised you? Perhaps it was a nuclear family. Or maybe you were raised by a single parent, with or without the help of extended kin. More and more kids are being raised by same-sex couples--giving them two moms or two dads. Perhaps your extended kin acted as your parents. Or maybe you had a stepparent and/or step- or half-siblings in a blended family. Your own family may match none of these descriptions, or it may have had different descriptions at different times.

Although contemporary American families may seem amazingly diverse, other cultures offer family alternatives that Americans might have trouble understanding. Imagine a society in which someone doesn't know for sure, and doesn't care much about, who his actual mother was. Consider Joseph Rabe, a Betsileo man who was my field assistant in Madagascar. Illustrating an adoptive pattern common among the Betsileo, Rabe was given as a toddler to his childless aunt, his father's sister. He knew that his birth mother lived far away, but did not know which of two sisters in his birth mother's family was his actual

mother. His mother and her sister both died in his childhood (as did his father), so he didn't really know them. But he was very close to his father's sister, for whom he used the term for mother. Indeed, he had to call her that because the Betsileo have only one kin term, *reny,* that they use for both mother and any blood aunt. (They also use a single term, *ray,* for father and all uncles.) The difference between "real" (biologically based) and socially constructed kinship didn't matter to Rabe.

Contrast this Betsileo case with Americans' attitudes about kinship and adoption. On call-in shows, I've heard hosts distinguish between birth mothers and adoptive mothers, and between "sperm daddies" and "daddies of the heart." The latter may be adoptive fathers or stepfathers who have "been like fathers" to someone. American culture tends to promote the idea that kinship is, and should be, biological. It's increasingly common for adopted children to seek out their birth parents (which used to be discouraged as disruptive), even after a perfectly satisfactory upbringing in an adoptive family. The American emphasis on biology for kinship is seen also in the recent proliferation of DNA testing. Viewing our beliefs through the lens of cross-cultural comparison helps us appreciate that kinship and biology don't always converge, nor do they need to.

FAMILIES

The kinds of societies anthropologists have studied, including the examples considered in this chapter, have stimulated a strong interest in families, along with larger systems of kinship, descent, and marriage. Cross-culturally, the social construction of kinship illustrates considerable diversity. Understanding kinship systems has become an essential part of anthropology because

of the importance of those systems to the people we study. Let's take a closer look at the kinship systems that have organized human life during much of our history.

Ethnographers quickly recognize social divisions—groups—within any society they study. During fieldwork, they learn about significant groups by observing their activities and composition. People often live in the same community, or work, pray, or celebrate together because they are related in some way. To understand that society, an ethnographer must investigate such kin ties. For example, local groups may consist of descendants of the same grandfather. These people may live in neighboring houses, farm adjoining fields, and help each other in everyday tasks. Other sorts of groups, based on different or more distant kin links, get together less often.

One kind of kin group that is widespread is the *nuclear family,* consisting of parents and children, who normally live together in the same household. Other kin groups include extended families and descent groups. Extended families are those that include three or more generations. **Descent groups** include people who share common ancestry—they *descend* from the same ancestor(s). Descent groups typically are spread out among several villages, so that all their members do not reside together. Only some of them do—those who live in a given village. Descent groups tend to be found in societies with economies based on horticulture, pastoralism, or agriculture.

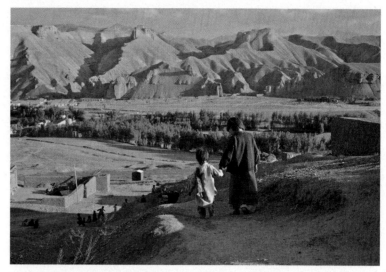

In Bamyan province, Afghanistan, older sister Aqila, 8, leads her 18-month-old brother, Abdul Wahid, down the hill toward their home village. Siblings play a prominent role in child-rearing in many societies. Do your siblings belong to your family of orientation or procreation?

Majority World/Getty Images

Nuclear and Extended Families

Most people belong to at least two nuclear families at different times in their lives. They are born into a family consisting of their parents and siblings. Reaching adulthood, they may establish a nuclear family that includes their spouse (or domestic partner) and eventually their children. Some people establish more than one family through successive marriages or domestic partnerships.

Anthropologists distinguish between the **family of orientation** (the family in which one is born and grows up) and the **family of procreation** (formed when one has children). From the individual's point of view, the critical relationships are with parents and siblings in the family of orientation and with spouse (or domestic partner) and children in the family of procreation.

In most societies, relations with nuclear family members (parents, siblings, and children) take precedence over relations with other kin. Nuclear family organization is widespread but not universal, and its significance varies from culture to culture. In a few societies, such as the classic Nayar case (described below), nuclear families are rare or nonexistent. In other societies, extended families and descent groups assume functions otherwise associated with the nuclear family.

The following example from Bosnia illustrates how an extended family can be the most important kinship unit, overshadowing the nuclear family. Among the Muslims of western Bosnia (Lockwood 1975), nuclear families did not exist as independent units. Rather, people lived in an extended family household called a *zadruga.* Heading this household were a senior man and his wife, the senior woman. Also living in the zadruga were their married sons and their wives and children, as well as unmarried sons and daughters. Each

married couple had a sleeping room, decorated and partly furnished from the bride's trousseau. However, possessions—even clothing items—were shared freely by zadruga members. Even trousseau items could be used by other zadruga members.

Within the *zadruga,* social interaction was more usual among its women, its men, or its children than between spouses, or between parents and children. When the *zadruga* was large, its members ate at three successive sittings: for men, women, and children, respectively. Traditionally, all children over age 12 slept together in boys' or girls' rooms. When a woman wanted to visit another village, she asked permission not from her husband, but from the male *zadruga* head. Although men may have felt closer to their own children than to those of their brothers, they were obliged to treat all of the *zadruga's* children equally. Any adult in the household could discipline a child. When a marriage broke up, children under age 7 went with the mother. Older children could choose between their parents. Children were considered part of the household where they were born even if their mother left. One widow who remarried had to leave her five children, all over age 7, in their father's *zadruga.*

Another example of how the extended family can overshadow the nuclear family is provided by the Nayars (or Nair), a large and powerful caste on the Malabar Coast of southern India (Figure 10.1). Their traditional kinship system was matrilineal (descent traced only through females). Nayar lived in matrilineal extended family compounds called *tarawads.* The *tarawad* was a residential complex with several buildings, its own temple, granary, well, orchards, gardens, and landholdings. Headed by a senior woman, assisted by her brother, the

descent group
A group based on belief in shared ancestry.

family of orientation
The nuclear family in which one is born and grows up.

family of procreation
The nuclear family established when one marries and has children.

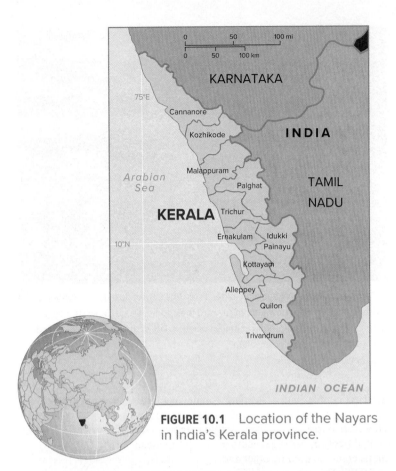

FIGURE 10.1 Location of the Nayars in India's Kerala province.

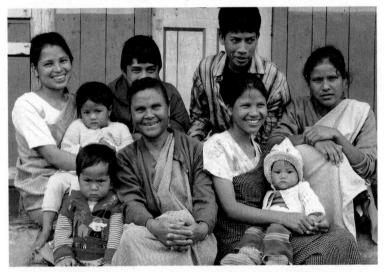

A matrilineal extended family of the Khasi ethnic group in India's northeastern city of Shillong. The Khasis trace descent through women, taking their maternal ancestors' surnames. Women choose their husbands; family incomes are pooled, and extended family households are managed by older women.

DINODIA/Dinodia Photo/age fotostock

tarawad housed her siblings, her children, her sisters' children, and other matrikin—matrilineal relatives (Gough 1959; Shivaram 1996).

Traditional Nayar marriage was barely more than a formality—a kind of coming-of-age ritual. A young woman would go through a marriage ceremony with a man, after which they might spend a few days together at her *tarawad.* Then the man would return to his own *tarawad,* where he lived with his mother, aunts, uncles, siblings, and other matrikin. Nayar men belonged to a warrior class, who left home regularly for military expeditions, returning permanently to their *tarawad* on retirement. Nayar women could have multiple sexual partners. Children became members of the mother's *tarawad;* they were not considered to be relatives of their biological father. Indeed, many Nayar children didn't even know who their father was. Child care was the responsibility of the *tarawad.* Nayar society therefore reproduced itself biologically without the nuclear family.

A third example of how the extended family can overshadow the nuclear family is provided by the Moso (also spelled Mosuo)—sedentary farmers who live in Yunnan province, southwestern China. Based on his many years of fieldwork among them, anthropologist Chuan-Kang Shih (2010) has described the unique Moso system of kinship and (insignificance of) marriage. Like the Nayars, the Moso are matrilineal and prefer to live in matrilocal extended family households. Although marriage exists and is practiced in some parts of the Moso territory, the dominant form of sexual and reproductive union is a visiting system called *tisese,* which means "walking back and forth" between the households of the lovers. *Tisese* relationships are neither binding nor exclusive, and all children produced by such a union belong to their mother's household. As among the Nayars, the biological father has no role in his child's family and no legal authority over his offspring. The Moso have no kinship terms for relatives on the father's side, or for in-laws (other than husband and wife, for those who are married). Paternity is recognized (only) when Moso marry.

Shih surmises that the *tisese* system has existed for at least a millennium. Marriage was introduced later, by members of a patrilineal group known as the Pumi, who established themselves as chiefs among the Moso in the 13th century. *Tisese* is still favored, and marriage remains a marginal practice. Those Moso who do marry live mostly in sparsely populated mountain areas where households are too far apart to make *tisese* practical. This is yet another example of how a society can reproduce itself biologically without the nuclear family.

Industrialism and Family Organization

The geographic mobility associated with an industrial economy works to fragment kinship groups larger than the nuclear family. As people move, often for economic reasons, they are separated from their parents and other kin. Eventually, most North Americans will enter a marriage or domestic partnership and establish a family of procreation. With only about 2 percent of the U.S. population now working in farming, relatively few Americans are tied to the land—to a family farm or estate. A nonfarming nation can be a mobile nation. Americans can move to places where jobs are available, even if they have to leave their hometown to do so. Individuals and married couples often live hundreds of miles from their parents. Usually, their jobs have played a major role in determining where they live (see Descartes and Kottak 2009). This pattern of postmarital residence, in which married couples establish a new place of residence away from their parents, is called **neolocality.** The prefix *neo* means new; the couple establishes a new residence, a "home of their own." For middle-class North Americans, neolocality is both a cultural preference and a statistical norm. That is, they both want to, and eventually do, establish homes and nuclear families of their own.

It should be noted, however, that there are significant differences involving kinship between middle-class and poorer North Americans. One example is the association between poverty and single-parent households. Another example is the higher incidence of *expanded family households* among Americans who are less well off. An **expanded family household** is one that includes a group of relatives other than, or in addition to, a married couple and their children. Expanded family households take various forms. When the expanded household includes three or more generations, it is an **extended family household,** like the Bosnian *zadruga* or the Nayar *tarawad.* Another type of expanded family household is the *collateral household,* which includes siblings and their spouses and children. Yet another form is a *matrifocal household,* which is headed by a woman and includes other adult relatives and children.

The higher proportion of expanded family households among poorer Americans has been explained as an adaptation to poverty (Stack

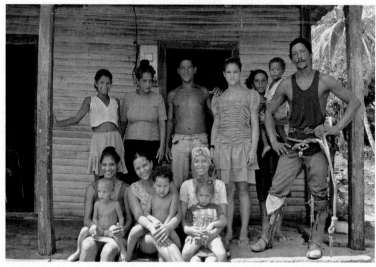

An extended family of *cocoteros,* workers on a coconut plantation in the rural town of Barigua in eastern Cuba. Try to guess the relationships among them.

James Quine/Alamy Stock Photo

1975). Unable to survive economically as independent nuclear family units, relatives band together in an expanded household and pool their resources (see Coles 2016; Hansen 2005). (This chapter's "Appreciating Diversity" shows how poor Brazilians use kinship, marriage, and fictive kinship as a form of social security.)

Changes in North American Kinship

Even in this age of "modern families," many Americans still think of the traditional nuclear family as the ideal family type. However, as we see in Table 10.1, nuclear families (married mom, dad, and kids under 18) now account for just 28 percent of American families (and a mere 18 percent of all American households).

neolocality
The living situation in which a couple establishes new residence.

expanded family household
A household that includes a group of relatives other than, or in addition to, a married couple and their children.

extended family household
A household with three or more generations.

TABLE 10.1 Household and Family Characteristics of the United States, 1970 versus 2019

	1970	2019
Numbers		
Total number of households	64 million	129 million
Total number of family households	52 million	83 million
Total number of non-family households	12 million	45 million
Percentage of non-family households	19%	35%
Percentage of single-person households	17%	28%
Number of people per household	3.1	2.5
For Family Households only:		
Families with own children under age 18	56%	41%
Married couples with children under 18	50%	28%
One parent families	6%	12%
Mother only families	6%	9%
Father only families	0%	3%

SOURCE: U.S. Census Bureau, Washington, DC, Table FM-1. Families by Presence of Own Children under 18: 1950 to present; Table HH-1. Households by Type: 1940 to Present; and Table HH-4. Households by Size: 1960 to Present.

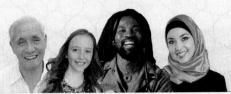

Social Security, Kinship Style

In all societies, people care for others. Sometimes, as in our own state-organized society, social security is a function of government as well as of the individual and the family. In other societies, such as Arembepe, as described here, social security has been part of systems of kinship, marriage, and fictive kinship.

My book *Assault on Paradise*, 4th edition (Kottak 2018), describes social relations in Arembepe, the Brazilian fishing community I've studied for many years. When I first studied Arembepe, I was struck by how similar its social relations were to those in the egalitarian, kin-based societies anthropologists have studied traditionally. The twin assertions "We're all equal here" and "We're all relatives here" were offered repeatedly as Arembepeiros' summaries of the nature and basis of local life. Like members of a clan (who claim to share common ancestry but who can't say exactly how they are related), most villagers couldn't trace precise genealogical links to their distant kin. "What difference does it make, as long as we know we're relatives?"

As in most nonindustrial societies, close personal relations were either based or modeled on kinship. A degree of community solidarity was promoted, for example, by the myth that everyone was kin. However, social solidarity was actually less developed in Arembepe than in societies with clans and lineages—which use genealogy to include some people, and exclude others from membership, in a given descent group. Intense social solidarity demands that some people be excluded. By asserting they all were related—that is, by excluding no one—Arembepeiros were actually weakening kinship's potential strength in creating and maintaining group solidarity.

Rights and obligations always are associated with kinship and marriage. In Arembepe, the closer the kin connection and the more formal the marital tie, the greater the rights and obligations. Couples could be married formally or informally. The most common union was a stable common-law marriage. Less common, but with more prestige, was legal (civil) marriage, performed by a justice of the peace and conferring inheritance rights. The union with the most prestige combined legal validity with a church ceremony.

The rights and obligations associated with kinship and marriage constituted the local social security system, but people had to weigh the benefits of the system against its costs. The most obvious cost was this: Villagers had to share in proportion to their success. As people (usually ambitious men) climbed the local ladder of success, they got more dependents. To maintain their standing in public opinion, and to guarantee that they could depend on others in old age, they had to share. However, sharing was a powerful leveling mechanism. It drained surplus wealth and restricted upward mobility.

How, specifically, did this leveling work? As is often true in stratified nations, Brazilian national cultural norms are set by the upper classes. Middle- and upper-class Brazilians frequently marry legally and in church. Even Arembepeiros knew this was the only "proper" way to marry. The most successful and ambitious local men copied the behavior of elite Brazilians. By doing so, they hoped to acquire some of their prestige.

However, legal marriage drained individual wealth, for example, by creating an obligation to offer financial assistance to one's in-laws. Responsibilities involving children also increased with income, because children had better survival chances in wealthier households than in poorer ones. Adequate incomes bought improved diets and provided the means and confidence to seek out better medical attention than was locally available. More living children meant more mouths to feed, and (since the heads of such households usually wanted a better education for their children) increased expenditures on schooling. Tomé, a fishing entrepreneur, envisioned a life of constant hard work if he was to feed, clothe, and educate his growing family. Unlike most Arembepeiros, Tomé and his wife had never lost a child. He recognized, however, that his growing family would, in the short run, be a drain on his resources. "But in the end, I'll have successful sons to help their mother and me, if we need it, in our old age."

Arembepeiros knew who could afford to share with others; success can't be concealed in a small community. Villagers based their expectations of others on this knowledge. Successful people had to share with more kin and in-laws, and with more distant kin, than did poorer people. Captains and boat owners were expected to buy beer for ordinary fishermen; store owners had to sell on credit. As in bands and tribes, any well-off person was expected to exhibit a corresponding generosity. With increasing wealth, people also were asked more frequently to enter ritual kin relationships. Through baptism—which took place twice a year when a priest visited, or which could be done outside—a child acquired two godparents. These people became the coparents (compadres) of the baby's parents. The fact that ritual kinship obligations increased with wealth was another factor limiting individual economic advance.

We see that kinship, marriage, and ritual kinship in Arembepe had costs and benefits. The costs were limits on the economic advancement of individuals. The primary benefit was social security—guaranteed help from kin, in-laws, and ritual kin in times of need. Benefits, however, came only after costs had been paid—that is, only to those who had lived "proper" lives, not deviating too noticeably from local norms, especially those about sharing.

Twelve percent of families are now headed by a single parent, usually the mother (9 percent of all families), but also increasingly the father (now 3 percent versus below one percent in 1970.)

From the child's perspective, between 1960 and 2019, the percentage of kids living with two married parents decreased from 88 percent to 65 percent. During that same period, the percentage of children living with only their *mother* nearly tripled from 8 to 22 percent, and the percentage living with only their *father* increased from 1 to 4 percent. The percentage of children not living with either parent also increased slightly, from 3 to 4 percent (U.S. Census Bureau 2019). A final group of children lived with their unmarried parents.

There are several reasons for these changing family statistics. Women increasingly have joined men in the cash workforce. Often, this removes them from their family of orientation while making it economically feasible to delay (or even forgo) marriage. The median age at first marriage for American women in 2019 was 28 years, compared with 21 years in 1970. For men the comparable ages were 30 and 23. Currently, more than a third (35 percent) of American men and 30 percent of American women have never married. Fewer than half (48 percent) of American women lived with a husband in 2019, compared with 65 percent in 1950. Only about half of U.S. adults are married and living with their spouse. About 36 million Americans now live alone, so that in 2019, about 28 percent of all households had just one resident, versus in 1970, when single-person households represented only 17 percent of all households.

Average family size has declined in both Canada (from 3.4 to 2.9 persons between 1980 and today) and in the U.S. (3.3 to 3.1) This trend toward smaller families also is detectable in Western Europe and other industrial nations. The entire range of kin attachments is narrower for contemporary North Americans and Western Europeans than it is for nonindustrial peoples. Although we recognize ties to grandparents, uncles, aunts, and cousins, we have less contact with, and depend less on, those relatives than people in other cultures do. We see this when we answer a few questions: Do we know exactly how we are related to all our cousins? How much do we know about our ancestors, such as their full names and where they lived? How many of the people with whom we associate regularly are our relatives?

Differences in the answers to these questions by people from industrial and those from nonindustrial societies confirm the declining importance of kinship in contemporary nations. Immigrants are often shocked by what they perceive as weak kinship bonds and lack of proper respect for family in contemporary North America. In fact, most of the people whom middle-class North Americans see every day are either household members or nonrelatives.

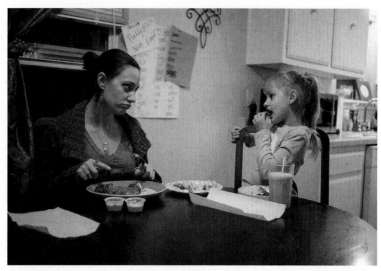

One among many kinds of American family. This 37-year-old divorced, now single, mother of two children, including Addison, 5, shown here, works as an office manager in Bastrop, Texas. What do you see as the main differences between nuclear families and single-parent families?

Ilana Panich-Linsman/Getty Images

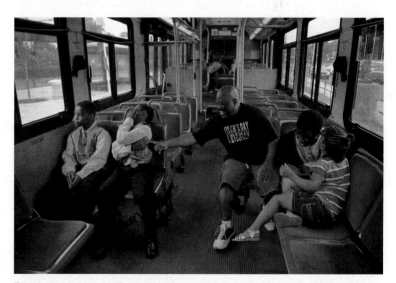

Tony Loring jokes with Tyrus, one of his 11-year-old twin sons, on a Metro bus ride to a school function in Washington, DC. The other twin, Tavon (left), takes in the passing view as sister Tiara (right) whispers to her older brother Tony II. Tony has raised five children as a single father since his marriage to their mother dissolved three years ago.

Jahi Chikwendiu/*The Washington* Post via Getty Images

One study (Qian 2013) found that the traditional American nuclear family was best represented among recent immigrants. Sociologist Zhenchao Qian describes several differences involving marriage and the family between recent immigrants and native-born Americans. Immigrants brought customs of their cultures of origin with them to the United States. One pattern was earlier marriage (especially of women) and marital stability. At every age, the immigrant marriage rate was greater than that of native-born

Americans, including American-born members of the immigrants' ethnic groups. Asian immigrants, for example, were twice as likely to marry as were U.S.-born Asian Americans. Compared with native-born marriages, those of immigrants also tended to be more ethnically homogeneous and less prone to divorce. About 30 percent of immigrant children lived in homes with a male breadwinner and a stay-at-home mother. This was nine percentage points higher than the figure for native-born Americans.

What does *family* mean in different cultures? Consider a striking contrast in the meaning of *family* between the United States and Brazil, the two most populous nations of the Western Hemisphere. Contemporary North American adults usually define their families as consisting of their spouse (or domestic partner) and their children. However, when Brazilians talk about their families, they mean their parents, siblings, aunts, uncles, grandparents, and cousins. Later they add their children, but rarely the spouse, who has his or her own family. The children are shared by the two families. Because middle-class Americans

normally lack a readily available extended family support system, marriage assumes more importance. The spousal relationship is supposed to take precedence over either spouse's relationship with his or her own parents. This places a significant strain on American marriages (see this chapter's "Appreciating Anthropology" for a study of American family life in the 21st century).

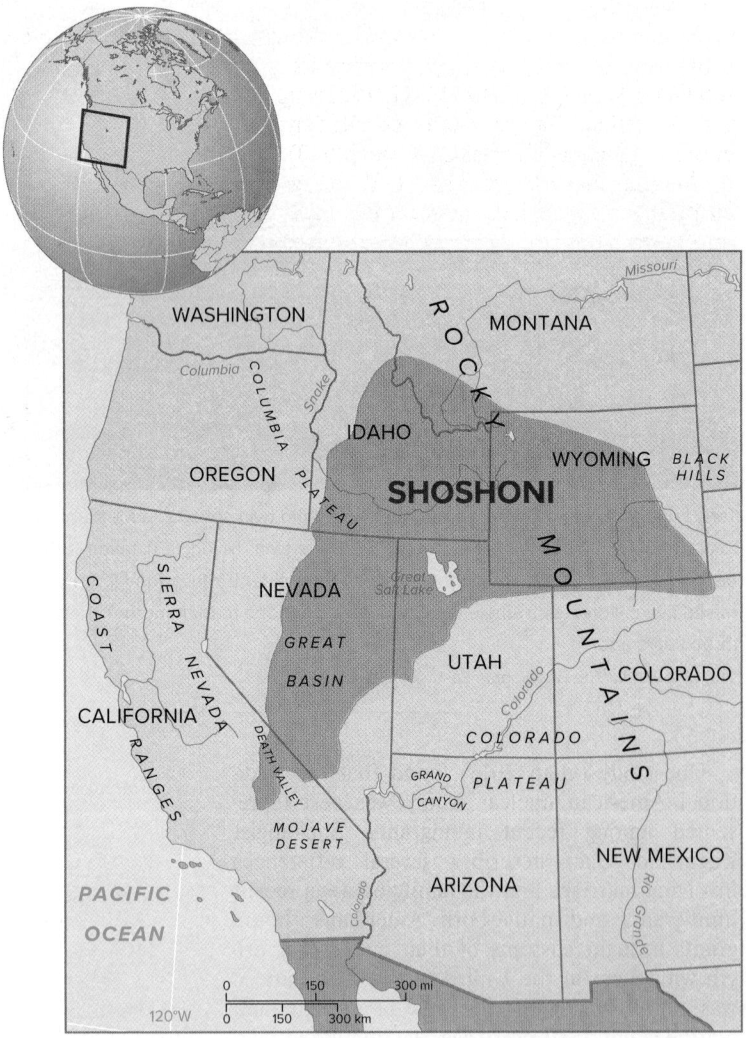

The Family among Foragers

Foraging societies are far removed from industrial nations in terms of population size and social complexity, but they do feature geographic mobility, which is associated with nomadic or seminomadic hunting and gathering. Here again, a mobile lifestyle favors the nuclear family as the most significant kin group, although in no foraging society is the nuclear family the only group based on kinship. The two basic social units of traditional foraging societies are the nuclear family and the band. Both are based on kinship ties.

Unlike middle-class couples in industrial nations, foragers don't usually reside neolocally. Instead, they join a band in which either the husband or the wife has relatives. However, couples and families may move freely from one band to another (see Hill et al. 2011). Although nuclear families are ultimately as impermanent among foragers as they are in any other society, they are usually more stable than bands are.

Many foraging societies lacked year-round band organization. The Native American Shoshoni of the Great Basin in Utah and Nevada (Figure 10.2) provide an example. The resources available to the Shoshoni were so meager that for most of the year nuclear families traveled alone through the countryside, hunting and gathering. In certain seasons such families got together to hunt cooperatively as a band; after just a few months together, they dispersed (see Fowler and Fowler 2008).

In neither industrial nor foraging societies are people tied permanently to the land. The mobility and the emphasis on small, economically self-sufficient family units promote the nuclear family as a basic kin group in both types of societies.

DESCENT

We've seen that the nuclear family is important in industrial nations and among foragers. The descent group, by contrast, is the key kinship group among nonindustrial farmers and herders. Descent groups, remember, are made up of people who share common ancestry—they *descend* from the same ancestor(s). Unlike nuclear families, descent groups are permanent. They last for generations. The group endures even as its individual members are born and die, move in and move out. Descent groups may take their names from an ancestor, or from a familiar animal, plant, or

FIGURE 10.2 Location of the Shoshoni.

natural feature. If a descent group is known as "Children of Abraham," there will be "Children of Abraham" generation after generation. Ditto for "Wolves," "Willow Trees," or "People of the Bamboo Houses." All of these are actual descent group names.

Attributes of Descent Groups

Descent groups frequently are *exogamous: Exogamy* means to marry outside one's own group. Members of a descent group must marry someone from another descent group. Often, descent group membership is determined at birth and is lifelong. Two common rules admit certain people as descent-group members while excluding others. With a rule of *matrilineal descent,* people belong to their mother's group automatically at birth and are life members. With *patrilineal descent,* people similarly are born into and have lifetime membership in the father's group. (In Figures 10.3 and 10.4, which show matrilineal and patrilineal descent groups, respectively, the triangles stand for males and the circles for females, and lineage members are shaded blue.) Matrilineal and patrilineal descent are types of **unilineal descent.** That means they use only *one* line of descent—either the male or the female line.

Members of any descent group believe that they are descended from a specific *apical ancestor.* That person stands at the apex, or top, of their common genealogy. For example, Adam and Eve, according to the Bible, are the apical ancestors of all humanity. Since Eve is said to have come from Adam's rib, Adam stands as the original apical ancestor for the patrilineal genealogies laid out in the Bible.

Lineages and clans are two types of descent group. Clans tend to be larger than lineages and can include lineages. A **lineage** is a descent group based on *demonstrated descent.* Members demonstrate how they descend from their common ancestor, by naming their forebears in each generation from the apical ancestor through the present. (This doesn't mean the genealogy is accurate, only that lineage members believe it is.) In the Bible the litany of men who "begat" other men demonstrates descent for a large patrilineage that ultimately includes Jews and Arabs (who share Abraham as their last common apical ancestor).

Unlike lineages, members of a clan do not demonstrate how they descend from their common ancestor. They merely claim, assert, or *stipulate* their common ancestry and descent. They don't try to specify actual genealogical links generation by generation, as members of a lineage do. A **clan,** then, is a descent group based on *stipulated descent.*

The Betsileo of Madagascar have both lineages and clans. They can demonstrate descent for the most recent 8 to 10 generations. Going further back than that, however, they can only stipulate their descent from particular ancestors. The stipulated founders of Betsileo clans can include vaguely defined foreign royalty or even mythical creatures, such as mermaids (Kottak 1980). Like the Betsileo, many societies have both lineages and clans. When this is true, the clan will have more members and cover a larger geographic area than

lineage
A unilineal descent group based on demonstrated descent.

clan
A unilineal descent group based on stipulated descent.

unilineal descent
Matrilineal or patrilineal descent.

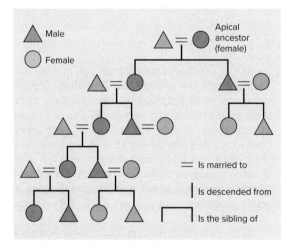

FIGURE 10.3 A Matrilineage Five Generations Deep.

Matrilineages are based on demonstrated descent from a female ancestor. Only the children of the group's women (blue) belong to the matrilineage. The children of the group's men are excluded; they belong to *their* mother's matrilineage.

NOTE: In this and other kin charts, *triangles* represent *males; circles* are *females;* an *equals* sign indicates *marriage;* a *vertical* line shows *descent;* and a *horizontal* line denotes a *sibling* relationship.

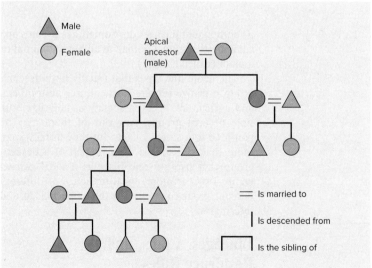

FIGURE 10.4 A Patrilineage Five Generations Deep.

Patrilineages are based on demonstrated descent from a male apical ancestor. With patrilineal descent, children of the group's men (blue) are included as descent-group members. Children of the group's women are excluded; they belong to *their* father's patrilineage.

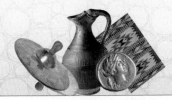

American Family Life in the 21st Century

Anthropologists today increasingly study daily life in the United States, including that of middle-class families. An excellent example is *Life at Home in the Twenty-First Century: 32 Families Open Their Doors* (Arnold et al. 2012), a study of home life in 32 middle-class, dual-income families in Los Angeles, focusing on physical surroundings and material culture, the items owned and used in daily life. The book's authors are three UCLA anthropologists—Jeanne Arnold, Anthony Graesch, and Elinor Ochs—and Italian photographer Enzo Ragazzini. All did research through UCLA's Center on Everyday Lives of Families (CELF), which was founded in 2001 and directed by Ochs (see also Ochs and Kremer-Sadlik 2013).

The families who participated in the study on which *Life at Home* was based were all middle-class and owned or were buying their homes. They varied in ethnicity, income level, and neighborhood. Same-sex couples were included. The authors took a systematic approach to their subjects. They videotaped the activities of family members, tracked their movements using positioning devices, measured their stress levels through saliva samples, and took almost 20,000 photographs (approximately 600 per family) of homes, yards, and activities. The researchers also asked family members to narrate tours of their homes and videotaped them as they did so. Over a 4-year period, the project generated 47 hours of family-narrated video home tours and 1,540 hours of videotaped family interactions and interviews (see Arnold et al. 2012; Feuer 2012; Ochs and Kremer-Sadlik 2013; Sullivan 2012).

A key finding of the study was the extent of clutter in those homes, a manifestation of a high degree of consumerism among dual-income American families. Never in human history, the researchers conclude, have families accumulated so many personal possessions. Hypothesizing that dealing with so much clutter would have psychological effects, the researchers collected saliva samples in order to measure diurnal cortisol, an indicator of stress. Mothers' saliva, it turned out, contained more diurnal cortisol than did fathers'. The researchers also noticed that, in their video tours, mothers often used words like "mess" and "chaotic" to describe their homes, while fathers rarely mentioned messiness. Author Anthony Graesch reasons that clutter bothers moms so much because it challenges deeply ingrained notions that homes should be tidy and well managed (see Feuer 2012). The role of domestic manager, of course, is traditionally a female one. For dads and kids, more than for moms, possessions appeared to be a source of pleasure, pride, and contentment rather than stress (Arnold et al. 2012; Feuer 2012).

Another finding was that children rarely went outside, despite the overall mild weather in Los Angeles. They used their possessions indoors, resulting in more clutter, including whole walls devoted to displays of dolls and toys. More than half of the 32 households had special rooms designed for work or schoolwork, but even in

its component lineages do. Sometimes a clan's apical ancestor is not a human at all but an animal or a plant (called a *totem*).

The economic types that usually have descent-group organization are horticulture, pastoralism, and agriculture. A given society usually has multiple descent groups. Any one of them may be confined to a single village, but they usually span more than one village. Any branch of a descent group that lives in one place is a *local descent group*. Two (or more) local branches of different descent groups may live in the same village and intermarry.

Lineages, Clans, and Residence Rules

As we've seen, descent groups, unlike nuclear families, are permanent units, with new members gained and lost in each generation. Members have access to the lineage estate, where some of them must live, in order to benefit from and manage that estate across the generations. To endure, descent groups need to keep at least some of their members at home. An easy way to do this is to have a rule about who belongs to the descent group and where they should live after they get married. Patrilineal and matrilineal descent, and the postmarital residence rules that usually accompany them, ensure that about half the people born in each generation will live out their lives on the ancestral estate.

With patrilineal descent, the typical postmarital residence rule is *patrilocality:* Married couples reside in the husband's father's community, so that the children will grow up in their father's village. It makes sense for patrilineal societies to require patrilocal postmarital residence. If the group's male members are expected to exercise their rights in the ancestral estate, it's a good idea to raise them on that estate and to keep them there after they marry.

home offices, kids' stuff tended to crowd parental items. The researchers speculate that guilt motivates dual-income parents to overbuy for their children. The parents in the study managed to spend, on an average weekday, no more than four hours with their kids, perhaps leading them to overcompensate with toys, clothes, and other possessions (Graesch quoted in Feuer 2012).

The study found that the kitchen was the center of home life. In this space, family members met, interacted, exchanged information, and socialized with their children. And in the kitchen, the refrigerator played a key role. Stuck on its doors and sides were pictures, displays of children's achievements, reminders, addresses, and phone lists (including many outdated ones). The typical refrigerator front panel held 52 objects. The most crowded refrigerator had 166 stick-ons. The refrigerator served as a compact representation of that family's history and activities (Feuer 2012; Sullivan 2012).

Researchers found a correlation between the number of objects on the refrigerator and the overall clutter in a home. The refrigerator thus

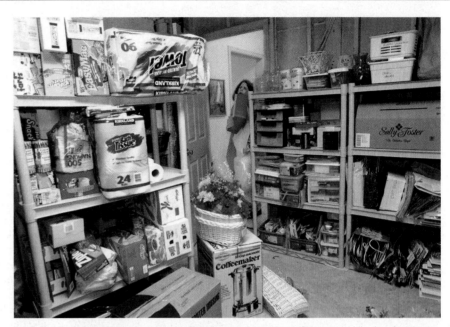

As studied by anthropologists in greater Los Angeles, the clutter that typifies many middle-class American homes reflects a high degree of consumerism, especially among dual-income families. Never in human history have non-elite families owned so many possessions.
The Washington Times/ZUMA Press/Newscom

served not only as a chronicler of family life but also as a measure of its degree of consumerism— and perhaps of stress. We might hypothesize that a high number of refrigerator stick-ons indicates that someone in the household needs to take up meditation to lower his or her blood pressure.

A less common postmarital residence rule, associated with matrilineal descent, is *matrilocality:* Married couples live in the wife's mother's community, and their children grow up in their mother's village. Together, patrilocality and matrilocality are known as *unilocal* rules of postmarital residence. Regardless of where one resides after marriage, one remains a member of one's original unilineal descent group for life. This means that a man residing in his wife's village in a matrilineal society keeps his membership in his own matrilineal descent group, and a woman residing in her husband's village is still a member of her own patrilineal descent group.

Ambilineal Descent

With unilineal descent, whether matrilineal or patrilineal, people at birth automatically become lifetime members of one—and only one—descent group. Unilineal descent admits some people while

clearly and definitely excluding others. Things aren't always so definite. Unilineal descent isn't the only descent rule known to anthropology. Ambilineal descent is a descent rule that offers more flexibility and choice. With **ambilineal descent,** group membership is neither automatic at birth nor fixed for life. Individuals have a choice about their descent group affiliation, and they can belong to more than one descent group. Ambilineal descent groups do not *automatically* exclude either the children of sons or those of daughters. People can choose the descent group they join (e.g., that of their father's father, father's mother, mother's father, or mother's mother). People also can change their descent-group membership, or belong to two or more groups at the same time.

Family versus Descent

There are rights and obligations associated with kinship and descent. Many societies have both

ambilineal descent
A flexible descent rule, neither patrilineal nor matrilineal.

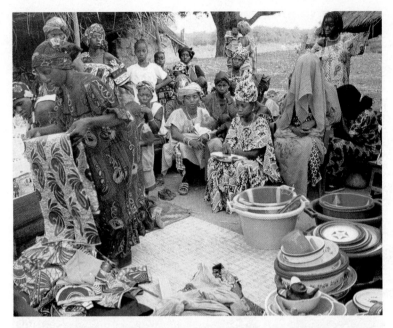

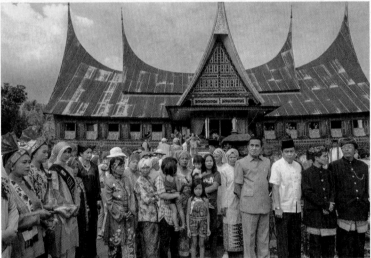

Most societies have a prevailing opinion about where couples should live after they marry; this is called a postmarital residence rule. A common rule is patrilocality: The couple lives with the husband's relatives, so that children grow up in their father's community. The top image shows a young Muslim bride (veiled in pink) in the West African country of Guinea Bissau. On the last day of her three-day wedding ceremony, she will collect laundry from her husband's family, wash it with her friends, and be taken to his village on a bicycle. In the bottom photo, members of a Minangkabau clan gather to celebrate a wedding in front of their traditional *rumah gadang* (big house). In this matrilineal society, postmarital residence is matrilocal, and ownership of these "big houses" passes from mother to daughter.

(top): Ami Vitale/Alamy Stock Photo; (bottom): Terry Allen/Alamy Stock Photo

kinship calculation
The relationships based on kinship that people recognize in a particular society, and how they talk about those relationships.

children, who will become members of her husband's group.

In a matrilineal society things are different. A man has obligations both to his family of procreation (his wife and children) and to his closest matrikin (his sisters and their children). The continuity of his own descent group depends on his sisters and their children, since descent is carried by females, and he has an obligation to look out for their welfare. He also has obligations to his wife and children. If a man is sure his wife's children are his own, he has more incentive to invest in them than when he has doubts.

Compared with patrilineal systems, matrilineal societies tend to have higher divorce rates and greater female promiscuity (Schneider and Gough 1961). According to Nicholas Kottak (2002), among the matrilineal Makua of northern Mozambique, a husband is concerned about his wife's potential promiscuity. A man's sister also takes an interest in her brother's wife's fidelity. She doesn't want her brother wasting time on children who may not be his, thus diminishing his investment in her children as their uncle (mother's brother). A confessional ritual that is part of the Makua birthing process demonstrates the sister's allegiance to her brother. When a wife is deep in labor, the husband's sister, who attends her, must ask, "Who is the real father of this child?" If the wife lies, the Makua believe the birth will be difficult, often ending in the death of the woman and/or the baby. This ritual serves as an important social paternity test. It is in both the husband's and his sister's interest to ensure that his wife's children are indeed his own.

KINSHIP CALCULATION

In addition to studying kin groups, anthropologists also are interested in **kinship calculation:** the relationships based on kinship that people recognize in different societies and how they talk about those relationships (see Sahlins 2013; Stone and King 2019). Who is, and who is not, considered to be a relative? Like race and gender, kinship is culturally constructed. This means that some genealogical kin are considered to be relatives, whereas others may not be. It also means that even people who aren't genealogical relatives can be socially recognized as kin. Kinship calculation, also known as *kinship classification,* is the system that people in a particular society use to recognize and categorize kinship relationships.

Cultures maintain varied beliefs about biological processes involving kinship, including the role of insemination in creating human life. We know that fertilization of an ovum by a single sperm is responsible for conception. Other cultures have different ideas about procreation. In some societies it is believed that spirits, rather than men, place babies in women's wombs. In others, people

families and descent groups. Obligations to one may conflict with obligations to the other—more so in matrilineal than in patrilineal societies. In a patrilineal society, a woman typically leaves home when she marries and raises her children in her husband's community. After leaving home, she has no primary or substantial obligations to her own descent group. She can invest fully in her

think that a fetus must be nourished by continuing insemination during pregnancy. People in many cultures believe that several acts of intercourse are needed to make a baby (see Beckerman and Valentine 2002; Shapiro 2009; Valentine et al. 2017). The Barí of Venezuela and their neighbors, for example, believe that multiple men can create the same fetus. When a Barí child is born, the mother publicly announces the names of the one or more men she believes to be the father(s). If those men accept paternity, they must provide care for the mother and child. Barí children with more than one official father turn out to be advantaged compared with those who have just one. Anthropologists report that 80 percent of Barí children with multiple dads survived to adulthood, compared with just 64 percent who had just one (Beckerman and Valentine 2002; Shapiro 2009).

Ethnographers strive to discover, in a given society, the specific genealogical relationships between "relatives" and the person who has named them—the **ego.** *Ego* means "I" (or "me") in Latin. It's who you, the reader, are in the kin charts that follow. It's your perspective looking out on your kin.

By posing the same questions to several local people, the ethnographer learns about the extent and direction of kinship calculation in a society. The ethnographer also begins to understand the relationship between kinship calculation and kin groups: how people use kinship to create and maintain personal ties and to join social groups. In the kinship charts that follow, the gray square labeled "ego" identifies the person (male or female) whose kinship calculation is being examined.

Kin Terms and Genealogical Kin Types

At this point, we may distinguish between *kin terms* (the words used for different relatives in a particular language) and *genealogical kin types.* **Kin terms** are the specific words used for different relatives in a particular culture and language. Kin terms are cultural, rather than biological, categories. *Genealogical kin types,* by contrast, refer to biology, to an actual genealogical relationship. Father's brother is a genealogical kin type, whereas *uncle* is a kin term (in English) that lumps together, or merges, multiple genealogical kin types, including father's brother, mother's brother, and often the husbands of "blood" aunts. Kin terms reflect the social construction of kinship in a given culture.

We designate genealogical kin types with the letters and symbols shown in Figure 10.5. As with *uncle,* a kin term may (and usually does) lump together multiple genealogical relationships. *Grandfather* includes mother's father and father's father. The term *cousin* lumps together several kin types. Even the more specific *first cousin* includes mother's brother's son (MBS), mother's brother's daughter (MBD), mother's sister's son (MZS),

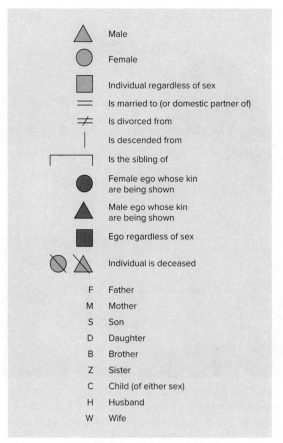

FIGURE 10.5 Kinship Symbols and Genealogical Kin Type Notation.

mother's sister's daughter (MZD), father's brother's son (FBS), father's brother's daughter (FBD), father's sister's son (FZS), and father's sister's daughter (FZD). *First cousin* thus lumps together at least eight genealogical kin types.

Even the key kin term *father,* which is used primarily for one kin type—the genealogical father—can be extended to an adoptive father or stepfather, and even to a priest or a "Heavenly Father."

We use *uncle* to include both mother's brother and father's brother because we perceive them as being the same sort of relative. Calling them *uncles,* we distinguish between them and another kin type, F, whom we call *Father, Dad,* or *Pop.* In many societies, however, it is common to call a father and a father's brother by the same term. Later we'll see why.

Kin Terms in America

It's reasonable for North Americans to distinguish between relatives who belong to their nuclear families and those who don't. We are more likely to grow up with our parents than with our aunts and uncles. We tend to see our parents more often than we see our uncles and aunts, who may live in different towns and cities. We often inherit from our parents, but our cousins have first claim to

ego
The position from which one views an egocentric genealogy.

kin terms
The words used for different relatives in a particular language and system of kinship calculation.

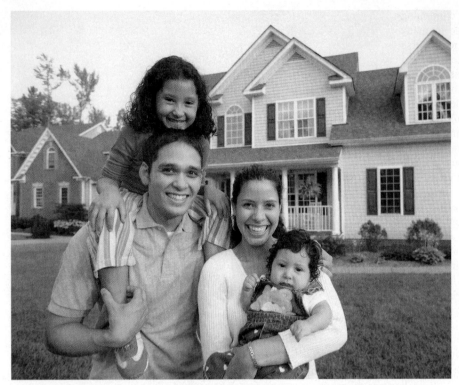

A neolocal American nuclear family in front of their (neolocal) home. The nuclear family's relative isolation from other kin groups in modern nations reflects geographic mobility within an industrial economy with sale of labor for cash. It's reasonable for North Americans to distinguish between relatives who belong to their nuclear families and those who don't.

Ariel Skelley/Blend Images

family visits, reunions, holidays, and extended family relations, than the husband does. This would tend to reinforce her kin network over his and thus favor matrilateral skewing.

Bilateral kinship means that people tend to perceive kin links through males and females as being similar or equivalent. This bilaterality is expressed in interaction with, living with or near, and rights to inherit from relatives. We don't usually inherit from uncles, but if we do, there's about as much chance that we'll inherit from the father's brother as from the mother's brother. We usually don't live with an aunt, but if we do, it might be either the mother's sister or the father's sister.

KINSHIP TERMINOLOGY

People perceive and define kin relations differently in different societies. In any culture, kinship terminology is a classification system, a taxonomy or typology. It is a *native taxonomy,* developed over generations by the people who live in a particular society. A native classification system is based on how people perceive similarities and differences in the things being classified.

However, anthropologists have discovered that there is a limited number of patterns or systems by which people classify their kin (see McConvell, Keen, and Hendery 2013). People who speak very different languages may use exactly the same system of kinship terminology. This section examines the four main ways of classifying kin on the parental generation: lineal, bifurcate merging, generational, and bifurcate collateral. We also consider the social correlates of these classification systems. (Note that each of the systems described here applies to the parental generation. There also are differences in kin terminology used to classify siblings and cousins. There are six such systems, which you can see diagrammed and discussed at the following websites: http://anthro.palomar.edu/kinship/kinship_5.htm and http://anthro.palomar.edu/kinship/kinship_6.htm.)

Kin terms provide useful information about social patterns. If two relatives are designated by the same term, we can assume that they are perceived as sharing socially significant attributes. Several factors influence the way people interact with, perceive, and classify relatives. For instance, do certain kinds of relatives customarily live together or apart? How far apart? What benefits do they derive from each other, and what are their obligations? Are they members of the same

inherit from our aunts and uncles. If our marriage is stable, we see our children daily as long as they remain at home. They are our heirs. We feel closer to them than to our nieces and nephews.

American kinship calculation and kin terms reflect these social features. Thus, the term *uncle* distinguishes between the kin types MB and FB on the one hand and the kin type F on the other. However, this term also lumps together kin types. We use the same term for MB and FB, two different kin types—one on the mother's side, the other on the father's side. We do this because American kinship calculation is **bilateral**—traced equally on both sides, through males and females, for example, father and mother. Both kinds of uncle are brothers of a parent. We think of both as roughly the same kind of relative.

"No," you may object, "I'm closer to my mother's brother than to my father's brother." That may be. However, in a representative sample of Americans, we would find a split, with some favoring one side and some favoring the other. We'd actually expect a bit of *matrilateral skewing*—a preference for relatives on the mother's side. This occurs for many reasons. When contemporary children are raised by just one parent, it's much more likely to be the mother than the father. Also, even with intact marriages, the wife tends to play a more active role in managing family affairs, including

bilateral kinship calculation

Kin ties calculated equally through both sexes.

descent group or of different descent groups? With these questions in mind, let's examine systems of kinship terminology.

Lineal Terminology

Our own system of kinship classification is called the *lineal system* (Figure 10.6). The number 3 and the color light blue stand for the term *uncle,* which we apply both to FB and to MB. **Lineal kinship terminology** is found in societies such as the United States and Canada in which the nuclear family is the most important group based on kinship.

Lineal kinship terminology gets its name from the fact that it distinguishes lineal relatives from collateral relatives. What does that mean? A **lineal relative** is an ancestor or a descendant, anyone on the direct *line* of descent that leads to and from ego (Figure 10.7). Thus, lineal relatives are one's parents, grandparents, great-grandparents, and other direct forebears. Lineal relatives also include children, grandchildren, and great-grandchildren. **Collateral relatives** are all other kin. They include siblings, nieces and nephews, aunts and uncles, and cousins. **Affinals** are relatives by marriage, whether of lineals (e.g., son's wife) or of collaterals (sister's husband).

Bifurcate Merging Terminology

Bifurcate merging kinship terminology (Figure 10.8) *bifurcates,* or splits, the mother's side from the father's side. But it also *merges* same-sex siblings—sisters with sisters and brothers with brothers. Thus, one's mother and mother's sister are lumped together or merged under the same term (1), while one's father and father's brother also are merged—into a common term (2). There are different terms for mother's brother (3) and father's sister (4).

Bifurcate merging kinship terminology is found in societies with unilineal descent groups. In such societies, its logic makes sense: One's mother and father always belong to different descent groups, so the terminology separates them. In a patrilineal society, it makes sense to use the same term for father and father's brother, because they belong to the same descent group, and they also share

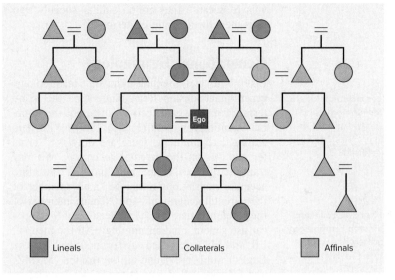

FIGURE 10.7 The Distinctions among Lineals, Collaterals, and Affinals as Perceived by Ego.

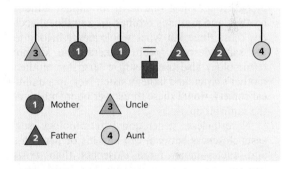

FIGURE 10.8 Bifurcate Merging Kinship Terminology.

the same gender and generation. Because patrilineal societies usually have patrilocal residence, the father and his brother live in the same local group. Because they share so many attributes that are socially relevant, ego regards them as social equivalents and calls them by the same kinship term—2. However, the mother's brother belongs to a different descent group, lives elsewhere, and has a different kin term—3.

What about mother and mother's sister in a patrilineal society? They belong to the same descent group, the same gender, and the same generation. Often they marry men from the same village and go to live there. These social similarities help explain the use of the same term—1—for both.

Similar observations apply to matrilineal societies. Consider a society with two matrilineal clans, the Ravens and the Wolves. Ego belongs to his or her mother's clan, the Raven clan. Ego's father belongs to the Wolf clan. Ego's mother and her sister are female Ravens of the same generation. If there is matrilocal residence, as there often is in matrilineal societies, they will live in the same

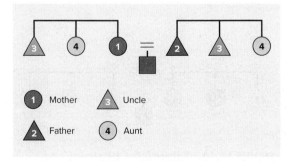

FIGURE 10.6 Lineal Kinship Terminology.

lineal kinship terminology
Four parental kin terms: M, F, FB=MB, and MZ=FZ.

lineal relatives
Ego's direct ancestors and descendants.

collateral relative
A relative outside ego's direct line, e.g., B, Z, FB, MZ.

affinals
Relatives by marriage.

bifurcate merging kinship terminology
Four parental kin terms: M=MZ, F=FB, MB, and FZ each stand alone.

village. Because they are so similar socially, ego calls them by the same kin term—1.

Generational Terminology

generational kinship terminology
Just two parental kin terms: M=MZ=FZ and F=FB=MB.

bifurcate collateral kinship terminology
Six separate parental kin terms: M, F, MB, MZ, FB, and FZ.

Like bifurcate merging kinship terminology, **generational kinship terminology** uses the same term for parents and their siblings, but the lumping is more complete (Figure 10.9). With generational terminology, there are only two terms for relatives on the parental *generation*. We may translate them as "father" and "mother," but more accurate translations would be "male member of the parental generation" and "female member of the parental generation." The Betsileo of Madagascar use generational terminology. All the men (F, FB, and MB) are called *ray* (pronounced like the English word "rye"), and all the women (M, MZ, and FZ) are called *reny* (sounds like "raynie" in English).

Generational kinship terminology does not distinguish between the mother's side and the father's side. It does not bifurcate, but it certainly does merge. It uses just one term for father, father's brother, and mother's brother. In a unilineal society, these three kin types would never belong to the same descent group. Generational kinship terminology also uses a single term for mother, mother's sister, and father's sister. Nor, in a unilineal society, would these three ever be members of the same group.

Nevertheless, generational terminology suggests closeness between ego and his or her aunts and uncles—much more closeness than exists between Americans and these kin types. How likely would you be to call your uncle "Dad" or your aunt "Mom"? We'd expect to find generational terminology in societies in which extended kinship is much more important than it is in our own but in which there is no rigid distinction between the father's side and the mother's side.

It makes sense, then, that generational kin terminology is found in societies with ambilineal descent, where descent-group membership is not automatic. People may choose the group they join, change their descent-group membership, or

belong to two or more descent groups simultaneously. Generational terminology fits these conditions. The use of intimate kin terms signals that people have close personal relations with all their relatives on the parental generation. People exhibit similar behavior toward their parents, aunts, and uncles, and may live for variable lengths of time with one or more of those relatives.

Generational terminology is also used in a series of band-organized societies, including the Kalahari San and several Native North American groups. Use of this terminology reflects certain similarities between foraging bands and ambilineal descent groups. In both kinds of society, people have a choice about their kin-group affiliation. Foragers always live with kin, but they often shift band affiliation and so may be members of several different bands during their lifetimes. Generational terminology among foragers helps maintain close personal relationships with several parental-generation relatives, whom ego may eventually use as a point of entry into different groups.

Bifurcate Collateral Terminology

Of the four kin classification systems, **bifurcate collateral kinship terminology** is the most specific. It has separate kin terms for each of the six kin types (mother, father, mother's sister, mother's brother, father's brother, and father's sister) on the parental generation (Figure 10.10). Bifurcate collateral terminology isn't as common as the other types. Many of the societies that use it are in North Africa and the Middle East, and many of them are offshoots of the same ancestral group.

Bifurcate collateral terminology also may develop when a child has parents of different ethnic backgrounds and uses terms for aunts and uncles derived from different languages. Thus, if you have a mother who is Latina and a father who is Anglo, you may call your aunts and uncles on your mother's side "tia" and "tio," while calling those on your father's side "aunt" and "uncle." And your mother and father may be "Mom" and "Pop." That's a modern form of bifurcate collateral kinship terminology. Recap 10.1 lists the types of kin group, the postmarital residence rule, and the economic type associated with the four types of kinship terminology.

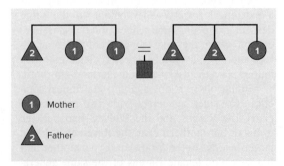

FIGURE 10.9 Generational Kinship Terminology.

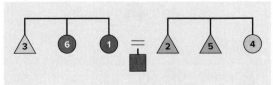

FIGURE 10.10 Bifurcate Collateral Kinship Terminology.

KINSHIP TERMINOLOGY	KIN GROUP	RESIDENCE RULE	ECONOMY
Lineal	Nuclear family	Neolocal	Industrialism, foraging
Bifurcate merging	Unilineal descent group—patrilineal or matrilineal	Unilocal—patrilocal or matrilocal	Horticulture, pastoralism, agriculture
Generational	Ambilineal descent group, band	Ambilocal	Agriculture, horticulture, foraging
Bifurcate collateral	Varies	Varies	Varies

It's All Relative

Defining "Close Family" Members

We've seen how the social construction of kinship varies widely among societies. Furthermore, even in a single country, there can be significant disagreement about kinship classification. Consider a travel ban announced by the Trump administration on June 29, 2017. Citizens of six Muslim-majority countries (Iran, Libya, Somalia, Sudan, Syria, and Yemen) would be denied visas to enter the United States as visitors or refugees unless they could demonstrate a "close family relationship" with an American citizen, or a connection with a school or business. Only the following family members of citizens were considered close enough to enter: parent, spouse, child, adult son or daughter, son-in-law, daughter-in-law, and sibling, as well as their stepfamily counterparts. The administration's definition of "close family member" excluded grandparents, grandchildren, uncles, aunts, cousins, and fiancés/fiancées.

When I, an anthropologist and a grandfather, first read the list, I was astonished. Grandparents are considered close relatives in every culture I've ever read about. Why should a stepbrother, who is an affinal relative, have preference over a grandfather, who is a lineal relative, I wondered? I was not alone in my bewilderment. Lawyers argued in court that fiancés/fiancées, grandparents, grandchildren, brothers-in-law, sisters-in-law, aunts, uncles, nieces, nephews, and cousins of U.S. citizens should also be exempt from the ban.

On July 14, 2017, U.S. district judge Derrick K. Watson agreed, ruling that the government's list was too "narrowly defined" and that grandparents and other extended relatives should be exempt from the travel ban. "Common sense . . . dictates that close family members be defined to include grandparents," he wrote. "Indeed, grandparents are the epitome of close family members" (see Zapotosky 2017). The U.S. Supreme Court later reaffirmed Judge Watson's wider definition of kinship.

Relatives whose status remained unclear included a fiancé's/fiancée's family (future in-laws), a half sibling's other parent, a stepchild's other parent, a stepsibling's parent, and any other "extended" family members of a U.S. citizen. Who

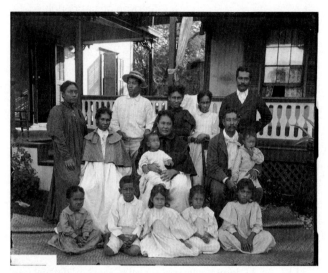

A historic photo of a Hawaiian extended family. Hawaiians traditionally used generational kinship terminology for the parental generation.

Archive PL/Alamy Stock Photo

might that be? We see how the social construction of kinship has moved beyond your anthropology textbook into our systems of law and border control. How do you define your close family members?

Relationships Queried in the 2020 Census

Figure 10.11 replicates a question about relationships asked in the 2020 U.S. census. For each household, the census first establishes "Person 1" as "someone living here who pays the rent or owns this residence." If the owner or rent payer doesn't reside in that household, then "list any adult living here as Person 1." Once Person 1 has been established, each additional person living in that household is asked to indicate how they are related to Person 1. Figure 10.11 shows the 16 options offered by the census, starting with "opposite-sex husband/wife/spouse," ending with "other nonrelative," and including "biological son or daughter," "adopted son or daughter," "stepson or stepdaughter," "roommate or housemate," and "foster child." Do you notice anything missing? Is there anything that is included that surprises you?

3. How is this person related to Person 1? *Mark* **X** *ONE box.*

☐ Opposite-sex husband/wife/spouse   ☐ Father or mother

☐ Opposite-sex unmarried partner   ☐ Grandchild

☐ Same-sex husband/wife/spouse   ☐ Parent-in-law

☐ Same-sex unmarried partner   ☐ Son-in-low or daughter-in-law

☐ Biological son or daughter   ☐ Other relative

☐ Adopted son or daughter   ☐ Roommate or housemate

☐ Stepson or stepdaughter   ☐ Foster child

☐ Brother or sister   ☐ Other nonrelative

FIGURE 10.11 Relationship Question in 2020 U.S. Census. Asks how each additional person living in that household is related to Person 1.

for REVIEW

summary

1. In nonindustrial societies, kinship, descent, and marriage organize social and political life. In studying kinship, we must distinguish between kin groups, whose composition and activities can be observed, and kinship calculation—how people identify and designate their relatives.

2. One widespread kin group is the nuclear family, consisting of a married couple and their children. There are functional alternatives to the nuclear family. That is, other groups may assume functions usually associated with the nuclear family. Nuclear families tend to be especially important in foraging and industrial societies. Among farmers and herders, other kinds of kin groups, particularly descent groups, often overshadow the nuclear family.

3. In contemporary North America, the nuclear family is a characteristic kin group for the middle class. Expanded households and sharing with extended family kin occur more frequently among the poor, who may pool their resources in dealing with poverty. Today, however, even in the American middle class, nuclear family households are declining as single-person households and other domestic arrangements increase.

4. The descent group is a basic kin group among nonindustrial farmers and herders. Unlike families, descent groups have perpetuity—they last for generations. Descent-group members share and manage a common estate: land, animals, and other resources. There are several kinds of descent groups. Lineages are based on demonstrated descent; clans, on stipulated descent. Descent rules may be unilineal or ambilineal. Patrilineal and matrilineal descent are associated, respectively, with patrilocal and matrilocal postmarital residence. Obligations to one's descent group and to one's family of procreation may conflict, especially in matrilineal societies.

5. A kinship terminology is a classification of relatives based on perceived differences and similarities. Comparative research has revealed a limited number of ways of classifying kin. Because there are correlations between kinship terminology and other social practices, we often can predict kinship terminology from other aspects of culture. The four basic kinship terminologies for the parental generation are lineal, bifurcate merging, generational, and bifurcate collateral. Industrial societies use lineal terminology, which is associated with nuclear family organization. Cultures with unilocal residence and unilineal descent tend to have bifurcate merging terminology. Generational terminology correlates with ambilineal descent and also occurs in certain foraging societies.

key terms

1. Why is kinship so important to anthropologists? How might the study of kinship be useful for research in fields of anthropology other than cultural anthropology?

2. What are some examples of alternatives to nuclear family arrangements considered in this chapter? What might be the impact of new (and increasingly accessible) reproductive technologies on domestic arrangements?

3. Although the nuclear family remains the cultural ideal for many Americans, other domestic arrangements now outnumber the "traditional" American household more than five to one. What are some reasons for this? Do you think this trend is good or bad? Why?

4. To what sorts of family or families do you belong? Have you belonged to other kinds of families? How do the kin terms you use compare with the four classification systems discussed in this chapter?

5. Cultures with unilineal descent tend to have bifurcate merging terminology, whereas ambilineal descent is associated with generational terminology. Why does this make sense? How might the terminology used for the parental generation be applied to your own generation?

think like an anthropologist

Design Elements: Understanding Ourselves: muha/123RF (rock paintings); Focus on Globalization: janrysavy/Getty Images (globe); Appreciating Diversity (left to right): Floresco Productions/age footstock; Hero/Corbis/Glow Images, Hill Street Studios/Blend Images, Billion Photos/Shutterstock; Understanding Ourselves : Hemera Technologies/Alamy (Cymbal), LACMA - Los Angeles County Museum of Art (Trefoil Oinochoe), Ingram Publishing/SuperStock (Coin), ChuckSchugPhotography/Getty Images (Rug).

credits

Marriage

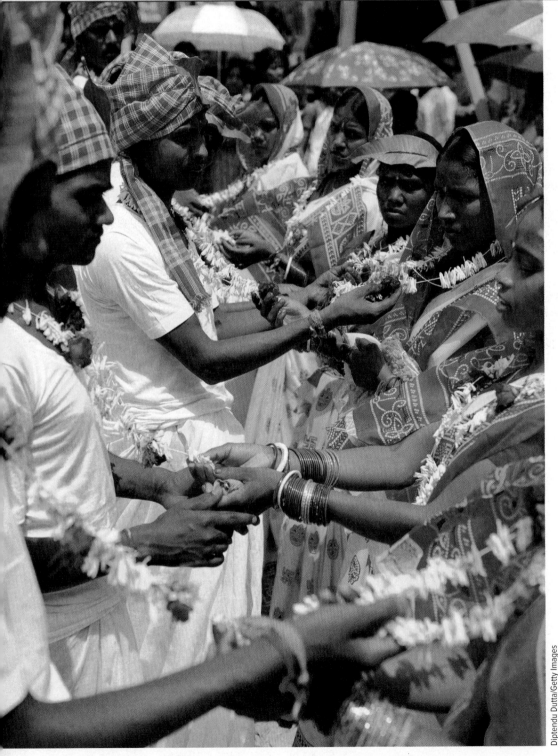

▶ How is marriage defined and regulated, and what rights does it convey?

▶ What role does marriage play in creating and maintaining group alliances?

▶ What forms of marriage exist cross-culturally, and what are their social correlates?

Diptendu Dutta/Getty Images

In North Bengal, India, these brides and grooms, members of the indigenous Adivasi ethnic group, take part in a mass marriage ceremony. The organizers of the ceremony enabled 51 couples, unable to pay for individual weddings, to marry.

understanding OURSELVES

chapter outline

According to the late radio call-in psychologist (and undergraduate anthropology major) Dr. Joy Browne, parents' job is to give their kids "roots and wings." Roots, she often stated, are the easier part. In other words, it's easier to raise children than to let them go. Lending support to her point, more young Americans aged 18 to 34 now live with their parents than with a spouse or romantic partner. Indeed, for the first time in more than a century, Americans in this age group are more likely to be housed in their parental home than in any other living arrangement (Cilluffo and Cohn 2017).

I suspect that both parents and children contribute to this trend. Parents have more trouble letting go, and their kids have more trouble finding the means to live independently. I've heard comments about today's "helicopter parents" hovering over even their college-aged kids, using cell phones, texting, e-mail, and GPS devices to follow their progeny more closely than in prior generations. Do you have any experience with such a pattern? Do you think you'll be living with your parents when you turn 30?

It can be difficult to make the transition between the family that raised us (our family of orientation) and the family we form if we have children (our family of procreation). In contemporary America, we usually get a head start by "leaving home" long before we establish a family of procreation. If we are lucky, we go off to college or find a job that enables us to support ourselves. In either case, we often live independently or with roommates.

In nonindustrial societies, people (especially women) may leave home abruptly when they marry. Often, a woman must leave her home village and her own kin and move in with her husband and his relatives. This can be an unpleasant and alienating transition. Many women complain about feeling isolated, or being mistreated, in their husband's village.

In contemporary North America, although neither women nor men typically have to adjust to living with in-laws full time, conflicts with in-laws aren't at all uncommon. Just read "Dear Abby" or similar columns for a week. Even more of a challenge is learning to live with a spouse. Marriage always raises issues of accommodation and adjustment. Initially, the married couple is just that, unless there are children from a previous marriage. If there are, adjustment issues will involve stepparenthood—and a prior spouse—as well as the new marital relationship. Once a couple has its own child, the family-of-procreation mentality takes over. In the United States, family loyalty shifts, but not completely, from the family of orientation to the family that includes spouse and child(ren). Given our bilateral kinship system, we maintain relations with our sons and daughters after they marry, and grandchildren theoretically are as close to one set of grandparents as to the other set. In practice, grandchildren tend to be a bit closer to their mother's than to their father's families. Can you speculate about why that might be? How is it for you? Are you closer to your paternal or maternal grandparents? How about your uncles and aunts on one side or the other? Why is that?

DEFINING MARRIAGE

"Love and marriage," "marriage and the family": These familiar phrases show how we link the romantic love of two individuals to marriage and how we link marriage to reproduction and family creation. But marriage is an institution with significant roles and functions in addition to reproduction. What is marriage, anyway?

Marriage is notoriously difficult to define because of the varied forms it can take in different societies. Consider the following definition from *Notes and Queries on Anthropology:*

> Marriage is a union between a man and a woman such that the children born to the woman are recognized as legitimate offspring of both partners. (Royal Anthropological Institute 1951, p. 111)

This definition isn't universally valid for several reasons. First, in many societies, marriage unites more than two spouses. Here we speak of *plural marriages,* as when a man weds two (or more) women, or a woman weds a group of brothers—an arrangement called *fraternal polyandry* that is characteristic of certain Himalayan cultures.

Second, some societies (even traditional ones) recognize various kinds of same-sex marriages. In South Sudan, for example, a Nuer woman could take a wife if her father had no sons, who were necessary for the survival of his patrilineage. That father could ask his daughter to stand as a fictive son in order to take a bride. This daughter would become the socially recognized husband of another woman (her wife). This was a symbolic and social relationship rather than a sexual one. The "wife" had sex with a man or men (whom her female "husband" approved) until she became pregnant. The children born to the wife were accepted as the offspring of both the female husband and the wife. Although the female husband was not the actual **genitor,** the biological father of the children, she was their **pater,** or socially recognized father. What's important in this Nuer case is *social* rather than *biological paternity.* We see again how kinship is socially constructed. The bride's children were considered the legitimate offspring of her female "husband," who was biologically a woman but socially a man, and the patrilineal descent line continued.

A third objection to the definition of marriage offered earlier is that it focuses on marriage's role in legitimizing children. Does this mean that people who marry after childbearing age, or who do not plan to have children, are not actually married?

In fact, marriage has roles in society beyond legitimating children. The British anthropologist Edmund Leach (1955) observed that, depending on the society, several different kinds of rights and benefits are allocated by marriage. According to Leach, marriage can, but doesn't always, accomplish the following:

- Establish legal parentage.

- Give either or both spouses a monopoly on the sexuality of the other.

- Give either or both spouses rights to the labor of the other.

- Give either or both spouses rights over the other's property.

- Establish a joint fund of property—a partnership—for the benefit of the children.

- Establish a socially significant "relationship of affinity" between spouses and their relatives.

EXOGAMY AND INCEST

In nonindustrial societies, a person's social world includes two main categories—friends and strangers. Strangers are potential or actual enemies. Marriage is one of the primary ways of converting strangers into friends, of creating and maintaining personal and political alliances. **Exogamy,** the custom and practice of seeking a mate outside one's own group, has adaptive value, because it links people into a wider social network that can nurture, help, and protect them in times of need. Incest restrictions (prohibitions on sex with relatives) reinforce exogamy by pushing people to seek their mates outside the local group. Most societies discourage sexual contact involving close relatives, especially members of the same nuclear family.

Incest refers to sexual contact with a relative, but cultures define their kin, and thus incest, differently. In other words, incest, like kinship, is socially constructed. For example, some U.S. states permit marriage, and therefore sex, with first cousins, while others ban those practices as incestuous. Cross-culturally, sex and marriage between first cousins may or may not be considered incestuous, depending on context and the kin type of the first cousin. Many societies distinguish between two types of first cousins: cross cousins and parallel cousins. The children of two brothers or two sisters are **parallel cousins.** The children of a brother and a sister are **cross cousins.** Your mother's sister's children and your father's brother's children are your parallel cousins. Your father's sister's children and your mother's brother's children are your cross cousins.

The American kin term *cousin* doesn't distinguish between cross and parallel cousins, but in many societies, especially those with unilineal descent, the distinction is essential. As an example, consider a community with only two descent groups. This exemplifies what is known as *moiety* organization—from the French *moitié,* which means "half." Descent bifurcates the community so that everyone belongs to one half or the other.

exogamy
Marriage outside one's own group.

incest
Sexual relations with a close relative.

genitor
A child's biological father.

pater
One's socially recognized father; not necessarily the genitor.

parallel cousins
Children of two brothers or two sisters.

cross cousins
Children of a brother and a sister.

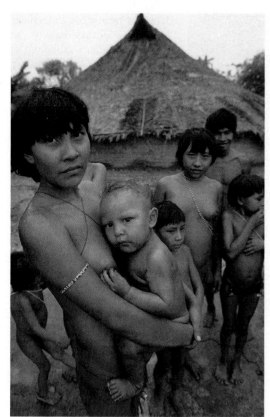

Among the Yanomami of Venezuela and Brazil (shown here), sex with (and marriage to) cross cousins is proper, but sex with parallel cousins is considered incestuous. With unilineal descent, sex with cross cousins isn't incestuous because cross cousins never belong to ego's descent group.

Nigel Dickinson/Alamy Stock Photo

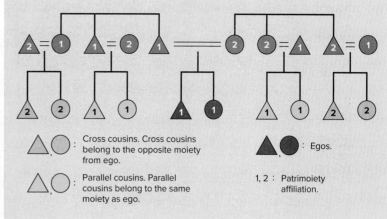

FIGURE 11.1 Parallel and Cross Cousins and Patrilineal Moiety Organization.

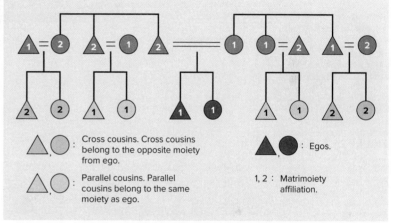

FIGURE 11.2 Parallel and Cross Cousins and Matrilineal Moiety Organization.

Some societies have patrilineal moieties; others have matrilineal moieties.

In Figures 11.1 and 11.2, notice that cross cousins always are members of the opposite moiety and parallel cousins always belong to your (ego's) own moiety. With patrilineal descent (Figure 11.1), people take the father's descent-group affiliation; in a matrilineal society (Figure 11.2), they take the mother's affiliation. You can see from these diagrams that your mother's sister's children (MZC) and your father's brother's children (FBC) always belong to your group. Your cross cousins—that is, FZC and MBC—belong to the other moiety.

Parallel cousins belong to the same generation and the same descent group as ego does, and they are like ego's brothers and sisters. They are called by the same kin terms as brothers and sisters are. Defined as close relatives, parallel cousins, like siblings, are excluded as potential mates; cross cousins are not.

In societies with unilineal moieties, cross cousins always belong to the opposite group. Sex with cross cousins isn't incestuous, because they aren't considered relatives. In fact, in many unilineal societies, people must marry either a cross cousin

or someone from the same descent group as a cross cousin. A unilineal descent rule ensures that the cross cousin's descent group is never one's own. With moiety exogamy, spouses must belong to different moieties.

Among the Yanomami of Venezuela and Brazil (Chagnon 2013a), boys anticipate eventual marriage to a cross cousin by calling her "wife." They call their male cross cousins "brother-in-law." Yanomami girls call their male cross cousins "husband" and their female cross cousins "sister-in-law." Here, as in many other societies with unilineal descent, sex with cross cousins is proper but sex with parallel cousins is incestuous.

If cousins can be classified as nonrelatives, how about even closer biological kin types? When unilineal descent is very strongly developed, the parent who belongs to a different descent group from your own isn't considered a relative. Thus, with strict patrilineality, the mother is not a relative but a kind of in-law who has married a member of your own group—your father. With strict matrilineality, the father isn't a relative because he belongs to a different descent group.

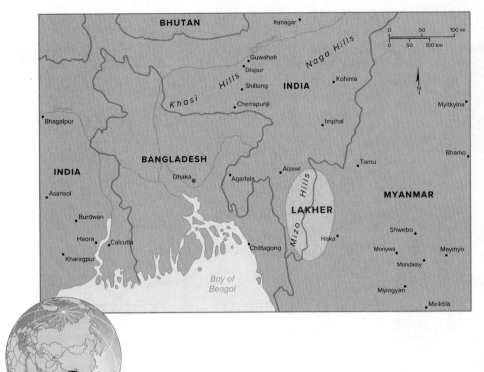

FIGURE 11.3　Location of the Lakher.

daughter by a second marriage. A Lakher always belongs to his or her father's group, all of whose members (one's *agnates,* or *patrikin*) are considered relatives, because they belong to the same descent group. Ego can't have sex with or marry his father's daughter by the second marriage, just as in contemporary North America it's illegal for half-siblings to have sex and marry. However, unlike our society, where all half-siblings are restricted, sex between our Lakher ego and his *maternal* half-sister would be nonincestuous. She isn't ego's relative because she belongs to her own father's descent group rather than ego's. The Lakher illustrate very well that definitions of relatives, and therefore of incest, vary from culture to culture.

INCEST AND ITS AVOIDANCE

We know from primate research that adolescent males (among monkeys) or females (among apes) often move away from the group in which they were born (see Chapais 2008; Martin 2019; Rodseth et al. 1991). This emigration reduces the frequency of incestuous unions, but it doesn't stop them. DNA testing of wild chimps has confirmed incestuous unions between adult sons and their mothers, when residing in the same group. Human behavior with respect to mating with close relatives may express a generalized primate tendency, in which we see both urges and avoidance.

The Occurrence of Incest

A cross-cultural study of 87 societies (Meigs and Barlow 2002) suggested that incest occurred in several of them (see also Wolf 2014). It's not clear, however, whether the authors of the study controlled for the social construction of incest. They report, for example, that incest occurs among the Yanomami, but they may be considering cross-cousin marriage to be incestuous, when it is not so considered by the Yanomami. Another society in their sample is the Ashanti, for whom the ethnographer Meyer Fortes reports, "In the old days it [incest] was punished by death. Nowadays the culprits are heavily fined" (Fortes 1950, p. 257). This suggests that there really were violations of Ashanti incest restrictions, and that such violations were, and still are, punished. More strikingly, among 24 Ojibwa individuals from whom he

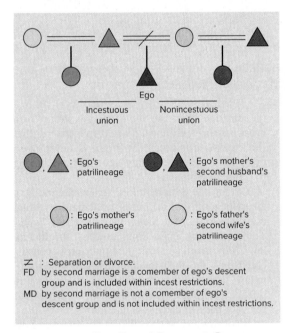

FIGURE 11.4　Patrilineal Descent-Group Identity and Incest among the Lakher.

The Lakher of Southeast Asia (Figure 11.3) are strictly patrilineal (Leach 1961). Using the male ego (the reference point, the person in question) in Figure 11.4, let's suppose that ego's father and mother get divorced. Each remarries and has a

obtained information about incest, A. Irving Hallowell found 8 cases of parent–child incest and 10 cases of brother–sister incest (Hallowell 1955, pp. 294-95). Because reported cases of actual parent–child and sibling incest are very rare in the ethnographic literature, questions about the possibility of social construction arise here too. In many cultures, including the Ojibwa, people use the same terms for their mother and their aunt, their father and their uncle, and their cousins and siblings. Could the siblings in the Ojibwa case actually have been cousins, and the parents and children, uncles and nieces?

In ancient Egypt, sibling marriage apparently was allowed for both royalty and commoners, in some districts at least. Based on official census records from Roman Egypt (first to third centuries C.E.), 24 percent of all documented marriages in the Arsinoites district were between "brothers" and "sisters." The rates were 37 percent for the city of Arsinoe and 19 percent for the surrounding villages. These figures are much higher than any other documented levels of inbreeding among humans (Scheidel 1997). Again one wonders if the relatives involved were as close biologically as the kin terms would imply.

According to Anna Meigs and Kathleen Barlow (2002), for Western societies with nuclear family organization, "father–daughter incest" is much more common with stepfathers than with biological fathers. But is it really incest if they aren't biological relatives? American culture is unclear on this matter. Incest also happens with biological fathers, especially those who were absent or did little caretaking of their daughters in childhood. In a carefully designed study, Linda M. Williams and David Finkelhor (1995) found father–daughter

incest to be least likely when fathers played a strong role in parenting their daughters. This experience enhanced the father's feelings of nurturance, protectiveness, and identification with his daughter, thus reducing the chance of incest.

Incest Avoidance

A century ago, early anthropologists speculated that societies ban incest because humans have an instinctive horror of mating with close relatives (Hobhouse 1915; Lowie 1920/1961). But why, one wonders, if humans really do have an instinctive aversion to incest, would a formal prohibition be necessary? No one would even *want* to have sexual contact with a relative. Yet as social workers, judges, psychiatrists, and psychologists are well aware, incest is more common than we might suppose.

Why do societies discourage incest? Is it because incestuous unions tend to produce abnormal offspring, as the early anthropologist Lewis Henry Morgan (1877/1963) suggested (see also

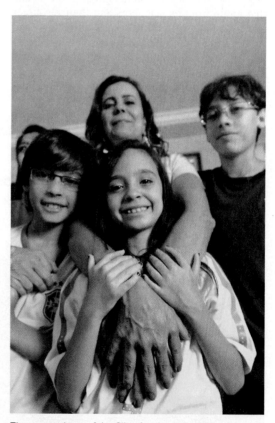

These members of the Silva family, posing here in their home in Brasília on June 21, 2014, were all born with twelve fingers. Such genetically determined traits as polydactylism (extra fingers) may show up when there is a high incidence of endogamy. Despite the biological effects of inbreeding, marriage preferences and prohibitions are based on specific cultural beliefs rather than universal concerns about future biological anomalies.

Evaristo Sa/Getty Images

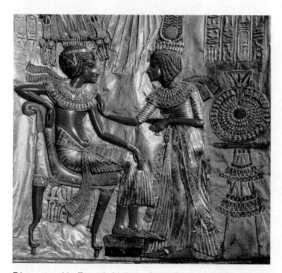

Discovered in Egypt's Valley of the Kings, a gold and silver inlaid throne from the tomb of Tutankhamun is now on display in Cairo's Egyptian Museum. Sibling marriage was allowed not only for ancient Egyptian royalty but also for commoners in some regions.

Kenneth Garrett/National Geographic Creative

Pipatti 2019)? Laboratory experiments with animals that reproduce faster than humans do (such as mice and fruit flies) have been used to investigate the effects of inbreeding: A decline in survival and fertility does accompany brother–sister mating across several generations. However, despite the potentially harmful biological results of systematic inbreeding, human marriage patterns are based on specific cultural beliefs rather than universal concerns about a decline in fertility several generations in the future. Biological concerns certainly cannot explain why so many societies promote marriage of cross cousins but not of parallel cousins.

In most societies, people avoid incest by following rules of exogamy, which force them to mate and marry outside their kin group (Lévi-Strauss 1949/1969; Tylor 1889; White 1959). Exogamy is adaptively advantageous because it creates new social ties and alliances. Marrying a close relative, with whom one already is on peaceful terms, would be counterproductive. There is more to gain by extending peaceful relations to a wider network of groups. Marriage within the group would isolate that group from its neighbors and their resources and social networks, and might ultimately lead to the group's extinction. Exogamy helps explain human adaptive success. Besides its sociopolitical function, exogamy also ensures genetic mixture between groups and thus maintains a successful human species.

endogamy

Marriage of people from the same social group.

ENDOGAMY

Exogamy pushes social organization outward, establishing and preserving alliances among groups. In contrast, rules of **endogamy** dictate mating or marriage within a group to which one belongs. Formal endogamic rules are less common but are still familiar to anthropologists. Indeed, most societies *are* endogamous units, although they usually don't need a formal rule requiring people to marry someone from their own society. In our own society, classes and ethnic groups are quasi-endogamous groups. Members of an ethnic or religious group often want their children to marry within that group, although many of them do not do so. Out-marriage rates vary among such groups, with some more committed to endogamy than others are.

Homogamy means to marry someone similar, as when members of the same social class intermarry. In modern societies, there's a correlation between socioeconomic status (SES) and education. People with similar SES tend to have similar educational aspirations, to attend similar schools, and to pursue similar careers. For example, people who meet at an elite university are likely to have similar backgrounds and career prospects. Homogamous marriage can work to concentrate wealth in social classes and to reinforce the system of social stratification. In the United States, for example,

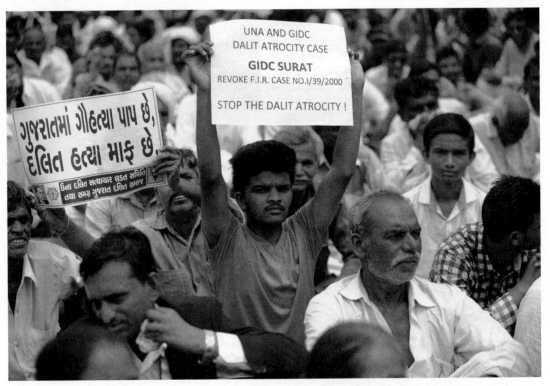

A member of India's Dalit ("untouchable") caste (center) holds a placard proclaiming (sarcastically): "In Gujarat, Cow Slaughter is a Sin while Killing Dalits is pardonable." This 2016 rally was organized to protest an attack on Dalit caste members in the town of Una, Gujarat state. The Dalits, who number some 200 million people, are denied access to temples, public wells, even barbershops, and are routinely subjected to violence.
Sam Panthaky/AFP/Getty Images

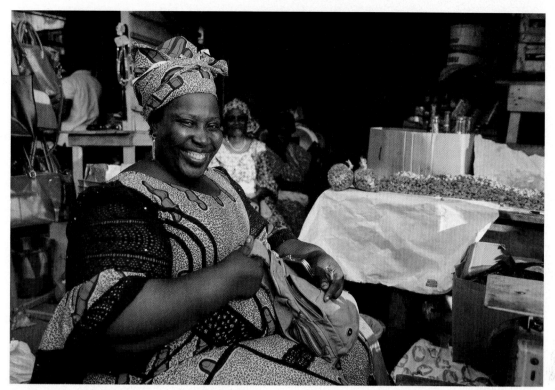

On August 10, 2019, in Abidjan, Ivory Coast, a vendor smiles for this photo in Adjeme Market. This market, whose name means "intersection" or "center," is open 24/7 and is considered the most important trade center in Central West Africa. Traditionally, in parts of West Africa, a prominent market woman might take a wife. By doing so, she would strengthen her social status and her household's economic clout.

Mahmut Serdar Alakus/Getty Images

the rise in female employment, especially in professional careers, when coupled with homogamy, has dramatically increased household incomes in the upper classes. This pattern has been one factor in sharpening the contrast in household income between the richest and poorest quintiles (top and bottom 20 percent) of Americans.

Caste

An extreme example of endogamy is India's caste system, which was formally abolished in 1949, although its structure and effects linger. Castes are stratified groups in which membership is determined at birth and is lifelong. Indian castes are grouped into five major categories, or *varna*. Each is ranked relative to the other four, and these categories extend throughout India. Each *varna* includes a large number of subcastes (*jati*), each of which includes people within a region who may intermarry. All the *jati* in a single *varna* in a given region are ranked, just as the *varnas* themselves are ranked.

Occupational specialization often sets off one caste from another. A community may include separate castes of agricultural workers, merchants, artisans, priests, and sweepers. The Dalit *varna* (outcastes or untouchables), found throughout India, includes subcastes whose ancestry, ritual status, and occupations are considered so impure

that higher-caste people consider even casual contact with Dalits to be defiling.

The Indian system fosters the belief that sexual relations between members of different castes brings ritual impurity to the higher-caste partner. A man who has sex with a lower-caste woman can restore his purity with a bath and a prayer. However, a woman who has intercourse with a man of a lower caste has no such recourse. Her defilement cannot be undone. Because women have the babies, these differences help ensure the pure ancestry of high-caste children.

Although Indian castes are endogamous groups, many of them are internally subdivided into exogamous lineages. Traditionally this meant that Indians had to marry a member of another descent group from the same caste. This shows that rules of exogamy and endogamy can coexist in the same society.

Royal Endogamy

Royal endogamy, based in a few societies on brother–sister marriage, is similar to caste endogamy. Inca Peru, ancient Egypt, and traditional Hawaii all allowed royal brother–sister marriages. In ancient Peru and Hawaii, such marriages were permitted despite the restrictions on sibling incest that applied to commoners in those societies.

Hawaiians (and other Polynesians) believed in an impersonal force called *mana*. Mana could exist in things or people, in the latter case marking them off from other people and making them sacred. The Hawaiians believed that no one had as much mana as the ruler. Mana depended on genealogy. The person whose own mana was exceeded only by the king's was his sibling. The most appropriate wife for a king, therefore, was his own full sister. Their marriage guaranteed that royal heirs would be as manaful, or sacred, as possible, and no one could question their right to rule.

If the king had married someone other, and with less mana, than his sister, his sister's children eventually could cause problems. Both sets of children could assert their sacredness and right to rule. Royal sibling marriage limited conflicts about succession by reducing the number of people with claims to rule. Furthermore, by limiting the number of heirs, royal sibling marriage also helped keep estates intact. Power often rests on wealth, and royal endogamy tended to ensure that royal wealth remained concentrated in the same line. Royal sibling marriage had similar results in ancient Egypt and Peru. Other kingdoms, including European royalty, also have practiced endogamy, but based on cousin marriage rather than sibling marriage.

SAME-SEX MARRIAGE

What about same-sex marriage? Such unions, of various sorts, have been recognized in many different historical and cultural settings (see Ball 2016; Thompson 2015). The Nuer of South Sudan allowed a woman whose father lacked sons to take a wife and

be socially recognized as her husband and as the father (pater, although not genitor) of her children. In situations in which women, such as prominent market women in West Africa, are able to amass property and other forms of wealth, they may take a wife. Such marriages allow the prominent woman to strengthen her social status and the economic importance of her household (Amadiume 1987).

Sometimes, when same-sex marriage is allowed, one of the partners is of the same biological sex as the spouse, but is considered to belong to a different, socially constructed gender. Several Native American groups had figures known as "Two-Spirit," representing a gender in addition to male or female (Murray and Roscoe 1998; Roscoe 1998). Sometimes, the Two-Spirit was a biological man who assumed many of the mannerisms, behavior patterns, and tasks of women. Such a Two-Spirit might marry a man and fulfill the traditional wifely role. Also, in some Native American cultures, a marriage of a "manly hearted woman" (a third or fourth gender) to another woman brought the traditional male–female division of labor to their household. The manly woman hunted and did other male tasks, while the wife played the traditional female role (see Roscoe 1998).

Beginning in the Netherlands in 2001, the legalization of same-sex marriage in modern nations has snowballed throughout the world. As of this writing, same-sex marriage is legal in 31 countries: Argentina, Australia, Austria, Belgium, Brazil, Canada, Colombia, Costa Rica, Denmark, Ecuador, England and Wales, Finland, France, Germany, Greenland, Iceland, Ireland, Luxembourg, Malta, the Netherlands, New Zealand, Northern Ireland,

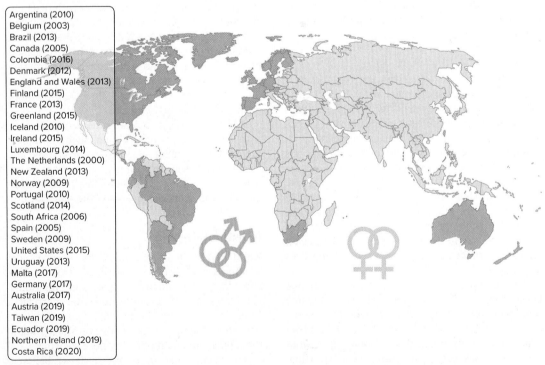

Argentina (2010)
Belgium (2003)
Brazil (2013)
Canada (2005)
Colombia (2016)
Denmark (2012)
England and Wales (2013)
Finland (2015)
France (2013)
Greenland (2015)
Iceland (2010)
Ireland (2015)
Luxembourg (2014)
The Netherlands (2000)
New Zealand (2013)
Norway (2009)
Portugal (2010)
Scotland (2014)
South Africa (2006)
Spain (2005)
Sweden (2009)
United States (2015)
Uruguay (2013)
Malta (2017)
Germany (2017)
Australia (2017)
Austria (2019)
Taiwan (2019)
Ecuador (2019)
Northern Ireland (2019)
Costa Rica (2020)

FIGURE 11.5 Countries Allowing Same-Sex Marriage (as of 2020).

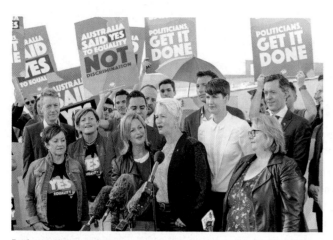

Professor Kerryn Phelps speaks to the media as her wife, Jackie Stricker-Phelps, looks on. Along with other supporters of same-sex marriage, they gathered in front of Parliament House in Canberra on December 7, 2017, ahead of the (favorable) parliamentary vote on Same Sex Marriage.

Sean Davey/AFP/Getty Images

Norway, Portugal, Scotland, South Africa, Spain, Sweden, Taiwan, the United States, and Uruguay. (Figure 11.5 is a map showing these countries and the year in which same-sex marriage was legalized.) Twenty-first-century North America has witnessed a rapid and dramatic shift in public and legal opinions about same-sex marriage.

Canada legalized same-sex marriage in 2005, but the United States delayed marriage equality for another decade. The legalization of same-sex marriage throughout the United States in June 2015 was achieved despite considerable opposition. In 1996, the U.S. Congress had approved the Defense of Marriage Act (DOMA), which denied federal recognition and benefits to same-sex couples. Voters in at least 29 U.S. states passed measures defining marriage as an exclusively heterosexual union. On June 26, 2013, the U.S. Supreme Court struck down a key part of DOMA and granted to legally married same-sex couples the same federal rights and benefits received by any legally married couple. In June 2015, the Supreme Court upheld the legality of same-sex marriage throughout the United States. Although opposition continues (often on religious grounds), public opinion has followed the judicial shift toward approval of same-sex marriage. (This chapter's "Appreciating Anthropology" discusses how anthropological knowledge could have informed the 2015 Supreme Court decision legalizing same-sex marriage.)

ROMANTIC LOVE AND MARRIAGE

In our society, we think of marriage as an individual matter. Although the bride and groom usually seek their parents' approval, the final choice (to live together, to marry, to divorce) lies with the couple. Contemporary Western societies stress the notion that romantic love is necessary for a good marriage.

Increasingly, this idea characterizes other cultures as well. The mass media and human migration spread Western ideas about the importance of love for marriage.

Just how widespread is romantic love, and what role should it play in marriage? A study by anthropologists William Jankowiak and Edward Fischer (1992) found romantic ardor to be very common cross-culturally. Previously, anthropologists had tended to ignore evidence for romantic love in other cultures, probably because arranged marriages were so common. Surveying ethnographic data from 166 cultures, Jankowiak and Fischer (1992) found evidence for romantic love in 147 of them—89 percent (see also Jankowiak 1995, 2008).

Furthermore, diffusion of Western ideas about the importance of love for marriage has influenced marital decisions in other cultures. Among villagers in the Kangra valley of northern India, as reported by anthropologist Kirin Narayan (quoted in Goleman 1992; see also Narayan 2016), even in the traditional arranged marriages, the partners might eventually fall in love. In that area nowadays, however, the media have spread the idea that young people should choose their own spouse based on romantic love, and elopements now rival arranged marriages.

The same trend away from arranged marriages toward love matches has been noted among Native Australians. Traditionally in the Australian Outback, marriages were arranged when children were very young. Missionaries disrupted that pattern, urging that marriage be postponed to adolescence. Before the missionaries, according to anthropologist Victoria Burbank (1988), all girls married before puberty, some as early as age 9; nowadays the average female age at marriage is 17 years. Parents still prefer the traditional arrangement

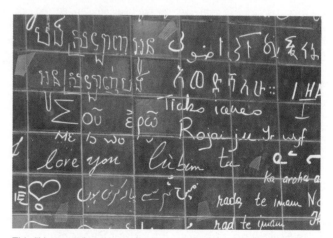

This "I love you" wall is on display in an open area of Monmartre, Paris, France. It shows how to say "I love you" in various languages. Is romantic love a cultural universal?

Conrad P. Kottak

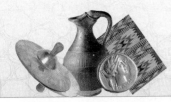

What Anthropologists Could Teach the Supreme Court about the Definition of Marriage

A majority of Americans today, especially the younger ones, have no trouble accepting the practice and legalization of same-sex marriage. However, opinions on this issue have evolved very rapidly. As recently as 2004, then-president George W. Bush was calling for a constitutional amendment banning gay marriage.

Eleven years later, on June 26, 2015, the U.S. Supreme Court issued one of its most socially significant rulings—legalizing same-sex marriage throughout the United States. In the landmark case *Obergefell v. Hodges,* the Court ruled, in a 5–4 decision, that the right to marry is guaranteed to same-sex couples by both the due process clause and the equal protection clause of the 14th Amendment to the U.S. Constitution.

In his strong dissent to that ruling, Chief Justice John Roberts asked, "Just who do we think we are?"—to so enlarge the definition of marriage. Roberts faulted the court for endorsing "the transformation of a social institution that has formed the basis of human society for millennia, for the Kalahari Bushmen and the Han Chinese, the Carthaginians and the Aztecs."

If Roberts knew more about anthropology, he would realize that these four societies don't really support his claim that marriage has universally been a union between one man and one woman. Although the "Kalahari Bushmen" (San peoples) do have exclusively heterosexual marriages, they also divorce and remarry at will. Nor, in Han period China, was marriage a lifetime union between one man and one woman. Han men were allowed to divorce, remarry, and consort with concubines. Within the Roman Empire, Carthaginian women who were Roman citizens were allowed to marry and divorce freely. Many members of the final society cited by Roberts—the Aztecs—were polygamists. The Aztecs used matchmakers to arrange marriages and asked widows to marry a brother of

dowry
Substantial gifts to the husband's family from the wife's group.

in which a girl's mother chooses a boy from the appropriate kin group. But more and more girls now choose to elope and get pregnant, thus forcing a marriage to someone they love. In the group Burbank studied, most marriages had become love matches (see Burbank 1988; Goleman 1992).

Love remains Americans' top reason to marry (see Figure 11.6). In a 2013 Pew Research Center survey, 88 percent of Americans ranked "love" highest among reasons to get married, ahead of making a lifelong commitment (81 percent) and companionship (76 percent). Notice that fewer than half (49 percent) of respondents listed '"having children" as a "very important reason" to marry.

MARRIAGE: A GROUP AFFAIR

Whether or not they are cemented by passion, marriages in nonindustrial societies remain the concern of social groups rather than mere individuals. The scope of marriage extends from the social to the political—alliance formation. Strategic marriages are tried-and-true ways of establishing alliances between groups.

Gifts at Marriage

Gifts at marriage are common among the world's cultures. A marital gift known as **dowry** occurs when the bride's family or kin group provides substantial gifts when their daughter marries. Ernestine Friedl (1962) describes a form of dowry in rural Greece, in which the bride gets a wealth transfer from her mother, to serve as a kind of trust fund during her marriage. More commonly, however, the dowry goes

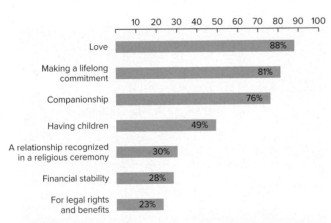

FIGURE 11.6 Percentage of Americans Citing Each of the Following as a Very Important Reason to Get Married.

SOURCE: Gretchen Livingston and Andrea Caumont, "5 Facts on Love and Marriage in America," *Pew Research Center,* February 13, 2017. http://www.pewresearch.org/fact-tank/2017/02/13/5-facts-about-love-and-marriage/

their deceased husband (Joyce 2015). I doubt that Chief Justice Roberts intended to endorse frequent divorce, consorting with mistresses and concubines, and polygamy as aspects of "a social institution that has formed the basis of human society for millennia."

Roberts went on to argue that marriage "arose in the nature of things to meet a vital need: ensuring that children are conceived by a mother and father committed to raising them in the stable conditions of a lifetime relationship." Here the focus is on the role of marriage in procreation and raising children. As we have seen, however, marriage confers socially significant rights and obligations other than raising children. Nor is procreation necessary for or within marriage. Is a childless marriage any less legitimate than one with children? Is legal adoption of a child less legitimate than conception of the child by a married heterosexual couple? Every day in contemporary societies, men and women marry without expecting to conceive and raise children.

As John Borneman and Laurie Kain Hart (2015) observe, marriage is an elastic institution whose meaning and value vary from culture to culture and evolve over time. Consider the many examples of families, kinship groups, and marriage types considered in this book. From the Bosnian *zadruga,* Nayar *tarawad,* and Moso *tisese* system, to matrilineal and patrilineal clans, lineages, local descent groups, and extended families, children have been raised in, and have managed to survive and even flourish in, all kinds of kin groups. If we go back millennia, as Chief Justice Roberts would like to trace marriage, we would find "love, marriage, and the baby carriage" to be the exception rather than the rule. That is, the combination of romantic love, marriage, procreation, and raising children mainly, or even exclusively, within a nuclear family is a relatively recent—rather than a universal or ages-old—development.

Finally, consider the different forms of marriage that have been considered in this chapter: woman-marriage-to-a-woman among the Nuer, cross-cousin marriage, Lakher marriage to a half-sibling, serial monogamy, and other forms that violate the idea that marriage is a lifetime union of one man and one woman.

I would hope, therefore, that the next time a member of the Supreme Court attempts to justify a practice using terms like "for millennia," "ages-old," "universal," or "basic human," he or she will first consult an anthropologist.

to the husband's family, and the custom is correlated with low female status. In this form of dowry, best known from India, women are perceived as burdens. When a man and his family take a wife, they expect to be compensated for the added responsibility.

In many societies with patrilineal descent, it is customary for the husband's group to present a substantial gift—before, at, or soon after the wedding—to his bride's group. The BaThonga of Mozambique call such a gift *lobola,* and the custom of giving something like **lobola** is widespread in patrilineal societies (Radcliffe-Brown 1924/1952). This gift compensates the bride's group for the loss of her companionship and labor. More important, it makes the children born to the woman full members of her husband's descent group. In matrilineal societies, children are members of the mother's group, and there is no reason for a lobola-like gift.

Lobola-like gifts exist in many more cultures than dowry does, but the nature and quantity of transferred items differ. Among the BaThonga of Mozambique, whose name—*lobola*—I will extend for this widespread custom, the gift consists of cattle. Use of livestock (usually cattle in Africa, pigs in Papua New Guinea) for lobola is common, but the number of animals given varies from society to society. We can generalize, however, that the larger the gift, the more stable the marriage. Lobola is insurance against divorce.

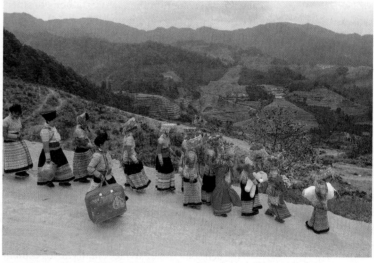

In southwest China's Sichuan Province, on February 21, 2017, a bride (4th right) walks with her companions carrying dowry to her groom's house during a traditional wedding ceremony of the Lisu ethnic group.
Xinhua/Alamy Stock Photo

Imagine a patrilineal society in which a marriage requires the transfer of about 25 cattle from the groom's descent group to the bride's. When Michael, a member of descent group A, marries Sarah from group B, he has to give lobola cattle to her group. His relatives help him assemble

lobola

A substantial marital gift from the husband and his kin to the wife and her kin.

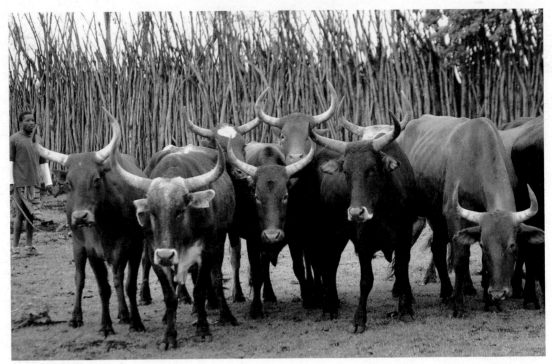

A few of the 100 lobola cattle presented prior to the (October 2013) wedding of Khulubuse Zuma and Swazi princess Fikisiwe Dlamini. Zuma is a South African businessman and nephew of former South African President Jacob Zuma. The wedding, held at the royal palace in Ludzudzini, Swaziland, and attended by 5,000 people, followed several years of courtship and lobola negotiations.

Khaya Ngwenya/Getty Images

that lobola. He gets the most help from his close patrikin—his older brother, father, father's brother, and closest patrilineal cousins. The distribution of the cattle once they reach Sarah's group mirrors the manner in which they were assembled. Sarah's father, or her oldest brother if the father is dead, receives her lobola. He keeps most of the cattle to use as lobola for his sons' marriages. However, a share also goes to everyone who will be expected to help when Sarah's brothers marry.

When Sarah's brother David gets married, many of the cattle go to a third group: C, which is David's wife's group. Thereafter, those same cattle may be transmitted as lobola to still other groups. Men continually use their sisters' lobola cattle to acquire their own wives. In a decade, the cattle given when Michael married Sarah will have been exchanged widely.

In such societies, marriage entails an agreement between descent groups. If Sarah and Michael try to make their marriage succeed but fail to do so, both groups may conclude that the marriage can't last. Here it becomes especially obvious that such marriages are relationships between groups as well as between individuals. If Sarah has a younger sister or niece (her older brother's daughter, for example), the concerned parties may agree to Sarah's replacement by a kinswoman.

However, incompatibility isn't the main problem that threatens marriage in societies with lobola customs. Infertility is a more important concern. If Sarah has no children, she and her group have not fulfilled their part of the marriage agreement. If the relationship is to endure, Sarah's group must furnish another woman, perhaps her younger sister, who can have children. If this happens, Sarah may choose to stay on in her husband's village as his wife. Perhaps she will someday have a child. If she does stay on, her husband will have established a plural marriage with more than one wife.

Durable Alliances

Also illustrating the group-alliance nature of marriage is another common practice: continuation of marital alliances when one spouse dies.

Sororate

What happens if Sarah dies young? Michael's group will ask Sarah's group for a substitute, often her sister. This custom is known as the **sororate** (Figure 11.7). If Sarah has no sister or if all her sisters are already married, another woman from her group may be available. Michael marries her, there is no need to return the lobola, and the alliance continues. The sororate exists in both matrilineal and patrilineal societies. In a matrilineal society with matrilocal postmarital residence, a widower may remain with his wife's group by marrying her sister or another female member of her matrilineage.

sororate
A custom in which a widower marries the sister of his deceased wife.

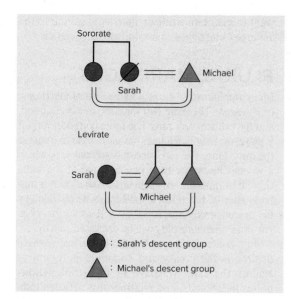

FIGURE 11.7 Sororate and Levirate.

Levirate

What happens if the husband dies? In many societies, the widow may marry his brother. This custom is known as the **levirate**. Like the sororate, it is a continuation marriage that maintains the alliance between descent groups, in this case by replacing the husband with another member of his group. The implications of the levirate vary with age. One study found that in African societies, the levirate, though widely permitted, rarely involves cohabitation of the widow and her new husband. Furthermore, widows don't automatically marry the husband's brother just because they are allowed to. Often, they prefer to make other arrangements (Potash 1986).

DIVORCE

Ease of divorce varies depending on the culture. What factors work for and against divorce cross-culturally? As we've seen, marriages that are political alliances between groups are more difficult to dissolve than are marriages that are more individual affairs, of concern mainly to the married couple and their children. We've seen that a substantial lobola gift may decrease the divorce rate for individuals and that replacement marriages (levirate and sororate) also work to preserve group alliances. Divorce tends to be more common in matrilineal than in patrilineal societies. When residence is matrilocal (in the wife's place), the wife may simply send off a man with whom she's incompatible.

Among the Hopi of the American Southwest, houses were owned by matrilineal clans, with matrilocal postmarital residence. The household head was the senior woman of that household, which also included her daughters and their husbands and children. A son-in-law had no important role there; he returned to his own mother's home for his clan's social and religious activities. In this matrilineal society, women were socially and economically secure, and the divorce rate was high.

Consider specifically the Hopi living in the Oraibi pueblo, northeastern Arizona (Levy with Pepper 1992; Titiev 1992). In a study of the marital histories of 423 Oraibi women, Mischa Titiev found that 35 percent had been divorced at least once. Jerome Levy found that 31 percent of 147 adult Oraibi women had been divorced and remarried at least once. Much of the instability of Hopi marriages was due to conflicting loyalties to matrikin versus spouse. Most Hopi divorces appear to have been matters of personal choice. Levy generalizes that, cross-culturally, high divorce rates are correlated with a secure female economic position. In Hopi society, women were secure in their homes and land ownership and in the custody of their children. In addition, there were no formal barriers to divorce.

Divorce is more difficult in a patrilineal society, especially when substantial lobola would have to be reassembled and repaid if the marriage failed. A woman residing patrilocally (in her husband's household and community) might be reluctant to leave him. In patrilineal-patrilocal societies, the children of divorce would be expected to remain with their father, as members of his patrilineage. From the women's perspective this is a strong impediment to divorce.

What about divorce in foraging societies? Among foragers, certain factors facilitate divorce, while other factors work to stabilize marriage. Facilitating divorce is the fact that the group-alliance functions of marriage are less important, because descent groups are not as characteristic of foragers as of food producers. Also facilitating divorce is the fact that marriages tend to last longer when a couple

levirate
A custom in which a widow marries the brother of her deceased husband.

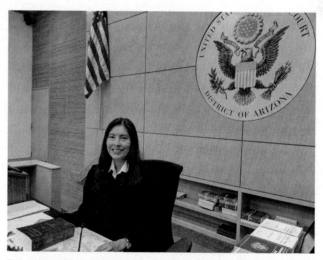

This photo of U.S. District Court Judge Diane Humetewa in her chambers at the federal courthouse in Phoenix, Arizona, was taken on January 17, 2020. Humetewa, who is Hopi, is one of only three Native Americans to have served as federal judges, and she is the first Native American woman to do so. Traditionally among the matrilineal-matrilocal Hopi, women were socially and economically prominent and secure (and the divorce rate was high).
Patty Talahongva/AP Images

shares—and would have trouble dissolving—a significant joint fund of property. This usually is not the case among foragers, who have minimal material possessions. Marital stability is favored, however, when the nuclear family is an important year-round unit with a gender-based division of labor, as is true of many foraging societies. Also favoring marital stability is the fact that foragers tend to have sparse populations, so that few alternative spouses are available if a marriage fails.

Many western societies have witnessed a decline in the prevalence and stability of marriage. In the United States, for example, continuing a decades-long trend, fewer than half (48 percent) of all adults were married in 2018, down from 70 percent in 1950. As marriage has declined, the number of Americans in cohabiting relationships (living with an unmarried partner) has increased (Cilluffo and Cohn 2017).

One interesting consequence of a declining marriage rate is a falling divorce rate. For example, the U.S. divorce rate has been dropping since the turn of the 21st century. In the year 2000, 4.0 out of every 1,000 Americans got divorced. By 2017, that rate had dropped to 2.9. Similarly, 8.2 Americans per 1,000 got married in the year 2000, falling to 6.9 in 2017.

Among married couples, when romance or attraction fail, so may the marriage. Or it may not fail, if other benefits associated with marriage are compelling. Economic ties and obligations to kids, along with other factors, such as concern about public opinion, or simple inertia, may keep marriages intact after sex, romance, and/or companionship fade. Also, even in modern nations, political leaders and other elites may

want to maintain strategic marriages similar to the arranged marriages of nonindustrial societies.

PLURAL MARRIAGES

Many nonindustrial societies allow **plural marriages,** or *polygamy.* There are two varieties; one is common, and the other is very rare. The more common variant is **polygyny,** in which a man has more than one wife at the same time. The rare variant is **polyandry,** in which a woman has more than one husband at the same time. If an infertile wife remains married to her husband after he has taken a substitute wife provided by her descent group, this is polygyny. Reasons for polygyny other than infertility will be discussed shortly.

In contemporary North America, where divorce is fairly easy and common, polygamy is against the law. Marriage in industrial nations unites individuals, and relationships between individuals can be severed more easily than can those between groups. As divorce grows more common, North Americans practice *serial monogamy:* Individuals may have more than one spouse but never, legally, more than one at the same time.

Polygyny

We must distinguish between the social approval of plural marriage and its actual frequency. Many cultures approve of a man's having more than one wife. However, even when polygyny is allowed or encouraged, most men are monogamous, and polygyny characterizes only a fraction of the marriages.

What factors promote, and discourage, polygyny? Polygyny is much more common in patrilineal than in matrilineal societies. The relatively high status that women enjoy in matrilineal societies tends to grant them a degree of independence from men that makes polygyny less likely. Nor is polygyny characteristic of most foraging societies, where a married couple and nuclear family often function as an economically viable team. Most industrial nations have outlawed polygyny.

An equal sex ratio tends to work against polygyny if marriage is an expectation for both men and women. In the United States, about 105 males are born for every 100 females. In adulthood, the ratio of men to women equalizes, and eventually it reverses. The average North American woman outlives the average man. In many nonindustrial societies as well, the male-biased sex ratio among children reverses in adulthood. In some societies, men inherit widows as their plural wives.

The custom of men marrying later than women promotes polygyny. Among the Kanuri people of Bornu, Nigeria, men got married between the ages of 18 and 30; women, between 12 and 14 (Cohen 1967). The age difference between spouses meant that there were more widows than widowers. Most of the widows remarried, some in polygynous unions. Among the Kanuri and in other

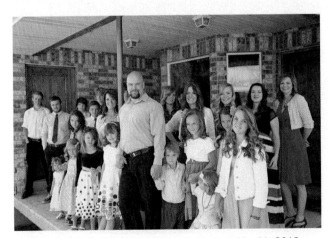

Modern-day North American polygyny is illustrated by this 2012 photo of the Darger family, standing in front of their home in Herriman, Utah. Their household includes Joe Darger, his three wives—Alina Darger, Valerie Kelsch, and Vicki Kelsch—and their 23 children. Aspects of the HBO series "Big Love" were inspired by this Mormon fundamentalist family, who have become public advocates for the legalization of plural marriage.

Peter Bohler/Redux Pictures

polygynous societies, widows made up a large number of the women involved in plural marriages (Hart, Pilling, and Goodale 1988). Polygyny is favored in situations in which having plural wives is an indicator of a man's household productivity, prestige, and social position. The more wives, the more workers. Increased productivity means more wealth. This wealth in turn attracts additional wives to the household. Wealth and wives bring greater prestige to the household and its head.

Polygyny also is supported when the existing spouses agree about when another one is to be added, especially if they are to share the same household. In certain societies, the first wife requests a second one to help with household chores. The second wife's status is lower than that of the first; they are senior and junior wives. The senior wife sometimes chooses the junior one from among her close kinswomen. Polygyny also can work when the co-wives live apart. Among the Betsileo of Madagascar, the different wives always lived in different villages. A man's first and senior wife, called "Big Wife," lived in the village where he cultivated his best rice field and spent most of his time. Polygynous men must be able to support multiple wives. High-status Betsileo men with multiple rice fields could have a wife and households near each field. Those men spent most of their time with the senior wife, but they visited the others throughout the year.

Polygyny also can be politically advantageous. Plural wives have played important political roles in nonindustrial states. The king of the Merina, a populous society in the highlands of Madagascar, had palaces for each of his 12 wives in different provinces. He stayed with them when he traveled through the kingdom, and they acted as his local agents, overseeing and reporting on provincial matters. The king of Buganda, the major precolonial state of Uganda, took hundreds of wives, representing all the clans in his nation. Everyone in the kingdom became the king's in-law, and all the clans had a chance to provide the next ruler. This was a way of giving the common people a stake in the government.

We see that there is no single explanation for polygyny. Its context and function vary from society to society and even within the same society. Some men are polygynous because they have inherited a widow from a brother (the levirate). Others have plural wives because they seek prestige or want to increase their household productivity. Still others use marriage as a political tool or a means of economic advancement. Men and women with political and economic ambitions cultivate marital alliances that serve their aims. In many societies, including the Betsileo of Madagascar and the Igbo of Nigeria, women arrange the marriages.

Like all institutions studied by anthropologists, customs involving plural marriage are changing

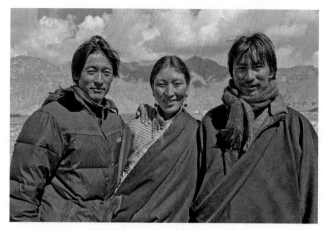

Fraternal polyandry: A Tibetan wife with her two husbands, who are brothers. They are shown here as pilgrims to the Potala Palace in Lhasa, Tibet.

John Henshall/Alamy Stock Photo

in the contemporary world and in the context of nation-states and globalization. For example, polygyny was legal in Turkey until 1926, mainly benefiting men who could afford multiple wives and many children. Although polygyny was banned officially, it persisted for years. After polygynous unions lost legal status, secondary wives found themselves without legal protections against a husband's mistreatment, neglect, or abandonment (Bilefsky 2006).

Polyandry

Polyandry is rare and is practiced under very specific conditions. Most of the world's polyandrous peoples live in South Asia—Tibet, Nepal, India, and Sri Lanka. In some of these areas, polyandry seems to be a cultural adaptation to mobility associated with customary male travel for trade, commerce, and military operations. Polyandry ensures there will be at least one man at home to accomplish male activities within a gender-based division of labor. Fraternal polyandry is also an effective strategy when resources are scarce. Brothers with limited resources (in land) pool their resources in expanded (polyandrous) households. They take just one wife. Polyandry restricts the number of wives and heirs. Less competition among heirs means that land can be transmitted with minimal fragmentation.

THE ONLINE MARRIAGE MARKET

People today shop for almost everything online, including romantic relationships, in what has been labeled the online "marriage market." There are huge differences in the marriage markets of industrial versus nonindustrial societies. In some of the latter, potential spouses may be limited to cross cousins or members of the opposite moiety. Sometimes there are set rules of exogamy, such that, for example, women of descent group A have to marry men from descent group B, while men from A must marry women from C. Often, marriages are arranged by relatives. In almost all cases, however, there is some kind of preexisting social relationship between any two individuals who marry and their kin groups.

Potential mates still meet in person in modern nations. Sometimes friends or relatives help arrange such meetings. In addition, the marriage market extends into schools, the workplace, bars, clubs, parties, churches, and hobby groups. Add the Internet, which has become a new place to seek out and develop "virtual" relationships, including romantic ones that may lead eventually to a face-to-face meeting. An early (2011) study done by the University of Oxford was the "Me, My Spouse, and the Internet" project. That survey, conducted by Bernie Hogan, Nai Li, and William Dutton (2011) gathered data from cohabiting couples in 18 countries. The researchers sampled 12,600 couples (25,200 individuals aged 18 and older), all with home Internet access. Respondents were asked about how they met their partners, their dating strategies, how they maintain their current relationships and social networks, and how they use the Internet.

Online dating has become a multibillion dollar industry and a growing component of today's marriage market (even more so in an era of social distancing). However, the Internet's role remains complementary to, rather than a substitute for, offline partner shopping. That is, people still seek and find partners in the old, familiar places, but they look online as well. One-third of the respondents in the Oxford study had some experience with online dating, and about 15 percent were in a relationship that had started online (Hogan et al. 2011).

Who benefits most from the new technology? Is it young, tech-savvy people who go online for almost everything? Or might it be people who are more socially isolated in the offline world, including divorced, older, and widowed people and others who feel alone in their local community? Interestingly, the Oxford researchers found that older people were more likely than younger ones to use online dating to find their current partner. About 36 percent of people over age 40 had done so, versus 23 percent of younger adults. A more recent survey of American adults produced different results.

Emily Vogels (2020b) describes the results of that 2019 survey by the Pew Research Center. As one might expect, never-married American adults were the most likely (52 percent of them) to report having used an online dating service. Of divorced, separated, or widowed Americans, 35 percent reported such use, compared with only 16 percent of married respondents. Overall, 30 percent of respondents reported experience with online dating—up from 15 percent in 2015 (see Figure 11.8). This survey found younger Americans to be most engaged in online dating. A full 65 percent of never-married Millennials (those born between 1981 and 1996) had done so. That statistic declined to 53 percent among never-married Gen Xers (born 1965-1980) and 29 percent among never-married Baby Boomers (born 1946-1964).

Lesbian, gay, and bisexual (LGB) adults were about twice as likely as others to have used online dating platforms (55 percent versus 28 percent [Vogels 2020a]). Overall, 12 percent of those surveyed had entered a committed relationship with, or married, someone they met through online

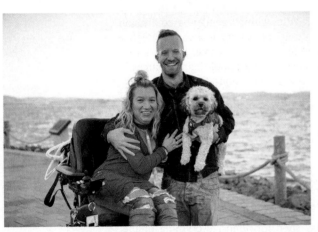
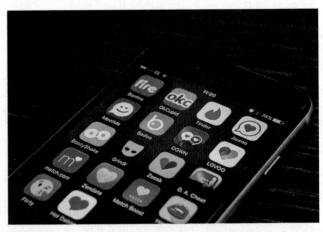

The photo on the left, taken in Brooklyn, New York on November 29, 2019, shows a married couple, Alyssa and Jimmy (with their dog) who met via a dating app. Alyssa, paralyzed since birth, but accustomed to overcoming obstacles, is an active user of social media to spread a message of positive thinking. In the photo on the right, taken in London, England in November, 2016, online dating apps fill up an entire mobile phone screen.

Left: Ruaridh Connellan/Getty Images; right: Leon Neal/Getty Images

dating. This figure was highest among LGB and younger adults (18 to 49 years). Offering a positive evaluation of online dating were 57 percent of respondents, while 43 percent considered their experience at least somewhat negative.

In Europe (returning to the Oxford study), the media-saturated nations of Northern Europe were most likely to use online dating, which benefits from a critical mass of Internet connectivity (the more people online, the larger the pool of potential contacts). Online Brazilians (who tend to be gregarious both on- and offline) were most likely to know someone who either began a relationship online or married someone first met online. Personal knowledge of an online romantic relationship was reported by 81 percent of the Brazilians in the sample versus less than 40 percent of Germans. Brazilians were most, while Britons and Austrians were least, likely to know someone whose partner had been met online.

The Internet enhances our opportunities to meet people and to form personal relationships. It lets us connect with old friends, new friends, groups, and individuals. But this accessibility also can be disruptive. It can spur jealousy, for example,

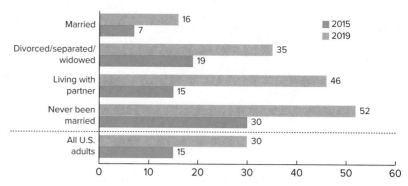

Note: 2019 data are from Pew Research Center's online American Trends Panel; 2015 data are from a telephone survey. Those who did not give an answer are not shown.

FIGURE 11.8 Percentage of Americans Who Have Ever Used a Dating Site or App, 2015 versus 2019, by Marital Status.
SOURCE: Pew Research Center, Survey of U.S. Adults Conducted October 16-28, 2019.

when a partner makes new friends or reconnects to old ones—and with good reason. The Oxford researchers found that many people disclosed intimate personal details in online settings with someone other than their spouse or partner (Hogan et al. 2011). Heavy media usage could endanger marital satisfaction (Oxford 2013).

for REVIEW

summary

1. Marriage, which usually is a form of domestic partnership, is difficult to define. Marriage conveys various rights. It establishes legal parentage, and it gives each spouse rights to the sexuality, labor, and property of the other. Marriage also establishes a "relationship of affinity" between each spouse and the other spouse's relatives.

2. Human behavior with respect to mating with close relatives may express generalized primate tendencies, but types, risks, and avoidance of incest also reflect specific kinship structures. The avoidance of incest promotes exogamy, which widens social networks.

3. Endogamic rules are common in stratified societies. One extreme example is India, where castes are the endogamous units. Certain ancient kingdoms encouraged royal incest while prohibiting incest by commoners.

4. In societies with descent groups, marriages are relationships between groups as well as between spouses. In patrilineal societies, the groom and his relatives often transfer wealth to the bride and her relatives. As the value of that transfer increases, the divorce rate declines. Examples of how marital customs create and maintain group alliances include the sororate and the levirate.

5. The ease and frequency of divorce vary across cultures. When marriage is a matter of intergroup alliance, divorce is less common. A large fund of joint property also complicates divorce.

6. Many societies permit plural marriages. The two kinds of polygamy are polygyny and polyandry. The former (and more common) involves multiple wives; the latter, multiple husbands.

7. The Internet, which reconfigures social relations and networks more generally, is an important addition to the marriage market in contemporary nations.

key terms

think like an anthro- pologist

1. What is homogamy? In countries such as the United States, what are the social and economic implications of homogamy (especially when coupled with other trends such as the rise of female education and employment)?

2. What is dowry? What customs involving gift giving typically occur with marriage in patrilineal societies? Do you have comparable customs in your society? Why or why not?

3. According to Edmund Leach (1955), depending on the society, several different kinds of rights are allocated by marriage. What are these rights? Which among these rights do you consider more fundamental than others in your definition of marriage? Which ones can you do without? Why?

4. Outside industrial societies, marriage is often more a relationship between groups than one between individuals. What does this mean? What are some examples of this?

5. How do you, personally, define marriage? Can you come up with a definition of marriage that would fit all the cases described in this chapter?

credits

Religion

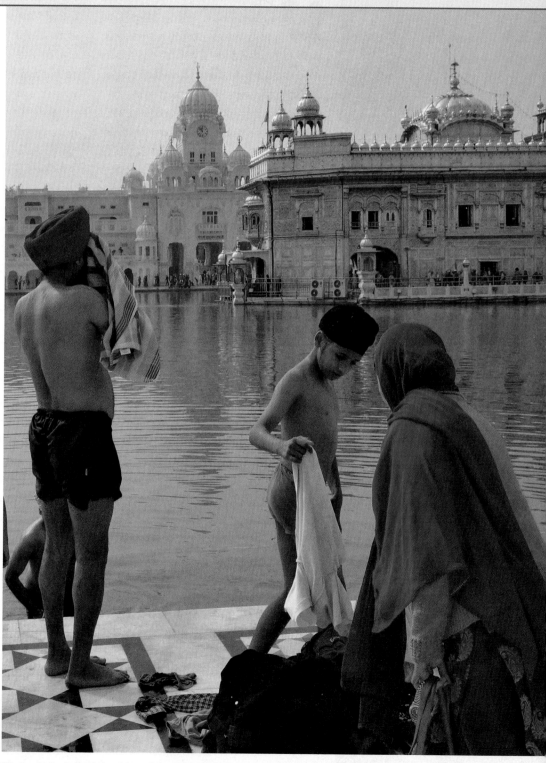

▶ What is religion, and what are its various forms, social correlates, and functions?

▶ What is ritual, and what are its various forms and expressions?

▶ What role does religion play in maintaining and changing societies?

Conrad P. Kottak

Pilgrims bathe in the holy waters of the Golden Temple in Amritsar, Punjab state, northwestern India. This is the chief house of worship of Sikhism and the Sikhs' most important pilgrimage site.

understanding **OURSELVES**

Did you ever notice the tradition of spitting by baseball players? Outside baseball—even among other male sports figures—spitting is considered impolite. Football players, with their customary headgear, don't spit, nor do basketball players, who might slip on the court. No spitting by tennis players, gymnasts, or swimmers, not even Mark Spitz (an Olympic swimmer turned dentist). But any baseball game played prior to COVID-19 would feature spitting galore. Because pitchers appear to be the spitting champions, the custom likely originated on the mound. It continues today as a carryover from the days when pitchers routinely chewed tobacco, believing that nicotine enhanced their concentration and effectiveness. The spitting custom spread to other players, who unabashedly spew saliva from the outfield to the dugout steps.

For the student of custom, ritual, and magic, baseball is an especially interesting game, to which lessons from anthropology are easily applied. The pioneering anthropologist Bronislaw Malinowski, writing about Pacific Islanders rather than baseball players, noted they had developed all sorts of magic to use in sailing, a hazardous activity. He proposed that when people face conditions they can't control (e.g., wind and weather), they turn to magic. Magic, in the form of rituals, taboos, and sacred objects, is particularly evident in baseball. Like sailing magic, baseball magic reduces psychological stress, creating an illusion of control when real control is lacking.

In several publications about baseball, the anthropologist George Gmelch makes use of Malinowski's observation that magic is most common in situations dominated by chance and uncertainty. All sorts of magical behaviors surround pitching and batting, which are full of uncertainty. There are fewer rituals for fielding, over which players have more control. (Batting averages of .350 or higher are very rare after a full season, but a fielding percentage below .900 is a disgrace.) Especially obvious are the rituals (like the spitting) of pitchers, who may tug their cap between pitches, spit in a particular direction, magically manipulate the resin bag, talk to the ball, or wash their hands after giving up a run. Batters have their rituals, too. Former outfielder Carlos Gomez, for example, was known for smelling or kissing his bat. Gomez noticed as a child that good hitters tend to use rituals as they approach the plate or between pitches. One of his rituals was to rotate his bat in front of his face while sniffing it—smelling it for hits! Another batter routinely would spit, then ritually touch his gob with his bat, to enhance his success at the plate.

Humans use tools to accomplish a lot, but technology still doesn't let us "have it all." To keep hope alive in situations of uncertainty, and for outcomes we can't control, all societies draw on magic and religion as sources of nonmaterial comfort, explanation, and control. What are your rituals?

WHAT IS RELIGION?

In his book *Religion: An Anthropological View,* Anthony F. C. Wallace (1966) defined **religion** as "belief and ritual concerned with supernatural beings, powers, and forces" (p. 5). By "supernatural," Wallace was referring to a nonmaterial realm beyond (but believed to impinge on) the observable world. The supernatural cannot be verified or falsified empirically. It cannot be explained in ordinary terms. It must be accepted "on faith." Supernatural *beings* (e.g., deities, ghosts, demons, souls, spirits) dwell outside our material world, which they may visit from time to time. There also are supernatural or sacred *forces,* some of them wielded by deities and spirits, others that simply exist. In many societies, people believe they can benefit from, become imbued with, or manipulate such forces (see Bielo 2015; Boddy and Lambek 2014; Bowen 2017; Eller 2015; Sidky 2015; Payne 2018; Stein and Stein 2017).

Wallace's definition of religion focuses on beings, powers, and forces within the supernatural realm. Émile Durkheim (1912/2001), one of the founders of the anthropology of religion, focused on the distinction between the sacred (the domain of religion) and the profane (the everyday world). Like the supernatural for Wallace, Durkheim's "sacred" was a domain set off from the ordinary, or the mundane. (Durkheim actually used the word *profane* for the ordinary, natural, nonsacred world). For Durkheim, although every society recognized a sacred domain, the specifics of that domain would vary from society to society. In other words, he saw religion as a cultural universal, while recognizing that specific religious beliefs and practices vary from society to society.

Durkheim believed that Native Australian societies had retained the most elementary, or basic,

forms of religion. He noted that their most sacred objects, including plants and animals that served as totems, were not supernatural at all. Rather, they were "real-world" entities (e.g., kangaroos, grubs) that had acquired religious meaning and became sacred objects for the social groups that "worshipped" them. Durkheim saw totemism as the most elementary or basic form of religion.

Durkheim (1912/2001) focused on groups of people—congregants—who gather together for worship, such as a group of Native Australians worshiping a particular totem. He stressed the collective, social, and shared nature of religion, the meanings it embodies, and the emotions it generates. He highlighted religious "effervescence," the bubbling up of collective emotional intensity generated by worship. As Michael Lambek (2008, p. 5) remarks, "good anthropology understands that religious worlds are real, vivid, and significant to those who construct and inhabit them."

Congregants who worship together share certain beliefs; they have accepted a particular set of doctrines concerning the sacred and its relationship to human beings. The word *religion* derives from the Latin *religare*—"to tie, to bind"—but it is not necessary for all members of a given religion to meet together as a common body. Subgroups meet regularly at local congregation sites. They may attend occasional meetings with adherents representing a wider region. And they may form an imagined community with people of similar faith throughout the world.

Verbal manifestations of religious beliefs include prayers, chants, myths, texts, and statements about

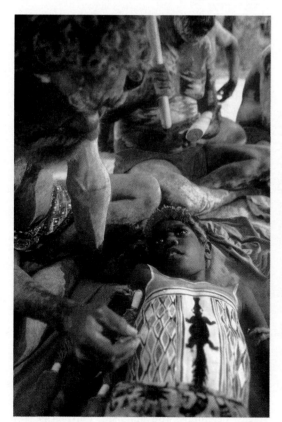

In Nangalala, Arnhem land, northern Australia, a father paints totemic symbols and clan motifs on his son in preparation for an initiation ceremony.

Penny Tweedie/Alamy Stock Photo

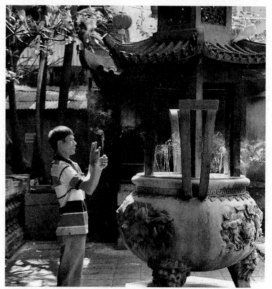

A man makes a burnt offering as he prays at a Taoist temple, the Jade Emperor Pagoda, in Ho Chi Minh City (formerly Saigon), Vietnam. Established in 1909 by the Cantonese (Chinese) community in Saigon, the pagoda remains a place of worship for Buddhists and Taoists; both religions are widely practiced in Vietnam.

Conrad P. Kottak

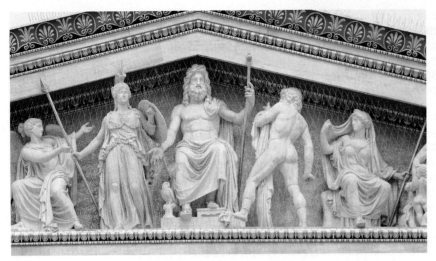

Illustrating polytheism, statues of ancient Greek gods (including a depiction of the birth of Athena) adorn the Academy of Athens, Greece's premier research establishment.

Ozgur Guvenc/123RF

ethics and morality (see Myers-Moro and Myers 2012; Stein and Stein 2017; Winzeler 2012). Other aspects of religion include notions about purity and pollution (including taboos involving diet and physical contact), sacrifice, initiation, rites of passage, vision quests, pilgrimages, spirit possession, prophecy, study, devotion, and moral actions (Lambek 2008, p. 9).

Like ethnicity and language, religion both unites and divides. Participation in common rites can affirm, and thus maintain, the solidarity of a group of adherents. Religious differences also can be associated with bitter enmity. Contacts and confrontations have increased between so-called world religions, such as Christianity and Islam, and the more localized forms of religion that missionaries typically lump together under the disparaging term *paganism.* Increasingly, ethnic, regional, and class conflicts come to be framed in religious terms. Contemporary examples of religion as a social and political force include the rise of the religious right in the United States, the worldwide spread of Pentecostalism, the Islamic State, and various other Islamic movements (see Lindquist and Handelman 2013).

Long ago, Edward Sapir (1928/1956) argued for a distinction between "a religion" and "religion." The former term would apply only to a formally organized religion, such as the world religions just mentioned. The latter—*religion*—is universal; it refers to religious beliefs and behavior, which exist in all societies, even if they don't stand out as a separate and clearly demarcated sphere. Indeed, many anthropologists (e.g., Asad 1983/2008) argue that such categories as *religion, politics,* and *the economy* are arbitrary constructs that apply best, and perhaps only, to Western, Christian, and modern societies. In such contexts, religion can be seen as a specific domain, separate from politics and the economy. By contrast, in nonindustrial societies,

religion typically is more embedded in society. Religious beliefs can help regulate the economy (e.g., astrologers determine when to plant) or permeate politics (e.g., divine right of kings).

Anthropologists agree that religion exists in all human societies; it is a cultural universal. However, we'll see that it isn't always easy to distinguish the sacred from the profane and that different societies conceptualize divinity, the sacred, the supernatural, and ultimate realities very differently.

EXPRESSIONS OF RELIGION

When and how did religion begin? No one knows for sure. There are suggestions of religion in Neandertal burials and on European cave walls, where painted stick figures may represent shamans, early religious specialists. Nevertheless, any statement about when, where, why, and how religion arose, or any description of its original nature, can be only speculative. Although such speculations are inconclusive, many have revealed important functions and effects of religious behavior. Several theories will be examined now.

Spiritual Beings

Another founder of the anthropology of religion was the Englishman Sir Edward Burnett Tylor (1871/1958; Tremlett et al. 2017). Religion arose, Tylor thought, as people tried to understand conditions and events they could not explain by reference to daily experience. Tylor believed that ancient humans—and contemporary nonindustrial peoples—were particularly intrigued with death, dreaming, and trance. People see images they remember when they wake up or come out of a trance state. Tylor concluded that attempts to explain dreams and trances led early humans to believe that two entities inhabit the body. One is active during the day, and the other—a double, or soul—is active during sleep and trance states. Although they never meet, they are vital to each other. When the double permanently leaves the body, the person dies. Death is departure of the soul. From *anima,* the Latin for "soul," Tylor named this belief animism. The soul was one sort of spiritual entity; people remembered various other entities from their dreams and trances— other spirits. For Tylor, **animism**, the earliest form of religion, was a belief in spiritual beings.

Tylor proposed that religion evolved through stages, beginning with animism. **Polytheism** (the belief in multiple gods) and then **monotheism** (the belief in a single, all-powerful deity) developed later. Because religion originated to explain things, Tylor thought it would decline as science

animism
The belief in spiritual beings, e.g., deities, ghosts, souls or doubles.

polytheism
The belief in multiple deities, who control aspects of nature.

monotheism
The belief in a single all-powerful deity.

generation after generation, rituals translate enduring messages, values, and sentiments into action.

Rituals are social acts. Inevitably, some participants are more committed than others are to the beliefs that lie behind the rites. However, just by taking part in a joint public act, the performers signal that they accept a common social and moral order, one that transcends their status as individuals.

Rites of Passage

Magic and religion, as Malinowski noted, can reduce anxiety and allay fears. Ironically, beliefs and rituals also can create anxiety and a sense of insecurity and danger (Radcliffe-Brown 1962/1965). Anxiety can arise because a rite exists. Indeed, participation in a collective ritual (e.g., circumcision of early teen boys, common among East African pastoralists) can produce stress, whose common reduction, once the ritual is completed, enhances the solidarity of the participants.

Rites of passage can be individual or collective. Traditional Native American vision quests illustrate individual **rites of passage** (customs associated with the transition from one place or stage of life to another). To move from boyhood to manhood, a youth would temporarily separate from his community. After a period of isolation in the wilderness, often featuring fasting and drug consumption, the young man would see a vision, which would become his guardian spirit. He would return then to his community as a socially recognized adult.

Contemporary rites of passage include confirmations, baptisms, bar and bat mitzvahs, initiations, weddings, and application for Social Security and Medicare. Passage rites involve changes in social status, such as from boyhood to manhood and from nonmember to sorority sister. More generally, a rite of passage can mark any change in place, condition, social position, or age.

All rites of passage have three phases: separation, liminality, and incorporation. In the first phase, people withdraw from ordinary society. In the third phase, they reenter society, having completed a rite that changes their status. The second, or liminal, phase is the most critical and interesting. It is the limbo, or "time-out," during which people have left one status but haven't yet entered or joined the next (Downey, Kinane, and Parker 2016; Turner 1969/1995).

Liminality always has certain characteristics. Liminal people exist apart from ordinary distinctions and expectations; they are living in a time out of time (see this chapter's "Appreciating Anthropology" for liminal aspects of the coronavirus pandemic). A series of contrasts demarcate liminality from normal social life. For example, among the Ndembu of Zambia, a chief underwent a rite of passage prior to taking office. During the liminal period, his past and future positions in society

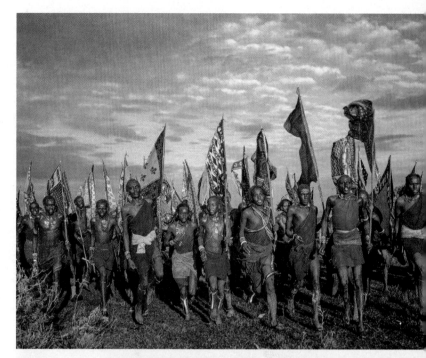

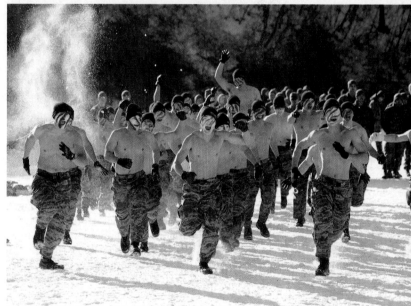

Passage rites are often collective. A group—such as these Maasai warriors in Kenya or these marines in South Korea—passes through the rites as a unit. Such liminal people experience the same treatment and conditions and must act alike. They share communitas, an intense community spirit, a feeling of great social solidarity or togetherness.

Top: Nigel Pavitt/John Warburton-Lee Photography Ltd/Aurora Photos/Cavan Images; bottom: Chung Sung-Jun/Getty Images News/Getty Images

were ignored, even reversed. He was subjected to a variety of insults, orders, and humiliations.

Passage rites often are collective. Several individuals—boys being circumcised, fraternity or sorority initiates, men at military boot camps, football players in summer training camps, women becoming nuns—pass through the rites together as a group. Recap 12.1 summarizes

rites of passage
Rites marking transitions between places or stages of life.

liminality
The in-between phase of a rite of passage.

LIMINALITY	NORMAL SOCIAL STRUCTURE
Transition	State
Homogeneity	Heterogeneity
Communitas	Structure
Equality	Inequality
Anonymity	Names
Absence of property	Property
Absence of status	Status
Nakedness or uniform dress	Dress distinctions
Sexual continence or excess	Sexuality
Minimization of sex distinctions	Maximization of sex distinctions
Absence of rank	Rank
Humility	Pride
Disregard of personal appearance	Care for personal appearance
Unselfishness	Selfishness
Total obedience	Obedience only to superior rank
Sacredness	Secularity
Sacred instruction	Technical knowledge
Silence	Speech
Simplicity	Complexity
Acceptance of pain and suffering	Avoidance of pain and suffering

SOURCE: Victor W. Turner, *The Ritual Process: Structure and Anti-Structure.* Chicago: Aldine de Gruyter, 1969, 106–107.

communitas
An intense feeling of social solidarity.

the contrasts, or oppositions, between liminality and normal social life. Most notable is the social aspect of collective liminality called **communitas**—an intense community spirit, a feeling of great social solidarity, equality, and togetherness (Turner 1967). Liminal people experience the same treatment and conditions and must act alike. Liminality can be marked ritually and symbolically by reversals of ordinary behavior. For example, sexual taboos may be intensified; conversely, sexual excess may be encouraged. Liminal symbols, such as special clothing or body paint, mark the condition as extraordinary—beyond ordinary society and everyday life.

Liminality is basic to all passage rites. Furthermore, in certain societies, including our own, liminal symbols can be used to set off one (religious) group from another—and from society as a whole. Such "permanent liminal groups" (e.g., sects, brotherhoods, and cults) are found most characteristically in nation-states. Such liminal features as humility, poverty, equality, obedience, sexual abstinence, and silence may be required for all sect or cult members. Those who join such a group agree to its rules. As if they were undergoing a passage rite—but in this case a never-ending one—they may have to abandon their previous possessions and social ties, including those with family members. Is liminality compatible with Facebook?

totem
An animal, a plant, or a geographic feature associated with a specific social group, to which that totem is sacred or symbolically important.

Members of a sect or cult often wear uniform clothing. Often they adopt a common hairstyle (shaved head, short hair, or long hair). Liminal groups submerge the individual in the collective. This may be one reason Americans, whose core values include individuality and individualism, are so fearful and suspicious of "cults."

Not all collective rites are rites of passage. Most societies have occasions on which people come together to worship or celebrate and, in doing so, affirm and reinforce their solidarity. Rituals such as the totemic ceremonies described in the next section are *rites of intensification:* They intensify social solidarity. The ritual creates communitas and produces emotions (the collective spiritual effervescence described by Durkheim [1912/2001]) that enhance social solidarity.

Totemism

Totemism was a key ingredient in the religions of the Native Australians. **Totems** could be animals, plants, or geographic features. In each tribe, groups of people had particular totems. Members of each totemic group believed themselves to be descendants of their totem, which they customarily neither killed nor ate. However, this taboo was suspended once a year, when people assembled for ceremonies dedicated to the totem. Only on that

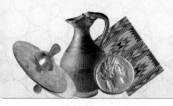

appreciating ANTHROPOLOGY

Rituals in a Pandemic's Shadow

Nothing in my life, and almost certainly nothing in yours, has affected society in the same way and to the same extent as the coronavirus pandemic that reached the United States in 2020. COVID-19 impacted all aspects of our lives—social, economic, linguistic, and religious. Socially, millions of us had to self-isolate in our homes for weeks or even months. With schools closed, co-resident family members saw much more of each other. Our interactions with others, if in person at all, were regulated by new norms of social distancing. Our children, grandchildren, and friends postponed visits, both planned and spontaneous, although we could still see their faces and hear their voices via FaceTime, Zoom, or a similar app.

Linguistically, a series of new expressions entered our vocabulary. From "coronavirus" itself arose words and expressions for its impact, including "social distancing," "flattening the curve," and "red zone." We were warned about spewing "droplets" and touching our face.

The economic change was pervasive and immense. Millions were suddenly unemployed, while millions of luckier others could work remotely from home. TV newscasters and late-night hosts did the same—worked, that is broadcasted, from home. Global supply chains were disrupted, even as remote communication was booming. Zoom became the new normal, and its increased use seemed likely to continue long past the pandemic's peak. Who wants to travel hours to attend a one- or two-hour meeting after seeing how easily it can be done remotely from home or office?

The effects of the coronavirus on our rituals and religious life were profound as well.

Important rites of passage, including weddings, graduation ceremonies, baptisms, and christenings, were postponed, abandoned, or truncated. Victims of the pandemic died in isolation—apart from loved ones who would never again see their faces or hold their hands. In the hardest hit areas, such as New York City and northern Italy, bodies accumulated too fast for proper burial or cremation. Funerary practices were disrupted. Graveside ceremonies were prohibited, or limited perhaps to a single priest, preacher, or rabbi, while family members of the deceased looked on from automobiles or attended remotely. Last rites were sometimes administered by phone. Ordinary gatherings for religious fellowship at houses of worship were discouraged. Remote and drive-in services replaced them. Religion traditionally is a collective phenomenon: people meet, physically, to worship and partake jointly in the same rituals. Religious fellowship and communion are intrinsically incompatible with social distancing.

We have experienced this pandemic together—all of us who have survived. Yet this common, shared experience is like none other we have endured. COVID-19 united us under its shadow even as it divided us physically. During the pandemic we experienced liminality: our usual behavior and expectations were suspended as we lived through a time out of time. The once ordinary (even something as mundane as buying toilet paper) became difficult or impossible. Although we had millions of fellow passengers through liminality, our physical separation prevented us from developing the intense communitas that typically marks rites of passage. Nor did we even get news about the

crisis from the same sources. Now more than ever, our politics dictates our media choices, so that the information we received about the virus was not uniform. This divisiveness helps explain why the coronavirus pandemic did not create the social solidarity that arose from the attacks waged against the United States on September 11, 2001, or Pearl Harbor Day in 1941. Those events—attacks by identifiable human outsiders—truly united us. It was easy for us all to perceive a common enemy.

As one might expect, given the liminality and uncertainty induced by the coronavirus, some new rituals did develop, both individually and collectively. People dressed differently in public, donning masks and gloves and standing six feet apart. Through social media, apartment dwellers coordinated balcony events, ranging from sing-alongs and libations at a set time of day to clapping and cheering on healthcare workers and first responders. Anthropologist Dimitris Xygalatas (2020) reminds us that stressful events often lead to spikes in ritual activity. As Malinowski explained, when people face uncertainty and danger they often turn to magic and ritual. Performing a ritual can give us a sense of control. We can do the ritual properly even if we can't control the troubling event that inspired it.

Did your own ritual behavior change as a result of COVID-19? Did you somehow, perhaps remotely, meet with others and engage in ritualized behavior—toasting from your balcony with a nightly or weekly "quarantini," for example. Do you have religious, or even personal, rituals that you found yourself performing more diligently during the pandemic?

occasion were they allowed to kill and eat their totem. These annual rites were believed to be necessary for the totem's survival and reproduction.

Totemism uses nature as a model for society. The totems usually are animals and plants, which

are part of nature. People relate to nature through their totemic association with natural species. Because each group has a different totem, social differences mirror natural contrasts. Diversity in the natural order becomes a model for diversity in the social order. However, although totemic plants and animals occupy different niches in nature, on another level they are united because they all are part of nature. The unity of the human social order is enhanced by symbolic association with and imitation of the natural order (Durkheim 1912/2001; Lévi-Strauss 1963; Radcliffe-Brown 1962/1965).

cosmology
A system, often religious, for imagining and understanding the universe.

Totemism is one form of **cosmology**—a system, in this case a religious one, for imagining and understanding the universe. Claude Lévi-Strauss, a prolific French anthropologist and a key figure in the anthropology of religion, is well known for his studies of myth, folklore, totemism, and cosmology. Lévi-Strauss believed that one role of religious rites and beliefs is to affirm, and thus maintain, the solidarity of a religion's adherents. Totems are sacred emblems symbolizing common identity. This is true not just among Native Australians but also among Native American groups of the North Pacific Coast of North America, whose totem poles are well known. Their totemic carvings, which commemorated and told visual stories about ancestors, animals, and spirits, were also associated with ceremonies. In totemic rites, people gather together to honor their totem. In so doing, they use ritual to maintain the social oneness that the totem symbolizes.

Totemic principles continue to demarcate groups, including clubs, teams, and universities, in modern societies. Badgers and Wolverines are animals, and (it is said in Michigan) Buckeyes are some kind of nut (more precisely, buckeye nuts come from the buckeye tree). Differences between natural species (e.g., Lions and Tigers and Bears) distinguish sports teams, and even political parties (donkeys and elephants). Although the modern context is more secular, one can still witness, in intense college football rivalries, some of the effervescence Durkheim noted in Australian totemic religion and other rites of intensification.

RELIGION AND CULTURAL ECOLOGY

Another domain in which religion plays a role is cultural ecology. Behavior motivated by beliefs in supernatural beings, powers, and forces can help people survive in their material environment. Beliefs and rituals can function as part of a group's cultural adaptation to its environment.

The people of India revere zebu cattle, which are protected by the Hindu doctrine of *ahimsa,* a principle of nonviolence that forbids the killing of animals generally. Western economic development agents occasionally (and erroneously) cite the Hindu cattle taboo to illustrate the idea that religious beliefs can stand in the way of rational economic decisions. Hindus might seem to be irrationally ignoring a valuable food (beef) because of their cultural or religious traditions. Development agents also have asserted that Indians don't know how to raise proper cattle. They point to the scraggly zebus that wander around town and country. Western techniques of animal husbandry grow bigger cattle that produce more beef and milk. Western planners lament that Hindus are set in their ways. Bound by culture and tradition, they refuse to develop rationally.

However, these assumptions are both ethnocentric and wrong. Sacred cattle actually play an important adaptive role in an Indian ecosystem that has evolved over thousands of years (Harris 1974, 1978). Peasants' use of cattle to pull plows and carts is part of the technology of Indian agriculture. Indian peasants have no need for large, hungry cattle of the sort that Westerners prefer. Scrawny animals pull plows and carts well enough but don't eat their owners out of house and home. How could peasants with limited land and marginal diets feed super-steers without taking food away from themselves?

Indians use cattle manure to fertilize their fields. Not all the manure is collected, because peasants don't spend much time watching their cattle, which wander and graze at will during certain seasons. In the rainy season, some of the manure that cattle deposit on the hillsides washes down to the fields. In this way, cattle also fertilize the fields indirectly. Furthermore, in a country where fossil fuels are scarce, dry cattle dung, which burns slowly and evenly, is a basic cooking fuel.

Sacred cattle are essential to Indian cultural adaptation. Biologically adapted to poor pasture land and a marginal environment, the scraggly zebu provides fertilizer and fuel, is indispensable in farming, and is affordable for peasants. The Hindu doctrine of *ahimsa* puts the full power of organized religion behind the command not to destroy a valuable resource, even in times of extreme need.

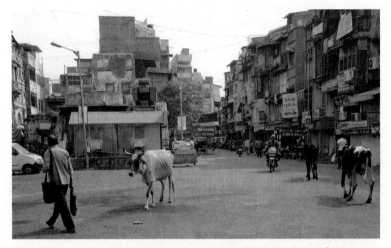

Cows freely walk the streets of any Indian city, including Ahmedabad, Gujarat, shown here. India's zebu cattle are protected by the doctrine of ahimsa, a principle of nonviolence that forbids the killing of animals generally.

Conrad P. Kottak

SOCIAL CONTROL

Religion helps people cope with adversity, fear, tragedy, and uncertainty (lack of control). Religion can offer hope that things will get better. Lives can be transformed through spiritual healing. Sinners can repent and be saved—or they can go on sinning and be damned. If the faithful truly internalize a system of religious rewards and punishments, their religion becomes a powerful influence on their attitudes and behavior, as well as what they teach their children.

Many people continue to engage in religious activity because it works for them. Prayers get answered. Healers heal. Native Americans in southwestern Oklahoma use faith healers at high monetary costs, not just because it makes them feel better about the uncertain, but because they believe it works (Lassiter 1998). Each year legions of Brazilians visit a church, Nosso Senhor do Bonfim, in the city of Salvador, Bahia. They vow to repay "Our Lord" (Nosso Senhor) if healing happens. Showing that the vows work, and are repaid, are the thousands of *ex votos,* plastic impressions of every conceivable body part, that adorn the church, along with photos of people who have been cured.

Religion can work by mobilizing emotions—joy, wrath, righteousness. People can feel a deep sense of shared joy, enlightenment, communion, belonging, and commitment to their religion. Religion affects action. When religions meet, they can coexist peacefully, or their differences can be a basis for enmity and disharmony, even battle. Throughout history, political leaders have used religion to promote and justify their views and policies.

How can leaders mobilize communities to support their own policies? One way is by persuasion; another is by hatred or fear. Consider witchcraft accusations. Witch hunts can be powerful means of social control by creating a climate of danger and insecurity that affects everyone. No one wants to seem deviant, to be accused of being a witch. Witch hunts often aim at socially marginal people who can be accused and punished with the least chance of retaliation. During the great European witch craze, during the 15th, 16th, and 17th centuries (Harris 1974), most accusations and convictions were against poor women with little social support.

Accusations of witchcraft are ethnographic as well as historical facts. Witchcraft beliefs are common in village and peasant societies, where people live close together and have limited mobility. Such societies often have what anthropologist George Foster (1965) called an "image of limited good"—the idea that resources are limited, so that one person can profit disproportionately only at the expense of others. In this context, the threat of witchcraft accusations can serve as a leveling mechanism if it motivates wealthier villagers to be especially generous or else face shunning and social ostracism. Similarly, we saw in Chapter 9, on gender, that Etoro women who wanted too much sex, as well as boys who grew too rapidly, could be shunned as witches who were depleting a man's limited lifetime supply of semen.

To ensure proper behavior, religions offer rewards (e.g., the fellowship of the religious community) and punishments (e.g., the threat of being cast out, or excommunicated). Religions, especially the formal, organized ones found in state societies, often prescribe a code of ethics and morality to guide behavior. Moral codes are ways of maintaining order and stability that are reinforced continually in sermons, catechisms, and the like. They become internalized psychologically. They guide behavior and produce regret, guilt, shame, and the need for forgiveness, expiation, and absolution when they are not followed.

KINDS OF RELIGION

Although religion is a cultural universal, religions exist in particular societies, and cultural differences show up systematically in religious beliefs and practices. For example, the religions of stratified, state societies differ from those of societies with less marked social contrasts—societies without kings, lords, and subjects. Churches, temples, and other full-time religious establishments, with their monumental structures and hierarchies of officials, must be supported in some consistent way, such as by tithes and taxes. What kinds of societies can support such hierarchies and architecture?

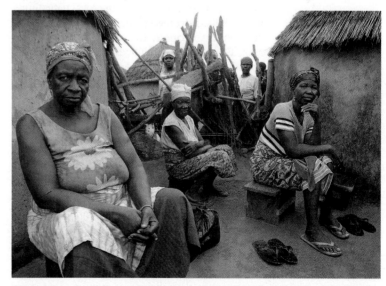

Witchcraft accusations persist in today's world, with women disproportionately targeted. Hundreds of alleged witches, including these women, are confined to five isolated "witch camps" in northern Ghana. Witchcraft accusations there tend to follow disputes over inheritance rights, or a husband's death that leaves a widow perceived to be a burden on her husband's family or her own.

Markus Matzel/ullstein bild via Getty Images

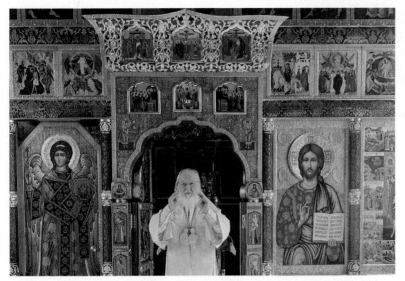

Representing an ecclesiastical religion, Russian Orthodox Patriarch Kirill conducts his Easter eve service in his official residence outside Moscow. The photo was taken on April 18, 2020, during a strict lockdown designed to stop the spread of the novel coronavirus COVID-19. All churches in Moscow were closed to worshippers that night.
Sergei Zaikin/Getty Images

Religious Specialists and Deities

All societies have religious figures—those believed capable of mediating between humans and the supernatural. More generally, all societies have medico-magico-religious specialists. Modern societies can support both priesthoods and health care professionals. Lacking the resources for such specialization, foraging societies typically have only part-time specialists, who often have both religious and healing roles. **Shaman** is the general term encompassing curers ("witch doctors"), mediums, spiritualists, astrologers, palm readers, and other independent diviners. In foraging societies, shamans usually are part time; that is, they also hunt or gather.

Societies with productive economies (based on agriculture and trade) and large, dense populations—that is, nation-states—can support full-time religious specialists—professional priesthoods. Like the state itself, priesthoods are hierarchically and bureaucratically organized. Anthony Wallace (1966) describes the religions of such stratified societies as "ecclesiastical" (pertaining to an established church and its hierarchy of officials) and Olympian, after Mount Olympus, home of the classical Greek gods. In such religions, powerful anthropomorphic gods have specialized functions, for example, gods of love, war, the sea, and death. Such *pantheons* (collections of deities) were prominent in the religions of many nonindustrial nation-states, including the Aztecs of Mexico, and several African and Asian kingdoms. Greco-Roman religions also were polytheistic, featuring many deities—the Olympian gods.

In monotheism, all supernatural phenomena are believed to be manifestations of, or under the control of, a single eternal, omniscient, omnipotent, and omnipresent being. In the ecclesiastical monotheistic religion known as Christianity, a single supreme being is manifest in a trinity. Robert Bellah (1978, 2011) viewed most forms of Christianity as examples of "world-rejecting religion." According to Bellah, the first world-rejecting religions arose in ancient civilizations, along with literacy and a specialized priesthood. These religions are so named because of their tendency to reject the natural (mundane, ordinary, material, secular) world and to focus instead on a higher (sacred, transcendent) realm of reality. The divine is a domain of exalted morality to which humans can only aspire. Salvation through fusion with the supernatural is the main goal of such religions.

Protestant Values and Capitalism

Notions of salvation and the afterlife dominate Christian ideologies. However, most varieties of Protestantism lack the hierarchical structure of earlier monotheistic religions, including Roman Catholicism. With a diminished role for the priest (minister), salvation is directly available to individuals. Regardless of their social status, Protestants have unmediated access to the supernatural. The individualistic focus of Protestantism offers a close fit with capitalism and with American culture.

In his influential book *The Protestant Ethic and the Spirit of Capitalism,* the social theorist Max Weber (1904/2011) linked the spread of capitalism to the values preached by early Protestant leaders. Weber saw European Protestants (and eventually their American descendants) as more successful financially than Catholics. He attributed this difference to the values stressed by their religions. Weber saw Catholics as more concerned with immediate happiness and security. Protestants were more entrepreneurial, and future oriented, he thought.

Capitalism, said Weber, required that the traditional attitudes of Catholic peasants be replaced by values befitting an industrial economy based on capital accumulation. Protestantism placed a premium on hard work, an ascetic life, and profit seeking. Early Protestants saw success on Earth as a sign of divine favor and probable salvation. According to some Protestant credos, individuals could gain favor with God through good works. Other sects stressed predestination, the idea that only a few mortals have been selected for eternal life and that people cannot change their fates. However, material success, achieved through hard work, could be a strong clue that someone was predestined to be saved.

Weber also argued that rational business organization required the removal of industrial production from the home, its setting in peasant societies. Protestantism made such a separation possible by emphasizing individualism: Individuals, not

shaman
The general term encompassing curers ("witch doctors"), mediums, spiritualists, astrologers, palm readers, and other independent diviners.

families or households, would be saved or not. Interestingly, given the connection that is usually made with morality and religion in contemporary American discourse about family values, the family was a secondary matter for Weber's early Protestants. God and the individual reigned supreme.

Today, of course, in North America, as throughout the world, people of many religions and with diverse worldviews are successful capitalists. Furthermore, traditional Protestant values often have little to do with today's economic maneuvering. Still, there is no denying that the individualistic focus of Protestantism was compatible with the severance of ties to land and kin that industrialism demanded. These values remain prominent in the religious background of many of the people of the United States.

WORLD RELIGIONS

Information on the world's major religions in 2015 and projected for 2050 is provided in Figure 12.1, based on the most recent comprehensive studies by the Pew Research Center (2015b, 2015c, 2017a). Considering data from more than 230 countries, researchers estimated that 84 percent of the world's population had some religious affiliation.

In 2015, there were approximately 2.3 billion Christians (31.2 percent of the world's population), 1.8 billion Muslims (24.1 percent), 1.1 billion Hindus (15.1 percent), about 500 million Buddhists (6.9 percent), and 14 million Jews (0.2 percent). In addition, about 400 million people (5.7 percent) practiced folk or traditional religions of various sorts. Around 60 million people,

a bit less than 1 percent of the world's population, belonged to other religions, including Baha'i, Jainism, Sikhism, Shintoism, Taoism, Tenrikyo, Wicca, and Zoroastrianism.

About 1.2 billion people—16 percent of the world's population—lacked any religious affiliation. The unaffiliated therefore constitute the third-largest group worldwide with respect to religious affiliation, behind Christians and Muslims. There are about as many unaffiliated people as Roman Catholics in the world. Many of the unaffiliated actually hold some religious or spiritual beliefs, even if they don't identify with a particular religion (Pew Research Center 2012, 2015b, 2015c).

Worldwide, Islam is growing at a rate of about 2.9 percent annually, compared with 2.3 percent for Christianity. Within Christianity, the growth rate is much higher for "born-again" Christians (e.g., Evangelicals/Pentecostals) than for either Catholics or mainline Protestants (see Coleman and Hackett 2015). Demographic projections by the Pew Research Center (2017a) suggest that by 2060 there will be almost as many Muslims (31.1 percent) as Christians (31.8 percent) in the world. In Europe, Muslims will constitute about 10 percent of the population, compared with about 6 percent today.

How about church and state? The Pew Research Center (2017) determined that about 40 percent of the 199 countries it surveyed favored one religion over others—either as an official, government-endorsed religion, or as one receiving preferential treatment. Islam was the most common state religion, endorsed by 27 countries, mostly in the Middle East and North Africa. Only 13 countries (including 9 in Europe) made Christianity, or some

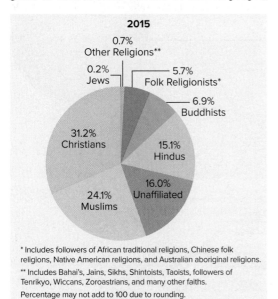

2015

0.7% Other Religions**

0.2% Jews

5.7% Folk Religionists*

6.9% Buddhists

31.2% Christians

15.1% Hindus

16.0% Unaffiliated

24.1% Muslims

* Includes followers of African traditional religions, Chinese folk religions, Native American religions, and Australian aboriginal religions.

** Includes Bahai's, Jains, Sikhs, Shintoists, Taoists, followers of Tenrikyo, Wiccans, Zoroastrians, and many other faiths.

Percentage may not add to 100 due to rounding.

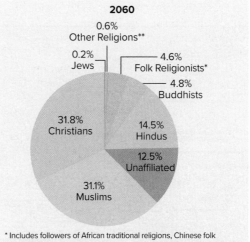

2060

0.6% Other Religions**

0.2% Jews

4.6% Folk Religionists*

4.8% Buddhists

31.8% Christians

14.5% Hindus

12.5% Unaffiliated

31.1% Muslims

* Includes followers of African traditional religions, Chinese folk religions, Native American religions, and Australian aboriginal religions.

** Includes Bahai's, Jains, Sikhs, Shintoists, Taoists, followers of Tenrikyo, Wiccans, Zoroastrians, and many other faiths.

Percentage may not add to 100 due to rounding.

FIGURE 12.1 Major World Religions by Percentage of World Population, 2015, and Projected for 2060.

SOURCE: Pew Research Center. The Changing Global Religious Landscape. April 5, 2017. https://www.pewforum.org/2017/04/05/the-changing-global-religious-landscape/

cargo cults
Postcolonial, acculturative religious movements in Melanesia.

Christian denomination, their state religion. However, 40 more governments unofficially favored a single religion, usually a form of Christianity. The governments of 10 countries either tightly regulated all religious activities or were hostile to religion in general. These countries included China, Cuba, North Korea, Vietnam, and several former Soviet republics. More than 100 countries and territories had no favored religion. Among them were countries like the United States, which may offer privileges to certain religious groups, but generally without formally favoring one group over others.

RELIGION AND CHANGE

Like political organization, religion helps maintain social order. And like political mobilization, religious energy can be harnessed not just for change but also for revolution. Reacting to conquest or to actual or perceived foreign domination, for instance, religious leaders may seek to alter or revitalize their society.

Revitalization Movements

revitalization movements
Social movements aimed at altering or revitalizing a society.

Revitalization movements are social movements that occur in times of change, in which religious leaders emerge and undertake to alter or revitalize a society. Christianity originated as a revitalization movement. Jesus was one of several prophets who preached new religious doctrines while the Middle

East was under Roman rule. It was a time of social unrest, when a foreign power ruled the land. Jesus inspired a new, enduring, and major religion. His contemporaries were not so successful.

Revitalization movements known as **cargo cults** have arisen in colonial situations in which local people have regular contact with outsiders but lack their wealth, technology, and living standards. Cargo cults attempt to explain European domination and wealth and to achieve similar success magically by mimicking European behavior and manipulating symbols of the desired lifestyle. The cargo cults of Melanesia and Papua New Guinea (see Figure 12.2) are hybrid creations that weave Christian doctrine with indigenous beliefs. They take their name from their focus on cargo—European goods of the sort natives have seen unloaded from the cargo holds of ships and airplanes.

In one early cult, members believed that the spirits of the dead would arrive one day in a ship. Those ghosts would bring manufactured goods for the natives and would kill all the whites. More recent cults replaced ships with airplanes (Worsley 1959/1985). Many cults have used elements of European culture as sacred objects. The rationale is that Europeans (or Americans) use these objects, have wealth, and therefore must know the "secret of cargo." By mimicking how Europeans use or treat objects, natives hope also to come upon the secret knowledge needed to get cargo for themselves.

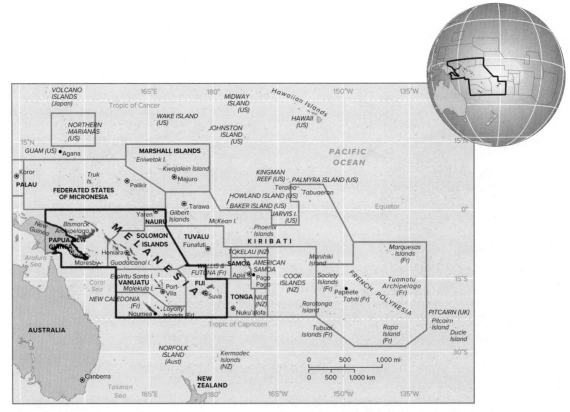

FIGURE 12.2 Location of Melanesia.

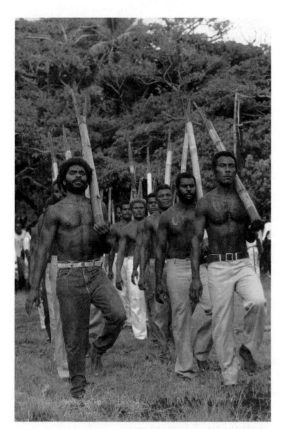

On the island of Tanna, in Vanuatu, Melanesia, members of the John Frum cargo cult stage their annual military parade. The young men, who carry fake guns and have "USA" painted on their bodies, see themselves as an elite force within the American army.

Thierry Falise/Getty Images

For example, having seen Europeans' reverent treatment of flags and flagpoles, the members of one cult began to worship flagpoles. They believed the flagpoles were sacred towers that could transmit messages between the living and the dead. Other natives built airstrips to entice planes bearing canned goods, portable radios, clothing, wristwatches, and motorcycles.

Some cargo cult prophets proclaimed that success would come through a reversal of European domination and native subjugation. The day was near, they preached, when natives, aided by God, Jesus, or native ancestors, would turn the tables. Native skins would turn white, and those of Europeans would turn brown; Europeans would die or be killed.

Syncretisms are cultural, especially religious, mixes that emerge from acculturation. Cargo cults are syncretisms that blend Aboriginal and Christian beliefs. Melanesian myths told of ancestors shedding their skins and changing into powerful beings and of dead people returning to life. Christian missionaries also preached resurrection. The cults' preoccupation with cargo is related to traditional Melanesian big-man systems. A Melanesian big man

was expected to be generous. People worked for the big man, helping him amass wealth, but eventually he had to host a feast and give away all that wealth.

Because of their experience with big man systems, Melanesians believed that all wealthy people eventually had to give away their wealth. For decades, they had attended Christian missions and worked on plantations. All the while they expected Europeans to return the fruits of their labor as their own big men did. When the Europeans refused to distribute the wealth or even to let natives know the secret of its production and distribution, cargo cults developed.

Like arrogant big men, Europeans would be put in their place or leveled, by death if necessary. However, natives lacked the physical means of doing what their traditions said they should do. Thwarted by well-armed colonial forces, natives resorted to magical leveling. They called on supernatural beings to intercede, to kill or otherwise deflate the European big men and redistribute their wealth.

Cargo cults are religious responses to the expansion of the world capitalist economy. However, this religious mobilization had political and economic results. Cult participation gave Melanesians a basis for common interests and activities and thus helped pave the way for political parties and economic interest organizations. Previously separated by geography, language, and customs, Melanesians started forming larger groups as members of the same cults and followers of the same prophets. The cargo cults paved the way for political action through which the indigenous peoples eventually regained their autonomy.

Religious Changes in the United States

Because the U.S. Census doesn't gather information on religion, there are no official statistics on Americans' religious affiliations. To help fill this gap, the Pew Research Center, based in Washington, D.C., carried out "Religious Landscape Studies" in 2007 and 2014. These comprehensive surveys of more than 35,000 adults revealed significant and ongoing changes in Americans' religious affiliations (see Pew Research Center 2015a). More recent information on Americans' religious preferences come from smaller surveys that Pew conducted in 2009 and 2019 (see Pew Research Center 2019). Results of these various surveys are incorporated below.

As of 2019, 65 percent of American adults described themselves as Christians, a falloff of 12 percentage points since 2009. Both Protestants and Catholics are losing share. In 2019, 43 percent of U.S. adults identified as Protestants, down from 51 percent in 2009. The percentage of Catholics also fell—from 23 percent to 20 percent. Meanwhile, the percentage of religiously unaffiliated Americans, a group also known as religious "nones," rose to 26 percent (from 17 percent in 2009).

syncretisms
Cultural, especially religious, mixes, emerging from acculturation.

Among them are self-identified atheists (now 4 percent of U.S. adults), agnostics (5 percent), and those who describe themselves as "nothing in particular" (17 percent). Membership in non–Christian religions (e.g., Jews, Muslims, Hindus) also has risen modestly to 7 percent of American adults (Pew Research Center 2019).

The earlier and more comprehensive "Religious Landscape Studies" conducted by Pew in 2007 and 2014 documented a decline in the number of mainline Protestants—Methodists, Baptists, Lutherans, Presbyterians, and Episcopalians (from 41 million in 2007 to 36 million in 2014). During that same period, the number of Americans (around 16 million) affiliated with historically Black Protestant churches remained stable. America's 62 million Evangelicals were the only group of Protestants whose numbers were rising, but even their share of the U.S. population had declined slightly.

The most notable (and ongoing) trend since 2007 has been the rise in the unaffiliated category. These 61 million religious "nones" now outnumber both Catholics and mainline Protestants (Pew Research Center 2019). Unaffiliated Americans have a median age of 36 years, compared with 52 years for mainline Protestants. Men are much more likely than women to be unaffiliated. This is part of a larger gender gap that characterizes American religion. Women are less likely than men to be unaffiliated (23 percent versus 30 percent), and more likely to be regular worshipers (Pew Research Center 2019). Still, religiosity has been declining among American women as well as among American men.

One factor behind the growth in the unaffiliated category may be the decline in religious in-marriage or endogamy. Of the Americans who have married since 2010, 39 percent were in a religiously mixed marriage, compared with 19 percent before 1960. When parents have different religions, it may be easier to raise unaffiliated children than to choose between faiths.

It is increasingly common for Americans to change, or give up, religion. Over one-third (34 percent) of Americans have a religious identity (or lack thereof) different from the one in which they were raised. If switching from one Protestant church to another, for example, from mainline to Evangelical, is also included, this figure rises to 42 percent.

Along with affiliation, religious attendance also is declining. In 2009, regular worshipers (once or more monthly) outnumbered occasional and non-worshipers 52 to 47 percent. By 2019, that ratio had reversed, with occasional and nonworshipers at 54 percent, compared with regular worshipers at 45 percent (Pew Research Center 2019).

In the context of this increasing U.S. religious diversity, the established religions themselves are also becoming more diverse. Minorities now constitute 41 percent of American Catholics, 24 percent of Evangelicals, and 14 percent of mainline Protestants. These trends are likely to continue. Have you changed religions?

New and Alternative Religious Movements

The previous section described religious changes in the United States, including significant growth in the unaffiliated category. This trend toward nonaffiliation, whether as atheist, agnostic, or "nothing in particular" can also be detected in Canada, Western Europe, China, and Japan. In addition to increasing nonaffiliation, contemporary industrial societies also feature new religious trends and forms of spiritualism. The New Age movement, which emerged in the 1980s, draws on and blends cultural elements from multiple traditions. It advocates change through individual personal transformation. In the United States and Australia, respectively, some people who are not Native Americans or Native Australians have appropriated the symbols, settings, and purported religious practices of Native Americans and Native Australians for New Age religions. Native American activists decry the appropriation and commercialization of their spiritual beliefs and rituals, as when "sweat lodge" ceremonies are held on cruise ships, with wine and cheese served. They see the appropriation of their ceremonies and traditions as theft. Some Hindus feel similarly about the popularization of yoga.

New religious movements have varied origins. Some have been influenced by Christianity, others by Eastern (Asian) religions, still others by mysticism and spiritualism. Religion also evolves in

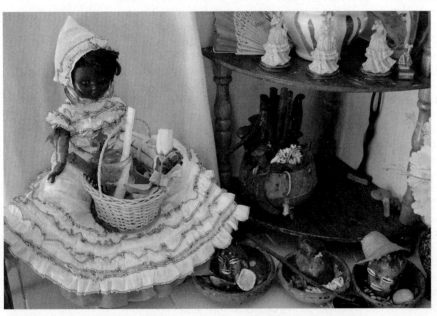

A Santeria shrine in the Alamar Neighborhood Housing Projects, Havana, Cuba.
Lissa Harrison

tandem with science and technology. For example, the Raelian movement, a religious group centered in Switzerland and Montreal, promotes cloning as a way of achieving eternal life (see http://www.rael.org/home).

Many contemporary nations contain unofficial religions. One example is *Yoruba religion,* a term applied to perhaps 15 million adherents in Africa as well as to millions of practitioners of syncretic, or blended, religions (with elements of Catholicism and spiritism) in the Western Hemisphere. Forms of Yoruba religion include *santeria* (in the Spanish Caribbean and the United States), *candombl*é (in Brazil), and *vodoun* (in the French Caribbean). Yoruba religion, with roots in precolonial nation-states of West Africa, has spread far beyond its region of origin, as part of the African diaspora. It remains an influential, identifiable religion today, despite suppression, such as by Cuba's communist government.

There are perhaps 3 million practitioners of santeria in Cuba, plus another 800,000 in the United States. At least 1 million Brazilians participate in candomblé, also known as *macumba.* Voodoo (vodoun) has an estimated 3 million practitioners. many (perhaps most) of whom would name something else, such as Catholicism, as their official religion (Ontario Consultants 2011).

RELIGION AND CULTURAL GLOBALIZATION

Evangelical Protestantism and Pentecostalism

The rapid and ongoing spread of Evangelical Protestantism, which originated in Europe and North America, constitutes a highly successful form of contemporary cultural globalization. A century ago, more than 90 percent of the then approximately 80 million Evangelicals in the world lived in Europe and North America (Pew Research Center 2011). Today, there are more than 600 million Evangelicals worldwide. Most now live in Latin America, Asia, sub-Saharan Africa, and the Middle East and North Africa (see Coleman and Hackett 2015).

The growth and spread of Evangelical Protestantism has been particularly explosive in Brazil—traditionally (and still) the world's most Catholic country. In 1980, when Pope John Paul II visited the country, 89 percent of Brazil's population claimed to be Roman Catholic, compared with just 51 percent in a 2019-2020 survey (see Lima 2020). This decline is due mainly to Evangelical Protestantism, which has spread like wildfire in Brazil. Having made small inroads during the first half of the 20th century, Evangelical Protestantism grew exponentially in Brazil during the second half. Protestants accounted for less than 5 percent of the population through the 1960s. By 2000, Evangelical Protestants constituted more than 15 percent of Brazilians affiliated with a church. Based on the 2019-2020 survey, the current Evangelical share of Brazil's population has risen to 31 percent and is still growing. Among the factors that have worked in Brazil against Catholicism are these: a declining and mainly foreign priesthood, sharply contrasting political agendas of many of its clerics, and its reputation as mainly a women's religion.

Evangelical Protestantism stresses conservative morality, biblical authority, and a personal ("born-again") conversion experience. Most Brazilian Evangelicals are Pentecostals, who also embrace glossolalia (speaking in tongues) and beliefs in faith healing, spirits, exorcism, and miracles.

In its focus on ecstatic and exuberant worship, Pentecostalism has been heavily influenced by—and shares features with—African American Protestantism. In Brazil it shares features with candomblé, which also features chanting and spirit possession (Casanova 2001; Meyer 1999).

Peter Berger (2010) thinks that modern Pentecostalism may be the fastest-growing religion in human history and focuses on its social dimensions to explain why. According to Berger, Pentecostalism promotes strong communities while offering practical and psychological support to people whose circumstances are changing. My own experience in Brazil supports Berger's hypothesis; most new Pentecostals I encountered came from underprivileged, poor, and otherwise marginalized groups in areas undergoing rapid social change.

The British sociologist David Martin (1990) argues that Pentecostalism is spreading so rapidly because its adherents embody Max Weber's Protestant ethic—valuing self-discipline, hard work,

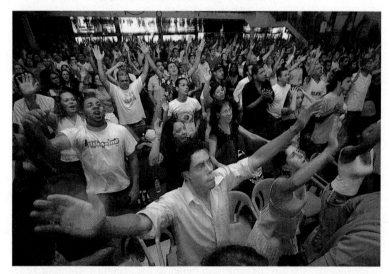

In São Paulo, Brazil, Evangelicals pray inside the Bola de Neve Church. Popular with youths, this church sponsors activities such as surfing, skating, and rock 'n' roll and reggae music with religious lyrics. Is Evangelical Protestantism Brazil's major religion?

Caetano Barreira/Reuters/Newscom

and thrift. Others see Pentecostalism as a kind of cargo cult, built on the belief that magic and ritual activity can promote material success (Freston 2008; Meyer 1999). Berger (2010) suggests that today's Pentecostals probably include both types—Weberian Protestants working to produce material wealth as a sign of their salvation along with people who believe that magic and ritual will bring them good fortune.

Converts to Pentecostalism are expected to separate themselves both from their pasts and from the secular social world that surrounds them. In Arembepe, Brazil, for example, the *crentes* ("true believers," as members of the local Pentecostal community are called) set themselves apart by their beliefs, behavior, and lifestyle (Kottak 2018). They worship, chant, and pray. They dress simply and forgo such worldly temptations (seen as vices) as tobacco, alcohol, gambling, and extramarital sexuality, along with dancing, movies, and other forms of popular culture.

Pentecostalism strengthens family and household through a moral code that respects marriage and prohibits adultery, gambling, drinking, and fighting. These activities were valued mainly by men in preconversion culture. Pentecostalism has appeal for men, however, because it solidifies their authority within the household. Although Pentecostal ideology is strongly patriarchal, with women expected to subordinate themselves to men, women tend to be more active church members than men are. Pentecostalism promotes services and prayer groups by and for women. In such settings women develop leadership skills, as they also extend their social-support network beyond family and kin (Burdick 1998).

Homogenization, Indigenization, or Hybridization?

Any cultural form that spreads from one society to another—be it a Starbucks, McDonald's, or a form of religion—has to fit into the country and culture it enters. We can use the rapid spread of Pentecostalism as a case study of the process of adaptation of foreign cultural forms to local settings.

Joel Robbins (2004) has examined the extent to which what he calls Pentecostal/charismatic Christianity preserves its basic form and core beliefs as it spreads and adapts to various national and local cultures. Pentecostalism is a Western invention: Its beliefs, doctrines, organizational features, and rituals originated in the United States, following the European rise and spread of Protestantism. The core doctrines of acceptance of Jesus as one's savior, baptism with the Holy Spirit, faith healing, and belief in the second coming of Jesus have spread across nations and cultures without losing their basic shape.

Scholars have argued about whether the global spread of Pentecostalism is best understood as (1) a process of Western cultural domination and homogenization (perhaps supported by a right-wing political agenda) or (2) a process in which diffused cultural forms respond to local needs and are differentiated and indigenized. Joel Robbins (2004) takes a middle-ground position, viewing the spread of Pentecostalism as a form of cultural hybridization. He argues that global and local features appear with equal intensity within these Pentecostal cultures. Churches retain certain core Pentecostal beliefs and behaviors while responding to the local culture and being organized at the local level.

Reviewing the literature, Robbins (2004) finds little evidence that a Western political agenda is propelling the global spread of Pentecostalism. It is true that foreigners (including American pastors and televangelists) have helped introduce Pentecostalism to countries outside North America. There is little evidence, however, that overseas churches are largely funded and ideologically shaped from North America. Pentecostal churches typically are staffed with locals, who run them as organizations that are attentive and responsive to local situations. Conversion is typically a key feature of that agenda. Once converted, a Pentecostal is expected to be an active evangelist, seeking to bring in new members. This evangelization is one of the most important activities in Pentecostal culture and certainly aids its expansion.

Pentecostalism spreads as other forces of globalization displace people and disrupt local lives (Martin 1990). To people who feel socially adrift, Pentecostal evangelists offer tightly knit communities and a weblike structure of personal connections within and between Pentecostal communities. Such networks can facilitate access to health care, job placement, educational services, and other resources.

Unlike Catholicism, which is hierarchical, Pentecostalism is egalitarian. Adherents need no special education—only spiritual inspiration—to preach or to run a church. Based on his research in Brazil, John Burdick (1993) notes that many Afro-Brazilians are drawn to the Pentecostal community because others who are socially and racially like them are in the congregation, some serving as preachers. Opportunities for participation and leadership are abundant, for example, as lay preachers, deacons, and leaders of various men's, women's, and youth groups. The churches fund outreach to the needy and other locally relevant social services.

The Spread of Islam

Islam—whose 1.8 billion followers constitute almost a quarter of the world's population—is another rapidly spreading global religion that can be used to illustrate cultural globalization. The globalization of Islam also illustrates cultural hybridization. Islam has adapted successfully to the many nations and cultures it has entered, adopting architectural styles, linguistic practices, and even religious beliefs from host cultures.

For example, although Mosques (Islamic houses of worship) all share certain characteristics (e.g., they face Mecca and have some common architectural features), they also incorporate architectural and decorative elements from their national settings. Arabic is Islam's liturgical language, used for prayer, but most Muslims' discussion of their faith occurs in their local language. In China, Islamic concepts have been influenced by Confucianism. In India and Bangladesh, the Islamic idea of the prophet has blended with the Hindu notion of the avatar, a deity who takes mortal form and descends to Earth to fight evil and guide the righteous. Islam entered Indonesia by means of Muslim merchants who devised devotional exercises that fit in with preexisting religions—Hinduism and Buddhism in Java and Sumatra and animism in the eastern islands, which eventually became Christian. In Bali, Hinduism survived as the dominant religion. Both Pentecostalism and Islam, we have learned, hybridize and become locally relevant as they spread globally. Although certain core features endure, local people always assign their own meanings to the messages and social forms they receive from outside, including religion. Such meanings reflect their cultural backgrounds, experiences, and prior belief systems. We must consider the processes of hybridization and indigenization in examining and understanding any form of cultural diffusion or globalization.

Antimodernism and Fundamentalism

Antimodernism is the rejection of the modern in favor of what is perceived as an earlier, purer, and better way of life. This viewpoint first arose out of disillusionment with the Industrial Revolution and with subsequent developments in science, technology, and consumption patterns. Antimodernists typically consider the use of modern technology to be misguided or think technology should have a lower priority than religious and cultural values. (A related example would be the avoidance of many machines by the Old Order Amish or Pennsylvania Dutch in the United States.)

Religious **fundamentalism** describes antimodernist movements in various religions, including Christianity, Islam, and Judaism (see Methenitis 2019). Not only do fundamentalists feel strongly alienated from modern secular culture, but they also have separated from a larger religious group, whose founding principles, they believe, have been corrupted or abandoned. Fundamentalists advocate return and strict fidelity to the "true" (fundamental) religious principles of the larger religion.

Exemplifying their antimodernism, fundamentalists also seek to rescue religion from absorption into modern, Western culture. In Christianity, fundamentalists are "born-again Christians" as opposed to "mainline Protestants." In Islam, they are *jama'at* (in Arabic, communities based on close fellowship) engaged in *jihad* (struggle) against a Western culture hostile to Islam and the God-given (*shariah*) way of life. In Judaism they are *Haredi*, "Torah-true" Jews. All these fundamentalists see a sharp divide between themselves and other religions, as well as between their own "sacred" view of life and the modern "secular" world (see Antoun 2008).

Both Pentecostalism and Christian fundamentalism preach ascetic morality, the duty to convert others, and respect for the Bible. Fundamentalists, however, tend to cite their success in living a moral life as proof of their salvation, whereas Pentecostals find assurance of their salvation in exuberant, ecstatic experience. Fundamentalists also seek to remake the political sphere along religious lines, whereas Pentecostals tend to have less interest in politics (Robbins 2004).

Recent Religious Radicalization

What motivates people to join militant groups like al Qaeda and the Islamic State (also known as IS, ISIS, ISIL, and Daesh)? The growth of such extremist groups is part of a process of political globalization that has accompanied economic globalization. Political globalization reflects the need, in a fragmented world, for some form of attachment to a larger community. Among those most likely to feel this need are displaced and alienated people. Among them are refugees, migrants, and marginalized groups—individuals who feel adrift and apart from, perhaps even despised by, the society or nation-state that surrounds them. One French militant whom anthropologist Scott Atran interviewed traced his radicalization to a childhood incident in which a Frenchman spat at his sister and called her a "dirty Arab" (Atran quoted in Reardon 2015).

Atran is the foremost anthropologist working on the topic of religious radicalization. He and his multinational team of researchers have interviewed members of radical movements in several countries, including members of ISIS in Kirkuk, Iraq, and potential members in Barcelona, Spain, and Paris, France. Atran's team also worked in Casablanca, Morocco, in two neighborhoods sympathetic to militant jihad. One of those neighborhoods had produced five of the seven 2004 Madrid train bombers. The other had sent dozens of volunteers, including suicide bombers, to Iraq and Syria. The researchers got to know the families and friends of the militants, learning how they lived and gaining insight into their beliefs.

Atran characterizes militants and terrorists as "devoted actors" (Atran 2016; Atran et al.

antimodernism
Rejecting the modern for a presumed earlier, purer, better way of life.

fundamentalism
Advocating strict fidelity to a religion's presumed founding principles.

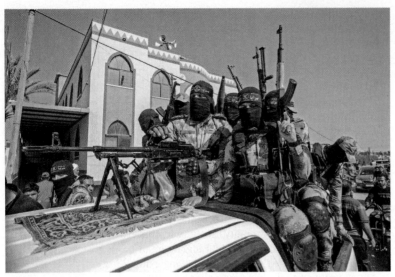

Devoted actors? Palestinian Islamic Jihad militants en route to the funeral of a comrade in the southern Gaza Strip on November 14, 2019. A ceasefire between Israel and Palestinian militants took hold that day after two days of fighting triggered by an Israeli strike that left 34 Palestinians dead.

Said Khatib/Getty Images

2014)—individuals who are willing to kill and die for values and beliefs they consider to be sacred and unquestionable. One key value of ISIS has been the need to establish a caliphate ruled by sharia law and led by a successor to the prophet Mohammed. Devoted actors will sacrifice themselves, their families, and all else for their cause (Atran 2016). The researchers found that militants, almost always young men, tend to form groups of three to four like-minded friends who forge themselves into a family-like unit, becoming a "band of brothers" in arms, devoted to one another. Like members of a cult, they share a collective sense of righteousness and special destiny. As potential martyrs, they require strong inspiration. Their commitment to a common cause, combined with family-like relationships, provides that inspiration.

These militant groups are not part of an organized global network based on top-down control. Rather, they tend to be decentralized and self-organizing. Such locally dispersed groups can, however, connect via the Internet to form a larger community of alienated youth seeking heroic sacrifice.

Although most recruits to ISIS and al Qaeda are Muslims, many have little prior knowledge of the religious teachings of Islam. What inspires them is not so much religious doctrine as the wish to pursue a thrilling cause—one that promises glory, esteem, respect, and remembrance. ISIS has even attracted "jihad tourists"—people who have visited Syria over school breaks or holidays seeking a brief adventure and then returned to their routine jobs in the West.

SECULAR RITUALS

In concluding this chapter on religion, we can recognize some problems with the definition of religion given at the beginning of this chapter. The first problem: If we define religion with reference to supernatural beings, powers, and forces, how do we classify ritual-like behavior that occurs in secular contexts? Some anthropologists believe there are both sacred and secular rituals. Secular rituals include formal, invariant, stereotyped, earnest, repetitive behavior and rites of passage that take place in nonreligious settings (see Bilgrami 2016).

A second problem: If the distinction between the supernatural and the natural is not consistently made in a society, how can we tell what is religion and what isn't? The Betsileo of Madagascar, for example, view witches and dead ancestors as real people who play roles in ordinary life. However, their occult powers are not empirically demonstrable.

A third problem: The behavior considered appropriate for religious occasions varies tremendously from culture to culture. One society may consider drunken frenzy the surest sign of faith, whereas another may encourage quiet reverence among the faithful. Who is to say which is "more religious"?

It is possible for apparently secular settings, things, and events to acquire intense meaning for individuals who have grown up in their presence. For example, identities and loyalties based on fandom, football, baseball, and soccer can be powerful, indeed. Rock stars and bands can mobilize many. Long overdue World Series wins led to celebrations across a "Red Sox Nation" in 2004 and among Cubs fans everywhere in 2016. Italians and Brazilians are rarely, if ever, as unified, nationally and emotionally, as they are when their teams are competing in the World Cup. The collective effervescence that Durkheim found so characteristic of religion can equally well describe what Brazilians experience when their country wins a World Cup.

In the context of comparative religion, the idea that the secular can become sacred isn't surprising. Long ago, Durkheim (1912/2001) pointed out that almost everything, from the sublime to the ridiculous, has in some societies been treated as sacred. The distinction between sacred and profane doesn't depend on the intrinsic qualities of the sacred symbol. In Australian totemic religion, for example, sacred beings include such humble creatures as ducks, frogs, and grubs, whose inherent qualities could hardly have given rise to the religious sentiment they inspire.

Many Americans believe that recreation and religion are separate domains. From my fieldwork in Brazil and Madagascar and my reading about other societies, I believe that this separation is

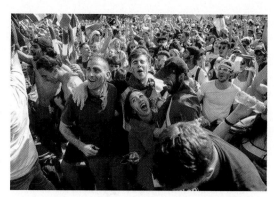 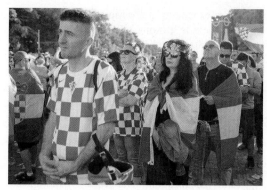

The thrill of victory and the agony of defeat: (Left) Football (soccer) fans in Paris celebrate as France scores its first goal against Croatia in the FIFA 2018 World Cup Final match (July 15, 2018). (Right) Croatian fans react to their team's loss in the same game. How is fandom similar to religion?

Left: Jack Taylor/Getty Images; right: Gregor Fischer/Getty Images

both ethnocentric and false. Madagascar's tomb-centered ceremonies are times when the living and the dead are joyously reunited, when people get drunk, gorge themselves, and enjoy sexual license.

Perhaps the gray, sober, ascetic, and moralistic aspects of many religious events in the United States, in taking the "fun" out of religion, force us to find our religion in fun.

for REVIEW

1. Religion, a cultural universal, consists of belief and behavior concerned with supernatural beings, powers, and forces. Religion also encompasses the feelings, meanings, and congregations associated with such beliefs and behavior. Anthropological studies have revealed many aspects and functions of religion.

2. Tylor considered animism—the belief in spirits or souls—to be religion's earliest and most basic form. He focused on religion's explanatory role, arguing that religion would eventually disappear as science provided better explanations. Besides animism, yet another view of the supernatural occurs in nonindustrial societies. This sees the supernatural as a domain of raw, impersonal power or force (called mana in Polynesia and Melanesia). People can manipulate and control mana under certain conditions.

3. When ordinary technical and rational means of doing things fail, people may turn to magic. Often they use magic when they lack control over outcomes. Religion offers comfort and psychological security at times of crisis. However, rites also can create anxiety. Rituals are formal, invariant, stylized, earnest acts in which people subordinate their particular beliefs to a social collectivity. Rites of passage have three phases:

separation, liminality, and incorporation. Such rites can mark any change in social status, age, place, or social condition. Collective rites often are cemented by communitas, a feeling of intense solidarity.

4. Besides their psychological and social functions, religious beliefs and practices play a role in the adaptation of human populations to their environments. The Hindu doctrine of *ahimsa*, which prohibits harm to living things, makes cattle sacred and beef a tabooed food. The taboo's force stops peasants from killing their draft cattle, even in times of extreme need.

5. Religion establishes and maintains social control through a series of moral and ethical beliefs, and real and imagined rewards and punishments, internalized in individuals. Religion also achieves social control by mobilizing its members for collective action. Religion helps maintain social order, but it also can promote change. Revitalization movements blend old and new beliefs and have helped people adapt to changing conditions.

6. Protestant values have been important in the United States, as they were in the rise and spread of capitalism in Europe. The world's major religions vary in their growth rates, with

summary

Islam expanding more rapidly than Christianity. There is growing religious diversity in the United States and Canada. Religious trends in contemporary North America include religious diversification, declining affiliation with organized religions, rising secularism, and new religions, some inspired by science and technology, some by spiritism. There are secular as well as religious rituals.

7. The spread of Evangelical/Pentecostal Protestantism worldwide illustrates contemporary cultural globalization. Evangelical Protestantism stresses conservative morality, the authority of the Bible, and a personal ("born-again") conversion experience. To people who feel socially adrift, Pentecostalism offers tightly knit communities and a weblike structure of personal connections. The rapid spread of Islam also illustrates cultural globalization and hybridization. Although certain core features endure, local people always assign their own meanings to the messages and social forms they receive from outside, including religion.

8. Antimodernism is the rejection of the modern, including globalization, in favor of what is perceived as an earlier, purer, and better way of life. Religious fundamentalism describes antimodernist movements in Christianity, Islam, and Judaism. Militant extremism in the name of religion also appeals to people, primarily young men, who feel alienated from, or despised by, the society that surrounds them. These radicals form "bands of brothers" united by common values and willing to kill and die for a cause.

key terms

animism 240

antimodernism 255

cargo cults 250

communitas 244

cosmology 246

fundamentalism 255

liminality 243

magic 241

mana 241

monotheism 240

polytheism 240

religion 238

revitalization movements 250

rites of passage 243

ritual 242

shaman 248

syncretisms 251

taboo 241

totem 244

think like an anthropologist

1. How did anthropologist Anthony Wallace define religion? After reading this chapter, what problems do you think there are with his definition?
2. Describe a rite of passage you (or a friend) have been through. How did it fit the three-phase model given in the text?
3. From the news or your own knowledge, can you provide additional examples of revitalization movements, new religions, or liminal cults?
4. Religion is a cultural universal. But religions are parts of particular cultures, and cultural differences show up systematically in religious beliefs and practices. How so?
5. This chapter notes that many Americans see recreation and religion as separate domains. Based on my fieldwork in Brazil and Madagascar and my reading about other societies, I believe that this separation is both ethnocentric and false. Do you agree with this? What has been your own experience?

credits

Arts, Media, and Sports

▶ What are the arts, and how have they varied historically and cross-culturally?

▶ How does culture influence the media, and vice versa?

▶ How are culture and cultural contrasts expressed in sports?

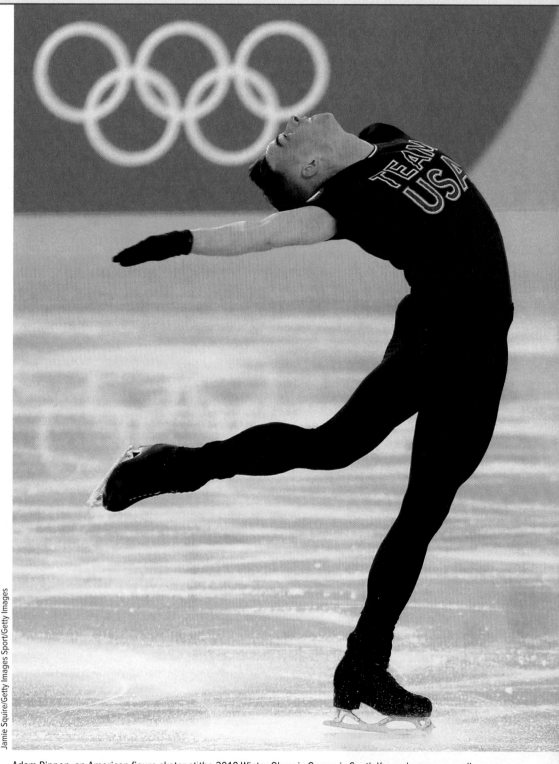

Jamie Squire/Getty Images Sport/Getty Images

Adam Rippon, an American figure skater at the 2018 Winter Olympic Games in South Korea, became a media favorite, based on his skill, artistry, and personality.

understanding OURSELVES

Imagine a TV series attracting over 50 percent of a nation's viewers. That has happened repeatedly in Brazil as a popular telenovela draws to a close. (Telenovelas are prime-time serial melodramas that run for about 150 episodes.) It happened in the United States in 1953, when 72 percent of all sets were tuned to *I Love Lucy* as Lucy Ricardo went to the hospital to give birth to Little Ricky. It happened even more impressively in 1956, when 83 percent of all sets tuned to *The Ed Sullivan Show* to watch Elvis Presley's TV debut. A single broadcast's largest audience share in more recent years occurred in 1983, when 106 million viewers, representing an audience share of 77 percent, watched the final episode of *M*A*S*H*.

The media, of course, have honed Americans' interest in sports. Football, in particular, is a powerful viewing magnet. In the 21st century, eight successive Super Bowls (2010–2017) topped the viewership, but never the audience share, of the *M*A*S*H* finale. The 2015 Super Bowl (XLIX) between Seattle and New England set an as-yet unbroken record, with 114.4 million viewers, but the half-time show that year, starring Katy Perry, did even better, attracting 118.5 million viewers. That Super Bowl also drew a 71 audience share, which means that 71 percent of people who were watching TV that Sunday were watching the Super Bowl. After 2017, Super Bowl viewership declined, with the 2018, 2020, and 2019 games (in that order) all trailing the *M*A*S*H* finale. Still, 29 of the 30 most watched broadcasts ever on American TV have been Super Bowls.

One notable development in the United States over the past few decades has been a shift from mass culture to segmented cultures. An increasingly differentiated nation recognizes and caters to diversity. The mass media and marketing join—and intensify—this trend, measuring and addressing various "demographics." Products and messages are aimed less at the masses than at particular segments—target audiences.

As one example, consider the evolution of sports coverage. From 1961 to 1998, ABC offered a weekly sports anthology titled *Wide World of Sports*. On a given Saturday afternoon, Americans might see bowling, track and field, skating, college wrestling, gymnastics, curling, swimming, diving, or another of many sports. It was like having a mini-Olympics running throughout the year. Today, dozens of specialized (often pay-for-view) sports channels cater to every taste, including Major League Baseball, the National Football League, golf, and international soccer. Think of the choices now available through WiFi, cable and satellite, smartphones, tablets, DVRs, the remote control, and myriad apps and websites. Target audiences have access to a multiplicity of channels, featuring all kinds of music, sports, games, news, comedy, science fiction, soaps, movies, cartoons, old TV sitcoms, programs in Spanish and various other languages, nature shows, travel shows, adventure shows, histories, biographies, and home shopping. News channels (e.g., Fox News or MSNBC) even cater to particular political interests.

It seems likely there is a connection between these media developments and the "special interests" and "divisiveness" about which politicians perpetually complain. Do you think people might agree more—and Americans be less polarized—if everyone still watched the same TV programs?

WHAT ARE THE ARTS?

For most of us, the media, which include print, radio, TV, digital media, the Internet, and everything they convey, provide access to a wide world of performance and storytelling as well as information. We rely on the media for much of our access to sports and various arts. The **arts** include music, performance arts, visual arts, storytelling, and literature (oral and written, poetry and prose). These manifestations of human creativity sometimes are called **expressive culture.** People express themselves in dance, music, song, painting, sculpture, pottery, cloth, storytelling, verse, prose, drama, and comedy. When we watch *Game of Thrones, Stranger Things,* and even *SpongeBob SquarePants,* we are experiencing scripted, visual, performed storytelling, usually enhanced by music. The efforts and competitions that comprise sports are not just played; they also are staged, managed, and performed.

Many cultures lack terms that can be translated easily as "art" or "the arts." Yet even without a word for art, people everywhere do associate an aesthetic experience—a sense of beauty, appreciation, harmony, and pleasure—with sounds, patterns, objects, and events that have certain qualities (see Bertram 2019; Garcia Canclini 2014; Laine 2018). Among the Yoruba of Nigeria, the word for art, *ona,* encompasses the designs made on objects, the art objects themselves, and the profession of the creators of those works. For two Yoruba lineages of leather workers, Otunisona and Osiisona, the suffix *-ona* in their names denotes art (Abiodun 2014; Adepegba 1991).

A dictionary defines **art** as "the quality, production, expression, or realm of what is beautiful or of more than ordinary significance; the class of objects subject to aesthetic criteria" (*Random House College Dictionary* 1982, p. 76). According to the same dictionary, **aesthetics** involves "the qualities perceived in works of art . . . in relation to the sense of beauty" (p. 22). A more recent definition sees art as "something that is created with imagination and skill and that is beautiful or that expresses important ideas or feelings" (*Merriam-Webster* 2016). We know, however, that a work of art can attract attention, have special significance, and demonstrate imagination and skill without being considered beautiful. Pablo Picasso's *Guernica,* a famous painting of the Spanish Civil War, comes to mind as a scene that, while not beautiful, is indisputably moving and thus a work of art.

In many societies, art isn't viewed as a separate, special activity. But this doesn't stop individuals from being moved by sounds, patterns, objects, and events in a way that we would call aesthetic. Our own society provides a fairly well-defined role for the connoisseur of the arts (see Fillitz and van der Grijp 2017). We also have sanctuaries—concert halls, theaters, and museums—where people go to appreciate performances, representations, objects, and displays (see Burt 2013).

art
An object, event, or other expressive form that evokes an aesthetic reaction.

aesthetics
The appreciation of qualities perceived in art.

arts
For example, music, performance arts, visual arts, storytelling, and literature (written and oral).

expressive culture
A term used to describe manifestations of human creativity, such as dance, music, painting, sculpture, pottery, cloth, stories, drama, and comedy.

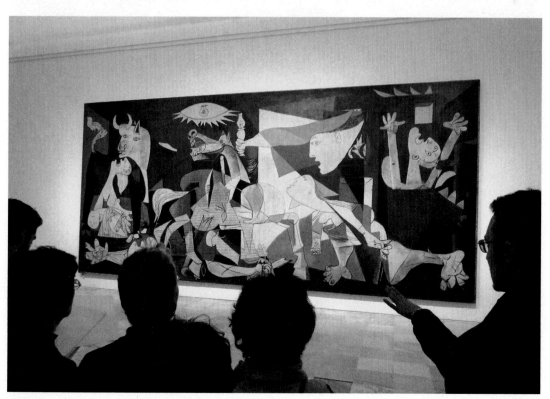

Onlookers learn about Pablo Picasso's painting *Guernica* at the Reina Sofia museum in Madrid.
Cristina Quicler/AFP/Getty Images

Western culture tends to compartmentalize art as something apart from everyday life. This reflects a more general modern separation of institutions like government and the economy from the rest of society. All these fields are treated as distinct domains, with their own personnel and academic specialists. In non-Western societies, however, the production and appreciation of art are part of everyday life, just as popular culture is in our own society.

This chapter will not attempt to provide a systematic survey of all the arts. Rather, the general approach will be to examine topics and issues that apply to expressive culture and performances generally. The term *art* will be used to encompass all the arts, including print and film narratives. In other words, the observations to be made about art are intended to apply to music, theater, film, television, books, stories, and lore, as well as to painting and sculpture. Expressive culture also encompasses such creative forms as jokes, storytelling, dance, children's play, sports, games, and festivals. Anthropologists have written about all of these.

That which is aesthetically pleasing is perceived by the senses. Usually, when we think of art, we have in mind something that can be seen or heard. But others might define art more broadly to include things that can be smelled (scents, fragrances), tasted (recipes), or touched (cloth textures). How enduring must art be? Architecture, visual works, and written compositions, including music, may last for centuries. Can a single noteworthy event, such as a feast, which is not in the least eternal, except in memory, be a work of art? How about a single culinary creation, such as an elaborate wedding cake, or even a pizza? An individual performance, whether in a theater or at a sporting event, can be called "a thing of beauty." Nowadays, such performances often are captured on film; otherwise, they would be as ephemeral as a "feast fit for a king."

Art and Religion

Some of the issues raised in the discussion of religion in Chapter 12 also apply to the arts. Definitions of both art and religion mention the "more than ordinary" or the "extraordinary." Religious scholars may distinguish between the sacred (religious) and the profane (secular). Similarly, art scholars may distinguish between the artistic and the ordinary.

If we adopt a special attitude or demeanor when confronting a sacred object, do we display something similar when experiencing a work of art? According to the anthropologist Jacques Maquet (1986), an artwork is something that stimulates

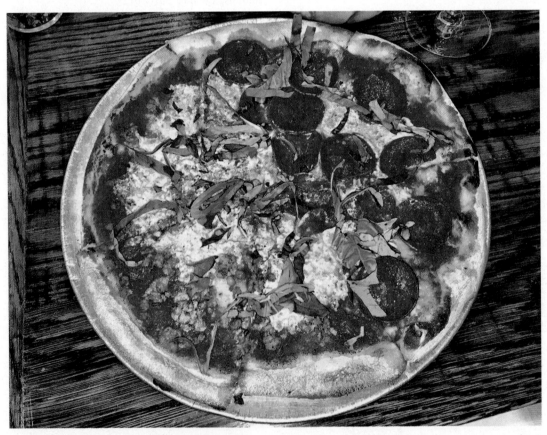

Can a pizza be a work or art? What could make it so?

Conrad P. Kottak

and sustains contemplation. It compels attention and reflection. *Guernica,* although unbeautiful, certainly meets these criteria. Maquet stresses the importance of the object's form in producing such contemplation. But other scholars stress feeling and meaning in addition to form. The experience of art involves feelings, such as being moved, as well as appreciation of form, such as balance or harmony.

Such an artistic attitude can be combined with and used to bolster a religious attitude. Many of the high points of Western art and music had religious inspiration, or were done in the service of religion, as a visit to a church or a large museum will surely illustrate. Bach and Handel are as well known for their church music as Michelangelo is for his religious painting and sculpture. The buildings (churches and cathedrals) in which religious music is played and in which visual art is displayed may themselves be works of art. Some of the major architectural achievements of Western art are religious structures (see Lucas 2020; Yaneva 2020).

Art may be created, performed, or displayed outdoors in public or in special indoor settings. Just as churches demarcate religion, museums and theaters set art off from the ordinary world, making it special, while inviting spectators in. Buildings dedicated to the arts help create the artistic atmosphere. Architecture may accentuate the setting as a place for works of art to be presented (see Ingold 2013).

The settings of rites and ceremonies, and of art, may be temporary or permanent. State societies have permanent religious structures: churches and temples. So, too, may state societies have buildings and structures dedicated to the arts. Nonstate societies tend to lack such permanently demarcated settings. Both art and religion are more "out there" in society. Still, in bands and tribes, religious settings can be created without churches. Similarly, an artistic atmosphere can be created without museums. At particular times of the year, ordinary space can be set aside for a visual art display or a musical performance. Such special occasions parallel the times set aside for religious ceremonies. In fact, in tribal performances, the arts and religion often mix. For example, masked and costumed performers may imitate spirits. Rites of passage often feature special music, dance, song, bodily adornment, and other manifestations of expressive culture.

Among tribes of the North Pacific Coast of North America, various art forms combined to create a ceremonial atmosphere. Masked and costumed dancers reenacted spirit encounters with human beings, which

are part of the origin myths of villages, clans, and lineages. Sometimes, dancers devised intricate patterns of choreography. Their esteem was measured by the number of people who followed them when they danced.

Non-Western art is often, but wrongly, assumed to have an inevitable connection to ritual. In fact, non-Western societies have art for art's sake, just as Western societies do. Even when acting in the service of religion, there is room for individual creative expression (see Osborne and Tanner 2007). In the oral arts, for example, the audience is much more interested in the delivery and performance of the artist than in the particular god for whom the performer may be speaking.

Locating Art

Aesthetic value is one way of distinguishing art. Another way is to consider placement. If something is displayed in a museum, someone must think it's art. Although tribal societies lack museums, they may have special areas where artistic expression takes place. The Tiwi of North Australia, for example, traditionally commissioned the manufacture of commemorative burial poles after a death. The pole artists were sequestered in a work area near the grave. That area was taboo to everyone else. The artists were freed temporarily from the daily food quest. Other community members served as their patrons, supplying the artists with the hard-to-get materials needed for their work (Goodale and Koss 1971).

The boundary between what's art and what's not isn't always sharp. The American artist Andy

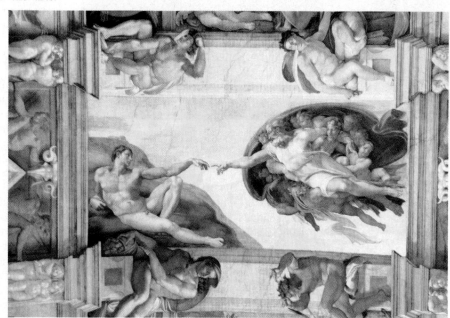

Many of the high points of Western art had religious inspiration or were done in the service of religion. Consider *The Creation of Adam* (and other frescoes painted from 1508 to 1512) by Michelangelo, on the ceiling of the Sistine Chapel in Vatican City, Rome, Italy.
Alex Segre/Alamy Stock Photo

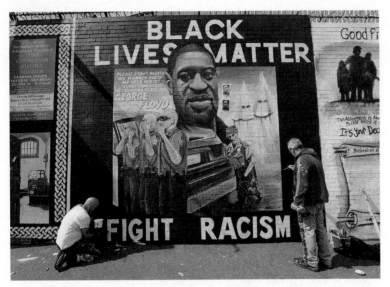

The transformation of urban space into art: Artists Lyonsie (Marty Lyons – left) and Micky Doc (Micky Doherty – right) apply finishing touches to a mural commemorating George Floyd on the International Wall in Belfast, Northern Ireland. The mural offers a portrait of the 46-year-old African-American, whose killing by Minneapolis police sparked protests and demonstrations across the U. S. and globally.

Brian Lawless//Getty Images

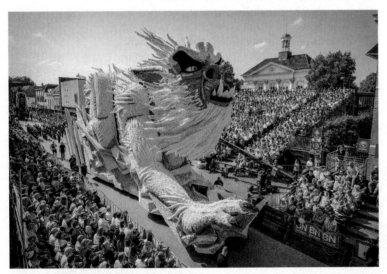

Zundert, a small town in the southern Netherlands, hosts an annual flower parade festival. The event takes over the streets with gigantic floats, all made with flowers. Shown here is "The Last Yeti" float during the 2018 parade. Is a float a work of art?

Nacho Calonge/Getty Images

Warhol is famous for transforming Campbell's soup cans, Brillo pads, and images of Marilyn Monroe into art. Many recent artists have tried to erase the distinction between art and ordinary life by converting the everyday into a work of art. Objects never intended as art, such as an Olivetti typewriter, may be transformed into art by being placed in a museum, such as New York's Museum of Modern Art. Jacques Maquet (1986) distinguishes such "art by transformation" from art created and intended to be art, which he calls "art by destination."

In state societies, we have come to rely on critics, judges, and experts to tell us what's art and what isn't. A play titled *Art* is about conflict that arises among three friends when one of them buys an all-white painting. They disagree, as people often do, about the definition and value of a work of art. Such variation in art appreciation is especially common in contemporary society, with its professional artists and critics and great cultural diversity. We'd expect more uniform standards and agreement in less diverse, less stratified societies.

We should avoid applying our own standards about what art is to the products of other cultures. Sculpture is art, right? Not necessarily. Previously, we challenged the view that non–Western art always has some kind of connection to religion. The Kalabari case to be discussed now makes the opposite point: that religious sculpture is not always art.

The Kalabari of southern Nigeria (Figure 13.1) carve wooden sculptures for religious, rather than aesthetic, reasons. They produce these sculptures not as works of art, but to serve as "houses" for spirits (Horton 1963). The sculptures will be placed in a cult house, where the spirits can dwell in them. Kalabari sculptures are created to manipulate and control spirits. The Kalabari do have standards for the carvings, but those standards are not aesthetic; beauty is not a goal. What is required is that a sculpture must be sufficiently complete to represent its spirit, and carvers must base their work on past models. Each spirit has a known image associated with it, and it's risky to deviate too much from that image. Offended spirits may retaliate. As long as they observe these standards of completeness and established images, carvers are free to express themselves. But these images are considered repulsive rather than beautiful.

Art and Individuality

Discussions of Western art tend to emphasize *individual* artistic production, whereas those who work with non–Western art have been criticized for ignoring the individual artist and focusing too much on the social nature and context of art. When art objects from Africa or Papua New Guinea are displayed in museums, often only the name of the tribe and of the Western donor are given, rather than that of the artist. This kind of presentation can create the impression that art is produced collectively, rather than by an individual. Sometimes it is; sometimes it isn't.

To some extent, there *is* more collective production of art in non–Western societies. In a tribal setting, an artist usually gets more feedback during the creative process than is the case in our own society. In Western societies, the feedback often comes too late, after the product is complete, rather than during production, when it can still be changed. During his fieldwork among Nigeria's Tiv people, Paul Bohannan (1971) found only a

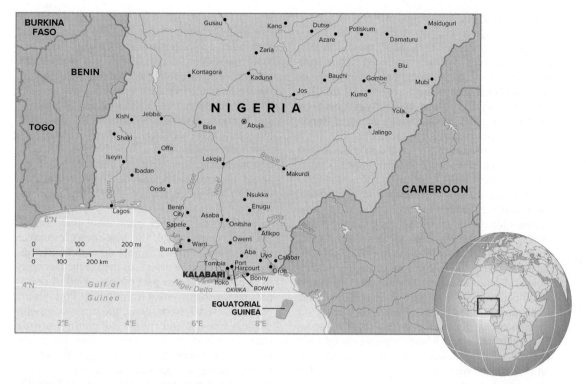

FIGURE 13.1 Location of the Kalabari of Nigeria.

few skilled artists, and those individuals preferred to work in private. Mediocre artists, however, typically worked in public, where they routinely got comments from onlookers (critics). Based on suggestions, an artist might change a design, such as a carving, in progress. There was yet another way in which Tiv artists worked socially rather than individually. Sometimes, when artists put their work aside, someone else would pick it up and start working on it. The Tiv did not recognize the same kind of connection between individuals and their art that we do.

Even in more modern societies, however, artistic creation can be an open and responsive process. Consider the production of Brazilian telenovelas (mentioned in this chapter's "Understanding Ourselves"). As a telenovela progresses, writer(s) typically pay close attention to audience reaction, measured in various ways, from surveys to informal conversations in such locales as beauty salons and other places where people congregate and have the Brazilian equivalent of "water-cooler conversations." Writers then modify, or even change the direction of, a telenovela in view of audience response.

The Tiv example notwithstanding, there *are* well-known individual artists in many non-Western societies. They are recognized as such by other community members, and perhaps by outsiders as well. Their artistic labor may even be conscripted for special displays and performances, including ceremonies, or palace arts and events (see Schneider 2017; Schneider and Wright 2013).

In Western societies, focus on the individual artist is common, even in collective displays and performances, where, for example, a conductor may be as well, or better, known than the orchestra. Haapala (1998) argues that an artist and his or her works become inseparable: "By creating works of art a person creates an artistic identity for himself. He creates himself quite literally into the pieces he puts into his art. He exists in the works he has created." In this view, Picasso created many Picassos, and he continues to exist in and through those works, as do William Shakespeare, Jane Austen, and Meryl Streep.

Sometimes, even in Western societies, little is known or recognized about the individual artist responsible for an enduring artwork. We are more likely, for example, to know the name of the recording artist than that of the writer of familiar songs. Sometimes we fail to acknowledge art individually because the artwork was created collectively. To whom should we attribute a pyramid or a cathedral? Should it be the architect, the ruler or leader who commissioned the work, or the master builder who implemented the design?

The Work of Art

The word *opera* is the plural of *opus,* which means a work. For the artist, at least, art is work, albeit creative work. In nonstate societies, artists may have to hunt, gather, herd, fish, or farm in order to eat, but they still manage to find time to work on their art. In state societies, artists are more typically specialists—professionals who have chosen careers as artists, musicians, writers, or actors. If they manage to support themselves from their art, they may be full-time professionals. If not, they do their art part-time while earning a living from another activity. Sometimes artists associate in professional groups, such as medieval guilds or contemporary unions. Actors Equity in New York, a labor union, is a modern guild, designed to protect the interests of its artist members.

Just how much work is needed to make a work of art? In the early days of French impressionism, many experts viewed the paintings of Claude Monet and his colleagues as too sketchy and spontaneous to be true art. Established artists and critics were accustomed to more formal and classic studio styles. The French impressionists got their name from their sketches—*impressions* in French—of natural and social settings. They took advantage of technological innovations, particularly the availability of oil paints in tubes, to take their palettes, easels, and canvases into the field. There they made the pictures of changing light and color that hang today in so many museums, where they are now fully recognized as art. But before impressionism became an officially recognized "school" of art, its critics perceived such works as crude and unfinished.

For familiar genres, such as painting or music, societies tend to have standards by which they judge whether an artwork is complete or fully realized. Most people would doubt, for instance, that an all-white painting could be a work of art. Prevailing standards may pose obstacles to unorthodox or renegade artists and, thus, to innovation. But like the impressionists, such artists may eventually succeed. Some societies tend to reward conformity, an artist's skill with traditional models and techniques. Others encourage breaks with the past, innovation. Standards may be maintained informally in society, or by specialists, such as art critics.

An interesting feature of contemporary society is that we have all become potential critics. Through the Internet, ordinary individuals are able to express their opinions about a huge variety of topics, including arts, media, and sports. Websites that provide information about movies, for example, now include viewers' comments and reviews, as well as those of "professional critics." Criticism is no longer reserved for the elites, whose opinions may vary significantly from those of "ordinary people" or "viewers like you." A common American expression is "that's just your opinion"—suggesting that anyone's opinion is as valid as anyone else's. The Internet provides an open forum in which to air such opinions by anyone wishing to post online.

ART, SOCIETY, AND CULTURE

Around 100,000 years ago, some of the world's first artists occupied Blombos Cave, located on a cliff facing the Indian Ocean at the tip of what is now South Africa. They hunted game and ate fish from the waters below them. In terms of body and brain size, these ancient Africans were anatomically modern humans. They also were turning animal bones into finely worked tools and weapon points. Furthermore, they were engraving artifacts with symbolic marks—manifestations of abstract and creative thought (Wilford 2002b). The most impressive bone tools are three sharp instruments. The bone appears first to have been shaped with a stone blade, then finished into a symmetrical shape and polished for hours. These ancient cave dwellers also processed red ocher, presumably for body painting.

In Europe, art goes back more than 30,000 years. Cave paintings, the best-known examples of Upper Paleolithic art, were done in true caves, located deep in the bowels of the Earth. They may have been painted as part of some kind of rite of passage involving retreat from society. Portable art objects carved in stone, bone, and ivory, along with musical whistles and flutes, also confirm artistic expression throughout the Upper Paleolithic (see Insoll 2017; Lesure 2011). The Upper Paleolithic cave paintings are unusual because of their inaccessibility. Art usually is more public. Typically, it is exhibited, evaluated, performed, and appreciated in society. It has spectators or audiences. It isn't just for the artist or the gods (see Pink and Abram 2015).

Ethnomusicology

Ethnomusicology is the comparative study of the musics of the world and of music as an aspect of culture and society. The field of ethnomusicology thus unites music and anthropology. The music side involves the study and analysis of the music itself and the instruments used to create it. The anthropology side views music as a way to explore a culture, to determine the role that music plays in that society, and the specific social and cultural features that influence how music is created and performed.

Ethnomusicology studies non-Western music, traditional and folk music, and even contemporary popular music from a cultural perspective (see Harris and Pease 2015; Rice 2014; Wade 2013). To do this there has to be fieldwork—firsthand study of particular forms of music, their social functions and cultural meanings, within particular societies. Ethnomusicologists talk with local musicians, make recordings in the field, and learn about the place of musical instruments, performances, and performers in a given society (Kirman 1997). Nowadays, given globalization, diverse cultures and musical styles easily meet and mix (Cicchelli et al. 2020). Music that draws on a wide range of cultural instruments and styles is called World Fusion, World Beat, or World Music—another topic within contemporary ethnomusicology (see Rommen et al. 2020; Wade 2020).

ethnomusicology The comparative study of the musics of the world and of music as an aspect of culture and society.

Because music is a cultural universal, and because musical abilities seem to run in families, it has been suggested that a predisposition for music may have a genetic basis (Crenson 2000). Could a "music gene" that arose tens, or hundreds, of thousands of years ago have conferred an evolutionary advantage on those early humans who possessed it? The fact that music has existed in all known cultures suggests that it arose early in human history. Providing direct evidence for music's antiquity is an ancient carved bone flute from a cave in Slovenia. This "Divje Babe flute," the world's oldest known musical instrument, dates back more than 43,000 years.

Exploring the possible biological roots of music, Sandra Trehub (2001) noted striking similarities in the way mothers worldwide sing to their children—with a high pitch, a slow tempo, and a distinctive tone. All cultures have lullabies, which sound so much alike they cannot be mistaken for anything else (Crenson 2000). Trehub speculates that music might have been adaptive in human evolution because musically talented mothers had an easier time calming their babies. Calm babies who fell asleep easily and rarely made a fuss might have been more likely to survive to adulthood. Their cries would not attract predators; they and their mothers would get more rest; and they would be less likely to be mistreated. If a gene conferring musical ability appeared early in human evolution, given a selective advantage, musical adults would pass their genes to their children.

Music is among the most social of the arts, because it typically unites people in groups, such as choirs, symphonies, ensembles, and bands. Could it be that early humans with a biological

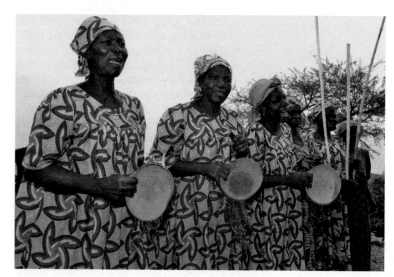

Music is among the most social of the arts, because it so often unites people in groups. Shown here, women in the village of Rhumsiki, Cameroon, Central Africa, offer a folkloristic musical performance.
imageBROKER/Alamy Stock Photo

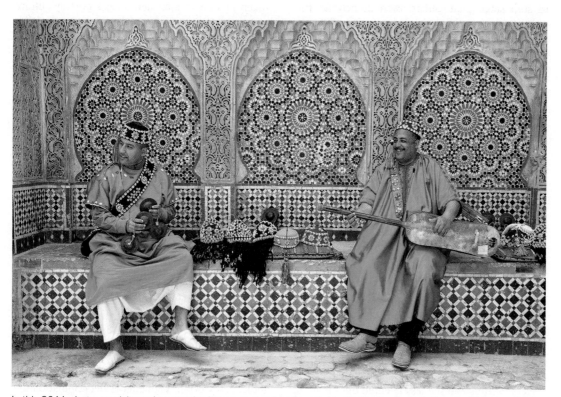

In this 2011 photo, musicians play carcaba (iron castanets) and gambri (guitar) in the Kasbah, Tangier, Morocco. For whose pleasure do you suppose this performance is being given? Nowadays, such performances attract tourists as well as local people.

Nico Tondini/Robert Harding World Imagery/Corbis

folk

Of the people; e.g., the art, music, and lore of ordinary people.

penchant for music were able to live more effectively in social groups—another possible adaptive advantage?

Originally coined for European peasants, **folk** art, music, and lore are the expressive culture of ordinary people, as contrasted with the "high" art, or "classic" art, of the European elites. When folk music is performed, the combination of costumes, music, and often song and dance is supposed to say something about local culture and about tradition. Tourists and other outsiders often perceive rural and folk life mainly in terms of such performances. Community residents themselves often use such performances to display and enact their local culture and traditions for outsiders.

In Planinica, a Muslim village in (prewar) Bosnia, Yvonne Lockwood (1983) studied folksong, which could be heard there day or night. The most active singers were unmarried females aged 16 to 26 (maidens). The social transition from girl to maiden (marriageable female) was signaled by active participation in public song and dance. Adolescent girls were urged to sing along with women and performing maidens. This was part of a rite of passage by which a little girl (*dite*) became a maiden (*cura*). Marriage, in contrast, moved most women from the public to the private sphere; public singing generally stopped. Married women sang in their own homes or among other women. Only occasionally would they join maidens in public song. After age 50, wives tended to stop singing altogether, even in private. For women, singing thus signaled a series of transitions between age grades: girl to maiden (public singing), maiden to wife (private singing), and wife to elder (no more singing).

Singing and dancing were common at Bosnian *prelos* attended by males and females. In Planinica, the Serbo-Croatian word *prelo*, usually defined as "spinning bee," meant any occasion for visiting. *Prelos* were especially common in winter. During the summer, villagers worked long hours, and *prelos* were few. The *prelo* offered a context for play, relaxation, song, and dance. All gatherings of maidens, especially *prelos*, were occasions for song. Married women encouraged them to sing, often suggesting specific songs. If males were also present, a singing duel might occur, in which maidens and young men teased each other. A successful *prelo* was well attended, with much singing and dancing.

Public singing was traditional in many other contexts among prewar Bosnian Muslims. After a day of cutting hay on mountain slopes, parties of village men would congregate at a specific place on the trail above the village. They formed lines according to their singing ability, with the best singers in front and the less talented ones behind. They proceeded to stroll down to the village together, singing as they went, until they reached the village center, where they dispersed. According to Lockwood, whenever an activity brought together a group of maidens or young men, it usually would end with public singing. The inspiration for parts of *Snow White* and *Shrek* (the movies) can be traced back to such customs of the European countryside.

Representations of Art and Culture

The creative products and images of folk, rural, and non-Western cultures are increasingly spread—and commercialized—by the media and tourism (see Wilkinson-Weber and DeNicola 2016). A result is that many Westerners have come to think of "culture" in terms of colorful customs, music, dancing, and adornments: clothing, jewelry, and hairstyles. A bias toward the arts and religion, rather than the more mundane economic and social aspects of culture, shows up on TV's Discovery Channel, and even in many anthropological films (see Grimshaw and Ravetz 2009; Schneider and Pasqualino 2014; Vannini 2020). Many ethnographic films start off with music, often drumbeats: "Bonga, bonga, bonga, bonga. Here in [whatever the place or society being depicted], the people are very religious." Such presentations just reinforce the previously critiqued assumption that the arts of nonindustrial societies are always linked to religion. This may create a false impression that non-Western peoples spend much of their time wearing colorful clothes, singing, dancing, and practicing religious rituals. Taken to an extreme, such images portray culture as recreational and ultimately not serious, rather than as something that ordinary people live every day of their lives—not just when they have festivals.

Art and Communication

Art also functions as a form of communication between artist and community or audience. Sometimes, however, there are intermediaries between the artist and the audience. Actors, for example, translate the works and ideas of other artists (writers and directors) into performances. Musicians play and sing compositions of other people along with music they themselves have composed. Using music written by others, choreographers plan and direct patterns of dance, which dancers then execute for audiences.

How does art communicate? We need to know what the artist intends to communicate and how the audience reacts. Often, the audience communicates right back to the artist. Live performers, for instance, get immediate feedback, as may writers and directors by viewing a performance of their own work. Contemporary artists, like businesspeople, are well aware that they have target audiences. Certain segments of the population are more likely to appreciate certain forms of art than are other segments.

Art can transmit several kinds of messages. It can convey a moral lesson or tell a cautionary tale.

It can teach lessons the artist, or society, wants told. Like the rites that induce, then dispel, anxiety, the tension and resolution of drama can lead to **catharsis,** intense emotional release, in the audience. Art can move emotions, make us laugh, cry, feel up or down. Art appeals to the intellect as well as to the emotions. We may delight in a well-constructed, nicely balanced, well-realized work of art.

Often, art is meant to commemorate and to last, to carry an enduring message. Like a ceremony, art may serve a mnemonic function, making people remember. Art may be designed to make people remember either individuals or events, such as the AIDS or COVID-19 pandemics or the cataclysmic events of September 11, 2001.

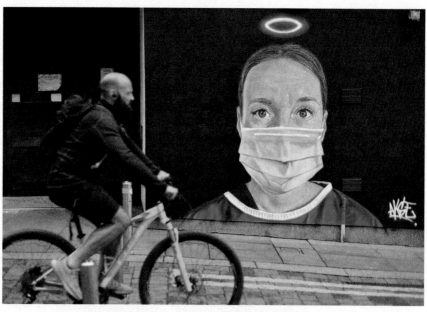

Coronavirus-inspired art: A man rides a bike past street art by the artist @akse_p19, depicting a nurse in scrubs and a face mask, but with an Angel's halo above her head, in Manchester, northern England, on June 3, 2020.
Paul Ellis/Getty Images

Art and Politics

To what extent should art serve society? Art can be self-consciously prosocial. It can be used to either express or challenge community sentiment and standards. Decisions about what counts as a work of art, or about how to display art, may be political and controversial. Museums have to balance concern over community standards with a wish to be as creative and innovative as the artists and works they display.

Much art that is valued today was received with revulsion in its own time. Children were prohibited from seeing paintings by Matisse, Braque, and Picasso when those works first were displayed in New York in the Armory Show of 1913. Almost a century later, the City of New York and then mayor Rudolph Giuliani took the Brooklyn Museum to court over its 1999–2000 "Sensation" exhibit. After religious groups protested Chris Ofili's *Holy Virgin Mary,* a collage that included elephant dung, Giuliani deemed the work sacrilegious. At the ensuing court trial, art advocates spoke out against the mayor's actions. The museum won the case, but Ofili's work again came under attack when a man smuggled paint inside the Brooklyn exhibition and tried to smear it on the *Virgin* (see Reyburn 2015). According to art professor Michael Davis, Ofili's collage is "shocking," because it deliberately provokes and intends to jolt viewers into an expanded frame of reference. The mayor's reactions may have been based on the narrow definition that art must be beautiful and an equally limited stereotype of a Virgin Mary as depicted in Italian Renaissance paintings.

Today, no museum director can mount an exhibit without worrying that it will offend some politically organized segment of society. In the United States there has been an ongoing battle

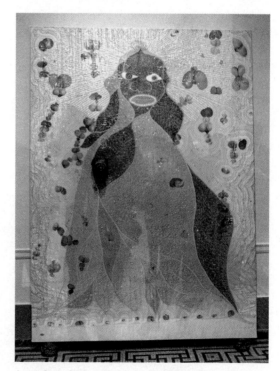

Artist Chris Ofili's controversial work The Holy Virgin Mary is seen in the Brooklyn Museum of Art as part of the 1999 Sensation exhibit in New York City. The work shows an African Virgin Mary covered with elephant dung.
Doug Kanter/AFP/Getty Images

between liberals and conservatives involving the National Endowment for the Arts. Artists have been criticized as being aloof from society, as creating only for themselves and for elites, as being

catharsis
Intense emotional release.

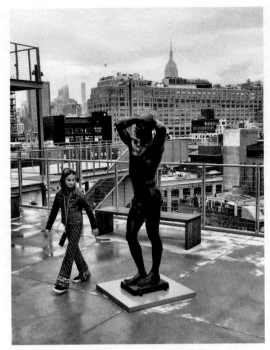

A girl glances at a male nude sculpture displayed outdoors at New York's Whitney Museum of American Art. Art appreciation must be learned, the earlier the better. How does the placement of art in museums, including this display at the Whitney, affect art appreciation?

Conrad P. Kottak

out of touch with conventional and traditional aesthetic values, and even as mocking the values of ordinary people.

The Cultural Transmission of the Arts

Appreciation of the arts reflects one's cultural background. Watch Japanese tourists try to interpret what they are seeing in a Western art museum. Conversely, the form and meaning of a Japanese tea ceremony, or a demonstration of origami (Japanese paper folding), will be alien to a foreign observer. Appreciation of the arts is learned, in particular cultural settings.

Music with certain tonalities and rhythm patterns pleases some people but alienates others. In a study of traditional Navajo music, McAllester (1954) found that it reflected the overall culture of that time in three main ways. First, individualism was a key Navajo cultural value: It was up to the individual to decide what to do with his or her songs. Second, the Navajo saw foreign music as dangerous and rejected it. (This second point is no longer true; there are now Navajo rock bands.) Third, a general stress on proper form applied to music. There was, in Navajo belief, a right way to sing every kind of song (see Figure 13.2 for the location of the Navajo).

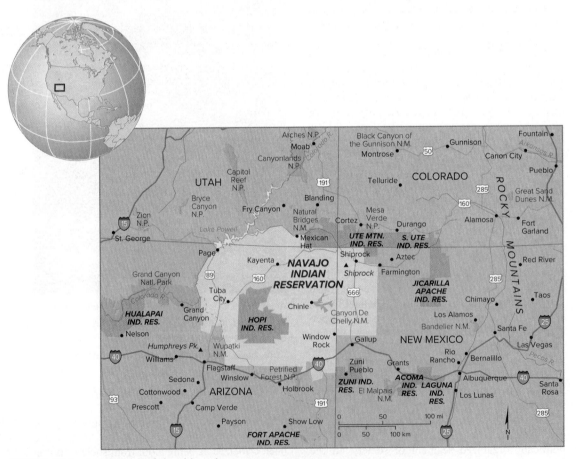

FIGURE 13.2 Location of the Navajo.

People learn to appreciate certain kinds of music and other art forms, just as they learn to hear and decipher a foreign language. Unlike Londoners and New Yorkers, Parisians don't flock to musicals. Despite its multiple French origins, even the musical *Les Misérables,* a huge hit in London, New York, and dozens of cities worldwide, bombed in Paris. Humor, too, a form of verbal art, depends on cultural background and setting. What's funny in one culture may not translate as funny in another. When a joke doesn't work, an American may say, "Well, you had to be there at the time." Jokes, like aesthetic judgments, depend on context.

Anthropology's approach to the arts contrasts with the traditional humanities' focus on "fine arts," as in art history, "Great Books," and classical music. Anthropology has extended the definition of "cultured" well beyond the elitist meaning of "high" art and culture (see Sansi-Roca 2015). For anthropologists, everyone acquires culture through enculturation. In academia today, growing acceptance of the anthropological definition of culture has helped broaden the study of the humanities from fine art and elite art to "folk" and non-Western arts, as well as to the creative expressions of popular culture.

In many societies, myths, legends, folk tales, and the art of storytelling play important roles in the transmission of culture. Oral traditions may preserve details of history and genealogy, as in many parts of West Africa. Storytelling and music may be combined for drama and emphasis (see lower photo, below), much as they are in films and theater.

At what age do children start learning the arts? In some cultures, they start early. Contrast the photo of the violin class (upper photo) with the photo of the Tusipono Embera community gathering (lower photo). The violin scene shows formal instruction. Teachers take the lead in showing students how to play the violin. The lower photo shows a more informal local scene in which children are learning about the arts as part of their overall enculturation. Many of the violin students are learning the arts because their parents want them to, rather than because they have an artistic temperament they are eager to express. In the United States, performance, often associated with schools, has a strong social, and usually competitive, component. Kids perform with their peers. In the process, they learn to compete, whether for a first-place finish in a sports event or for a first chair in the school orchestra or band.

Continuity and Change

The arts go on changing, although certain art forms, such as the Upper Paleolithic cave paintings, have survived from the distant past. Monumental architecture, along with sculpture, ornamental pottery, and written music, literature, and drama, have survived from early civilizations (see Burt 2013; Ingold 2013).

Classic Greek theater is still read in college courses and performed on stages from Athens to New York. In today's world, the dramatic arts are part of a huge "arts and leisure" industry (encompassing arts, media, and sports), which links Western and non–Western art forms in a global network that has both aesthetic and commercial dimensions (see Root 1996; Schneider 2017). Non-Western musical traditions and instruments have joined this network. Folk musicians routinely perform for outsiders, including tourists who increasingly visit their villages.

And "tribal" instruments such as the Native Australian didgeridoo, a very long, wooden wind instrument, are now exported worldwide. At least one shop in Amsterdam, the Netherlands, sells

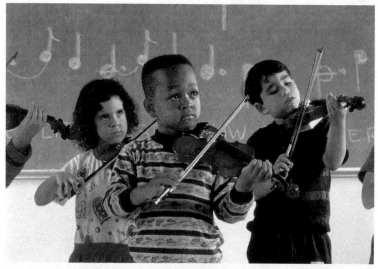

Young music students. Does this scene illustrate education, enculturation, or both?
Zephyr Picture/Getty Images

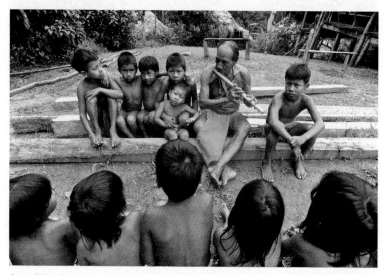

A traditional musician and storyteller performs with local children in Panama's Tusipono Embera community. Are there comparable figures in your society? Does this scene illustrate education, enculturation, or both?
Kike Calvo/National Geographic Creative

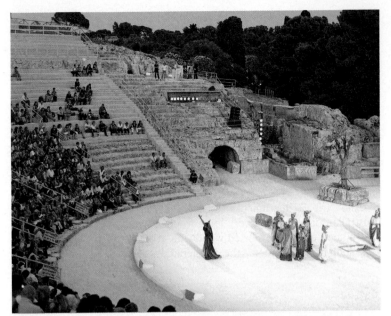

In an ancient amphitheater at Syracuse, Sicily, ancient Greek theater (*Medea*) is being performed for a contemporary audience. Theater is typically a multimedia experience, with visual, aural, and often musical attributes.

Ingolf Pompe/AGE Fotostock

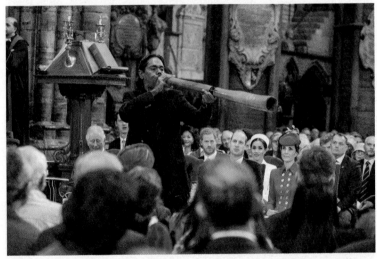

International didgeridoo player William Barton performs at the Westminster Abbey Commonwealth Day service on March 11, 2019 in London, England. The year 2019 marked the 70th anniversary of the modern British Commonwealth--a global network of almost 2.4 billion people living in 53 countries, including Australia, where the didgeridoo originated.

Richard Pohle/Getty Images

text
A cultural product that is processed and assigned meaning by anyone exposed to it.

only didgeridoos. Stores in any world capital hawk "traditional" arts, including musical instruments, from dozens of non-Western countries (see Fillitz and van der Grijp 2017; Wilkinson-Weber and DeNicola 2016).

Countries and cultures are known for particular contributions, including the arts. The Balinese are known for dance; the Navajo for sand paintings, jewelry, and weaving; and the French for making

cuisine an art form. Thanks to globalization, ingredients and flavors from all over the world now combine in modern cuisine. So, too, are elements from many cultures and epochs woven into our contemporary arts and expressive culture, including in modern media.

MEDIA AND CULTURE

Today's mass culture, or popular culture, features cultural forms that have appeared and spread rapidly because of major changes in the material conditions of contemporary life—particularly work organization, transportation, and communication, including the media. Sports, movies, TV shows, video games, digital media, amusement parks, and fast-food restaurants have become powerful elements of national (and international) culture (see Pertierra 2018; Sanjek and Tratner 2016). They offer a framework of common expectations, experiences, and behavior overriding differences in region, class, formal religious affiliation, political sentiment, gender, ethnic group, and place of residence.

Using the Media

Any media-borne image or message can be analyzed in terms of its nature, including its symbolism, and its effects. It also can be analyzed as a **text**—something that can be received, processed, interpreted, and potentially appreciated by anyone exposed to it. Such a text doesn't have to be written; the term can refer to a film, an image, or an event. "Readers"—users of the text—make their own interpretations and derive their own feelings from it. "Readers" of media messages constantly produce their own meanings.

According to media scholar John Fiske (2011), any individual's use of popular culture is a personal creative act (an original "reading" of a "text"). A particular celebrity, movie, game, or TV show means something different to each fan. Fiske argues that the personal meanings one finds in popular culture are most pleasurable when they relate directly and practically to that person's everyday life (Fiske 2011; see also Fiske and Hartley 2003).

Consumers actively select, evaluate, and interpret media in ways that make sense to them. People use media for all sorts of reasons: to validate beliefs, to indulge fantasies, to find messages unavailable in the local setting, to locate information, to make social comparisons, to relieve frustrations, to chart social courses, and to formulate life plans. Popular culture (from hip-hop to comedy) can be used to express discontent and resistance by groups that are or feel powerless or oppressed.

In Ibirama, a town in southern Brazil, anthropologist Alberto Costa found that women and young adults of both sexes were particularly attracted to telenovelas, melodramatic nightly programs often compared to American soap operas, usually featuring sophisticated urban settings (see Kottak 2009; Pace and Hinote 2013). Women and young men used the (socially more liberal) content of telenovelas to challenge conservative local norms. In Brazil, elites, intellectuals, educators, the clergy, and older men have tended to be more suspicious and dismissive of mass media than are less powerful people. Often, these groups view media messages as threatening or subverting their traditional authority as guardians of power or cultural capital.

During our fieldwork in a middle-class Michigan town, Lara Descartes and I found that parents selected media messages that supported and reinforced their own opinions and life choices (Descartes and Kottak 2009). Media images of work and family gave parents the chance to identify, or contrast themselves, with media figures. Townfolk compared themselves with people and situations from the media as well as with people in their own lives. We also found, as in Brazil, that some people (traditionalists) were much more dismissive of, distrustful of, or hostile to media than others were.

When people seek certain messages and can't easily find them in their home communities, they are likely to look somewhere else. The media, especially modern social media, offer instant access to a web of connections that can provide contact, information, entertainment, and potential social validation. In Brazil, we've found that greater use of all media is part of an external orientation, a general wish for information, contacts, models, and support beyond those that are locally and routinely available. For some of the parents (especially mothers) in our Michigan study, media offered a welcome gateway to a wider world. Others, however, were comfortable with, and even sought to enhance, their isolation, limiting both media exposure and the outside social contacts of themselves and their children.

Connection to a wider world, real or imagined, on- or offline, is a way to move beyond local standards and expectations, even if the escape is only temporary and vicarious. David Ignatius (2007) describes the escapist value of 19th-century English novels, whose strong heroines pursued "free thought and personal freedom," rejecting the "easy comforts and arranged marriages of their class" in a quest for something more. Despite (and/or because of) their independent or rebellious temperaments, characters such as Elizabeth Bennett in Jane Austen's *Pride and Prejudice* almost always found a happy ending. Nineteenth-century readers found such a heroine's success "deeply satisfying," because there were so few opportunities in real life (the local community) to see such behavior and choices (all quotes from Ignatius 2007, p. A21).

Another role of the media is to provide social cement—a basis for sharing—as families or friends watch favorite programs, play *Jeopardy,* or attend events together. The media also can provide common ground for much larger groups, nationally and internationally. Brazilian and French audiences can be just as excited, at the same moment but with radically different emotions, by a soccer goal scored in a World Cup match. And they can remember the same winning goal for decades. The common information and knowledge that people acquire through exposure to the same media illustrate *culture* in the anthropological sense (see also Askew and Wilk 2002; Ginsburg, Abu-Lughod, and Larkin 2002; Lange 2019).

Assessing the Effects of Television

My co-researchers and I first got the idea that TV might be influencing family planning in Brazil from a brief article in *The New York Times.* Based on interviews with Brazilians, that report suggested that TV (along with other factors) was influencing Brazilians to have smaller families. Fortunately, our research project on media impact in rural Brazil had provided us with the quantitative data we needed to test that hypothesis.

Our findings already had confirmed many other studies showing that the strongest predictor of (smaller) family size is a woman's educational level. However, it turned out that two television variables—current viewing level and especially the number of years of TV presence in the home—were better predictors of (smaller) family size than were many other potential predictors, including income, class, and religiosity.

In the four towns in our study with the longest exposure to television, the average woman had had a TV set in her home for 15 years and had had 2.3 pregnancies. In the three communities where TV had arrived most recently, the average woman had had a home set for 4 years and had had 5 pregnancies. Thus, length of site exposure was a useful predictor of reproductive histories. Of course, television exposure at a site is an aspect of that site's increasing overall access to external systems and resources, which usually include improved methods of contraception. But the impact of longer home TV exposure showed up not only when we compared sites but also within sites, within age cohorts, and among individual women in our total sample.

What social mechanisms were behind these correlations? Family planning opportunities (including contraception) are greater in Brazil now than they used to be. However, experience in Africa, Asia, and Latin America has shown that mere access to contraception does not ensure family planning. Rather, popular demand for contraception must be created. Often, as in India (see photo on the next page), this is done through "social marketing," including planned multimedia campaigns. In Brazil, however, there has been little direct use of TV to get people to limit their offspring. How, then, has television influenced Brazilians to plan smaller families?

The families Brazilians see on TV tend to have fewer children than traditional small-town Brazilians do. Narrative form and production costs limit the number of actors in each telenovela (nightly soap opera) to about 50 characters. Telenovelas usually are gender-balanced and include three-generation extended families of different social classes, so that some of the main characters can "rise in life" by marrying up. These narrative conventions limit the number of young children per TV family.

People's ideas about proper family size are influenced as they see, day after day, nuclear families smaller than the traditional ones in their towns. Furthermore, the aim of commercial television is to sell products and lifestyles. Brazilian TV families routinely are shown enjoying consumer goods and lives of leisure, to which viewers learn to aspire. Telenovelas may convey the idea that viewers can achieve such lifestyles by emulating the apparent family planning of TV characters. The effect of Brazilian television on family planning seems to be a corollary of a more general, TV-influenced shift from traditional toward more liberal social attitudes. Anthropologist Janet Dunn's (2000) further fieldwork in Brazil has demonstrated how TV exposure actually works to influence reproductive choice and family planning.

Online Access and Connectivity

For generations, anthropologists have stressed the linking social functions (alliance creation) of such ages-old institutions as marriage and trade. Today's world offers new ways to link socially. Aaron Sorkin chose *The Social Network* as the title for his movie about the founding of Facebook, which is precisely that—a social networking site, where people go to connect in cyberspace. Modern media offer local people a new form of connectivity that provides contacts, information, entertainment, and potential social validation.

The Internet's International Spread

The Internet's spread is now global. A 2019 Pew Research Center survey examined Internet access in 34 countries. On average, 77 percent of respondents in those countries reported at least occasional Internet use, either by computer, tablet, or smartphone. Those most likely to use digital technology were younger, higher-income, and living in wealthier countries. Smartphone ownership varied substantially by country, ranging from 32 percent in India and 36 percent in Kenya to highs of 97 percent in South Korea and 88 percent in Lebanon (Schumacher and Kent 2020).

Internet penetration now exceeds 70 percent in Brazil. Among Brazilians, as we saw previously,

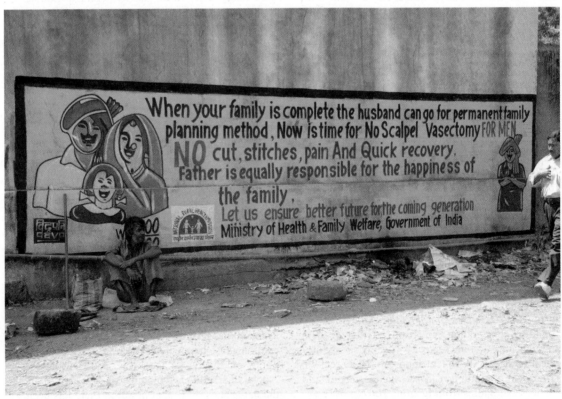

In some countries, popular demand for birth control has been created through multimedia campaigns, illustrated by this poster in Panaji, Goa, India.
Stuart Forster/Alamy Stock Photo

heavy media use reflects an external orientation, a general wish for connectivity—a social network—beyond what is locally and routinely available. Internet access has spread across the vastness of Brazil, although it remains least reliable in small communities along the Amazon and in poorer rural areas. With 149 million Internet users as of 2020, Brazil is the largest Internet market in Latin America, and the fifth largest Internet market in the world (behind China, India, the United States, and Indonesia). Offline, Brazilians are inherently social people, and they seem to be transferring that sociability to the online world. Brazilians have become heavy Internet users; 85 percent of those with access go online daily.

Most Brazilians use Facebook, which has been offered free of charge on Brazilian smartphones since 2010. Brazil ranks fourth globally in number of Facebook users (after India, the United States, and Indonesia). Despite its popularity, Facebook is no longer the most popular social media site/app in Brazil. That distinction belongs to Whats-App, used by over 90 percent of online Brazilians, compared with Facebook (86 percent) and Instagram (60 percent).

Americans' Internet Use

How do these Brazilian social media choices compare with preferences in the United States? In 2019, YouTube and Facebook were the favored sites of online Americans (used by 73 percent and 69 percent respectively). Other popular sites/apps were Instagram (37 percent), Pinterest (28 percent), LinkedIn (27 percent), Snapchat (24 percent), Twitter (22 percent) and WhatsApp (20 percent) (see Perrin and Anderson 2019).

About 90 percent of American adults (aged 18 and over) routinely go online, using a computer, a tablet, and/or (increasingly) a smartphone. About 81 percent of American adults owned a smartphone in 2019, up from 77 percent the year before. The smartphone has become, for those who own one, a preferred means of accessing the Internet. In 2019, 46 percent of smartphone owners said they accessed the Internet mostly on their phone, up from 34 percent in 2013. Simultaneously, the percentage of smartphone owners using a computer or a tablet as their primary means of going online fell from 53 percent to 30 percent (Anderson 2019). (The rest reported using their smartphone and computer/tablet about equally.)

Although Americans' smartphone ownership is widespread, there is more noticeable variation in access to broadband. The 36-point gap in broadband availability between higher- and lower-income groups is much larger than the 24-point gap in smartphone ownership between those groups. The overall share of Americans with home broadband service stood at 73 percent in 2019, up from 65 percent the previous year. Comparing income groups, 92 percent of adults in households earning over $75,000 a year had broadband

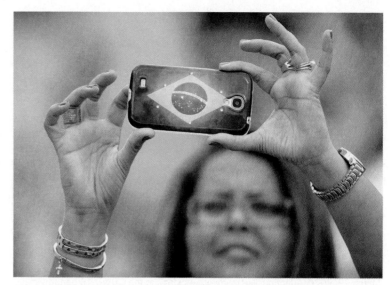

At the start of a World Cup soccer game played in Salvador da Bahia, Brazil, on June 16, 2014, a fan uses her smartphone, decorated with the Brazilian flag, to photograph some memories.
dpa picture alliance/Alamy Stock Photo

Internet, versus 56 percent when household income fell below $30,000. Stratification in access by educational level follows a similar pattern (Anderson 2019).

Nonusers

About 10 percent of the U. S. population does not use the Internet (Anderson et al. 2019). The size of this group has changed little over the past few years, despite government and social service programs to encourage Internet adoption in underserved areas. That nonuse percentage, however, has fallen considerably since 2000, when almost half (48 percent) of American adults did not use the Internet.

Nonusers are disproportionately older, lower-income, and less well-educated. Of Americans aged 65 and older, 27 percent still do not use the Internet. Of non–high-school graduates, 29 percent were nonusers in 2019, an improvement over 35 percent in 2018. Of adults in homes earning less than $30,000 a year, 18 percent lacked access, compared with just 2 percent of the most affluent.

Use of smartphones and social media also declines in older age groups. While 59 percent of Americans between the ages of 65 and 74 owned smartphones in 2019, only 40 percent of those aged 75 and older did (Anderson 2019). In terms of social media use, in most countries surveyed, there was a gap of at least 50 percent between the youngest (most active) users and the oldest (least active) users. Nearly all young Lithuanians (95 percent), for example, reported social media use, compared with only 28 percent of those aged 50 and older. In only seven of 34 countries surveyed did most users aged 50 or older report social media use (Schumacher and Kent 2020).

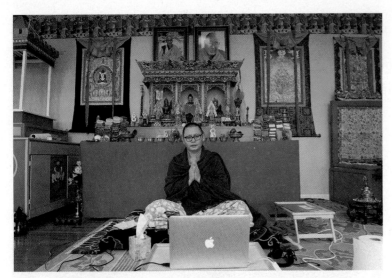

March 29, 2020: Adapting, like many other clergy, to the COVID-19 pandemic, Buddhist temple leader Lhoppön Rinpoche offers his first online meditation from Mipham Shedra temple in Westminster, Colorado. The service was live-streamed in real time on Facebook. Rinpoche planned to continue live streaming every Sunday morning until the pandemic is under control.

Helen H. Richardson/Getty Images

Social Media and Trust

How does all this access affect our feelings about our fellow humans? The Pew Research Center has done a series of studies investigating how Americans' social media use is related to their levels of trust and social support (see Hampton et al. 2011; Pink and Abram 2015). These studies have found consistently that participation in social media enhances social connectivity, rather than (as some had feared) isolating people and truncating their social relationships. Specifically, as social media use increases, so do measures of trust, sociability, and political engagement.

When queried, Internet users were twice as likely as nonusers to say people can be trusted. Facebook users were especially trusting and socially oriented. The more one used Facebook, the more likely one was to say that most people can be trusted. Of course, Facebook users routinely reveal personal and family details online, so it's not surprising they would be more trusting. Finally, Internet users, especially those on Facebook, were found to be more politically engaged than nonusers. They were much more likely than nonusers to attend political meetings, to vote, and to try to influence someone else's vote. Here again, heavy Facebook users stood out as most likely to do those things.

SPORTS AND CULTURE

We now turn to the cultural context of sports and the cultural values expressed in them. We can recognize links among sports, media, and the arts.

Like many artists and media personalities, sports figures are performers, some with celebrity status, who must meet cultural expectations and standards regarding performance and conduct. Because so much of what we know about sports comes from the media, a discussion of sports inevitably provides further illustration of the pervasive role of the mass media in contemporary life. This section mainly describes how sports and the media *reflect* culture. Sports and the media also *influence* culture, as we saw in the discussion of how Brazilian television modifies social attitudes and family planning. Does it surprise you that the influence of media (and sports) on culture and vice versa are reciprocal?

American Football

On fall Saturdays, hordes of Americans travel to and from college football games. Smaller congregations meet in high school stadiums. Millions of Americans watch televised football. Indeed, nearly half the adult population of the United States watches the Super Bowl, which attracts people of diverse ages, ethnic backgrounds, regions, religions, political parties, jobs, social statuses, levels of wealth, and genders.

The popularity of football, particularly professional football, depends directly on the mass media. Is football, with its territorial incursion and hard hitting, popular because Americans are an especially violent people? Are football spectators vicariously realizing their own hostile and aggressive tendencies? The anthropologist W. Arens (1981) has discounted this interpretation, arguing that if American football were a particularly effective channel for expressing aggression, it would have spread (like soccer and baseball) to many other countries, where people have as many aggressive tendencies and hostile feelings as Americans do. He concludes reasonably that the explanation for football's popularity must lie elsewhere.

Arens contends that football is popular because it symbolizes certain key aspects of American life. In particular, it features teamwork based on division of labor, which is a pervasive feature of contemporary life. Susan Montague and Robert Morais (1981) take the analysis a step further. They link football's values, particularly teamwork, to those associated with business. Like good organization men and women, the ideal players are diligent and dedicated to the team. Within corporations, however, decision making is complicated, and workers aren't always rewarded for their dedication and job performance. Decisions are simpler and rewards are more consistent in football, these anthropologists contend, and this helps explain its popularity. Even if we can't figure out how a major corporation runs, any fan can become an expert on football's rules, teams, scores, statistics, and patterns of play. Even more important, football suggests that the values stressed by business really do pay off. Teams whose members work the hardest, show the most spirit, and best develop and coordinate their talents can be expected to win more often than other teams do.

What Determines International Sports Success?

Why do countries excel at particular sports? Why do certain nations pile up dozens of Olympic medals, while others win only a handful? It isn't simply a matter of rich and poor, developed and underdeveloped, or even governmental or other institutional support of promising athletes. It isn't even a question of a "national will to win," for although certain nations stress winning even more than Americans do, a cultural focus on winning doesn't necessarily lead to the desired result.

Cultural values, social forces, and the media influence international sports success. We can see this by contrasting the United States and Brazil, two countries with continental proportions and the largest, most physically and ethnically diverse populations in the Americas. Although each is its continent's major economic power and most populous nation, they offer revealing contrasts in Olympic success: In the 2016 Summer Olympics, held in Rio de Janeiro, the United States won 121 medals, including 46 gold medals, compared with 19 and 7, respectively, for Brazil, which even had "home field advantage."

Americans' interest in sports has been honed over the years by a proliferating media establishment, offering a steady stream of games, matches, playoffs, championships, and analyses. Cable and satellite TV offer almost constant sports coverage, including packages for every major sport and season. The Super Bowl is a national event. The Olympic games receive extensive coverage and attract significant audiences. Brazilian television, by contrast, traditionally has offered less sports coverage, with no nationally televised annual event comparable to the Super Bowl. The World (soccer) Cup, held every four years, is the only sports event that consistently draws huge national audiences (see Dolan and Connolly 2018; O'Brien et al. 2021).

In international competition, a win by a Brazilian team or the occasional nationally known individual athlete is felt to bring respect to the entire nation, but the Brazilian media are strikingly intolerant of losers. When the now legendary swimmer Ricardo Prado swam for his silver medal in the finals of the 400 individual medley (IM), during prime time on national TV in 1984, one newsmagazine observed that "it was as though he was the country with a swimsuit on, jumping in the pool in a collective search for success" (*Isto É* 1984). Prado's own feelings confirmed the magazine observation, "When I was on the stands, I thought of just one thing:

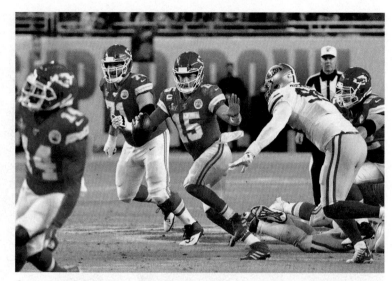

Quarterback Patrick Mahomes, #15 of the Kansas City Chiefs, scrambles away from the pressure as his team plays the San Francisco 49ers in Super Bowl LIV at Miami's Hard Rock Stadium on February 02, 2020. The Chiefs won the game 31-20. Is teamwork equally valued in other sports, such as baseball, basketball, or soccer?

Focus on Sport/Getty Images

what they'll think of the result in Brazil." After beating his old world record by 1.33 seconds, in a second-place finish, Prado told a fellow team member, "I think I did everything right. I feel like a winner, but will they think I'm a loser in Brazil?" Prado contrasted the situations of Brazilian and American athletes. The United States has, he said, so many world-class athletes that no single one has to summarize the country's hopes (*Veja* 1984a). Fortunately, Brazil did seem to value Prado's performance, which was responsible for "Brazil's best result ever in Olympic swimming" (*Veja* 1984a). Labeling Prado "the man of silver," the media never tired of characterizing his main event, the 400 IM, in which he once had held the world record, as the most challenging event in swimming. However, the kind words for Ricardo Prado did not extend to the rest of the Brazilian team. The press lamented their "succession of failures" (*Veja* 1984a). (Brazil finally got its [as yet only] Olympic gold medal in swimming at the 2008 games in Beijing, with César Cielo Filho winning the 50-meter freestyle race.)

Because Brazilian athletes are viewed as stand-ins for their entire country, and because team sports are emphasized, the Brazilian media focus too exclusively on winning. Winning, of course, is also an American cultural value, particularly for team sports, as in Brazil. American football coaches are famous for comments like "Winning isn't everything; it's the only thing" and "Show me a good loser and I'll show you a loser." However, and particularly for sports such as running, swimming, diving, gymnastics, and skating, which focus on the individual, and in which American athletes

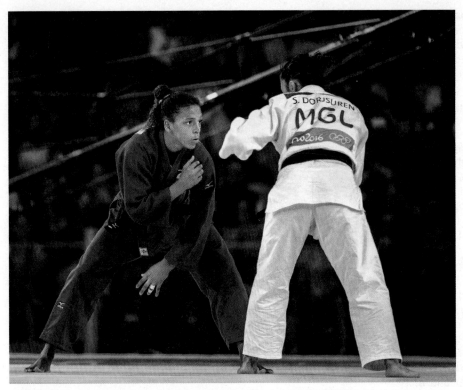

At the 2016 Summer Olympics in Rio de Janeiro, Brazilian judoist Rafaela Silva (blue) defeated Sumiya Dorjsuren of Mongolia to win a gold medal.

David Finch/Getty Images Sport/Getty Images

are more abundant, chances to achieve more numerous, and poverty less pervasive. American society has room for many winners. Brazilian society is more stratified; together the middle class and the small elite group at the top comprise just about half of the national population. Brazilian sports echo lessons from the larger society: Victories are scarce and usually reserved for the privileged few.

Being versus Doing

The factors believed to contribute to sports success belong to a larger context of cultural values. Particularly relevant is the contrast between ascribed and achieved status. An ascribed status (e.g., age) is based on what one *is* rather than what one *does.* Individuals have more control over their achieved statuses (e.g., student, golfer, tennis player). American culture emphasizes achieved over ascribed status: We are supposed to make of our lives the best we can. Success comes through achievement. An American's identity emerges as a result of what he or she *does.*

In Brazil, by contrast, identity rests not so much on doing as on being, on what one *is* from the start—a strand in a web of personal connections, originating in social class and the extended family. Social position and network membership contribute substantially to individual fortune, and all social life is hierarchical. High-status Brazilians don't stand patiently in line as Americans do. Important people expect their business to be attended to immediately, and social inferiors readily yield. A high-status Brazilian is as likely to say "Do you know who you're talking to?" as an American is to say "Who do you think you are?"—reflecting a more democratic and egalitarian value system (DaMatta 1991).

In sports reporting and commentary, American media typically focus on some aspect of doing, some special personal triumph or achievement. Often, this involves the athlete's struggle with adversity (illness, injury, pain, or the death of a parent, sibling, friend, or coach). The featured athlete is presented as not only successful but noble and self-sacrificing as well.

Given the Brazilian focus on ascribed status, the guiding assumption there is that one cannot do more than what one is. One year the Brazilian Olympic Committee sent no female swimmers to the Summer Olympics, because none had made arbitrarily established cutoff times. This excluded a South American record holder, while swimmers

usually do well, American culture also admires "moral victories," "personal bests," "comeback athletes," and "Special Olympics" and commends those who run good races without finishing first. In amateur and individual sports, American culture tells us that hard work and personal improvement can be as important as winning.

Americans are so accustomed to being told their culture overemphasizes winning that they may find it hard to believe other cultures value it even more. Brazil certainly does. Brazilian sports enthusiasts are preoccupied with world records, probably because only a win (as in soccer) or a best time (as in swimming) can make Brazil indisputably, even if temporarily, the best in the world at something. Prado's former world record in the 400 IM was mentioned constantly in the press prior to his Olympic swim. Such a best-time standard also provides Brazilians with a ready basis to fault a swimmer or runner for not going fast enough, when he or she doesn't make previous times. One might predict, accurately, that sports with more subjective standards would not be very popular in Brazil. Brazilians like to assign blame to athletes who fail them, and negative comments about gymnasts or divers are more difficult, because grace and execution can't be quantified as easily as time can.

Brazilians, I think, value winning so much because it is rare. In the United States, resources

with slower times were attending from other countries. No one seemed to imagine that Olympic excitement might spur swimmers to extraordinary efforts.

American culture, supposedly so practical and realistic, has a remarkable faith in the possibility of coming from behind. These values are those of an achievement-oriented society where (ideally) "anything is possible" compared with an ascribed-status society in which it's determined before it's begun. In American sports coverage, underdogs and unexpected results, virtually ignored by the Brazilian media, provide some of the "brightest" moments. Brazilian culture has little interest in the unexpected.

Athletes internalize these values. Brazilians assume that if you go into an event with a top seed time, as Ricardo Prado did, you've got a chance to win a medal. Prado's second-place finish made perfect sense back home, because his former world record had been bettered before the race began.

Given the overwhelming value American culture places on work, it might seem surprising that our media devote so much attention to unforeseen results and so little to the years of training, preparation, and competition that underlie Olympic performance. It probably is assumed that hard work is so obvious and fundamental that it goes without saying. Or perhaps the assumption is that by the time athletes actually enter Olympic competition all are so similar (the American value of equality) that only mysterious and chance factors can explain variable success. The American focus on the unexpected applies to losses as well as wins. Such concepts as chance, fate, mystery, and uncertainty are viewed as legitimate reasons for defeat.

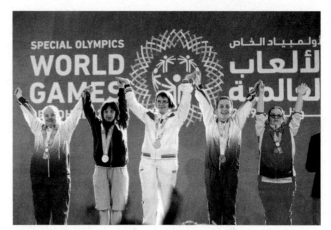

"Special Olympics" commend people who run exemplary races, without necessarily being the best in the world. Shown here, athletes show their emotions in receiving their medals at the Special Olympics Summer World Games in Abu Dhabi in 2019. These Games take place every 4 years. In 2019, 7,500 athletes from nearly 200 countries competed in 24 events.

Dominika Zarzycka/Getty Images

Runners and skaters fall; ligaments tear; a gymnast "inexplicably" falls off the pommel horse.

Brazilians place more responsibility on the individual. Less is attributed to factors beyond human control. When individuals who should have performed well don't do so, they are blamed for their failures. It is, however, culturally appropriate in Brazil to use poor health as an excuse for losing. The American media, by contrast, talk much more about the injuries and illnesses of the victors than those of the losers (see also Dolan and Connolly 2018).

for REVIEW

summary

1. The media, which include print, radio, TV, digital media, the Internet, and everything they convey, provide access to a wide world of performance and storytelling as well as information. We rely on the media for much of our access to sports and various arts.

2. Even if they lack a word for "art," people everywhere do associate an aesthetic experience with objects and events having certain qualities. The arts, sometimes called "expressive culture," include music, performance arts, visual arts, storytelling, and literature (written and oral). Some issues raised about religion also apply to art. If we adopt a special attitude or demeanor when confronting a sacred object, do we display something similar with art? Much art has been done in association with religion. In tribal performances, the arts and religion often mix. But non-Western art isn't always linked to religion.

3. The special places where we find art include museums, concert halls, opera houses, and theaters. However, the boundary between what's art and what's not may be blurred. Variation in art appreciation is especially common in contemporary society, with its professional artists and critics and great cultural diversity.

4. Those who work with non-Western art have been criticized for ignoring individual artists and for focusing too much on the social context and collective artistic production. Art is work, albeit creative work. In state societies, some people manage to support themselves as full-time

artists. In nonstates, artists are usually part-time. Typically, the arts are exhibited, evaluated, performed, and appreciated in society. Music, which often is performed in groups, is among the most social of the arts. Folk art, music, and lore are the expressive culture of ordinary, usually rural, people.

5. Art can stand for tradition, even when traditional art is removed from its original context. Art can express community sentiment, with political goals used to call attention to social issues. Often, art is meant to commemorate and to last. Growing acceptance of the anthropological definition of culture has guided the humanities beyond fine art, elite art, and Western art to the creative expressions of the masses and of many cultures. Myths, legends, tales, and the art of storytelling often play important roles in the transmission of culture.

6. The arts go on changing, although certain art forms have survived for thousands of years. Countries and cultures are known for particular contributions. Today, a huge "arts and leisure" industry links Western and non-Western art forms in an international network with both aesthetic and commercial dimensions.

7. Any media-borne message can be analyzed as a text, something that can be "read"—that is, processed, interpreted, and assigned meaning by anyone exposed to it. People use media to validate beliefs, indulge fantasies, seek out messages, make social comparisons, relieve frustrations, chart social courses, and resist unequal power relations. The media can provide common ground for social groups. Length of home TV exposure is a useful measure of the impact of television on values, attitudes, and beliefs. The effect of Brazilian television on family planning seems to be a corollary of a more general TV-influenced shift from traditional toward more liberal social attitudes. Use of online social media correlates with overall social connectivity and sociability, including measures of trust, companionship, and political involvement.

8. As in the arts and media, performance is a key feature of sports. Much of what we know about sports comes from the media. Like the arts, both sports and the media reflect and influence culture. Football symbolizes and simplifies certain key aspects of American life and values (e.g., hard work and teamwork). Cultural values, social forces, and the media influence international sports success. In amateur and individual sports, American culture tells us that hard work and personal improvement can be as important as winning. Other cultures, such as Brazil, may value winning even more than Americans do. The factors believed to contribute to sports success belong to a larger context of cultural values. Particularly relevant is the contrast between ascribed and achieved status: being versus doing. An American's identity emerges as a result of what he or she does. In Brazil, by contrast, identity rests on being: what one is from the start—a strand in a web of personal connections, originating in social class and the extended family.

key terms

aesthetics 261
art 261
arts 261
catharsis 269

ethnomusicology 266
expressive culture 261
folk 268
text 272

think like an anthropologist

1. Recall the last time you were in an art museum. What did you like, and why? How much of your aesthetic tastes can you attribute to your education, to your culture? How much do you think responds to your own individual tastes? How can you make the distinction?

2. Think of a musical composition or performance you consider to be art, but whose status as such is debatable. How would you convince someone else that it is art? What kinds of arguments against your position would you expect to hear?

3. Can you think of a political dispute involving art or the arts? What were the different positions being debated?

4. Media consumers actively select, evaluate, and interpret media in ways that make sense to them. People use media for all sorts of reasons. What are some examples? Which are most relevant to the way you consume, and maybe even creatively alter and produce, media?

5. This chapter describes how sports and media *reflect* culture. Can you come up with examples of how sports and media *influence* culture?

credits

Design Elements: Understanding Ourselves: muha/123RF (rock paintings); Focus on Globalization: janrysavy/Getty Images (globe); Appreciating Diversity (left to right): Floresco Productions/age footstock; Hero/Corbis/Glow Images, Hill Street Studios/Blend Images, Billion Photos/Shutterstock; Understanding Ourselves : Hemera Technologies/Alamy (Cymbal), LACMA - Los Angeles County Museum of Art (Trefoil Oinochoe), Ingram Publishing/SuperStock (Coin), ChuckSchugPhotography/Getty Images (Rug).

The World System, Colonialism, and Inequality

▶ When and why did the world system develop, and what is it like today?

▶ When and how did European colonialism develop, and how is its legacy expressed in postcolonial studies?

▶ How do colonialism, neoliberalism, development, and industrialization exemplify intervention philosophies?

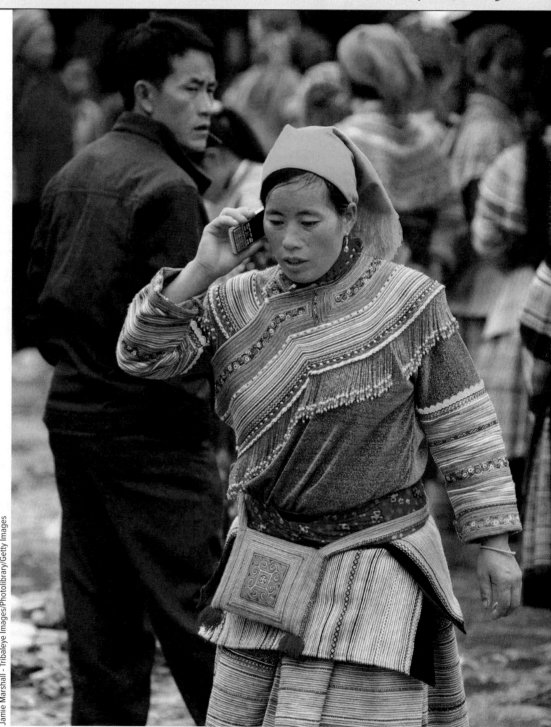

Jamie Marshall - Tribaleye Images/Photolibrary/Getty Images

The "Flower Hmong," known for their colorful clothing and market activity, are one of many subgroups of the Hmong ethnic group, which inhabits mountainous areas of Southeast Asia and southern China. Shown here, a Flower Hmong woman on a mobile telephone call in Bac Ha, Vietnam. The rapid diffusion of the cell phone has transformed communication throughout the world.

understanding OURSELVES

In our 21st-century world system, people are linked as never before by modern means of transportation and communication. Descendants of villages that hosted ethnographers a generation ago now live transnational lives. For me, some of the most vivid illustrations of this new transnationalism come from Madagascar. They begin in Ambalavao, a town in southern Betsileo country, where I rented a small house in 1966–1967.

By 1966, Madagascar had gained independence from France, but its towns still had foreigners to remind them of colonialism. Besides my wife and me, Ambalavao had at least a dozen world-system agents, including an Indian cloth merchant, Chinese grocers, and a few French people. Two young men in the French equivalent of the Peace Corps were there teaching school. One of them, Noel, lived across the street from a prominent local family. Since Noel often spoke disparagingly of the Malagasy, I was surprised to see him courting a young woman from this family. She was Lenore, the sister of Leon, a schoolteacher who became my good friend.

My next trip to Madagascar was a brief visit in February 1981. I had to spend a few days in Antananarivo, the capital. There I was confined each evening to the newly built Hilton hotel by a curfew imposed after a civil insurrection. I shared the hotel with a group of Russian military pilots, there to teach the Malagasy to defend their island, strategically placed in the Indian Ocean, against imagined enemies. Later, I went down to Betsileo country to visit Leon, my schoolteacher friend from Ambalavao, who had become a prominent politician. Unfortunately for me, he was in Moscow, participating in a three-month exchange program.

During my next visit to Madagascar, in summer 1990, I met Emily, the 22-year-old daughter of Noel and Lenore, whose courtship I had witnessed in 1967. One of her aunts brought Emily to meet me at my hotel in Antananarivo. Emily was about to visit several cities in the United States, where she planned to study marketing. I met her again just a few months later in Gainesville, Florida. She asked me about her father, whom she had never met. Noel, who had never married Lenore, had left the country before Emily was born. Emily had sent several letters to France, but Noel never responded.

Descendants of Ambalavao are dispersed globally. Emily, a child of colonialism, had aunts in France (Malagasy women married to French men) and another in Switzerland (a retired diplomat). Members of her family, which is not especially wealthy, have traveled to Russia, Canada, the United States, France, Germany, and West Africa. How many of your classmates, including perhaps you, yourself, have recent transnational roots? A descendant of a Kenyan village (although not born there himself) even grew up to become a twice-elected president of the United States.

THE WORLD SYSTEM

Although fieldwork in small communities is anthropology's hallmark, isolated groups are impossible to find today. Truly isolated human societies probably never have existed. For thousands of years, human groups have been in contact with one another. Local societies always have participated in a larger system, which today has global dimensions. We call it the *modern world system,* by which we mean a world in which nations are economically and politically interdependent.

A huge increase in international trade during and after the 15th century led to the **capitalist world economy** (Wallerstein et al. 2013), a single world system oriented toward production for sale or exchange, with the object of maximizing profits. **Capital** refers to wealth or resources available to invest in a business, with the intent of making a profit.

World-System Theory

World-system theory can be traced to the French social historian Fernand Braudel. In his three-volume work *Civilization and Capitalism, 15th–18th Century* (1981, 1982, 1992), Braudel argued that societies consist of interrelated parts assembled into a system. Societies themselves are subsystems of larger systems, with the world system the largest. The key claim of **world-system theory** is that all the countries of the world belong to a larger, global system, marked by differences in wealth and power. This world system, based on capitalism, has existed at least since the late 15th century, when the Old World established sustained contact with the Americas.

World-system theory assigns particular countries to one of three different positions, based on their economic and political clout: core, semiperiphery, and periphery (see also Wallerstein 2004). The **core** consists of the wealthiest and most powerful nations, which have the most productive economies and the greatest concentration of capital. The core monopolizes the most profitable activities, especially the control of world finance (Arrighi 2010). The **semiperiphery** is intermediate between the core and the periphery. Nations of the semiperiphery are industrialized. Like core nations, they produce and export both industrial goods and commodities, but they lack the power and economic dominance of core nations. Thus, Brazil, a semiperiphery nation, exports automobiles to Nigeria (a periphery nation) and auto engines, orange juice extract, coffee, and shrimp to the United States (a core nation). The **periphery** includes the world's poorest and least privileged countries. Economic activities there are less mechanized than in the semiperiphery, although some degree of industrialization has reached even periphery nations. The periphery produces mainly raw materials, agricultural commodities, and, increasingly, human labor for export to the core and the semiperiphery (Shannon 1996).

In the United States and Western Europe today, immigration—legal and illegal—from the periphery and semiperiphery supplies cheap labor for agriculture. U.S. states as distant as California, Michigan, and South Carolina make significant use of farm labor from Mexico. The availability of relatively cheap workers from non-core nations such as Mexico (in the United States) and Turkey (in Germany) benefits farmers and business owners in core countries while supplying remittances to families in the semiperiphery and the periphery. As a result of 21st-century telecommunications technology, cheap labor doesn't even need to migrate to the United States.

capitalist world economy
A profit-oriented global economy based on production for sale or exchange.

capital
Wealth invested with the intent of producing profit.

world-system theory
The idea that a discernible social system, based on wealth and power differentials, transcends individual countries.

core
The dominant position in the world system; nations with advanced systems of production.

semiperiphery
The position in the world system intermediate between the core and the periphery.

periphery
The weakest structural and economic position in the world system.

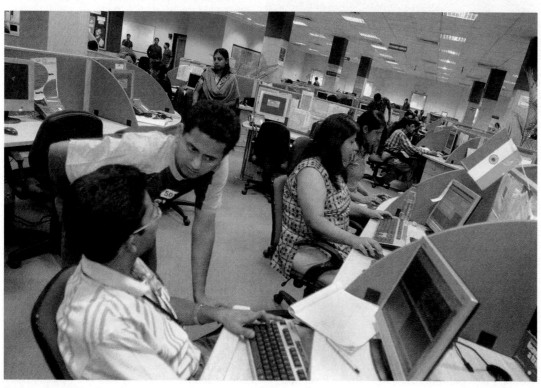

Outsourcing: Indian men and women working at a call center in New Delhi, India.

Fredrik Renander/Alamy Stock Photo

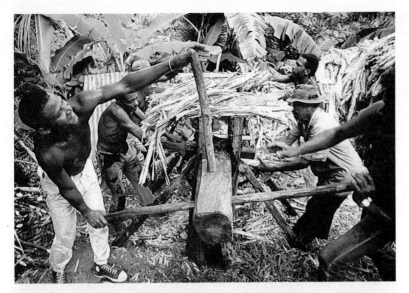

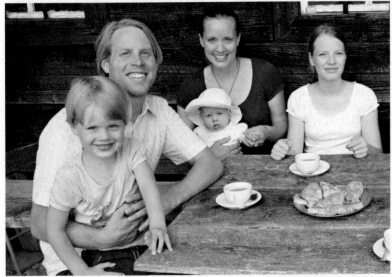

From producer to consumer, in the modern world system. The top photo, taken in the Caribbean nation of Dominica, shows the hard labor required to extract sugar using a manual press. In the bottom photo, an English middle-class family enjoys afternoon tea, sweetened with imported sugar. Which of the ingredients in your breakfast today were imported?

Top: Bruce Dale/National Geographic Creative; bottom: Henglein and Steets/Getty Images

in navigation, mapmaking, and shipbuilding fueled the geographic expansion of trading networks. Europe established regular contact with Asia, Africa, and eventually the Caribbean and the Americas. Christopher Columbus's first voyage from Spain to the Bahamas and the Caribbean in 1492 was soon followed by additional voyages. These journeys opened the way for sustained contact and major exchanges between the hemispheres, as the Old and New Worlds were forever linked (Crosby 2003, 2015; Diamond 1997/2017; Mann 2012; Marks 2020). The *Columbian exchange* is the term for the spread of people, resources, products, ideas, and diseases between Eastern and Western Hemispheres after contact.

Previously in Europe as throughout the world, rural people had produced mainly for their own needs, growing their own food and making clothing, furniture, and tools from local products. People produced beyond their immediate needs in order to pay taxes and to purchase trade items, such as salt and iron. As late as 1650, the English diet, like diets in much of the world today, was based on locally grown starches (Mintz 1985). In the 200 years that followed, however, the English became extraordinary consumers of imported goods. One of the earliest and most popular of those goods was sugar (Mintz 1985).

Sugarcane, originally domesticated in Papua New Guinea, was first processed in India. Reaching Europe via the eastern Mediterranean, it was carried to the Americas by Columbus (Mintz 1985, 2007). The climate of Brazil and the Caribbean proved ideal for growing sugarcane, and Europeans built plantations there to supply the growing demand for sugar. This led to the development in the 17th century of a plantation economy based on a single cash crop—a system known as *monocrop* production.

The demand for sugar spurred the development of the trans-Atlantic slave trade and New World plantation economies based on the labor of enslaved people. By the 18th century, an increased English demand for raw cotton had led to rapid settlement of what is now the southeastern United States and the emergence there of another slave-based monocrop production system. Like sugar, cotton was a key trade item that fueled the growth of the world system.

Thousands of families in India and the Philippines, for example, are being supported as American companies "outsource" jobs—from telephone assistance to software engineering—to nations outside the core.

The Emergence of the World System

International trade is much older than the capitalist world economy. As early as 600 b.c.e., the Phoenicians/Carthaginians sailed around Britain on regular trade routes and circumnavigated Africa. Likewise, Indonesia, the Middle East, and Africa have been linked in Indian Ocean trade for at least 2,000 years. By the 15th century, advances

INDUSTRIALIZATION

By the 18th century the stage had been set for the **Industrial Revolution**—the historical transformation of "traditional" into "modern" societies through industrialization. The Industrial Revolution began, in Europe, around 1750. However, the seeds of industrial society had been planted well before then (Gimpel 1988). For example, a knitting machine invented in England in 1589 was so far ahead of its time that it played a profitable role in factories two and three centuries later.

The Industrial Revolution required capital for investment, and that capital came from trans-oceanic commerce, which generated enormous profits. Wealthy people invested in machines and engines to drive machines. New technology and techniques increased production in both farming and manufacturing.

European industrialization eventually replaced the *domestic system* of production, also known as the home-handicraft system. In this system, an organizer-entrepreneur supplied the raw materials to workers in their homes and collected finished products from them. This entrepreneur, whose sphere of operations might span several villages, owned the materials, paid for the work, and arranged the distribution of the final product.

Causes of the Industrial Revolution

The Industrial Revolution began with machines that manufactured cotton products, iron, and pottery. These were widely used items whose manufacture could be broken down into simple routine motions that machines could perform. As manufacturing moved from homes into factories, where machinery replaced handwork, agrarian societies evolved into industrial ones. The Industrial Revolution led to a dramatic increase in production, initially of cheap staple goods. Industrialization also fueled urban growth and created a new kind of city, with factories crowded together in places where coal and labor were cheap.

The Industrial Revolution began in England—for several reasons. More than other nations, England needed to innovate in order to meet a demand for staples—at home and from its far-flung colonies. As industrialization proceeded, Britain's population began to increase dramatically. It doubled during the 18th century (especially after 1750) and did so again between 1800 and 1850. This demographic explosion fueled consumption, but British entrepreneurs could not meet the increased demand with the traditional production methods. This spurred experimentation, innovation, further industrialization, and rapid technological change.

Also supporting early English industrialization were Britain's advantages in natural resources. Britain was rich in coal and iron ore and had navigable coasts and waterways. It was a seafaring island-nation located at the crossroads of international trade. These features gave Britain a favored position for importing raw materials and exporting manufactured goods. Another factor in England's industrial growth was the fact that much of its 18th-century colonial empire was occupied by English settler families, who looked to the mother country as they tried to replicate European civilization abroad. These colonies bought large quantities of English staples.

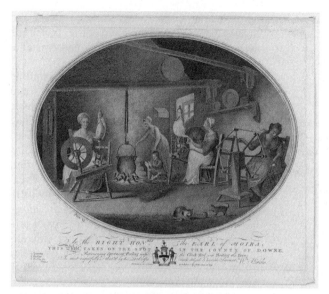

In the home-handicraft, or domestic, system of production, an organizer supplied raw materials to workers in their homes and collected their products. Family life and work were intertwined, as in this English scene. Is there a modern equivalent to the domestic system of production?

SOURCE: Library of Congress Prints and Photographs Division, LC-USZ62-4801

It also has been argued that particular cultural and religious factors contributed to industrialization. Many members of the emerging English middle class were Protestants, whose beliefs and values encouraged industry, thrift, the dissemination of new knowledge, inventiveness, and willingness to accept change (Weber 1904/2011). These cultural values were eminently compatible with the spirit of entrepreneurial innovation that propelled the Industrial Revolution.

Industrial Stratification

The socioeconomic changes associated with industrialization were mixed. English national income tripled between 1700 and 1815 and increased 30 times more by 1939. Standards of comfort rose, but prosperity was uneven. Initially, factory workers got decent wages, until owners started recruiting workers in areas where living standards were low and labor (including that of women and children) was cheap. Smoke and filth from factories polluted 19th-century cities. Housing was crowded and unsanitary. People faced disease outbreaks and rising death rates. This was the world of Ebenezer Scrooge, Bob Cratchit, Tiny Tim—and Karl Marx.

The Industrial Revolution created a new form of socioeconomic stratification. Based on his observations of 19th-century industrial capitalism in England, Karl Marx described this stratification as a sharp and simple division between two opposed classes: the bourgeoisie (capitalists) and the proletariat (propertyless workers) (Marx and Engels 1848/1976). The bourgeoisie traced its origins to overseas ventures, which had created a wealthy commercial class (White 2009).

Industrialization changed society by shifting production from farms and cottages to mills and factories, where mechanical power was available and where workers could be assembled to operate heavy machinery. The **bourgeoisie** owned the factories, mines, estates, and other means of production. Members of the **working class,** or **proletariat,** had to sell their labor to survive.

By promoting rural-to-urban migration, industrialization hastened the process of *proletarianization*—the separation of workers from the means of production. The bourgeoisie controlled not only factories but also schools, the press, and other key institutions. *Class consciousness* (personal identification and solidarity with one's economic group) was a vital part of Marx's view of class. He saw bourgeoisie and proletariat as having radically opposed interests. Marx viewed classes as powerful collective forces that could mobilize human energies to influence the course of history. Based on their common experience, workers, he thought, would develop class consciousness, which could lead to revolutionary change.

Although no proletarian revolution was to occur in England, workers did develop organizations to protect their interests and increase their share of industrial profits. During the 19th century, trade unions and socialist parties emerged, expressing a rising anticapitalist spirit. This early English labor movement worked to remove young children from factories and limit the hours during which women and children could work. The profile of stratification in industrial core nations gradually took shape. Capitalists controlled production, but labor was organizing for better wages and working conditions. By 1900, many governments had factory regulation and social welfare programs. Mass living standards in core nations rose as population grew.

Today, the existence of publicly traded companies complicates the division between capitalists and workers. Through pension plans and personal investments, some workers have become part-owners rather than propertyless workers. Today's key capitalist isn't the factory owner, who may have been replaced by stockholders, but the CEO or the chair of the board of directors, neither of whom may actually own the corporation.

The social theorist Max Weber faulted Karl Marx for an overly simple and exclusively economic view of stratification (see Kalberg 2017). Weber (1922/1968) looked beyond class and identified three (separate but correlated) dimensions of social stratification: wealth, power, and prestige. Weber also believed that social identities based on nationality, ethnicity, and religion could

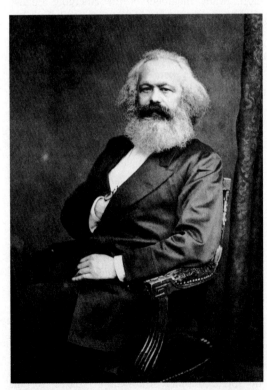

Karl Marx (1818–1883). Marx proposed a class-based view of social stratification, with a sharp separation between owners and workers.

Bettmann/Getty Images

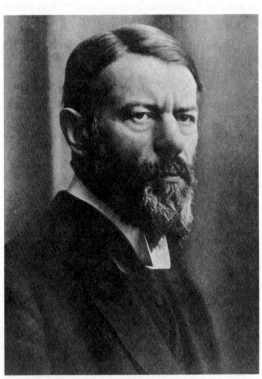

Max Weber (1864–1920). Did Weber improve on Marx's view of stratification?

source: General Collections, Prints and Photographs Division, Library of Congress, LC-USZ62-74580

take priority over class (social identity based on economic status). Supporting Weber's view, today's world system *is* crosscut by collective identities based on nationality, ethnicity, and religion. Class conflicts tend to occur within nations, and nationalism has impeded global class solidarity, particularly of proletarians.

Although the capitalist class dominates politically in most countries, growing wealth has made it easier for core nations to offer benefits to their workers. However, this improvement in core workers' living standards would not have occurred without the world system. The wealth that flows from periphery and semiperiphery to core has helped core capitalists maintain their profits while also satisfying the demands of core workers. In the periphery and semiperiphery, wages and living standards are lower. The current *world stratification system* features a substantial contrast between both capitalists and workers in the core nations, on the one hand, and workers in the periphery, on the other.

THE PERSISTENCE OF INEQUALITY

The sociologist Gerhard Lenski (1966) argued that social equality tends to increase in advanced industrial societies. The masses improve their access to economic benefits and political power. In Lenski's scheme, the shift of political power to the masses reflects the growth of the middle class, which reduces the polarization between owning and working classes. The proliferation of middle-class occupations creates opportunities for social mobility and a more complex stratification system (Atkinson 2020; Carrier and Kalb 2015; Giddens 1981).

Wealth Distribution in the United States

Most contemporary Americans claim to belong to the middle class, which they tend to perceive as a vast, undifferentiated group. There are, however, significant, and growing, socioeconomic contrasts within the middle class, and especially between the richest and the poorest Americans. Table 14.1 shows how income varied from the top to the bottom fifths (quintiles) of American households in 2019. In that table we see that the top fifth earned more than half (51.9 percent) of all income generated in the United States. Income has been rising much more significantly for the richest Americans than for everyone else. The top quintile earned 17 times the share of the bottom quintile in 2019, compared with a ratio of 14:1 in 2000 and 11:1 in 1970. Even more dramatically, the top 5 percent of Americans earned 29 times the share of the bottom fifth in 2019, compared with ratios of 24:1 in 2000 and 17:1 in 1970.

Incomes for the top 1 percent of Americans dropped sharply (about 36 percent) during the Great Recession of 2007–2009. By 2012, however, those incomes had rebounded by 31 percent. The incomes of the other 99 percent declined only 12 percent during the recession, but they recovered much more slowly. The top 1 percent benefited significantly more than anyone else from the income gains between 2009 and early 2020, before the COVID-19 recession began. Higher stock prices, home values, and corporate profits propelled that recovery among affluent Americans, while blue- and white-collar workers continued to feel the effects of unemployment, underemployment, and lower or stagnant wages (Goldstein 2017; Lowrey 2013).

Over the past three decades, America's most affluent families have been adding to their net worth, while those at the bottom have dipped into "negative wealth," meaning the value of their debts exceeds that of their assets. The share of U.S. wealth held by the nation's wealthiest peaked in the late 1920s, right before the Great Depression, then fell during the next three decades. Currently the nation's most affluent once again hold as large a wealth share as they did in the 1920s. America's top 1 percent holds more than half the national wealth invested in stocks and mutual funds. Most of the wealth of Americans in the bottom 90 percent

TABLE 14.1 U.S. National Income by Quintile, 2019

	PERCENT SHARE OF NATIONAL INCOME	MEAN HOUSEHOLD INCOME
Top 5 percent	23.0	$451,122
Top 20 percent	51.9	254,449
Second 20 percent	22.7	111,112
Third 20 percent	14.1	68,938
Fourth 20 percent	8.3	40,652
Bottom 20 percent	3.1	15,286

SOURCE: Semega, Jessica L., Kollar, Melissa A., Shrider, Emily A., and John F. Craemer "Table A-4. Selected Measures of Household Income Dispersion: 1967 to 2019. Income and Poverty in the United States: 2019," U.S. Census Bureau, *Current Population Reports*, P60-270. Washington, DC: U.S. Government Printing Office. https://www.census.gov/content/dam/Census/library/publications/2020/demo/p60-270.pdf

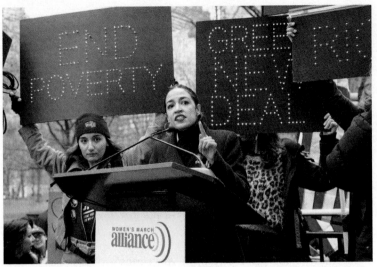

Alexandria Ocasio-Cortez ("AOC"), a media-savvy congresswoman from New York, kicks off the 3rd Annual Women's March in Manhattan on January 19, 2019. Among the causes championed by AOC are poverty reduction, immigration reform, and a Green New Deal to combat climate change.

Ira L. Black/Getty Images

comes from their principal residences, the asset category that took the biggest hit during the Great Recession. These Americans also hold almost three-quarters of America's debt.

Recognition of wealth disparities, and a growing realization that the rich have been getting richer and the poor, poorer, led to the Occupy movement of 2011 and fueled Bernie Sanders's 2016 and 2020 presidential campaign. Both the Occupy movement and the Sanders campaigns drew attention to the lagging economic recovery for a majority of Americans (see also Galbraith 2016; Piketty 2020).

Risky Living on the American Periphery

The nations on the periphery of the world system have the least economic development and political clout. Furthermore, within any given nation, certain regions and communities are similarly disadvantaged. One expression of this inequality is exposure to pollution and environmental hazards. Communities that are poorer and predominantly minority are more likely to be the victims of toxic waste exposure than are more affluent or even average (middle-class) communities.

News reports in 2015 and 2016 highlighted the plight of Flint, Michigan, whose water supply was seriously contaminated following a 2014 cost-cutting switch in its water source. The state of Michigan, which had seized control of Flint's city administration and budget from locally elected officials during a financial emergency, temporarily switched Flint's water source from Lake Huron and the Detroit River to the Flint River. The switch,

which took place in April 2014, was to be in effect until completion, in an estimated three years, of a new supply line from Lake Huron. The Flint River had a reputation for nastiness, and, soon after the switch, residents complained their water looked, smelled, and tasted funny (McLaughlin 2016).

Four months after the switch, Flint resident LeeAnne Walters, concerned about her family's deteriorating health, contacted Marc Edwards, a civil engineering professor and expert on water quality from Virginia Tech University. Walters previously had sought help from city and state officials, who told her nothing was wrong. However, when Edwards tested the water entering her home, he found lead levels he had never seen in 25 years of testing. Thereafter, Professor Edwards assembled a research team, which confirmed the overall toxicity of Flint's water supply, providing the scientific proof that ultimately led officials to abandon the Flint River (Kozlowski 2016).

The new water source had corroded the lead pipes that brought water into the city's homes. Residents complained about myriad health problems, including skin rashes, hair loss, nausea, dizziness, and pain. A local pediatrician found that lead levels in Flint toddlers had doubled, and in some cases tripled, since the switch. By the time the city switched back to the Detroit River and Lake Huron in October 2015, irreparable damage had been done not only to public health but also to the lead pipes. The state responded by handing out filters and bottled water (McLaughlin 2016). Arguments erupted about who should fund the replacement of Flint's water pipes. On January 5, 2016, then Michigan governor Rick Snyder declared Flint to be in a state of emergency. Soon thereafter, President Obama declared the city to be in a federal state of emergency, authorizing additional help from FEMA (the Federal Emergency Management Agency) and the Department of Homeland Security.

Residents of Flint have filed multiple lawsuits, faulting various agencies and individuals, including the city of Flint, the state's Department of Environmental Quality, and Governor Snyder, for violating the U.S. Safe Drinking Water Act. On January 21, 2020, the U.S. Supreme Court cleared the way for Flint water crisis victims to sue state and local government officials. This class action lawsuit includes thousands of Flint residents suing for damages from the 2014 incident.

Although millions in federal and state dollars have been allocated to Flint since the crisis, many Flint residents wonder if the fact that they live in one of the poorest cities in the nation is a reason why the process has moved so slowly, especially when they see the rapid recovery efforts carried out in places like Florida and Texas after hurricanes hit. They are right to wonder. That this story of toxic endangerment happened in one of Michigan's least affluent cities is no accident. Throughout the United States (as in many other nations), environmental hazards disproportionately endanger poor and minority communities. Flint's population is 54 percent African American. About 40 percent of its residents live below the poverty line, compared with state and national rates of 14 percent and 12 percent, respectively. One doubts that similar events would have played out in one of Michigan's affluent communities.

Research demonstrates that industries typically target minority and low-income neighborhoods when deciding where to locate polluting facilities (Erickson 2016). Environmental researchers Paul Mohai and Robin Saha (2015) analyzed 30 years of data on the placement of hazardous waste facilities in the United States. Their sample included 319 commercial hazardous waste treatment, storage, and disposal facilities built between 1966 and 1995. Their analysis revealed a clear pattern of racial and socioeconomic bias in the location of environmental hazards. Polluting facilities and other locally unwanted land uses were, and still are, located disproportionately in nonwhite and poor neighborhoods. These communities have fewer resources and political clout to oppose the location of such facilities.

The researchers also examined the demographic composition of neighborhoods at the time polluting facilities were built, as well as the demographic changes that followed the construction of a hazardous waste facility. They found that polluting facilities are often built in neighborhoods in transition. For a decade or two before the project arrived, whites had been moving out, and minorities and poor people moving in. Such demographic and social transition often is accompanied by the loss of community leaders and the weakening of social ties and civic organizations. Potential opposition to placement of hazardous facilities diminishes. Affluent communities, by contrast, are quick to mount organized resistance to environmental threats, and political leaders take them seriously. Industries choose to follow the path of least resistance and target communities with fewer resources and less political clout. Flint's story garnered headlines, but there are hundreds more stories waiting to be told about environmental threats on the American periphery.

COLONIALISM AND IMPERIALISM

The major forces influencing cultural interactions during the past 500 years have been commercial expansion, industrial capitalism, and the dominance of colonial and core nations (Wallerstein 2004; Wolf 1982). As state formation had done previously, industrialization accelerated local participation in larger networks. According to Bodley (2012), perpetual expansion is a distinguishing feature of industrial economic systems. That expansionist tendency fueled the growth of

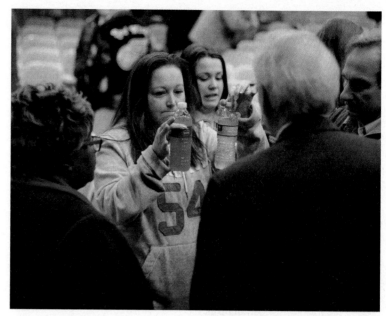

At a public meeting called to address her city's water crisis, Flint resident LeeAnne Walters displays water samples from her home to the city's new emergency manager.

Detroit Free Press/ZUMA Press/Alamy Stock Photo

European colonial empires during and after the 16th century.

Colonialism is the political, social, economic, and cultural domination of a territory and its people by a foreign power for an extended time. The colonial power establishes and maintains a presence in the dominated territory, in the form of colonists and administrative personnel (see Manjapra 2020; Stoler, McGranahan, and Perdue 2007). **Imperialism** refers to a conscious policy of extending the rule of a country or an empire over foreign nations and of taking and holding foreign colonies (see Burbank and Cooper 2010). Imperialism goes back to early states, including Egypt in the Old World and the Incas in the New. A Greek empire was forged by Alexander the Great, and Julius Caesar and his successors spread the Roman empire. More recent examples include the British, French, and Soviet empires (see Burbank and Cooper 2010).

If imperialism is almost as old as the state, colonialism can be traced back to the Phoenicians, who established colonies along the eastern Mediterranean 3,000 years ago. The ancient Greeks and Romans were avid colonizers as well as empire builders (see Pagden 2015; Stearns 2019).

The First Phase of European Colonialism: Spain and Portugal

The first phase of modern colonialism began with the European "Age of Discovery"—of the Americas and of a sea route to the Far East. During the 16th century, Spain, having conquered Mexico (the Aztec empire) and Peru-Bolivia (the Incas),

colonialism

The political, social, economic, and cultural domination of a territory and its people by a foreign power for an extended time.

imperialism

A conscious policy aimed at seizing and ruling foreign territory and peoples.

explored and colonized widely in the Caribbean, the southern portions of what was to become the United States, and Central and South America. In the Pacific, Spain extended its rule to the Philippines and Guam. The Portuguese colonial empire included Brazil, South America's largest colonial territory; Angola and Mozambique in Africa; and Goa, now in India.

Rebellions and wars aimed at independence ended the first phase of European colonialism by the early 19th century. Brazil declared independence from Portugal in 1822. By 1825, most of Spain's colonies had gained political independence. Spain held on to Cuba and the Philippines until 1898 but otherwise withdrew from the colonial field. During the first phase of colonialism, Spain and Portugal, along with Britain and France, were the major colonizing nations (see del Valle et al. 2020; Herzog 2015). The last two (Britain and France) dominated the second phase of colonialism.

Commercial Expansion and European Imperialism

A second phase of European colonialism occurred between 1875 and 1914. Europe's capitalists sought new markets and its nations competed for colonies and extended their imperial reach to Africa, Asia, and Oceania. During the second half of the 19th century, European imperial expansion was aided by improved transportation, which facilitated the colonization of vast areas of sparsely settled lands, e.g., in Australia. The new colonies purchased goods from Europe's industrial centers and shipped back wheat, cotton, wool, mutton, beef, and leather.

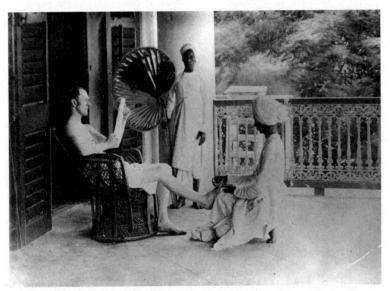

On January 1, 1900, a British officer in India receives a pedicure from a servant. What does this photo say to you about colonialism? Who gives pedicures today?

Hulton Archive/Getty Images

The British Colonial Empire

Like several other European nations, Britain had two stages of colonialism. The first began with the Elizabethan voyages of the 16th century. During the 17th century, Britain acquired most of the eastern coast of North America, Canada's St. Lawrence basin, islands in the Caribbean, ports in Africa, and interests in India.

The British shared the exploration and early European settlement of the New World with the Spanish, Portuguese, French, and Dutch. The British by and large left Mexico, along with Central and South America, to the Spanish and the Portuguese. The end of the Seven Years' War in 1763 forced a French retreat from most of Canada and India, where France previously had competed with Britain (Cody 1998). The American Revolution ended the first stage of British colonialism. India, Canada, and various Caribbean islands remained under British control.

The second stage of British colonialism—the British empire, on which the "sun never set," rose from the ashes of the first (see Black 2015; Levine 2020). Beginning in 1788, but intensifying after 1815, the British settled Australia. Britain had acquired Dutch South Africa by 1815. By 1819, Singapore anchored a British trade network that extended to much of South Asia and along the coast of China. By this time, the empires of Britain's traditional rivals, particularly Spain, had been severely diminished in scope. Britain's position as imperial power and the world's leading industrial nation was unchallenged.

Britain's colonial expansion continued during the Victorian Era (1837–1901). Under Queen Victoria, Prime Minister Benjamin Disraeli guided a foreign policy justified by a view of imperialism as shouldering "the white man's burden"—a phrase coined by the poet Rudyard Kipling. People in the empire were seen as incapable of governing themselves, so British guidance was needed to civilize and Christianize them. This paternalistic and racist doctrine was used to legitimize Britain's acquisition and control of parts of central Africa and Asia (Cooper 2014).

The British empire reached its maximum extent around 1914, when it covered a fifth of the world's land surface and ruled a fourth of its population (see Figure 14.1). After World War II, the British empire began to fall apart, with the rise of nationalist movements for independence. India gained its independence in 1947, as did the Republic of Ireland in 1949. The independence movement accelerated in Africa and Asia during the late 1950s (see Buettner 2016; Cooper 2019). Today, the ties that remain between Britain and its former colonies are mainly linguistic or cultural rather than political (Cody 1998).

French Colonialism

French colonialism also had two phases. The first began with the explorations of the early 1600s.

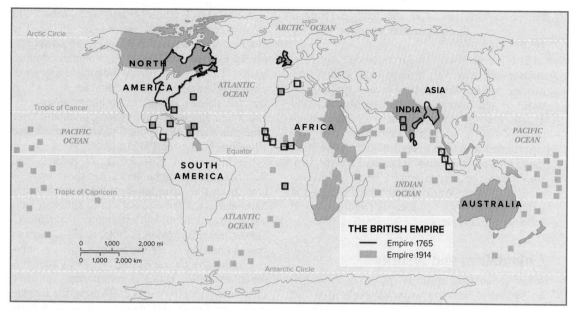

FIGURE 14.1 Map of British Empire in 1765 and 1914.

SOURCE: *Academic American Encyclopedia,* Vol. 3. 1998 Edition. Grolier, 1998.

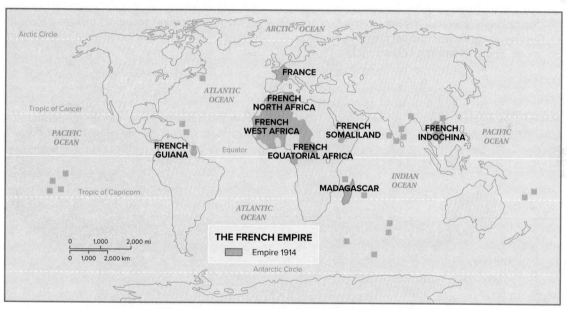

FIGURE 14.2 Map of the French Empire at Its Height around 1914.

SOURCE: *Academic American Encyclopedia,* Vol. 3. 1998 Edition. Grolier, 1998.

Prior to the French Revolution in 1789, missionaries, explorers, and traders carved out niches for France in Canada, the Louisiana Territory, several Caribbean islands, and parts of India, which were lost along with Canada to Great Britain in 1763 (Harvey 1980).

The foundations of the second French empire were established between 1830 and 1870. In Great Britain the drive for profit led expansion, but French colonialism was spurred more by the state, church, and armed forces than by pure business interests. France acquired Algeria and part of what eventually became Indochina (Cambodia, Laos, and Vietnam). By 1914, the French empire covered 4 million square miles and included some 60 million people (see Figure 14.2). By 1893, French rule had been fully established in Indochina. Tunisia and Morocco became French protectorates in 1883 and 1912, respectively (Harvey 1980).

To be sure, the French, like the British, had substantial business interests in their colonies, but they also sought, again like the British, international glory and prestige. The French promulgated a *mission civilisatrice,* their equivalent of Britain's "white man's burden." The goal was to implant

French culture, language, and religion (Roman Catholicism), throughout the colonies (Harvey 1980).

The French used two forms of colonial rule: *indirect rule,* governing through local leaders and existing political structures, in areas with long histories of state organization, such as Morocco and Tunisia; and *direct rule* by French officials in many areas of Africa, where the French imposed new government structures to control diverse societies, many of them previously stateless. Like the British empire, the French empire began to disintegrate after World War II. France fought long—and ultimately futile—wars to keep its empire intact in Indochina and Algeria.

Colonialism and Identity

Many geopolitical labels in the news today had no equivalent meaning before colonialism. Whole countries, along with social groups and divisions within them, were colonial inventions. In West Africa, for example, by geographic logic, several adjacent countries could be one (Togo, Ghana, Ivory Coast [Côte d'Ivoire], Guinea, Guinea-Bissau, Sierra Leone, Liberia). Instead, they are separated by linguistic, political, and economic contrasts promoted under colonialism (Figure 14.3).

Hundreds of ethnic groups and "tribes" are colonial constructions (see Ranger 1996). The Sukuma of Tanzania, for instance, were first registered as a single tribe by the colonial administration. Then missionaries standardized a series of dialects into a single Sukuma language, into which they translated the Bible and other religious texts, and which they taught in missionary schools. Over time this standardized the Sukuma language and ethnicity (Finnstrom 1997).

As in most of East Africa, in Rwanda and Burundi farmers and herders live in the same areas and speak the same language. Historically, they have shared the same social world, although their social organization is "extremely hierarchical," almost "castelike" (Malkki 1995, p. 24). There has been a tendency to see the pastoral Tutsis as superior to the agricultural Hutus. Tutsis have been presented as nobles, Hutus as commoners. Yet when distributing identity cards in Rwanda, the Belgian colonizers simply identified all people with more than 10 head of cattle as Tutsi. Owners of fewer cattle were registered as Hutus (Bjuremalm 1997). Years later, these arbitrary colonial registers were used systematically for "ethnic" identification during the mass killings (genocide) that took place in Rwanda in 1994 (as portrayed vividly in the film *Hotel Rwanda*).

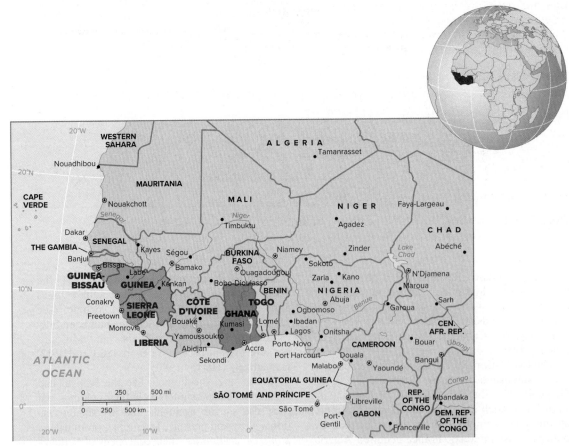

FIGURE 14.3 Small West African Nations Created by Colonialism.

Postcolonial Studies

In anthropology, history, and literature, the field of postcolonial studies has gained prominence since the 1970s (see Ashcroft, Griffiths, and Tiffin 2013; Nayar 2016). **Postcolonial** studies focus on the past and present interactions between European nations and the societies they colonized (mainly after 1800). In 1914, European empires ruled more than 85 percent of the world (see Streets-Salter and Getz 2016). The term *postcolonial* also has been used to describe the second half of the 20th century in general, the period following colonialism. Even more generically, *postcolonial* may be used to signify a position against colonialism, imperialism, and Eurocentrism (Buettner 2016; Sèbe and Stanard 2020; Stoler 2013). Eurocentrism refers to interpretations of the world that rely mainly or entirely on European or Anglo-American perspectives.

The former colonies (*postcolonies*) can be divided into settler, nonsettler, and mixed (Petraglia-Bahri 1996). The settler countries, with large numbers of European colonists and sparser native populations, include Australia, Canada, and the United States. Examples of nonsettler countries include India, Pakistan, Bangladesh, Sri Lanka, Malaysia, Indonesia, Nigeria, Senegal, and Madagascar. All these had substantial native populations and relatively few European settlers. Mixed countries include South Africa, Zimbabwe, Kenya, and Algeria. Such countries had significant European settlement despite having sizable native populations.

Given the varied experiences of such countries, *postcolonial* has to be a loose term. The United States, for instance, was colonized by Europeans and fought a war for independence from Britain. Is the United States a postcolony? It usually isn't perceived as such, given its current world-power position and its treatment of Native Americans (sometimes called settler colonialism). Research in postcolonial studies has been growing, permitting a wide-ranging investigation of power relations in varied contexts. Broad topics in the field include the formation of empires, the impact of colonization, and the state of the postcolony today (Petraglia-Bahri 1996; Stoler 2013).

DEVELOPMENT

During the Industrial Revolution, a strong current of thought viewed industrialization as a beneficial process of organic development and progress. Many economists still assume that industrialization increases production and income. They seek to create in "developing" countries a process like the one that first occurred spontaneously in 18th-century Great Britain.

We have seen that Britain used the notion of a white man's burden to justify its imperialist expansion and that France claimed to be engaged in a *mission civilisatrice,* a civilizing mission, in its

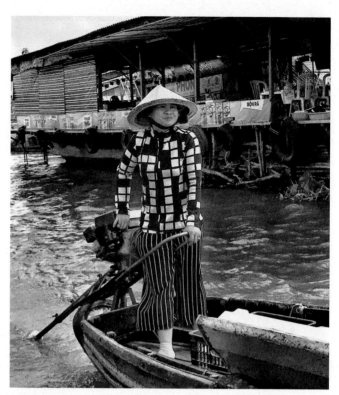

A postcolonial woman on the Mekong River in southern Vietnam, February 2018. Which European empire once ruled Vietnam?
Conrad P. Kottak

colonies. Both these ideas illustrate an **intervention philosophy,** an ideological justification for outsiders to guide native peoples in specific directions. Economic development plans also have intervention philosophies. John Bodley (2012) argues that the basic belief behind interventions—whether by colonialists, missionaries, governments, or development planners—has been the same for more than a century. This belief is that industrialization, Westernization, and individualism are desirable evolutionary advances and that development schemes that promote them will bring long-term benefits to local people.

Neoliberalism

One currently prominent intervention philosophy is neoliberalism, which encompasses a set of assumptions that have gained influence among planners during the past 30 years (see Carrier 2016). Neoliberal policies are being implemented in developing nations, including postsocialist societies (e.g., those of the former Soviet Union). **Neoliberalism** is the current form of the classic economic liberalism laid out in Adam Smith's famous capitalist manifesto *The Wealth of Nations,* published in 1776, soon after the Industrial Revolution. Smith advocated laissez-faire (hands-off) economics as the basis of capitalism: The government should stay out of its nation's economic affairs. Free trade, Smith argued, is the best way for a nation's economy to develop. There should

postcolonial
Describing relations between European nations and areas they colonized and once ruled.

intervention philosophy
An ideological justification for outsiders to guide or rule native peoples.

neoliberalism
The principle that governments shouldn't regulate private enterprise; free market forces should rule.

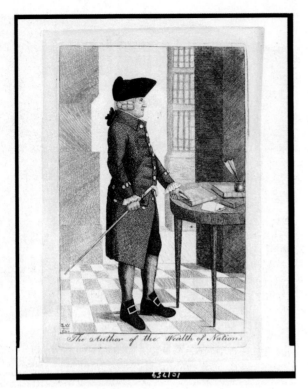

An engraving of Scottish political philosopher and economist Adam Smith (1723-1790) made by a contemporary artist of his time. In his famed capitalist manifesto, *The Wealth of Nations,* published in 1776, Smith advocated "free" enterprise and competition, with the goal of generating profits.

source: Library of Congress [LC-USZ62- 101759]

be no restrictions on manufacturing, no barriers to commerce, and no tariffs. This philosophy is called "liberalism" because it aimed at liberating or freeing the economy from government controls. Economic liberalism encouraged "free" enterprise and competition, with the goal of generating profits. (Ironically, Adam Smith's liberalism is closer to today's capitalist "conservatism" than to what is usually considered "liberalism" today.)

Economic liberalism prevailed in the United States until President Franklin Roosevelt's New Deal during the 1930s. The Great Depression produced a turn to Keynesian economics, which challenged liberalism. John Maynard Keynes (1927, 1936) insisted that full employment was necessary for capitalism to grow, that governments and central banks should intervene to increase employment, and that government should promote the common good (see Hayes 2019).

Especially since the fall of Communism (1989–1991), there has been a widespread revival of (neo) liberalism. Around the world, neoliberal policies have been imposed by powerful financial institutions such as the International Monetary Fund (IMF), the World Bank, and the Inter-American Development Bank (see Edelman and Haugerud 2005). Neoliberalism entails open (tariff- and

barrier-free) international trade and investment. Profits are increased by lowering costs, whether by improving productivity, automating, laying off workers, or seeking workers who accept lower wages. In exchange for loans, the governments of postsocialist and developing nations have been required to accept the neoliberal premise that deregulation leads to economic growth, which will eventually benefit everyone through a process sometimes called "trickle down." Accompanying the belief in free markets and the idea of cutting costs is a tendency to impose austerity measures that cut government expenses. This can entail reduced public spending on education, health care, and other social services, as has happened in recent years with imposed austerity in Greece and elsewhere (see Donnelly 2019; Kozaitis 2021).

In the United States, the Trump administration has departed from neoliberal policies traditionally favored by his Republican Party. Trump's suspicion of unfettered trade and "unfair trade deals" led his administration to (1) impose tariffs on goods imported from China and other countries and (2) abandon or modify trade agreements designed to facilitate freer trade among partners to the pact. One example of such a pact is NAFTA, the North American Free Trade Agreement. Signed in 1992, NAFTA was to gradually eliminate most tariffs and other trade barriers on products and services passing between the United States, Canada, and Mexico.

Neoliberalism and NAFTA's Economic Refugees

Most Americans know about large-scale Mexican migration to the United States since the 1990s. Most are unaware, however, that the direction of migration has shifted in recent years. Since 2008, more Mexicans have returned to Mexico than have entered the United States. Americans also are familiar with rhetoric (e.g., during the 2016 presidential campaigns and thereafter under President Trump) about negative effects of trade agreements on American workers.

Much less common is knowledge about how NAFTA has been harmful to Mexico. Anthropologist Ana Aurelia López (2011) has argued convincingly that international forces, including new technologies and NAFTA, have destroyed traditional Mexican farming systems, degraded agricultural land, and displaced Mexican farmers and small-business people—thereby fueling the migration of millions of undocumented Mexicans to the United States. The following account summarizes her findings.

For thousands of years, Mexican farmers grew corn (maize, which was originally domesticated in what is now Mexico) in a sustainable manner. Generation after generation, farmers selected diverse strains of corn well adapted to a huge variety of specific microclimates. Mexico became a repository of corn genetic diversity for the world. When corn grown elsewhere developed disease or pest susceptibility or was of poor quality, Mexico provided other countries with genetically superior plants.

Before NAFTA, Mexico supported its farmers by buying a portion of their harvest each year at an elevated cost through price supports. This corn went to a countrywide chain of successful CONASUPO (Compañia Nacional de Subsistencias Populares) stores, which sold corn and other staple foodstuffs below market price to the urban and rural poor. Tariffs protected Mexican farmers from the entrance of foreign corn, such as that grown in the United States.

The first assault on Mexico's sustainable farming culture began in the 1940s when "Green Revolution" technologies were introduced, including seeds that required chemical inputs (e.g., fertilizer). The Mexican government encouraged farmers to replace their traditional, genetically diverse *maíz crillo* ("creole corn") with the genetically homogenized *maíz mejorado* ("improved corn"), a hybrid from the United States. Agrochemical companies initially supplied the required chemical inputs free of charge.

Company representatives visited rural villages and offered free samples of seeds and agrochemicals to a few farmers. As news of unusually large first-year crops spread, other farmers abandoned their traditional corn strains for the "improved," chemically dependent corn. As the transition accelerated, the price of both the new seeds and the associated chemical inputs began to rise, and kept on rising. Eventually, farmers no longer could afford either the seeds or the required agrochemicals. When cash-strapped farmers tried to return to planting their former *maíz criollo* seeds, the plants would grow but corn would not appear. Only the hybrid seeds from the United States would produce corn on the chemically altered soils. Today over 60 percent of Mexico's farmland has been degraded by the spread of agrochemicals—chemical fertilizers and pesticides.

NAFTA, which went into effect in 1994, proved to be another major assault on the Mexican farming system. The agreement forced Mexico to restructure its economy along neoliberal lines. The government had to end its price supports for corn grown by small-scale farmers. Also ended were Mexico's CONASUPO food stores, which had benefited the rural and urban poor.

These terminations caused considerable harm to Mexico's farmers and its urban and rural poor. American agricultural industries, by contrast, have benefited from NAFTA. Prior to NAFTA, Mexico's border tariffs made the sale of U.S. corn in Mexico unprofitable. Under NAFTA, Mexico's corn tariffs were phased out, and corn from the United States began flooding the Mexican markets.

The NAFTA economy offered Mexico's small-scale corn farmers few options: (1) stay in rural Mexico and suffer, (2) look for work in a Mexican city, or (3) migrate to the United States in search of work. NAFTA did not create a common labor market (i.e., the ability of Mexicans, Americans, and Canadians to move freely across each country's borders and work legally anywhere in North America). Nor did NAFTA make provisions for the predicted 15 million Mexican corn farmers who would be forced off the land as a result of the trade agreement. As could have been expected

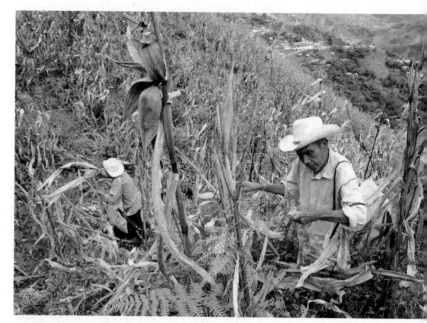

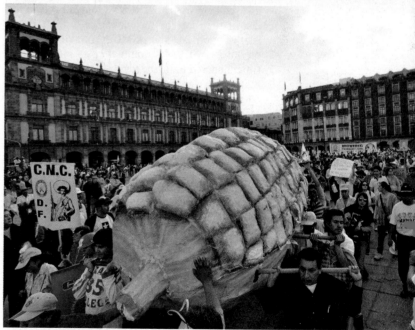

On the top, farmers harvest native corn in Oaxaca, Mexico. These are some of the many varieties that were first cultivated in Mesoamerica around 8,000 years ago. On the bottom, demonstrators in Mexico City protest NAFTA's removal of import tariffs on farm goods, especially corn and beans, entering Mexico from the United States and Canada.

Top: Philippe Psaila/Science Source; bottom: Eduardo Verdugo/AP Images

(and planned for), millions of Mexicans seeking a livelihood migrated to the United States.

As a result of NAFTA, Mexican corn farmers have fled the countryside, and U.S.-subsidized corn has flooded the Mexican market. A declining number of traditional farmers remain to plant and conserve Mexico's unique corn varieties. Between one-third and one-half of Mexico's corn now is imported from the United States, much of it by U.S.-based Archer-Daniels-Midland, the world's largest corporate corn exporter. NAFTA also has facilitated the entrance of other giant U.S. corporations into Mexico: Walmart, Dow Agribusiness, Monsanto, and Coca-Cola. These multinationals, in turn, have displaced many small Mexican businesses, creating yet another wave of immigrants—former shopkeepers and their employees—to the United States.

We can summarize the impact of NAFTA on the Mexican economy: destroying traditional small-scale farming, degrading farmland, displacing farmers and small-business people, and fueling massive migration to the United States. In migrating, these millions of economic refugees have faced daunting challenges, including separation from their families and homeland, dangerous border crossings, and the ever-present possibility of deportation from the United States.

As of this writing, under President Trump, their fate has become even more uncertain. In 2018 the United States, Mexico, and Canada agreed to modify NAFTA, renaming it the United States–Mexico–Canada Agreement, or USMCA. Final ratification of this modified trade pact was assured in March 2020, when Canada became the last of the three partner countries to give it legislative approval. The USMCA entered into force on July 1, 2020. Its eventual costs and benefits (intended and unintended) to Mexico, the United States, and Canada remain to be seen.

As contemporary forces transform rural landscapes worldwide, rural–urban and transnational migration have become global phenomena. Over and over again, Green Revolution technologies have converted subsistence into cash economies, fueling a need for money to acquire foreign inputs while hooking the land on chemicals, reducing genetic diversity and sustainability, and forcing the poorest farmers off the land. Few Americans are aware, specifically, of NAFTA's role in ending a 7,000-year-old sustainable farming culture and displacing millions of Mexicans and, more generally, that comparable developments are happening all over the world.

COMMUNISM, SOCIALISM, AND POSTSOCIALISM

Communism

The two meanings of communism involve how it is written, whether with a lowercase (small) or an uppercase (large) *c*. Small-*c* **communism** is a

social system in which property is owned by the community and in which people work for the common good. Large-*C* **Communism** was a political movement and doctrine seeking to overthrow capitalism and to establish a form of Communism such as that which prevailed in the Soviet Union (UssR) from 1917 to 1991. The heyday of Communism was a 40-year period from 1949 to 1989, when more Communist regimes existed than at any time before or after. Today only five Communist states remain—China, Cuba, Laos, North Korea, and Vietnam, compared with 23 in 1985.

Communism, which originated with Russia's Bolshevik Revolution in 1917 and took its inspiration from Karl Marx and Friedrich Engels, was not uniform over time or among countries. All Communist systems were *authoritarian* (promoting obedience to authority rather than individual freedom). Many were *totalitarian* (banning rival parties and demanding total submission of the individual to the state). The Communist Party monopolized power in every Communist state, and relations within the party were highly centralized and strictly disciplined. Communist nations had state ownership, rather than private ownership, of the means of production. Finally, all Communist regimes, with the goal of advancing communism, cultivated a sense of belonging to an international movement (Brown 2001).

Social scientists have tended to refer to such societies as socialist rather than Communist. Today research by anthropologists is thriving in *postsocialist* societies—those that once emphasized bureaucratic redistribution of wealth according to a central plan (Gevorkyan 2018; Giordano, Ruegg, and Boscoboinik 2014; Verdery 2001). In the postsocialist period, states that once featured planned economies have been following the neoliberal agenda, by divesting themselves of state-owned resources in favor of privatization and marketization. Some of them have moved toward formal liberal democracy, with political parties, elections, and a balance of powers (see Gudeman and Hann 2015).

Postsocialist Transitions

Socialism is a sociopolitical organization and economic system in which the means of production are owned and controlled by the government, rather than by individuals or corporations. Because of their state ownership, Communist nations were also socialist, and their successors are referred to as postsocialist. Neoliberal economists assumed that dismantling and privatizing the Soviet Union's planned economy would raise gross domestic product (GDP) and living standards. The goal was to enhance production by substituting a free market system and providing incentives through privatization. In October 1991, Boris Yeltsin, who had been elected president of Russia that June, announced a program of radical market-oriented reform, pursuing a postsocialist changeover to capitalism.

socialism
A sociopolitical organization and economic system in which the means of production are owned and controlled by the government, rather than by individuals or corporations.

communism
A social system in which property is owned by the community and people work for the common good.

Communism
A political movement aimed at replacing capitalism with Soviet-style Communism.

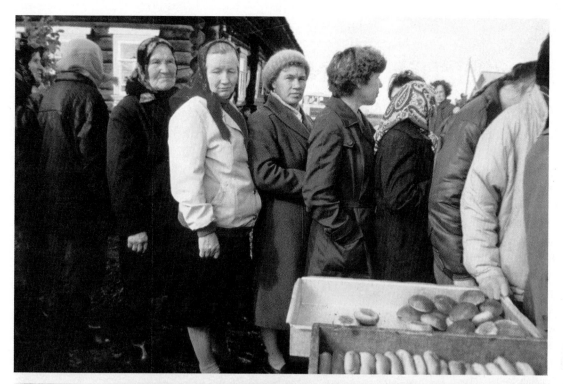

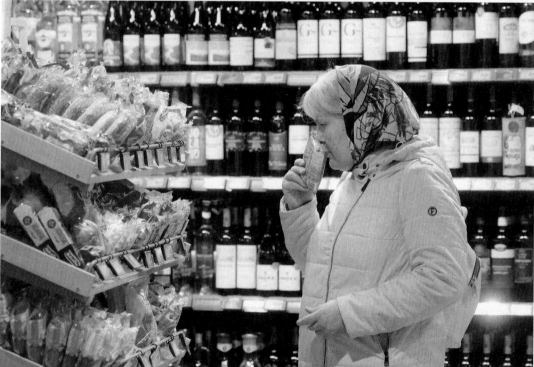

(Top) As the former Soviet Union was nearing its end, villagers in the Kirov region lined up to buy rolls on May Day eve, 1990. (Bottom) A customer chooses bread in a Pyaterochka store in Moscow in November, 2019. Pyaterochka is a popular Russian chain of more than 15,000 convenience stores.

Top: Sovfoto/Univeral Images Group/Getty Images; bottom: Sergei Savostyanov/Getty Images

Yeltsin's program of "shock therapy" cut subsidies to farms and industries and ended price controls.

During the 1990s, postsocialist Russia endured a series of disruptions, leading to declines in its GDP, average life expectancy, and birth rate, as well as increased poverty. In 2008–2009, Russia shared in the global recession after 10 years of economic growth, but its economy recuperated rapidly and was growing again by 2010, as were its birth rate and average life expectancy. The poverty rate has fallen substantially since the late 1990s, and Moscow is said to be home to more billionaires

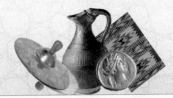

appreciating **ANTHROPOLOGY**

When the Mills Shut Down: An Anthropologist Looks at Deindustrialization

Since the year 2000, over 5.5 million manufacturing jobs have been lost in the United States, continuing a trend that started in the 1970s and intensified in the 1980s and thereafter. This industrial decline has affected hundreds of towns and cities, particularly in the Rust Belt states of Illinois, Wisconsin, Michigan, and Pennsylvania. As described by Elizabeth Svoboda (2017), Christine Walley, an anthropology professor at MIT, focuses on the human effects of factory closures on laid-off workers, their families, and communities.

Walley was raised in a steel-working family in Southeast Chicago. Returning to her childhood neighborhood as a participant observer, she has been gathering stories that reveal the trauma that displaced industrial workers have suffered. In her book *Exit Zero: Family and Class in Postindustrial Chicago* (2013) and her film *Exit Zero: An Industrial Family Story* (2014), Walley describes how her father, Chuck, lost his job at Wisconsin Steel when that mill closed in 1980. Other mill closures followed, devastating Walley's family and community.

Southeast Chicago's mills were still churning out steel when Christine Walley was born in 1965. Every morning, her dad headed to his job at Wisconsin Steel, the area's oldest mill. The work was hazardous, but it paid enough to support the Walley family of five, and it promised Chuck a generous pension when he retired.

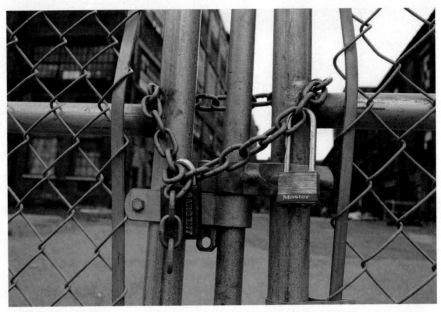

Bethlehem Steel's massive five furnace industrial complex in Bethlehem, Pennsylvania, produced American steel for 120 years, employing tens of thousands of workers. After it closed for good in 1995, the city redeveloped the area as a tourist attraction, park, and community arts center.

Andrew Lichtenstein/Getty Images

Along with more than 3,000 other Wisconsin Steel workers, Chuck was laid off in 1980, when Christine Walley was 14 years old. For years, the mill's corporate owners had neglected its upkeep, and its final owner was suspected of deliberately squeezing some terminal profits out of the mill before declaring bankruptcy. Chuck lost not only his job but also his promised pension. Henceforth, the lives of the Walley family would be divided sharply into "before" and "after" the mill shut down.

Following his layoff, Chuck Walley pursued a series of odd jobs, including janitorial work and truck driving. Those jobs paid very little, and Chuck's wife had to start working as well. No longer able to support his family, Chuck suffered chronic depression and despair—lying on his couch and smoking cigarettes. He died of

than New York City or London (Rapoza 2012). In recent years, rising wages have been offset by rising living costs and galloping inflation.

THE WORLD SYSTEM TODAY

The spread of industrialization continues today, although nations have shifted their positions within the world system. Recap 14.1 summarizes

those shifts. By 1900, the United States had become a core nation within the world system and had overtaken Great Britain in iron, coal, and cotton production. In a few decades (1868–1900), Japan had changed from a medieval handicraft economy to an industrial one, joining the semiperiphery by 1900 and moving to the core between 1945 and 1970. India and China have joined Brazil as leaders of the semiperiphery. Figure 14.4 is a map showing the modern world system.

lung cancer in 2005, still shaken by his inability to find satisfactory employment. Of the 3,400 men and women who once worked for Wisconsin Steel, about one-quarter were dead just eight years later. They fell victim to addiction, depression, and suicide. Around them, the layoffs continued. The nearby U.S. Steel South Works production plant, which once employed more than 20,000 Chicagoans, shut down in 1992 (Svoboda 2017).

As an adult and an anthropologist, Christine Walley has sought to understand what happened—not just to her family and community but throughout the Rust Belt. Her Exit Zero Project, which combines film, writing, and collaboration with a local historical museum, tells the story of her family's postindustrial demise. Walley brings in other voices as well; she conversed with and interviewed people in her old neighborhood who shared her family's experience and its sense of displacement and alienation. The social and psychological impacts of industrial closures have been profound. Former workers lost both their livelihoods (financial security) and the work that gave their lives meaning and value. Churches, restaurants, and other local gathering spots closed along with the mills, depriving laid-off workers of familiar networks of social support.

Deindustrialization continues today for three main reasons: (1) global competition, (2) automation, and (3) corporate decisions and government policies. Some manufacturing jobs have been shifted to other countries, or lost to foreign competition. Even more significant is automation, as machines do more and more jobs—a trend that will continue. As automation—increasingly powered by artificial intelligence—continues, white-collar workers, too, will face the same displacement and anxiety that blue-collar workers have experienced for decades.

Also important have been federal laws that have facilitated corporate decisions to close factories. A trend toward looser regulation began in the 1970s and accelerated during the 1980s. Corporations could merge, acquire, and dispose of new companies with little interference. Federal laws permitted investors to buy up older factories and milk them for profits while neglecting pension funds, and eventually allowing the enterprises to go bankrupt. This is exactly what happened at Wisconsin Steel. With further deregulation under the Trump administration, workers are likely to be even more at the mercy of corporate schemes.

Examples from other countries demonstrate that industrial decline is not an inevitable result of global competition. As American mills and factories were failing, something very different was happening in Canada. Government policies were encouraging companies to modernize and funnel profits back into mill upkeep. As a result, not a single Canadian steel mill closed during this period of American industrial decline. Germany, too, has managed to maintain a robust industrial economy even with global competition (see Svoboda 2017).

During the 2016 U.S. presidential primaries and election, both the eventual winner, Donald Trump, and Vermont senator Bernie Sanders, who calls himself a democratic socialist, drew significant support from Rust Belt blue-collar workers. Trump mainly faulted trade agreements and immigrants, promising to bring back jobs and "make America great again." Sanders blamed "millionaires and billionaires," including corporations and Wall Street, for the country's ills. Both promised more radical solutions than their rivals. As President, in March, 2018, Trump announced that he would impose a tariff of 25 percent on imported steel. When Christine Walley analyzed election data from her old neighborhood, she found that Trump voters there tended to be swing voters, rather than core Trump supporters. She speculates that they may well abandon Trump if his policies fail to bring back jobs. The overriding concern of these Southeast Chicago voters was to challenge an economic system that had failed them (see Svoboda 2017).

From Walley's work, we learn how industrial workers and their families have experienced their loss of, and how they wish to recapture, the sense of dignity and self-worth that comes from work that is productive and meaningful. Walley advocates closer scrutiny of laws and policies that have facilitated the wave of mill closures. Along with social scientists, policy makers need to pay more concerted attention to what future work should look like, and to mitigating laws and policies that favor corporate interests over workers' well-being. Is this a pipe dream, or do you think it might really happen?

Twentieth-century industrialization added hundreds of new industries and millions of new jobs. Production increased, often beyond immediate demand, spurring strategies, such as advertising, to sell everything industry could churn out. Mass production gave rise to a culture of consumption, which valued acquisitiveness and conspicuous consumption (see Menely 2018).

How do things stand today? Worldwide, young people are abandoning traditional subsistence pursuits and seeking cash. A popular song once queried "How're you gonna keep 'em down on the farm after they've seen Paree?" Nowadays most people *have* seen Paree—Paris, that is—along with other world capitals, maybe not in person but in print or on-screen. Young people today are better educated and wiser in the ways of the world than ever before. Increasingly they are exposed to the material and cultural promises of a better life away from the farm. They seek paying jobs, but work is scarce, spurring migration within and across national boundaries. If they can't get cash legally, they seek it illegally.

RECAP 14.1 Ascent and Decline of Nations within the World System

PERIPHERY TO SEMIPERIPHERY	SEMIPERIPHERY TO CORE	CORE TO SEMIPERIPHERY
United States (1800–1860)	United States (1860–1900)	Spain (1620–1700)
Japan (1868–1900)	Japan (1945–1970)	
Taiwan (1949–1980)	Germany (1870–1900)	
S. Korea (1953–1980)		

SOURCE: Shannon, Thomas R., *An Introduction to the World-System Perspective,* 2nd ed., Westview Press, 1989, 1996, 147.

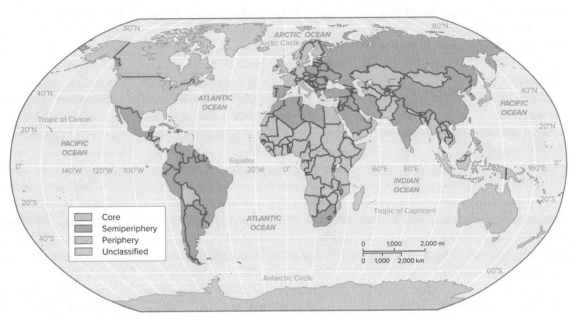

FIGURE 14.4 The World System Today.

In the aftermath of the global recession of 2007–2009, job opportunities diminished in core nations, including the United States and Western Europe. In a global economy, profitability doesn't necessarily come from hiring workers who are fellow citizens. Jobs in core nations continue to be transferred to machines and to be outsourced to the semiperiphery and the periphery. (This chapter's "Appreciating Anthropology" focuses on the human effects of factory closures on laid-off workers, their families, and communities.) Corporations, from airlines to banks, offer their customers incentives to bypass humans. Even outside the industrial world, but especially within it, the Internet allows an increasing number of people to buy and cancel plane tickets, rent cars, reserve hotel rooms, move money, or pay bills online. Amazon has become a virtual department store that has sent, or threatens to send, not only "mom and pop" shops but even national chains such as Barnes and Noble, Office Depot, and Sears into oblivion. Nowadays, when one does manage to speak by phone to a human, that person is as likely to be in Mumbai or Manila as Minneapolis or Miami.

Companies claim, with some justification, that labor unions limit their flexibility, adaptability, and profitability. American corporations (and the politicians who represent them) have become more ideologically opposed to unions and more aggressive in discouraging unionization. Unions still bring benefits to their workers. Median weekly earnings for union members—$1,095 in 2019—remain higher than those of nonunion workers—$892. Still, union membership in the United States keeps falling. The unionized percentage of the American workforce was 10.3 percent in 2019, down from 20.1 percent in 1983 and a high of 35 percent during the mid-1950s. The number of unionized private-sector workers increased from 7.1 million in 2010 to 7.5 million in 2019, while the number of public-sector union members declined from 7.6 million to 7.1 million. This mainly reflected growth in private-sector jobs, while jobs in the public sector were being reduced. The union membership rate of public-sector workers (33.6 percent) remains more than five times higher than that of private-sector workers (6.2 percent) (All 2019 figures are from the U.S. Bureau of Labor Statistics [2020]). What jobs do you know that are unionized? How likely is it that you will join a union?

1. Local societies increasingly participate in wider systems—regional, national, and global. The capitalist world economy depends on production for sale, with the goal of maximizing profits. The key claim of world-system theory is that an identifiable social system, based on wealth and power differentials, extends beyond individual countries. That system is formed by a set of economic and political relations that has characterized much of the globe since the 16th century. World capitalism has political and economic specialization at the core, semiperiphery, and periphery.

2. Columbus's voyages opened the way for a major exchange between the Old and New Worlds. Seventeenth-century plantation economies in the Caribbean and Brazil were based on sugar. In the 18th century, plantation economies based on cotton arose in the southeastern United States.

3. The Industrial Revolution began in England around 1750. Transoceanic commerce supplied capital for industrial investment. Industrialization hastened the separation of workers from the means of production. Marx saw a sharp division between the bourgeoisie and the proletariat. Class consciousness was a key feature of Marx's view of this stratification. Weber believed that social solidarity based on ethnicity, religion, race, or nationality could take priority over class. Today's capitalist world economy maintains the contrast between those who own the means of production and those who don't, but the division is now worldwide. There is a substantial contrast between not only capitalists but also workers in the core nations versus workers on the periphery.

4. Inequality in measures of income and wealth has been increasing in the United States. Another aspect of inequality is in exposure to environmental risks such as pollution and hazardous waste facilities. Communities that are poorer and predominantly minority, such as Flint, Michigan, are most likely to be the victims of toxic waste exposure.

5. Imperialism is the conscious policy of extending the rule of a nation or an empire over other nations and of taking and holding foreign colonies. Colonialism is the domination of a territory and its people by a foreign power for an extended time. European colonialism had two main phases. The first started in 1492 and lasted through 1825. For Britain this phase ended with the American Revolution. For France it ended when Britain won the Seven Years' War, forcing the French to abandon Canada and India. For Spain it ended with Latin American independence. The second phase of European colonialism extended approximately from 1850 to 1950. The British and French empires were at their height around 1914, when European empires controlled 85 percent of the world. Britain and France had colonies in Africa, Asia, Oceania, and the New World.

6. Many geopolitical labels and identities that were created under colonialism had little or nothing to do with existing social demarcations. The new ethnic or national divisions were colonial inventions, sometimes aggravating conflicts.

7. Like colonialism, economic development has an intervention philosophy that provides a justification for outsiders to guide native peoples toward particular goals. Development usually is justified by the idea that industrialization and modernization are desirable evolutionary advances. Neoliberalism revives and extends classic economic liberalism: the idea that governments should not regulate private enterprise and that free market forces should rule. This intervention philosophy currently dominates aid agreements with postsocialist and developing nations. Neoliberal policies, new technologies, and the North American Free Trade Agreement (NAFTA) have endangered traditional Mexican farming systems, degraded agricultural land, and displaced Mexican farmers and small-business people—thereby fueling the migration of millions of undocumented Mexicans to the United States.

8. Spelled with a lowercase c, communism is a social system in which property is owned by the community and in which people work for the common good. Spelled with an uppercase C, Communism indicates a political movement and doctrine seeking to overthrow capitalism and to establish a form of communism such as that which prevailed in the Soviet Union from 1917 to 1991. The heyday of Communism was between 1949 and 1989. The fall of Communism can be traced to 1989–1990 in eastern Europe and 1991 in the Soviet Union. Postsocialist states have followed the neoliberal agenda, through privatization, deregulation, and democratization.

9. By 1900, the United States had become a core nation. Mass production had given rise to a culture, now global in scope, that valued acquisitiveness and conspicuous consumption.

key terms

think like an anthropologist

1. According to world-system theory, societies are subsystems of bigger systems, with the world system as the largest. What are the various systems, at different levels, in which you participate?

2. How does world-system theory help explain why companies hire thousands of workers in India while laying off an equivalent number in Europe and the United States?

3. What were the causes and socioeconomic consequences of the Industrial Revolution? How might knowledge of early industrialization be relevant for an anthropologist interested in investigating the dynamics of industrialization today?

4. Think of a recent case in which a core nation has intervened in the affairs of another nation. What was the intervention philosophy used to justify the action?

5. To what extent is the following statement still true: "The wealth that flows from periphery and semiperiphery to core has helped core capitalists maintain their profits while satisfying the demands of core workers." Are core workers still satisfied? What factors might diminish their level of satisfaction?

credits

Anthropology's Role in a Globalizing World

- ▶ What is global climate change, and how can anthropologists study it, along with other environmental threats?

- ▶ What is cultural imperialism, and what forces work to favor and oppose it?

- ▶ What are indigenous peoples, and how and why has their importance increased in recent years?

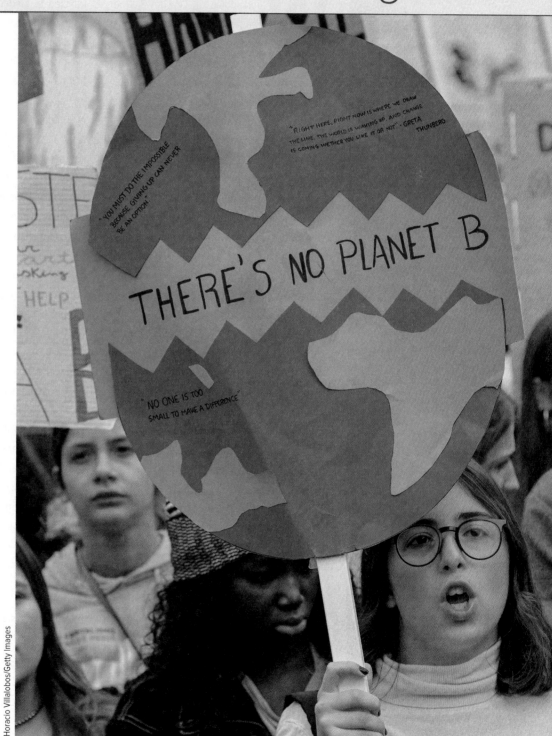

Horacio Villalobos/Getty Images

This rally supporting action on climate change was held in Lisbon, Portugal on November 29, 2019. It was part of a global school strike preceding the United Nations Conference on Climate Change, which began in Madrid, Spain on December 2, 2019.

understanding OURSELVES

What's your favorite science fiction movie or TV show? What images of other planets, or of a future Earth, stand out in your memory? Can you visualize various planets in the *Star Wars* galaxy? Movie images probably are more familiar to you than those of real planets. Think, too, about how extraterrestrials have been portrayed in movies. On the one hand are *ET*'s harmless plant collectors and *Avatar*'s endangered Na'vi. More typical are Earth's would-be conquerors, as shown in two *Independence Day* films, three *Starship Troopers* movies, and a hundred others. Still other films, most notably *The Day the Earth Stood Still* (either the 1951 or the 2008 version), feature omnipotent, omniscient guardians of the galaxy and interplanetary affairs.

If some of our most vivid perceptions of other planets come from fiction, modern technology makes it easier than ever for us to perceive the Earth as both a planet and our world. Anthropologists can use Google Earth to locate communities they have studied in remote corners of the world. My colleagues and I have even used space images to choose communities to study on Earth. Interested in the causes of deforestation in Madagascar, we examined a series of satellite images taken in successive years to determine areas where the forest

cover had diminished significantly. Then we traveled to Madagascar to study those areas on the ground. It's interesting to imagine what an alien might "see" in similar images. If those aliens were (as the more benevolent science fiction movies imagine) interested in studying life on Earth, rather than conquering, controlling, or even eating its inhabitants, they would have a lot to interpret. In my work abroad, I've been impressed by two major global trends: population increase and the shift from subsistence to cash economies. These trends have led to agricultural intensification, resource depletion (including deforestation), and emigration and have made it increasingly harder to not think globally when asking ourselves who we are.

I'm struck by the growing number of young people worldwide who have abandoned traditional subsistence pursuits. They seek jobs for cash, but work is scarce, spurring migration within and across national boundaries. In turn, transnational migration increases cultural diversity, while also generating heated political debates, in the United States and Europe. Every day we encounter people whose ancestral countries and cultures have been studied by anthropologists for generations—making cultural anthropology all the more relevant to our daily lives in an increasingly interconnected world.

This chapter applies an anthropological perspective to contemporary global issues. Let's begin by reviewing two different meanings of the term *globalization*. As used in this book, the primary meaning of globalization is worldwide connectedness. Modern systems of transportation, communication, and finance are global in scope. There are

interlinked systems of production, distribution, and consumption that extend across all nations and regions. A second meaning of globalization is political; it has to do with ideology, policy, and neoliberalism (see Hosseini et al. 2020; Kotz 2015). In this more limited sense, globalization refers to efforts by international financial powers to create a global free market for goods and services. This second, political meaning of globalization has generated and continues to generate significant opposition. In this book, *globalization* is a neutral term for the fact of global connectedness and linkages, rather than any kind of political position (see also Eriksen 2014; Ervin 2014; Lechner and Boli 2019).

The fact that certain practices and risks have global implications warrants a discussion of energy consumption and environmental degradation, including climate change, or global warming. Also considered in this chapter are the threats that deforestation and emerging diseases pose to global biodiversity and human life. The second half of this chapter turns from ecology to the contemporary flows of people, technology, finance, information, messages, images, and ideology that contribute to a global culture of consumption. Part of globalization is intercultural communication, through the media, travel, and migration, which increasingly brings people from different societies into direct contact. Finally, we'll consider how such contacts and external linkages affect indigenous peoples, as well as how those groups have organized to confront and deal with national and global issues.

It would be impossible in a single chapter (or even book) to do a complete review of all the global issues that are salient today and that anthropologists have studied. Many such issues (e.g., war, displacement, terrorism, non-govermental organizations, the media) have been considered in previous chapters, and throughout this book a series of boxes have a "focus on globalization". For anthropological analysis of a range of global issues, see books by John Bodley (2012, 2015, 2017), Shirley Fedorak (2014), and Richard Robbins (2014).

ENERGY CONSUMPTION AND INDUSTRIAL DEGRADATION

One result of industrial expansion has been the ongoing destruction of indigenous economies, ecologies, and populations. Two centuries ago, as industrialization was developing, 50 million people still lived in politically independent bands, tribes, and chiefdoms. Around 1800, those non-industrial societies controlled half the globe and constituted 20 percent of its population (Bodley 2015). Industrialization tipped the balance in favor of state-organized societies (see Hornborg and Crumley 2007).

Industrialization entailed a shift from reliance on renewable resources to the use of fossil fuels. Earth's supply of oil, gas, and coal is being depleted to support previously unknown levels of consumption. Table 15.1 compares energy

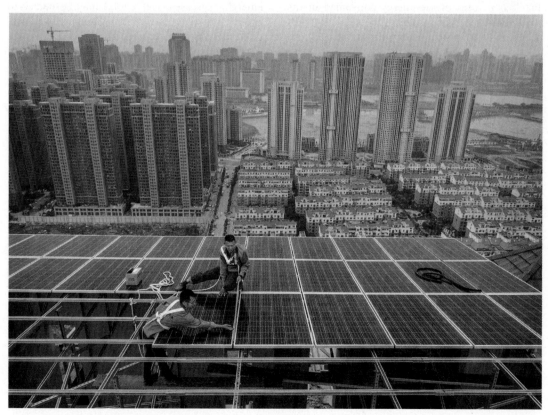

On May 14, 2017, workers install solar panels on the roof of a 47-story building in Wuhan, China. That nation produces two-thirds of the world's solar energy.
Kevin Frayer/Getty Images News/Getty Images

TABLE 15.1 Energy Consumption for the Top 12 Countries, 2018

	TOTAL (MTOE)	SHARE OF WORLD ENERGY CONSUMPTION (PERCENT)	RATE OF ANNUAL INCREASE (PERCENT)	PER-CAPITA ENERGY CONSUMPTION (GIGAJOULES)
World	13,865	100.0	2.9	76
China	3,274	23.6	4.3	97
United States	2,301	16.6	3.5	295
India	809	7.9	5.8	25
Russia	721	5.2	3.8	210
Japan	454	3.3	−0.2	150
Canada	344	2.5	0.2	390
Germany	324	2.3	−3.0	165
South Korea	301	2.2	1.3	246
Brazil	298	2.1	1.3	59
Iran	286	2.1	5.0	146
Saudi Arabia	259	1.9	−1.4	323
France	243	1.7	2.2	156

Note: MTOE—million tons of oil equivalent. 1 gigajoule—1 billion joules.

SOURCE: BP. 2019. BP Statistical Review of World Energy, 68th ed. https://www.bp.com/content/dam/bp/business-sites/en/global/corporate/pdfs/energy-economics/statistical-review/bp-stats-review-2019-full-report.pdf.

consumption, total and per capita, in the United States and the other eleven countries that use the most total energy. The United States, ranking second among those countries, is responsible for 16.6 percent of the energy consumed in the world each year. China ranks first, accounting for 23.6 percent of global energy consumption. However, among those 12 countries, North Americans—Canadians and Americans—rank first and third, respectively, in per-capita consumption. The average American consumes 3 times the energy used by the average Chinese and 12 times the energy used by the average citizen of India. In 2018, global energy demand and carbon emissions from energy use grew at their fastest rate since 2010/11, departing significantly from goals set by the Paris climate accord of 2015 (*BP Statistical Review of World Energy, 2019*). In terms of energy consumption per capita, only Germany, Saudi Arabia, and Japan had decreases in 2018, while India, Iran, and China had the largest increases.

Many contemporary nations are repeating—at an accelerated rate—the process of resource depletion that began in Europe and the United States during the Industrial Revolution. Fortunately, however, today's world has some environmental watchdogs that did not exist in that earlier time. Given the appropriate political will, leading to national and international cooperation and sanctions, the modern world may yet benefit from the lessons of the past.

There are, however, new dangers in today's world, some of which have become worldwide in scope. Accompanying globalization are significant risks that can move rapidly from nation to nation.

Global connectedness facilitates the spread of almost everything. Most alarmingly, diseases (e.g., COVID-19) that break out in one part of the world can quickly become global threats. Furthermore, emerging diseases (e.g., ebola) may be perceived as such a threat even when they are fairly well confined to a particular region. Another global threat, which can spread even faster than a disease, is a cyberattack. We should fear cyber viruses as well as real ones. We have become so reliant on the Internet that anything that might disrupt the flow of information in cyberspace would have worldwide repercussions.

Such dangers that can affect people anywhere and everywhere on the planet are part of a *globalization of risk*. Risks are no longer merely local, like the Flint, Michigan, water crisis, or regional, like drought and raging wildfires in California or southeastern Australia. We face threats that are global in scope—most recently a deadly virus pandemic, but also threats associated with global climate change. People tend to worry more about immediate threats, like toxic water or a coronavirus, than about long-term, less immediately obvious, threats such as a changing planet.

GLOBAL CLIMATE CHANGE

The past decade was the hottest on record, and 2019 was the second-warmest year ever, just behind 2016. Since the 1960s, each decade has been significantly warmer than the previous one, with the years 2015–2019 the five hottest ever recorded (Fountain and Popovich 2020).

This global warming is not due to increased solar radiation. The causes are mainly **anthropogenic**—caused by humans and their activities. Each consumer of fossil fuels makes his or her individual contribution (that consumer's "carbon footprint") to global climate change, including global warming. The fact that there are today 7.8 billion of those "footprints" has major global significance. Who can reasonably deny that those *billions*, along with their animals, crops, machines, and increasing use of fossil fuels, have a greater environmental impact than the 5 *million* or so pre-Neolithic hunter-gatherers estimated to have lived on our planet 12,000 years ago?

Scientists prefer the more general and inclusive term **climate change** to *global warming*, because the phenomenon involves many and varied processes (see Recap 15.1). Contemporary aspects of global climate change include rising surface, atmospheric, and oceanic temperatures; melting glaciers; reduced snow cover; shrinking sea ice; rising sea levels; ocean acidification; increasing atmospheric water vapor; and changing storm patterns.

The **greenhouse effect** is a natural phenomenon that keeps the Earth's surface warm. Greenhouse gases, which trap heat, include water vapor (H_2O), carbon dioxide (CO_2), methane (CH_4), nitrous oxide (N_2O), halocarbons, and ozone (O_3). Without those gases, life as we know it wouldn't exist. Like a greenhouse window, those gases allow sunlight to enter the atmosphere and then trap heat, preventing it from escaping.

The amount of carbon dioxide in the atmosphere has fluctuated naturally in the past. Every time it increases, the Earth heats up, ice melts, and sea levels rise. Since the Industrial Revolution, humans have been pumping carbon dioxide (and other heat-trapping gases) into the air faster than nature ever did. The global atmospheric concentration of CO_2, caused in large part by the burning of fossil fuels, has now passed 400 parts per million. This buildup will continue without actions to curb emissions (Wuebbles et al. 2017).

Oceans are particularly sensitive to small fluctuations in the Earth's temperature. During the 19th century, as industrialization proceeded, sea levels began to rise, and they continue to do so. Globally, the average sea level has risen 7–8 inches since 1900. About 3 inches of that rise has occurred since 1993. Tidal flooding has accelerated in more than 40 coastal American cities. In the decade between 1955 and 1964, a tide gauge at Annapolis, Maryland, measured 32 days of flooding. Fifty years later, between 2005 and 2014, that figure jumped to 394 days. In Charleston, South Carolina, flood days increased from 34 in the earlier decade to 219 between 2005 and 2014 (Gillis 2016a). Rising sea levels send more ocean water into streets, sewers, and homes, as we see in the Charleston photo on the next page. Sea levels are

anthropogenic
Caused by humans and their activities.

climate change
Global warming, plus changing sea levels, precipitation, storms, and ecosystem effects.

greenhouse effect
Warming caused by trapped atmospheric gases, which, like a greenhouse window, allow sunlight to enter the atmosphere and then trap heat, preventing it from escaping.

RECAP 15.1   What Heats, What Cools, the Earth?

WARMING	
Carbon dioxide (CO_2)	Has natural and human sources; levels increasing due to burning of fossil fuels.
Methane (CH_4)	Has risen due to an increase in human activities, including livestock raising, rice growing, landfill use, and the extraction, handling, and transport of natural gas.
Ozone (O_3)	Has natural sources, especially in the stratosphere, where chemicals have depleted the ozone layer; ozone is also produced in the troposphere (lower part of the atmosphere) when hydrocarbons and nitrogen oxide pollutants react.
Nitrous oxide (N_2O)	Has been rising from agricultural and industrial sources.
Halocarbons	Include chlorofluorocarbons (CFCs), which remain from refrigerants in appliances made before CFC ban.
Aerosols	Some airborne particles and droplets warm the planet; black carbon particles (soot) produced when fossil fuels or vegetation are burned; generally have a warming effect by absorbing solar radiation.
COOLING	
Aerosols	Some cool the planet; sulfate (SO_4) aerosols from burning fossil fuels reflect sunlight back to space.
Volcanic eruptions	Emit gaseous sulfur dioxide (SO_2), which, once in the atmosphere, forms sulfate aerosol and ash; both reflect sunlight back to space.
Sea ice	Reflects sunlight back to space.
Tundra	Reflects sunlight back to space.
WARMING/COOLING	
Forests	Deforestation creates land areas that reflect more sunlight back to space (cooling); it also removes trees that absorb CO_2 (warming).

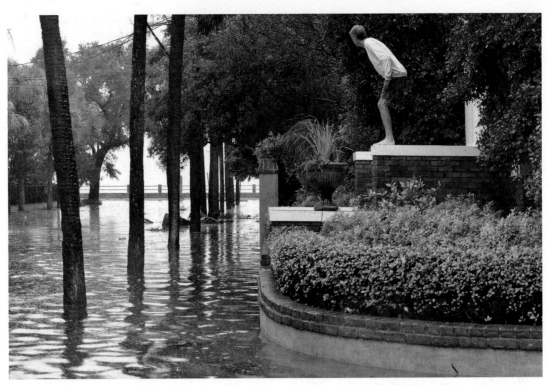

Flooding in downtown Charleston, South Carolina on October 15, 2015: A resident surveys his flooded street.

Mladen Antonov/AFP/Getty Images

projected to rise by several more inches in the next 15 years, and by 1–4 feet by 2100 (Wuebbles et al. 2017). For the United States, sea level rise is projected to be highest on the East and Gulf Coasts.

When Hurricane Harvey inundated parts of Houston, Texas, with over four feet of water in August 2017, the National Weather Service needed to add two new colors to its rainfall maps. Areas of dark purple and lavender now show amounts of rain from 20 to 30 inches, and above (Graef 2017). The intensity and destructiveness of the 2017 hurricane season (Hurricanes Harvey, Irma, and Maria) suggests the immediacy of climate change, as do huge wildfires in California and Australia. Previous predictions of extreme events have become a reality: In just a few weeks in 2017, the United States and the Caribbean experienced rapidly intensifying storms and record-breaking rainfall. Writing for Climate.gov, meteorologist Tom Di Liberto (2017) notes that climate change "does not, by itself, *cause* hurricanes . . . but it can certainly make a hurricane's impacts worse," because warmer seas and air increase the strength and intensity of storms (quoted in Graef 2017).

Global energy demand is the single greatest obstacle to slowing down climate change. Worldwide, energy consumption continues to grow with economic and population expansion. China produces more emissions than the United States and Europe combined, but the United States, with just 4.3 percent of the world's population, emits over 16 percent of global greenhouse gases (Bee 2020, p. 15).

India, which with China accounts for 37 percent of global population, continues its rapidly increasing use of fossil fuels and, consequently, its emissions. New Delhi is one of the world's most polluted cities. Pollution is a problem in Chinese cities as well. Among the alternatives to fossil fuels are nuclear power and renewable energy sources such as solar, wind, and biomass generators. What can *you* do to address the threat of global climate change?

In 2017, the American Anthropological Association (AAA) issued a "Statement on Humanity and Climate Change," which can be found at http://s3.amazonaws.com/rdcms-aaa/files/production/public/anthropology_and_climate_change.pdf. That statement makes several key points, including the following:

- Humans are the most important causes of the dramatic environmental changes that have taken place during the past 100 years. Two key factors influencing climate change are (1) reliance on fossil fuels as the primary energy source, and (2) an ever-expanding culture of consumerism.

- Climate change will accelerate migration, destabilize communities, and exacerbate the spread of infectious diseases.

- Most affected will be people living on coasts, in island nations, and in high-latitude (e.g., far north) and high-altitude (e.g., very mountainous) areas (see also Tehan 2017).

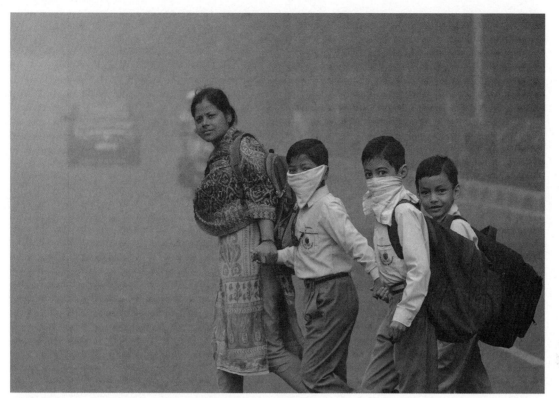

In the global economy, India (shown here) and China in particular have increased their use of fossil fuels and, consequently, their emissions of CO_2. This photo shows school children in New Delhi on November 3, 2016, when a blanket of heavy smog sent air pollution to dangerous levels. Some 16 million people had to breathe this toxic air. Experts warned of severe health problems for children forced to attend school. What's the most polluted place you've ever been to?

Arvind Yadav/*Hindustan Times* via Getty Images

- The tendency has been to address climate change at the international and national levels. We also need planning at the regional and local levels, because the impacts of climate change vary in specific locales. Affected communities, perhaps working with anthropologists, must be active participants in planning how to adapt to climate change—and in implementing those plans (see also Baer and Singer 2018; Singer 2019).

ENVIRONMENTAL ANTHROPOLOGY

Anthropology always has been concerned with how environmental forces influence humans and how human activities affect the environment. The 1950s–1970s witnessed the emergence of an area of study known as cultural ecology, or **ecological anthropology** (see Haenn et al. 2016). That field initially focused on how cultural beliefs and practices helped human populations adapt to their environments, as well as how people used elements of their culture to maintain their ecosystems. Ecological anthropologists showed that many indigenous groups had traditional ways of

categorizing resources and using them sustainably (see Blewitt 2018; Dagne 2015). The term **ethnoecology** describes a society's set of environmental perceptions and practices (see Vinyeta and Lynn 2013).

Given national and international incentives to exploit and degrade, ethnoecologies that once preserved local and regional environments increasingly are ineffective or irrelevant (see Dove et al. 2011). Anthropologists routinely witness threats to the people they study and their environments. Among such threats are commercial logging, mining, industrial pollution, and the imposition of external management systems on local ecosystems (see Johnston 2010). Today's ecological anthropology, now usually called *environmental anthropology,* attempts not only to understand but also to find solutions to environmental problems (see Kottak 1999).

Local people and their landscapes, ideas, values, and traditional management systems face attacks from all sides (see Hornborg, Clark, and Hermele 2011; Roothaan 2019). Outsiders attempt to remake native landscapes and cultures in their own image. The aim of many agricultural development projects, for example, seems to be to make the world as much like a midwestern American

ethnoecology
A culture's set of environmental perceptions and practices.

ecological anthropology
The study of cultural adaptations to environments.

agricultural state as possible (see Giugale 2017). Often, there is an attempt to impose mechanized farming and nuclear family ownership, even though these institutions may be inappropriate in areas far removed from the midwestern United States. Anthropologists know that development projects usually fail when they try to replace indigenous institutions with culturally alien concepts (Kottak 1990*b*).

Global Assaults on Local Autonomy

A clash of cultures related to environmental change may occur when development threatens indigenous peoples and their environments (see this chapter's "Appreciating Diversity"). A different kind of culture clash related to environmental change may occur when external regulation aimed at conservation impinges on indigenous peoples and their ethnoecologies. Like development projects, conservation schemes may ask people to change their ways in order to satisfy planners' goals rather than local goals. In places as different as Madagascar, Brazil, and the Pacific Northwest of the United States, people have been asked, told, or forced to abandon basic economic activities because to do so is good for "nature" or "the globe." "Good for the globe" has not played well in Brazil, whose Amazon has been a focus of international environmentalist attention. Brazilians complain that outsiders (e.g., Europeans and North Americans) promote "global needs" and "saving the Amazon" after having destroyed their own primary forests for economic growth. Conservation efforts always face local opposition when they promote radical changes without involving local people in planning and carrying out the policies that affect them. When people are asked to give up the basis of their livelihood, understandably they usually resist.

Consider the case of a man from the Tanosy ethnic group who lives on the edge of the Andohahela reserve in southeastern Madagascar. For years he has relied on rice fields and grazing land inside that reserve. Now external agencies are telling him to abandon that land for the sake of conservation. This man is a wealthy *ombiasa* (traditional sorcerer-healer). With four wives, a dozen children, and 20 head of cattle, he is an ambitious, hardworking, and productive peasant. With money, social support, and supernatural authority, he has mounted effective resistance against the park ranger who has been trying to get him to abandon his fields. The *ombiasa* claims he has already relinquished some of his fields, but he is waiting for compensatory land. His most effective resistance has been supernatural. The death of the ranger's young son was attributed to the *ombiasa*'s magic. After that, the ranger became less vigilant in his enforcement efforts.

The spread of environmentalism may reveal radically different notions about the "rights" and value of plants and animals versus humans. In Madagascar, many intellectuals and officials complain that foreigners seem more concerned about lemurs and other endangered species than about the people of Madagascar (the Malagasy). As a geographer there remarked to me, "The next time you come to Madagascar, there'll be no more Malagasy. All the people will have starved to death, and a lemur will have to meet you at the airport." Most Malagasy perceive human poverty as a more pressing problem than animal and plant survival.

On the other hand, who can reasonably doubt that conservation, including the preservation of biodiversity, is a worthy goal? The challenge for applied ecological anthropology is to devise culturally appropriate strategies to conserve biodiversity in the face of unrelenting population growth and commercial expansion. How does one get people to support conservation measures that may—in the short run, at least—diminish their access to resources? Like development plans in general, the most effective conservation strategies pay attention to the needs and wishes of the local people.

Deforestation

Anthropologists know that food producers (farmers and herders) typically do more to degrade the environment than foragers do. Population increase and agricultural expansion caused deforestation in many parts of the ancient Middle East and Mesoamerica (see Cairns 2015; Hornborg and Crumley 2007). Even today, many farmers think of trees as giant weeds to be removed and replaced with productive fields.

Often, deforestation is demographically driven—caused by population pressure. For example, Madagascar's human population almost quadrupled, from 7.6 million in 1975 to 27.7 million in 2020. Population growth propels migration, including rural–urban migration. When I left Madagascar's capital city, Antananarivo, in 1967 and moved to Ann Arbor, Michigan, I could joke that its entire population of 100,000 people could fit into the Michigan football stadium (known as the Big House). The stadium now seats 107,601, while Antananarivo's population is 3.4 million.

Urban growth causes deforestation if urbanites rely on fuelwood from the countryside, as is true in Madagascar. As forested watersheds disappear, crop productivity declines. Madagascar is known as the "great red island," after the color of its soil. On that island, the effects of soil erosion and water runoff are visible to the naked eye. From the look of its rivers, Madagascar appears to be bleeding to death. Increasing runoff of water no longer trapped by trees causes erosion of low-lying rice fields near swollen rivers as well as siltation in irrigation canals (Kottak 2007).

Globally, other causes of deforestation include commercial logging, road building, cash cropping, and clearing and burning associated with livestock and grazing. The fact that forest loss has several causes has a policy implication: Different deforestation scenarios require different conservation strategies.

What can be done? On this question applied anthropology weighs in, spurring policy makers to think about new conservation strategies. The traditional approach has been to restrict access to forested areas designated as parks or reserves, then employ park guards and punish violators. Modern strategies are more likely to consider the needs, wishes, and abilities of the people (often impoverished) living in and near the forest. Because effective conservation depends on the cooperation of the local people, their concerns must be addressed in devising conservation strategies.

Reasons to change behavior must make sense to local people. In Madagascar, the economic value of the forest for agriculture (as an anti-erosion mechanism and a reservoir of potential irrigation water) provides a much more powerful incentive against forest degradation than do such global goals as "preserving biodiversity." Most Malagasy have no idea that lemurs and other endemic species exist only in Madagascar. Nor would such knowledge provide much of an incentive for them to conserve the forests if doing so jeopardized their livelihoods.

To curb the global deforestation threat, we need conservation strategies that work. Laws and enforcement may help reduce commercially driven deforestation caused by burning and clear-cutting. But local people also use and abuse forested lands. A challenge for the environmentally oriented applied anthropologist is to find ways to make forest preservation attractive to local people and ensure their cooperation. Applied anthropologists must work to make "good for the globe" good for the people (see Cairns 2017; Jodoin 2017; Wasson et al. 2012).

Emerging Diseases

A number of potentially lethal infectious diseases have emerged and spread in the past few decades. These *emerging diseases* include HIV/AIDS, Ebola, West Nile, SARS (severe acute respiratory syndrome, caused by a coronavirus), Lyme disease, Zika, and, most recently, the coronavirus known as COVID-19. All these diseases have emerged as a result of human activity. Driven by factors including population increase, changing settlement patterns, and commercial expansion, humans have been encroaching on wild lands, particularly forests, and creating conditions that favor the spread of disease pathogens. In the Amazon, for example, one study showed that an increase in deforestation of just 4 percent produced a 50 percent increase in the incidence of malaria. This is because the mosquitoes that transmit malaria thrive in the right mix of sunlight and water in recently deforested areas (Robbins 2012).

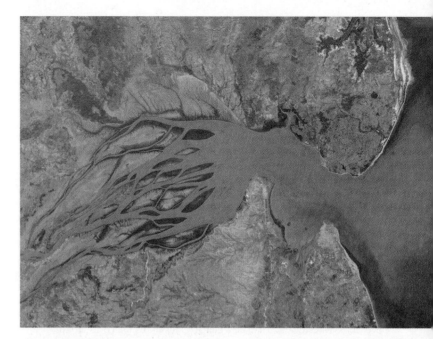

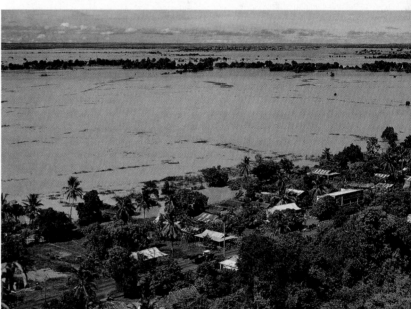

Erosion in Madagascar, known as the Great Red Island, turns its river waters red, so that from space, the island appears to be bleeding to death. In the top image of western Madagascar we see the Betsiboka River as it enters Bombetoka Bay, where it has created a delta. The bottom image is a closer look at the same river.

Top: Earth Science and Remote Sensing Unit/NASA Johnson Space Center/NASA; bottom: DEA/C. DANI I. JESKE/DeAgostini/Getty Images

Many–perhaps most–emerging diseases are *zoonotic*–they spread from animals to humans. The transmission of diseases from wild to domesticated animals and then to humans has been going on since the Neolithic, when animals first were domesticated. Zoonotic diseases pose a huge threat today because of human population increase and forces of globalization. Even before COVID-19, emerging diseases were killing more than 2 million people annually, and most of those diseases originate in animals (Robbins 2012).

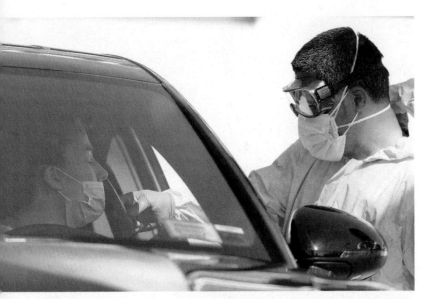

April 6, 2020: A health-care worker administers a coronavirus test at a drive-thru testing site in Jericho, New York. The World Health Organization declared the novel coronavirus COVID-19 to be a global pandemic on March 11, 2020.

Al Bello/Getty Images

Among the diseases that have jumped from woods and wildlife to humans through their domesticated animals is the Nipah virus, which began its migration from fruit bats to humans in South Asia. Because fruit bats have co-evolved with the Nipah virus for millions of years, it does little damage to their health. When the virus moves from bats into other species, however, it can be lethal. Fruit bats eat the pulp of fruit and spit out the residue. In rural Malaysia in 1999, an infected bat appears to have dropped a piece of

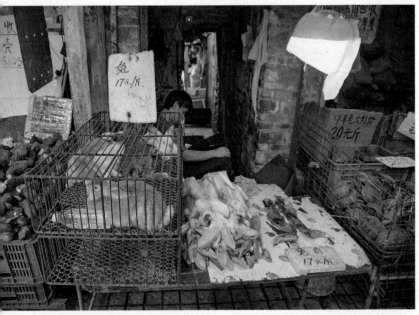

Ground zero for COVID-19 appears to have been a wholesale market in Wuhan, a city in central China. At this similar wet market in Guangzhou, China, we see rabbits for sale. To the left are live rabbits; in the middle, rabbit skins; and to the right, two halves of freshly-killed rabbit.

Nisa Maier/Getty Images

chewed fruit into the food supply of a swine herd (a scenario depicted in the movie *Contagion*). The virus then spread from those pigs to humans. Of 276 people infected in Malaysia, 106 died. Eleven more people died in Singapore, when the virus was exported there via live pigs. South Asia has experienced a dozen smaller Nipah outbreaks in recent years.

Ground zero for the 2020 coronavirus appears to have been a wholesale market in Wuhan, a city in central China. For sale there were live animals, including snakes, turtles, cicadas, guinea pigs, bamboo rats, badgers, hedgehogs, otters, palm civets, even wolf cubs. Both SARS (in 2002) and the 2020 coronavirus originated in such markets, which are common in China and feature animals packed in small cages in crowded stalls. This creates a perfect environment for breeding viruses that can enter human cells, then be spread through saliva, sputum, blood, or feces.

The 2002 SARS outbreak originated as a coronavirus that jumped from bats to Asian palm civets, a catlike creature considered a delicacy in southern China, and then to humans. COVID-19 appears also to have originated in bats and to have reached humans via a not-yet-identified mammal. Driving Chinese consumption of game are cultural factors, including beliefs about the supposed (but unproven) health and medicinal benefits of wildlife and the desire to show off wealth through exotic consumption. Wildlife also has been touted as an alternative source of protein, and of revenue in impoverished areas (Myers 2020).

Spillovers from wildlife to humans have quadrupled in the past half-century, reflecting increasing human encroachment on disease hotspots, especially in the tropics (Robbins 2012). The United Nations Environment Program estimates that a new animal disease that can also infect humans is discovered every four months. Modern air travel contributes to the potential for a transnational outbreak or even a pandemic. (A *pandemic* is an epidemic with global scope.) The zero patient for the HIV/AIDS pandemic (in North America, at least) is reputed to have been a flight attendant who flew internationally. HIV/AIDS originally jumped from chimpanzees to humans through bushmeat hunters in Africa, who kill and butcher chimps.

Biologists and health-care professionals are acutely aware of the threat posed by zoonotic diseases. One international project, called PREDICT, funded teams of veterinarians, conservation biologists, medical doctors, and epidemiologists to identify disease-causing organisms in wildlife before they spread to humans. PREDICT, which was financed by the United States Agency for International Development (USAID), attempted to "predict," spot, and prevent the spread of zoonotic diseases from world areas with high potential for disease transmission. Some 31 countries in Africa, Latin America, and Asia participated in the program. PREDICT scientists monitored areas where deadly viruses are known to exist and where humans have been encroaching. One such locale is the Interoceanic Highway, which now links the Atlantic and Pacific Oceans in South America, traversing Brazil and the Peruvian Andes.

PREDICT scientists also gathered blood, saliva, and other samples from wildlife species to create a "library" of viruses, to facilitate identification when a threat is imminent. This library focused on the animals most likely to carry diseases to people, such as primates, rats, and bats. PREDICT scientists also considered ways of preventing disease transmission. Some solutions can be remarkably simple. In Bangladesh, for example, outbreaks of the Nipah virus were contained by placing bamboo screens (which cost 8 cents each) over the containers used to collect date palm sap (Robbins 2012). Humans, by modifying the environment, and through their patterns of consumption, create the conditions that allow diseases to emerge and spread. Anthropologists can contribute by studying the cultural (including economic) causes of environmental encroachment and suggesting culturally appropriate and workable solutions.

In October 2019, the Trump administration announced the termination of the PREDICT program (see https://www.nytimes.com/2019/10/25/health/predict-usaid-viruses.html). That initiative, which ran for a decade, collected more than 140,000 biological samples from animals. Its scientists identified over 1,000 new viruses, including a new strain of Ebola. PREDICT trained some 5,000 people in over 30 African and Asian countries, and it built or strengthened 60 medical research laboratories, mostly in poor countries (McNeil 2019). As a rationale for ending the program, the administration argued that USAID's chief mission is supposed to be economic aid. The officials who terminated PREDICT may have considered it inappropriate for USAID to fund cutting-edge science in pursuit of exotic pathogens. Without PREDICT, however, the world has become more vulnerable to lethal pathogens (McNeil 2019). Can you think of any examples? Do pandemics have economic implications?

INTERETHNIC CONTACT

Since at least the 1920s, anthropologists have been interested in changes that take place where there is sustained contact between industrial and nonindustrial societies. The term *acculturation* refers to the cultural changes that occur when different societies come into continuous firsthand contact (Redfield, Linton, and Herskovits 1936). Most acculturation studies have focused on contact between Western and non-Western cultures. Often, this contact reflects Western domination over a non-Western society. In that case, the cultural patterns of the dominant Western society are more likely to be forced upon or accepted by the non-Western society than vice versa. However, the westerners who take up residence in a non-Western setting also will be affected by the cultural practices of that setting. In postcolonial times, people have been migrating from the former colonies to the former colonial nations. Inevitably, these migrants bring along their own cultural practices. It is not uncommon for their foods, music, art, and clothing styles to influence the cultural practices of the former colonial nation. If contact is sustained long enough, acculturation will be reciprocal—influencing both groups, even if one is influenced more than the other.

Acculturation is a form of cultural borrowing, or diffusion, that requires sustained firsthand contact. Diffusion, however, can also occur without direct, firsthand contact between the cultures involved. For example, most North Americans who eat hot dogs ("frankfurters") or hamburgers have never been to Frankfurt or Hamburg (Germany), nor have most North American Toyota owners or sushi eaters ever visited Japan. Although *acculturation* can be applied to any case of cultural contact and change, the term most often has described **Westernization**—the influence of Western expansion on indigenous peoples and their cultures. Thus, local people who wear store-bought clothes, learn Indo-European languages, and otherwise adopt Western customs are called "acculturated." Acculturation may be voluntary or forced, and there may be considerable resistance to the process.

Different degrees of destruction, domination, resistance, survival, adaptation, and modification of native cultures may follow interethnic contact. In the most destructive encounters, native and subordinate cultures face obliteration. When contact with powerful outsiders seriously threatens an indigenous culture, a "shock phase" often follows the initial encounter (Bodley 2012). Outsiders may attack or exploit the native people. Such exploitation may increase mortality, disrupt subsistence, fragment kin groups, damage social support systems, and inspire new religious movements. During the shock phase, there may be civil repression backed by military force. Such factors may lead to the group's cultural collapse (*ethnocide*) or physical extinction (*genocide*).

Cultural Imperialism and Indigenization

Cultural imperialism refers to the spread or advance of one culture at the expense of others, or its imposition on other cultures, which it modifies, replaces, or destroys—usually because of differential economic or political influence. Thus, children in the French colonial empire learned French history, language, and culture from standard textbooks also used in France. Tahitians, Malagasy,

Westernization
The acculturative influence of Western expansion on local cultures worldwide.

cultural imperialism
The spread or advance of one (dominant) culture at the expense of others, or its imposition on other cultures, which it modifies, replaces, or destroys.

Vietnamese, and Senegalese learned the French language by reciting from books about "our ancestors the Gauls."

Some commentators see the mass media as erasing cultural differences by spreading dominant products and brands globally. Others focus on how particular groups and cultures use media to express themselves, survive, and even spread (see Lule 2018; Pace ed. 2018). Across time and space, the Internet can and does transmit local and national happenings and expressions to a larger, perhaps global, audience. Think, for example, of YouTube's role in globalizing "Gangnam Style," a song and video originating in South Korea –and, more recently, in making Korean popular music (Kpop) and especially the hugely popular boy band BTS the global phenomena they became.

In Brazil, local practices, celebrations, and performances have changed in the context of outside forces, including the mass media and tourism (see Sharpley and Teller 2015). In the town of Arembepe, Brazil (Kottak 2018), TV coverage stimulated increased participation in a traditional annual performance, the Chegança. This is a danceplay that reenacts events during the Portuguese discovery of Brazil. Arembepeiros have traveled to the state capital to perform the Chegança before television cameras, for a TV program featuring traditional performances from many rural communities, and cameras have gone to Arembepe to record it. It can be seen on YouTube at the following link: https://www.youtube.com/watch?v=I6wpwW-Ofbc.

In several towns along the Amazon River, annual folk ceremonies now are staged lavishly for TV and video cameras. In the Amazon town of Parantíns, for example, boatloads of tourists arriving any time of year are shown video-recorded images of the town's annual Bumba Meu Boi festival. This is a costumed performance mimicking bullfighting, parts of which have been shown on national TV. This pattern, in which local communities preserve, revive, and intensify the scale of traditional ceremonies to perform for the media and tourists, is expanding. To see whether I could do so, I just managed to watch snippets of these two annual events in Arembepe and Parantíns on YouTube! (for the Parantíns festival see https://www.youtube.com/watch?v=3WBO1y5EoT8). (For more general discussions of media and tourism see Lundberg and Ziakis [2019] and Månsson et al. [2020]).

Brazilian TV also has aided the national spread of Carnaval beyond its traditional urban centers (Kottak 2009). Still, local reactions to the nationwide broadcasting of Carnaval and its trappings (elaborate parades, costumes, and frenzied dancing) are not simple or uniform responses to external stimuli. Rather than direct adoption of Carnaval, local Brazilians respond in various ways. Often, they don't take up Carnaval itself but modify their local festivities to fit Carnaval images. Others actively spurn Carnaval. One example is Arembepe, where Carnaval has never been important, probably because of its calendrical closeness to the main local festival, which is held in February to honor Saint Francis of Assisi. In the past, villagers couldn't afford to celebrate both occasions.

Now, not only do the people of Arembepe reject Carnaval; they also are increasingly hostile to their own main festival. Arembepeiros resent the fact that the Saint Francis festival has become "an outsiders' event," because it draws thousands of tourists to Arembepe each year. Arembepeiros now prefer the traditional June festivals honoring Saint John, Saint Peter, and Saint Anthony. Formerly, these were observed on a much smaller scale than was the Saint Francis celebration. Arembepeiros observe them now with a new vigor and enthusiasm. The national or the global can become that only if the local populace cooperates.

In the process of globalization, people continually make and remake culture as they assign their own meanings to the information, images, and products they receive from outside. **Indigenization** refers to the process by which people modify borrowed forms to make them fit into their local culture. Indigenization occurs in cultural domains as varied as fast food, music, movies, social media,

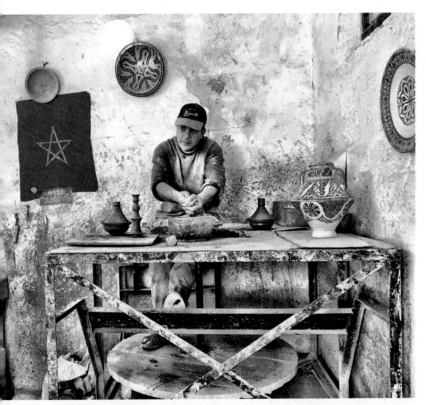

A potter plies his trade for a group of observers (including the author) in Fez, Morocco, in February 2015. Increasingly, local communities perform "traditional" activities, especially ceremonies, celebrations, and arts and crafts for TV and tourists.

Conrad P. Kottak

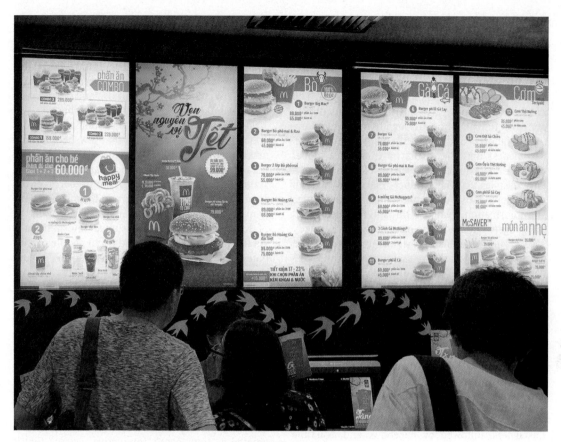

Illustrating both globalization and indigenization, McDonald's now routinely tailors its offerings to specific cultural appetites. The menus at this store in downtown Ho Chi Minh City (formerly Saigon) offer an expanded array of chicken preparations, reflecting the Vietnamese preference for that form of animal protein. Also, seasonal specials have been added for the Lunar New Year (Tet).
Conrad P. Kottak

housing styles, science, terrorism, celebrations, religion, and political ideas and institutions (Ellen, Lycett, and Johns 2013; Fiske 2011; Wilk 2006; Wilk and Barbosa 2012).

A Global System of Images

With globalization, more people in many more places imagine "a wider set of 'possible' lives than they ever did before. One important source of this change is the mass media" (Appadurai 1991, p. 197). The United States as a global media center has been joined by Canada, Japan, Western Europe, Brazil, Mexico, Nigeria, Egypt, India, and Hong Kong.

Like print (see Anderson 1991/2006), modern media can diffuse the cultures of countries within (and often beyond) their borders. Millions of Brazilians, for example, formerly were cut off (by geographic isolation or illiteracy) from urban, national, and international events and information; they now participate in a larger "mediascape" (Appadurai 1991) through mass media and the Internet (Kottak 1990a, 2009; Pace and Hinote 2013).

Brazil's most popular network (Rede Globo) relies heavily on its own productions, especially news and telenovelas (nightly serial programs often compared to American soap operas). Globo plays each night to one of the world's largest and most devoted audience. The programs that attract this horde are made by Brazilians, for Brazilians.

On August 21, 2017, for example, 49 million Brazilians watched Globo's one-hour national newscast, *Jornal Nacional.* That is the typical audience size for this program, which is broadcast nightly at 8:30, in a country with about 70 million TV homes. By contrast, the *combined* nightly viewership of the three network news broadcasts (ABC, CBS, and NBC) in the United States is around 16 million, in a country with twice the number of TV homes as Brazil (Ariens 2017).

Television and the Internet also play a prominent role in maintaining ethnic and national identities among people who lead transnational lives. Arabic-speaking Muslims, including migrants in several countries, follow the TV network Al Jazeera, based in Qatar. As groups move, they can stay linked to each other and to their homeland through global media. **Diasporas** (people who have spread out from an original, ancestral homeland) have enlarged the markets for media, communication, brands, and travel services targeted at specific ethnic, national, or religious groups who now live in various parts of the world.

diaspora
People who have spread out from an original, ancestral homeland.

A Global Culture of Consumption

Besides the media, other key global forces are production, commerce, and finance. As Arjun Appadurai (1991, p. 194) puts it, "money, commodities, and persons unendingly chase each other around the world." Residents of many Latin American communities now rely financially on outside cash, which their relatives who have migrated send back home. Also illustrating finance as a global force, the U.S. economy is increasingly influenced by foreign investment, especially from Britain, Canada, Germany, the Netherlands, Japan, and China. The American economy also has increased its dependence on foreign labor—through both the immigration of laborers and the outsourcing of jobs.

Business and the media have fueled a global culture of consumption, based on a craving for certain lifestyles and the products that go along with them. People also crave and consume knowledge and information, available through the media and the gadgets that allow media access (see Kennedy 2015). The media also provide connectivity and a forum for expressing shared sentiments. In the Middle East, for example, social media use exploded during the Arab Spring of 2011. In cyberspace, Middle Easterners found something missing from their ordinary, offline worlds: platforms permitting social connectivity and the collective airing of grievances. Since then, social media have entered the region commercially, in a big way. Almost 70 percent of Middle Easterners have Internet access, and most of them use social media regularly. WhatsApp is the number one social media site there, used by over 70 percent of Middle Easterners, followed by Facebook and YouTube (see Northwestern University in Qatar, 2017).

This rapidly rising Middle Eastern Internet presence is occurring in an area where youths (younger than 24 years) make up between 50 and 65 percent of the population. The smartphone is another key element in the Middle Eastern marketing mediascape. The United Arab Emirates lead the world in smartphone penetration. A global survey by Google found that 93 percent of smartphone users notice mobile ads, and 39 percent of those follow up with an online purchase.

As further illustration of the global reach of the consumer culture, consider that few people have never seen a T-shirt advertising a Western product (see Gould 2016). American and English rock stars' recordings blast through the streets of Rio de Janeiro, while taxi drivers from Toronto to Antananarivo listen to Brazilian music. The popularity of Korean pop music has spread internationally via the Internet. Peasants and tribal people participate in the modern world system not only because they have been hooked on cash but also because their products and images are appropriated by world capitalism. They are commercialized by others (like the Quileute nation in the *Twilight* series of books and movies). Furthermore, indigenous peoples also market their own images and products, through outlets like Cultural Survival.

PEOPLE IN MOTION

The linkages created through globalization have created a "translocal" "interactive system" that is "strikingly new" (Appadurai (1990, p. 1). Whether as refugees, migrants, tourists, students, pilgrims, proselytizers, laborers, businesspeople, development workers, politicians, terrorists, soldiers, sports figures, or media-borne images, people are on the move (despite a lull, likely temporary, caused by COVID-19). Migrants maintain their ties with home through social media, by phoning, emailing, texting, Skyping, WhatsApping, Facebooking, and FaceTiming. Frequently, they send money home; when possible, they also visit. In a sense, they live multilocally—in different places at once. Dominicans in New York City, for example, have been characterized as living "between two islands": Manhattan and the Dominican Republic (Grasmuck and Pessar 1991).

With so many people "in motion," the unit of anthropological study expands from the local community to the diaspora (see Margolis 2013; Wilson and Stierstorfer 2018). Anthropologists increasingly follow descendants of the villages we have studied as they move from rural to urban areas and across national boundaries. For an annual meeting of the American Anthropological Association held in Chicago, the anthropologist Robert Kemper once organized a session of presentations about long-term ethnographic fieldwork. Kemper's own long-time research focus was the Mexican village of Tzintzuntzan, which, with his mentor George Foster, he studied for decades. Eventually, their database expanded to include not only Tzintzuntzan but also its descendants all

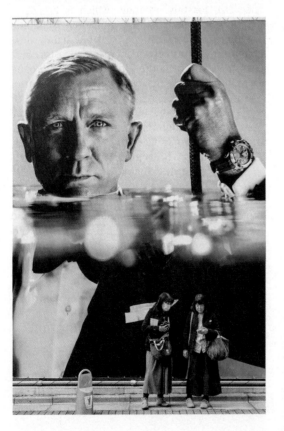

November 1, 2018: That's Craig, Daniel Craig, advertising Omega watches (Omega Seamaster Diver 300M) on a billboard in Tokyo, Japan. One mark of globalization is the transnational diffusion of brands—and celebrity.
Steve Vidler/Alamy Stock Photo

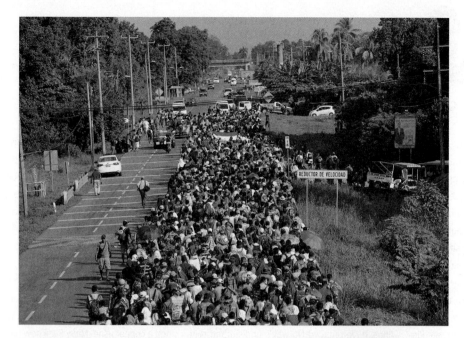

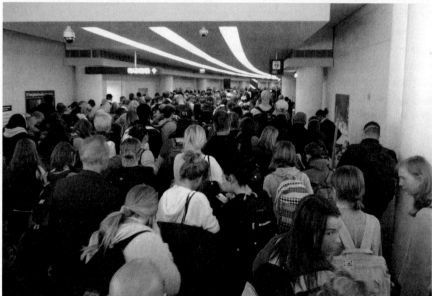

People on the move: On the top we see a "caravan" composed mostly of Central Americans entering Mexico from Guatemala on October 21, 2018. Fleeing dangers in their home countries, these refugees and would-be migrants hoped eventually to reach, and enter, the United States. The photo on the bottom taken, on March 14, 2020, shows other would-be entrants in the United States – international travelers (mostly returning American citizens) – waiting to go through customs at Chicago's O'Hare International Airport. About 3,000 Americans fleeing Europe in the wake of the coronavirus pandemic were stuck for hours that day inside this customs area.

First: John Moore/Getty Images; Second: Michael Sadler/AP Images

over the world. Given the Tzintzuntzan diaspora, Kemper was even able to use some of his time in Chicago to visit people from Tzintzuntzan who had established a colony there. In today's world, as people move, they take their traditions and their anthropologists along with them.

Postmodernity describes our time and situation: today's world in flux, these people on the move who have learned to manage multiple identities depending on place and context. In its most general sense, **postmodern** refers to the blurring and breakdown of established canons (rules or standards), categories, distinctions, and boundaries. The word is taken from **postmodernism**—a style and movement in architecture that succeeded modernism, beginning in the 1970s. Postmodern architecture rejected the rules, geometric order,

and austerity of modernism. Modernist buildings were expected to have a clear and functional design. Postmodern design is "messier" and more playful. It draws on a diversity of styles from different times and places—including popular, ethnic, and non-Western cultures. Postmodernism extends "value" well beyond classic, elite, and Western cultural forms. *Postmodern* is now used to describe comparable developments in music, literature, and visual art. From this origin, *postmodernity* describes a world in which traditional standards, contrasts, groups, boundaries, and identities are opening up, reaching out, and breaking down.

New kinds of political and ethnic units have emerged along with globalization. In some cases, cultures and ethnic groups have banded together in larger associations. There is a growing pan-Native

postmodernity
Time of questioning of established canons, identities, and standards.

postmodern
Marked by the breakdown of established canons, categories, distinctions, and boundaries.

postmodernism
A movement after modernism in architecture; now describes comparable developments in music, literature, and visual art.

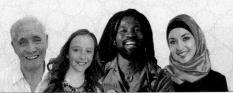

Diversity under Siege: Global Forces and Indigenous Peoples

Around the globe, diversity is under siege. In Alaska, which has been warming twice as fast as the rest of the United States, displaced villagers have become climate change refugees—forced to move as rising sea levels have eroded and flooded their settlements. In the South Pacific, Marshall Islanders also face rising seas, which render their villages increasingly uninhabitable and their land too salty for productive agriculture (Davenport and Haner 2015). In the Brazilian Amazon, outside settlers, including farmers, cattle herders, and commercial loggers, are illegally encroaching on areas reserved for indigenous groups. A combination of forces at work globally, including climate change and development, are threatening the lifestyles, livelihoods, and even the lives of indigenous peoples.

We focus now on the Norwegian Arctic, where a Sami (Lapp) population of about 100,000 traditional reindeer herders extends over a vast territory—northern areas of Norway, Sweden, Finland, and Russia's Kola Peninsula. Sami nomads once moved their herds seasonally across this expanse, paying little attention to national borders. Today, a mere one-tenth of the total Sami population, Western Europe's only indigenous Arctic group, continues to herd reindeer for a living. (The information in this box about the contemporary Sami comes mainly from Wallace [2016].)

The Sami way of life is being destroyed incrementally rather than by a major project or event. The cumulative effects of a series of smaller constructions, including roads and pipelines, have reduced Norway's undisturbed reindeer habitat by 70 percent in the past century. Like so many other indigenous peoples, the Sami must compete with powerful external interests for use of their traditional (grazing) lands. For generations, the Sami have lived under state organization. The state allows the Sami to graze their herds, but the land belongs to the national government. The Sami must deal with decisions made at the national level by planners, legislators, and the courts. What is good for the nation and business interests often takes precedence over what may be best for local people.

External inputs have been both positive and negative. The group benefits from the use of GPS collars and smartphone apps to track their animals, and snowmobiles and all-terrain vehicles to round them up. On the negative side, the steady encroachment of industrial infrastructure has reduced their range and freedom of movement. Current threats include dams, roads, live-fire military drills, high-voltage power lines, wind farms, and a copper mine. Many Sami now have to move their herds by truck and boat between summer and winter pastures—a costly operation. When courts approved large-scale projects that negatively affected the Sami, the herders received only a one-time payment as compensation for their losses.

Norway is proceeding with plans to extract more resources and build more industry in the Arctic. The Sami fear that their languages and culture, largely sustained by herding, will ultimately be sacrificed to benefit the larger society.

American identity and an international pantribal movement as well. Thus, in June 1992, the World Conference on Indigenous Peoples met in Rio de Janeiro concurrently with UNCED (the United Nations Conference on the Environment and Development). Along with diplomats, journalists, and environmentalists came 300 representatives of the tribal diversity that survives under globalization—from Lapland to Mali (see Maybury-Lewis 2002; Maybury-Lewis et al., 2009).

INDIGENOUS PEOPLES

All too often, conquest, annexation, colonialism, and development have been associated with genocide—the deliberate extermination of a specific ethnic group. Examples of genocide include the Holocaust, Rwanda in 1994, and Bosnia in the early 1990s. Bodley (2015) estimates that an average of 250,000 indigenous people perished annually between 1800 and 1950. The causes included warfare, outright murder, introduced diseases, slavery, land grabbing, and other forms of dispossession and impoverishment.

Remaining in the world today are more than 5,000 distinct groups of indigenous peoples, located in some 90 countries. Called Tribal Peoples, First Peoples, Native Peoples, and indigenous Peoples, these original inhabitants call themselves by many names in their more than 4,000 languages. They constitute more than 5 percent of the world's population, numbering between 370 and 500 million people. For a detailed and up-to-date (2019) report on indigenous peoples in 63 countries see the following website: https://www.iwgia.org/images/documents/indigenous-world/IndigenousWorld2019_UK.pdf. Indigenous groups are among the world's most vulnerable populations. Many of them struggle to hold on to their lands and natural resources (see this chapter's "Appreciating Diversity").

All the indigenous groups that survive now live within nation-states (see Ivison 2020). Often, they maintain a distinct ethnic identity, even if they have lost their ancestral languages and

The government has ambitious targets for renewable energy, including more hydroelectric and wind power projects. These projects, although possibly "good for the globe," negatively affect reindeer herding, as well as Arctic biodiversity, wilderness landscapes, and traditional subsistence activities. A proposed wind farm (now under judicial review) and associated power lines would encroach substantially on the summer grazing lands of a group of herders who still speak South Sami, a language listed by UNESCO as endangered.

In addition to the threats from development, the Sami have an ongoing conflict with the military. Since the Cold War, Norwegian soldiers have been a regular presence in Sami country, preparing for a possible Russian incursion across northern Scandinavia. These troops stage regular, often daily, war exercises, including live gunfire. Herders must be vigilant to avoid flying bullets as they go about their activities.

Even the most enlightened governments pursue policies that are incompatible with preserving the traditional activities and lifestyles

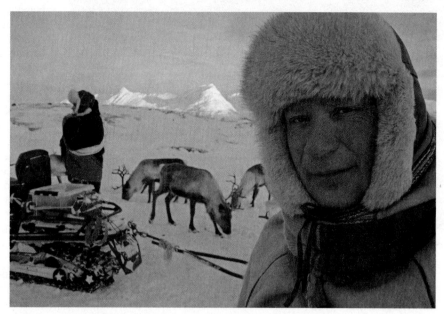

Sami herder Johann Anders Oskal and his brother tend their reindeer herd in Troms County, Norway.
Scott Wallace/Hulton Archive/Getty Images

of indigenous peoples. Like certain conservation schemes aimed at preserving biodiversity, efforts that are good for the globe, such as the development of green energy sources, may not be best for local people. Planners must be attentive to the need to seek a delicate balance between what's good for the globe and what's good for the people.

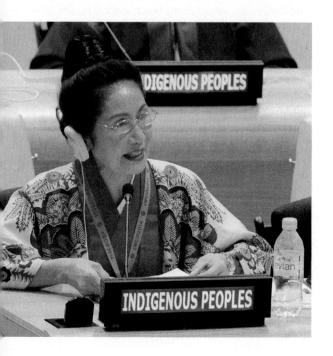

cultures to varying degrees. Many such groups aspire to autonomy. To describe these original inhabitants of their territories, the term *indigenous people* entered international law in 1982 with the creation of the United Nations Working Group on Indigenous Populations (WGIP). This group meets annually and has members from six continents. The United Nations General Assembly adopted its Declaration on the Rights of Indigenous Peoples in 2007. Convention 169, a

Okinawan Keiko Itokazu, a member of Japan's House of Councillors, speaks at the World Conference on Indigenous Peoples at U.N. headquarters in New York on Sept. 22, 2014. Delegates for indigenous peoples from around the world, including Ainu and Okinawans from Japan, attended this first U.N.-backed conference of its kind to discuss measures aimed at ensuring their political representation and freedom from discrimination. Kyodo/Newscom

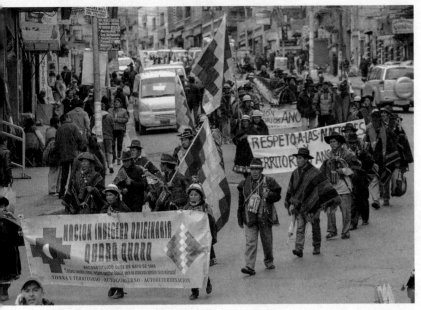

On March 18, 2019, following a 41-day march, a large group of indigenous people from Sucre (Bolivia's constitutional capital, located in southern Bolivia) arrive in La Paz, the seat of the national government. They traveled some 700 kilometers (435 miles) to demand recognition of their community's traditional territory.

Martin Alipaz/Alamy Stock Photo

territories. Other Andean "peasants" have experienced similar reindigenization as well. Brazil recognized 30 new indigenous communities in the northeast, a region previously seen as having lost its indigenous population. In Guatemala, Nicaragua, Brazil, Colombia, Mexico, Paraguay, Ecuador, Argentina, Bolivia, Peru, and Venezuela, constitutional reforms have recognized those nations as multicultural. Several national constitutions now recognize the rights of indigenous peoples to cultural distinctiveness, sustainable development, political representation, and limited self-government.

The indigenous rights movement exists in the context of globalization, including transnational movements focusing on human rights, women's rights, and environmentalism. Transnational organizations have helped indigenous peoples to influence legislation. Since the 1980s, there has been a (still imperfect) shift in Latin America from authoritarian to democratic rule. Despite this trend, inequality and discrimination against indigenous peoples persist.

Ceuppens and Geschiere (2005) comment on an upsurge, in several world areas, of the notion of *autochthony* (being native to, or formed in, the place where found), with an implicit call for excluding strangers. The terms *autochthony* and *indigenous* both go back to classical Greek history, with similar implications. *Autochthony* refers to self and soil. *Indigenous* literally means born inside, with the connotation in classical Greek of being born "inside the house." Both notions stress rights of first-comers to privileged status and protection versus later immigrants—legal or illegal (Ceuppens and Geschiere 2005; Hornborg et al. 2011).

During the 1990s, autochthony became an issue in many parts of Africa, inspiring violent efforts to exclude (European and Asian) "strangers." Simultaneously, autochthony became a key notion in debates about immigration and multiculturalism in Europe. European majority groups have claimed the label *autochthon*. This term highlights the prominence that the exclusion of strangers has assumed in day-to-day politics worldwide (Ceuppens and Geschiere 2005). Familiar contemporary examples include the rise of ethnonationalism in the United States, and the June 2016 Brexit vote (for Britain to leave the European Union).

Essentialism describes the process of viewing an identity (e.g., an ethnic label) as innate, real, and frozen, thus ignoring the historical processes within which that identity developed. Identities, however, are not fixed; they are fluid and multiple. People draw on particular, sometimes competing, self-labels and identities. Some Peruvian groups, for instance, self-identify as *mestizos* but still see themselves as indigenous. Identity is a fluid, dynamic process, and there are multiple ways of being indigenous. Neither speaking an indigenous language nor wearing "native" clothing is required to self-identify as indigenous (Jackson and Warren 2005).

essentialism
Viewing identities that have developed historically as innate and unchanging.

document supporting cultural diversity and indigenous empowerment, was approved by the International Labor Organization (ILO) in 1989. Such documents, along with the global work of the WGIP, have influenced governments, NGOs, and international agencies to adopt policies favorable to indigenous peoples. In May 2012, the United Nations sponsored a high-level commemoration of the fifth anniversary of the adoption of the Declaration on the Rights of Indigenous Peoples (see Doyle 2015; Drahos 2014). In September 2014, the United Nations hosted a World Conference on Indigenous Peoples, to reiterate the U.N.'s ongoing role in promoting and protecting the rights of indigenous peoples (see http://www.un.org/en/ga/69/meetings/indigenous/#&panel1-1). Social movements worldwide now use *indigenous people* as a self-identifying label in their quests for social, cultural, and political rights (Brower and Johnston 2007; de la Peña 2005).

In Spanish-speaking Latin America, social scientists and politicians now favor the term *indígena* (indigenous person) over *indio* (Indian), the colonial term that European conquerors used for Native Americans (de la Peña 2005). Until the mid- to late 1980s, Latin American public policy emphasized assimilation, rather than maintenance of indigenous identities. Since then, the emphasis has shifted dramatically from biological and cultural assimilation—*mestizaje*—to identities that value difference, especially as indigenous peoples.

In Ecuador, for example, groups seen previously as Quichua-speaking peasants are classified now as indigenous communities with assigned

ANTHROPOLOGY'S LESSONS

Anthropology teaches us that the adaptive responses of humans are more flexible than those of other species, because our main adaptive means are sociocultural. However, in the face of globalization, the cultural institutions of the past always influence subsequent adaptation, producing continued diversity in the actions and reactions of different groups as they indigenize global inputs. Anthropology offers a people-centered vision of social change for today's world. The existence of anthropology is itself a tribute to the continuing need to understand similarities and differences among human beings throughout the world.

Anthropology offers relevant, indeed powerful, ways of seeing how the world works. To benefit humanity, lessons of the past can and should be applied to the present and future. Anthropologists know that civilizations and world powers rise and fall, and that social transformations typically follow major innovations, such as the Neolithic and the Industrial Revolution. There is little chance that the current world system and the power relations within it will last forever. Whatever it may be, our social future will trace its origins to our social present. That is, future developments will need to build on, modify, and perhaps discard preexisting practices and institutions. What trends observable in the world today are most likely to transform society in the long run? Using your new knowledge of anthropology, try to imagine possible futures for humanity.

for REVIEW

summary

1. Fueling global warming are human population growth and increasing use of fossil fuels. The term *climate change* encompasses global warming along with changing sea levels, precipitation, storms, and ecosystem effects.

2. Anthropologists have studied how environmental forces influence humans and how human activities affect the Earth's atmosphere. An ethnoecology is a society's set of environmental practices and perceptions. Indigenous ethnoecologies increasingly are being challenged by global forces. A challenge for applied ecological anthropology is to devise culturally appropriate strategies for conservation in the face of population growth and commercial expansion.

3. Causes of deforestation include demographic pressure on subsistence economies, commercial logging, road building, cash cropping, urban expansion, and clearing and burning associated with livestock. Infectious diseases such as HIV/AIDS, Ebola, West Nile, SARS, Zika, and COVID-19 have emerged and spread because of things that people have done to their environments.

4. Cultural imperialism is the spread of one culture and its imposition on other cultures, which it modifies, replaces, or destroys—usually because of differential economic or political influence. Some critics worry that modern technology, including the mass media, is destroying traditional cultures. But others see an important role for new technology in allowing local cultures to express themselves.

5. As the forces of globalization spread, they are modified (indigenized) to fit into local cultures. Modern media can help diffuse a national culture within its own boundaries. The media also play a role in preserving ethnic and national identities among people who lead transnational lives.

6. People travel more than ever. But migrants also maintain ties with home, so they live multilocally. *Postmodernity* describes this world in flux, with people on the move who manage multiple social identities depending on place and context. New kinds of political and ethnic units are emerging as others break down or disappear.

7. Governments, NGOs, and international agencies have adopted policies designed to recognize and benefit indigenous peoples. Social movements worldwide have adopted the term *indigenous people* as a self-identifying and political label based on past oppression but now signaling a search for social, cultural, and political rights. In Latin America, several national constitutions now recognize the rights of indigenous peoples. Identity is a fluid, dynamic process, and there are multiple ways of being indigenous.

key
terms

think
like an
anthro-
pologist

1. What does it mean to apply an anthropological perspective to contemporary global issues? Can you come up with an anthropological research question that investigates such issues? Imagine you had a year (and the money!) to carry out this project. How would you spend your time and your resources?

2. The topic of global climate change has been hotly debated during the past few years. Why is there so much debate? Are you concerned about global climate change? Do you think everyone on the planet should be equally concerned and share the responsibility of doing something about it? Why or why not?

3. Consider majority and minority rights in the context of contemporary events involving religion, ethnicity, politics, and law. In pluralistic societies, what kind of rights should be granted on the basis of religion? What kinds of groups, if any, within a nation should have special rights? How about indigenous peoples?

4. Do you now live, or have you ever lived, multilocally? If so, how so?

5. What term do anthropologists use to describe the view that identities have developed historically as innate and unchanging? We know, however, that identities are not fixed; they are fluid and multiple. What does this mean? What implications does this have for understanding indigenous political movements?

credits

GLOSSARY

acculturation An exchange of cultural features between groups in firsthand contact.

achieved status Social status based on choices or accomplishments.

adaptive Favored by natural selection.

adaptive strategy Means of making a living; predominant system of production.

aesthetics The appreciation of qualities perceived in art.

affinals Relatives by marriage.

African American Vernacular English (AAVE) The rule-governed dialect spoken by some African Americans.

agency The actions of individuals, alone and in groups, that create and transform culture.

agriculture Cultivation using land and labor continuously and intensively.

ambilineal descent A flexible descent rule, neither patrilineal nor matrilineal.

animism The belief in spiritual beings, e.g., deities, ghosts, souls or doubles.

anthropogenic Caused by humans and their activities.

anthropological archaeology The study of human behavior through material remains.

anthropology The study of the humans around the world and through time.

anthropology and education The study of students in the context of their family, peers, and enculturation.

antimodernism Rejecting the modern for a presumed earlier, purer, better way of life.

applied anthropology The use of anthropology to solve contemporary problems.

art An object, event, or other expressive form that evokes an aesthetic reaction.

arts For example, music, performance arts, visual arts, storytelling, and literature (written and oral).

ascribed status Social status based on limited choice.

assimilation The absorption of minorities within a dominant culture.

association An observed relationship between two or more variables.

balanced reciprocity The midpoint on the reciprocity continuum, between generalized and negative reciprocity.

band The basic social unit among foragers; fewer than a hundred people; may split up seasonally.

bifurcate collateral kinship terminology Six separate parental kin terms: M, F, MB, MZ, FB, and FZ.

bifurcate merging kinship terminology Four parental kin terms: M=MZ, F=FB, MB, and FZ each stand alone.

big man A generous tribal entrepreneur with multivillage support.

bilateral kinship calculation Kin ties calculated equally through both sexes.

biocultural Combining biological and cultural approaches to a given problem.

biological anthropology The study of human biological variation through time and as it exists today.

bourgeoisie Owners of the means of production.

call systems Communication systems of nonhuman primates.

capital Wealth invested with the intent of producing profit.

capitalist world economy A profit-oriented global economy based on production for sale or exchange.

cargo cults Postcolonial, acculturative religious movements in Melanesia.

catharsis Intense emotional release.

chiefdom A society with permanent political structure, hereditary leaders, and social ranking but lacking class divisions.

cisgender Individuals who identify with the gender assigned to them at birth.

clan A unilineal descent group based on stipulated descent.

climate change Global warming, plus changing sea levels, precipitation, storms, and ecosystem effects.

collateral relative A relative outside ego's direct line, e.g., B, Z, FB, MZ.

colonialism The political, social, economic, and cultural domination of a territory and its people by a foreign power for an extended time.

communism A social system in which property is owned by the community and people work for the common good.

Communism A political movement aimed at replacing capitalism with Soviet-style communism.

communitas An intense feeling of social solidarity.

complex societies Large, populous societies (e.g., nations) with social stratification and central governments.

configurationalism The view of culture as integrated and patterned.

conflict resolution Means of settling disputes.

core The dominant position in the world system; nations with advanced systems of production.

core values Key, basic, or central values that integrate a culture.

correlation An association; when one variable changes, another does too.

cosmology A system, often religious, for imagining and understanding the universe.

cross cousins Children of a brother and a sister.

cultivation continuum A continuum of land and labor use running from horticulture (noncontinuous, non-intensive) to agriculture (continuous, intensive).

cultural anthropology The comparative, cross-cultural study of human society and culture.

cultural colonialism The internal domination by one group and its culture or ideology over others.

cultural consultants People who teach an ethnographer about their culture.

cultural imperialism The spread or advance of one (dominant) culture at the expense of others, or its imposition on other cultures, which it modifies, replaces, or destroys.

cultural materialism (Harris) The idea that cultural infrastructure determines structure and superstructure.

cultural relativism The idea that behavior should be evaluated not by outside standards but in the context of the culture in which it occurs.

cultural resource management Deciding what needs saving when entire archaeological sites cannot be saved.

cultural rights Rights vested in religious and ethnic minorities and indigenous societies.

cultural transmission Transmission through learning, basic to language.

culture Traditions and customs transmitted through learning.

curer One who diagnoses and treats illness.

daughter languages Languages sharing a common parent language, e.g., Latin.

descent Social identity based on ancestry.

descent group A group based on belief in shared ancestry.

development anthropology A field that examines the sociocultural dimensions of economic development.

diachronic (Studying societies) across time.

diaspora People who have spread out from an original, ancestral homeland.

differential access Favored access to resources by superordinates over subordinates.

diffusion Borrowing of cultural traits between societies.

diglossia A language with "high" (formal) and "low" (informal, familial) dialects.

discrimination Policies and practices that harm a group and its members.

disease A scientifically identified health threat caused by a known pathogen.

displacement Describing things and events that are not present; basic to language.

domestic–public dichotomy Work at home versus more valued work outside the home.

dowry Substantial gifts to the husband's family from the wife's group.

ecological anthropology The study of cultural adaptations to environments.

economizing The allocation of scarce means (resources) among alternative ends.

economy A system of resource production, distribution, and consumption.

egalitarian society A society with rudimentary status distinctions.

ego The position from which one views an egocentric genealogy.

emic A research strategy focusing on local explanations and meanings.

empire A mature state that is large, multiethnic, militaristic, and expansive.

enculturation The process by which culture is learned and transmitted across the generations.

endogamy Marriage of people from the same social group.

essentialism Viewing identities that have developed historically as innate and unchanging.

ethnic group One among several culturally distinct groups in a society or region.

ethnicity Identification with, and feeling part of, an ethnic group and exclusion from certain other groups because of this affiliation.

ethnocentrism Judging other cultures using one's own cultural standards.

ethnocide The deliberate suppression or destruction of an ethnic culture by a dominant group.

ethnoecology A culture's set of environmental perceptions and practices.

ethnography Fieldwork in a particular cultural setting.

ethnology The study of sociocultural differences and similarities.

ethnomusicology The comparative study of the musics of the world and of music as an aspect of culture and society.

ethnosemantics The study of lexical (vocabulary) categories and contrasts.

etic A research strategy emphasizing the ethnographer's explanations and categories.

exogamy Marriage outside one's own group.

expanded family household A household that includes a group of relatives other than, or in addition to, a married couple and their children.

expressive culture A term used to describe manifestations of human creativity, such as dance, music, painting, sculpture, pottery, cloth, stories, drama, and comedy.

extended family household A household with three or more generations.

family of orientation The nuclear family in which one is born and grows up.

family of procreation The nuclear family established when one marries and has children.

fiscal Pertaining to finances and taxation.

focal vocabulary A set of words describing particular domains (foci) of experience.

folk Of the people; e.g., the art, music, and lore of ordinary people.

food production An economy based on plant cultivation and/or animal domestication.

foraging An economy and a way of life based on hunting , gathering, and/or fishing.

functionalism An approach that focuses on the role (function) of sociocultural practices in social systems.

fundamentalism Advocating strict fidelity to a religion's presumed founding principles.

gender The cultural construction of whether one is female, male, or something else.

gender identity A person's identification by self and others as male, female, or something else.

gender roles The tasks and activities that a culture assigns to each sex.

gender stereotypes Oversimplified, strongly held views about the characteristics of males and females.

gender stratification The unequal distribution of social resources between men and women.

genealogical method The use of diagrams and symbols to record kin connections.

general anthropology Anthropology as a whole: cultural, archaeological, biological, and linguistic anthropology.

generality Culture pattern or trait that exists in some but not all societies.

generalized reciprocity Exchanges among closely related individuals.

generational kinship terminology Just two parental kin terms: M=MZ=FZ and F=FB=MB.

genitor A child's biological father.

genocide The deliberate elimination of a group through mass murder.

globalization The accelerating interdependence of nations in the world system today.

greenhouse effect Warming caused by trapped atmospheric gases, which, like a greenhouse window, allow sunlight to enter the atmosphere and then trap heat, preventing it from escaping.

health care systems Beliefs, customs, and specialists concerned with preventing and curing illness.

hegemony A stratified social order in which subordinates accept hierarchy as "natural."

historical linguistics The study of languages over time.

historical particularism (Boas) The idea that histories are not comparable; diverse paths can lead to the same cultural result.

holistic Encompassing past, present, and future; biology, society, language, and culture.

hominid Member of hominid family; any fossil or living human, chimp, or gorilla.

hominins Hominids excluding the African apes; all the human species that ever have existed.

honorifics Terms of respect; used to honor people.

horticulture Nonintensive, shifting cultivation with fallowing.

human rights Rights based on justice and morality beyond and superior to particular countries, cultures, and religions.

hypodescent Children of mixed unions assigned to the same group as their minority parent.

hypothesis A suggested but as yet unverified explanation.

illness A condition of poor health perceived or felt by an individual.

imperialism A conscious policy aimed at seizing and ruling foreign territory and peoples.

incest Sexual relations with a close relative.

increased equity Reduction in absolute poverty, with a more even distribution of wealth.

independent invention The independent development of a cultural feature in different societies.

indigenization The process by which borrowed forms are modified to fit the local culture.

Industrial Revolution In Europe, after 1750, the socioeconomic transformation through industrialization.

informed consent An agreement to take part in research—after having been informed about its purpose, nature, procedures, and possible impacts.

international culture Cultural traditions that extend beyond national boundaries.

interpretive anthropology (Geertz) The study of a culture as a system of meaning.

intersex Pertaining to a group of biological conditions reflecting a discrepancy between external and internal genitals.

intervention philosophy An ideological justification for outsiders to guide or rule native peoples.

interview schedule A form (guide) used to structure a formal, but personal, interview.

IPR Intellectual property rights; an indigenous group's collective knowledge and its applications.

key cultural consultants Experts on a particular aspect of local life.

kin terms The words used for different relatives in a particular language and system of kinship calculation.

kinesics The study of communication through body movements and facial expressions.

kinship calculation The relationships based on kinship that people recognize in a particular society, and how they talk about those relationships.

language The primary means of human communication, spoken and written.

law A legal code of a state-organized society, with trial and enforcement.

levirate A custom in which a widow marries the brother of her deceased husband.

lexicon Vocabulary; all the morphemes in a language and their meanings.

life history Of a key consultant; a personal portrait of someone's life in a culture.

liminality The in-between phase of a rite of passage.

lineage A unilineal descent group based on demonstrated descent.

lineal kinship terminology Four parental kin terms: M, F, FB=MB, and MZ=FZ.

lineal relatives Ego's direct ancestors and descendants.

linguistic anthropology The study of language and linguistic diversity in time, space, and society.

lobola A substantial marital gift from the husband and his kin to the wife and her kin.

longitudinal research Long-term study, usually based on repeated visits.

magic The use of supernatural techniques (e.g., offerings, spells, formulas, incantations) to accomplish specific ends.

mana A sacred, impersonal force, so named in Melanesia and Polynesia.

market principle Buying, selling, and valuation based on supply and demand.

mater The socially recognized mother of a child.

matrilineal descent Descent traced through women only.

means (factors) of production Major productive resources, e.g., land, labor, technology, capital.

medical anthropology The comparative, biocultural study of disease, health problems, and health care systems.

melanin "Natural sunscreen" produced by skin cells responsible for pigmentation.

mode of production A specific set of social relations that organizes labor.

monotheism The belief in a single all-powerful deity.

morphology The (linguistic) study of morphemes and word construction.

multiculturalism The view of cultural diversity as valuable and worth maintaining.

nation A society that shares a language, religion, history, territory, ancestry, and kinship.

nation-state An autonomous political entity; a country.

national culture Cultural features shared by citizens of the same nation.

nationalities Ethnic groups that have, once had, or want their own country.

natural selection Selection of favored forms through differential reproductive success.

negative reciprocity Potentially hostile exchanges among strangers.

neoliberalism The principle that governments shouldn't regulate private enterprise; free market forces should rule.

neolocality The living situation in which a couple establishes new residence.

nomadism (pastoral) The annual movement of an entire pastoral group with herds.

office A permanent political position.

overinnovation Trying to achieve too much change.

pantribal sodalities Non-kin-based groups with regional political significance.

parallel cousins Children of two brothers or two sisters.

participant observation Taking part in community life, participating in the events one is observing, describing, and analyzing.

particularity Distinctive or unique culture trait, pattern, or integration.

pastoralists Herders of domesticated animals.

pater One's socially recognized father; not necessarily the genitor.

patriarchy Political system ruled by men.

patrilineal descent Descent traced through men only.

patrilineal-patrilocal complex Male supremacy based on patrilineality, patrilocality, and warfare.

peasant A small-scale farmer with rent fund obligations.

periphery The weakest structural and economic position in the world system.

phenotype The expressed biological characteristics of an organism.

phoneme The smallest sound contrast that distinguishes meaning.

phonemics The study of significant sound contrasts (phonemes) in a language.

phonetics The study of speech sounds—what people actually say.

phonology The study of sounds used in speech in a particular language.

plural marriage Having more than two spouses simultaneously; polygamy.

plural society A society with economically interdependent ethnic groups.

political economy The web of interrelated economic and power relations in society.

polyandry A variant of plural marriage in which a woman has more than one husband at the same time.

polygyny A variant of plural marriage in which a man has more than one wife at the same time.

polytheism The belief in multiple deities, who control aspects of nature.

postcolonial A conscious policy aimed at seizing and ruling foreign territory and peoples.

postmodern Marked by the breakdown of established canons, categories, distinctions, and boundaries.

postmodernism A movement after modernism in architecture; now describes comparable developments in music, literature, and visual art.

postmodernity Time of questioning of established canons, identities, and standards.

potlatch A competitive feast on the North Pacific Coast of North America.

power The ability to exercise one's will over others.

prejudice Devaluing a group because of its assumed attributes.

prestige Esteem, respect, or approval.

productivity Creating new expressions that are comprehensible to other speakers.

protolanguage A language ancestral to several daughter languages.

public anthropology Efforts to extend anthropology's visibility beyond academia and to demonstrate its public policy relevance.

questionnaire A form used by sociologists to obtain comparable information from respondents.

race An ethnic group assumed to have a biological basis.

racial classification Assigning humans to categories (purportedly) based on common ancestry.

racism Discrimination against an ethnic group assumed to have a biological basis.

random sample A sample in which all population members have an equal statistical chance of inclusion.

reciprocity The principle governing exchanges among social equals.

reciprocity continuum A continuum running from generalized reciprocity (closely related/deferred return) to negative reciprocity (strangers/immediate return).

redistribution The flow of goods from the local level into a center, then back out; characteristic of chiefdoms.

refugees People who flee a country to escape persecution or war.

religion Belief and ritual concerned with supernatural beings, powers, and forces.

revitalization movements Social movements aimed at altering or revitalizing a society.

rickets Vitamin D deficiency marked by bone deformation.

rites of passage Rites marking transitions between places or stages of life.

ritual Formal, repetitive, stereotyped behavior; based on a liturgical order.

sample A smaller study group chosen to represent a larger population.

Sapir-Whorf hypothesis The theory that different languages produce different patterns of thought.

science A field of study that seeks reliable explanations, with reference to the material and physical world.

scientific medicine A health care system based on scientific knowledge and procedures.

semantics A language's meaning system.

semiperiphery The position in the world system intermediate between the core and the periphery.

sexual dimorphism Marked differences in male and female anatomy and temperament.

sexual orientation Sexual attraction to persons of the opposite sex, same sex, or both sexes.

shaman The general term encompassing curers ("witch doctors"), mediums, spiritualists, astrologers, palm readers, and other independent diviners.

social control Maintaining social norms and regulating conflict.

socialism A sociopolitical organization and economic system in which the means of production are owned and controlled by the government, rather than by individuals or corporations.

society Organized life in groups; shared with humans by monkeys, apes, wolves, mole rats, and ants, among other animals.

sociolinguistics The study of language in society.

sororate A custom in which a widower marries the sister of his deceased wife.

state A society with a central government, administrative specialization, and social classes.

status Any position, no matter what its prestige, that someone occupies in society.

stereotypes Fixed ideas—often unfavorable—about what members of a group are like.

stratification The presence of social divisions—strata—with unequal wealth and power.

stratified Class structured, with differences in wealth, prestige, and power.

style shifts Varying one's speech in different social contexts.

subcultures Different cultural traditions associated with subgroups in the same complex society.

subgroups (Linguistic) closely related languages.

subordinate The lower, underprivileged group in a stratified society.

superordinate The upper, privileged group in a stratified society.

superorganic (Kroeber) The special domain of culture, beyond the organic and inorganic realms.

survey research The study of society through sampling, statistical analysis, and impersonal data collection.

symbol Something, verbal or nonverbal, that stands for something else.

symbolic anthropology The study of symbols in their social and cultural context.

synchronic (Studying societies) at one time.

syncretisms Cultural, especially religious, mixes, emerging from acculturation.

syntax The arrangement and order of words in phrases and sentences.

taboo Sacred and forbidden; prohibition backed by supernatural sanctions.

text A cultural product that is processed and assigned meaning by anyone exposed to it.

theory A set of ideas formulated to explain something.

totem An animal, a plant, or a geographic feature associated with a specific social group, to which that totem is sacred or symbolically important.

transgender A gender identity that is socially constructed and individually performed by individuals whose gender identity contradicts their biological sex at birth and the gender identity assigned to them in infancy.

transhumance A system in which only part of a pastoral population moves seasonally with herds.

tribe A food-producing society with a rudimentary political structure.

tropics Zone between 23 degrees north (Tropic of Cancer) and 23 degrees south (Tropic of Capricorn) of the equator.

underdifferentiation Seeing less-developed countries as all the same; ignoring cultural diversity.

unilineal descent Matrilineal or patrilineal descent.

unilinear evolutionism The (19th-century) idea of a single line or path of cultural development.

universal Something that exists in every culture.

urban anthropology The anthropological study of cities and urban life.

variables Attributes that differ from one person or case to the next.

village head A local tribal leader with limited authority.

wealth All a person's material assets; basis of economic status.

Westernization The acculturative influence of Western expansion on local cultures worldwide.

working class (proletariat) People who must sell their labor to survive; for Karl Marx, workers in factories, mines, estates, etc.

world-system theory The idea that a discernible social system, based on wealth and power differentials, transcends individual countries.

BIBLIOGRAPHY

Abiodun, R.
2014   *Yoruba Art and Language: Seeking the African in African Art.* New York: Cambridge University Press.

Adamou, E., and Y. Matras, eds.
2020   *Routledge Handbook of Language Contact.* New York: Routledge.

Adepegba, C. O.
1991   The Yoruba Concept of Art and Its Significance in the Holistic View of Art as Applied to African Art. *African Notes* 15: 1-6.

Ahearn, L. M.
2017   *Living Language: An Introduction to Linguistic Anthropology.* Hoboken, NJ: Wiley.

Akmajian, A. et al.
2017   *Linguistics: An Introduction to Language and Communication,* 7th ed. Cambridge, MA: MIT Press.

Alexandrakis, O., ed.
2016   *Impulse to Act: A New Anthropology of Resistance and Social Justice.* Indianapolis: Indiana University Press.

Amadiume, I.
1987   *Male Daughters, Female Husbands.* Atlantic Highlands, NJ: Zed.

Amos, T. D.
2011   *Embodying Difference: The Making of the Burakumin in Modern Japan.* Honolulu: University of Hawaii Press.

Anderson, B.
2006   (orig. 1991) *Imagined Communities: Reflections on the Origin and Spread of Nationalism,* rev. ed. New York: Verso.

Anderson, M.
2019   Mobile Technology and Home Broadband 2019. Pew Research Center, June 13. https://www.pewresearch.org/internet/2019/06/13/mobile-technology-and-home-broadband-2019/.

Anderson, M. et al.
2019   10 percent of American Don't Use the Internet him. Who Are They? Pew Research Center, April 22. https://www.pewresearch.org/fact-tank/2019/04/22/some-americans-dont-use-the-internet-who-are-they/.

Anderson-Levitt, K. M., ed.
2012   *Anthropologies of Education: A Global Guide to Ethnographic Studies of Learning and Schooling.* New York: Berghahn Books.

Anderson-Levitt, K. M., and E. Rockwell, eds.
2017   *Comparing Ethnographies: Local Studies of Education across the Americas.* Washington: American Educational Research Association.

Andersson, R.
2014   *Inequality Inc.: Clandestine Migration and the Business of Bordering Europe.* Berkeley: University of California Press.
2019   *No Go World: How Fear Is Redrawing our Maps and Infecting our Politics.* Oakland: University of California Press.

Anemone, R. L.
2011   *Race and Human Diversity: A Biocultural Approach.* Upper Saddle River, NJ: Prentice Hall/Pearson.

Ansell, A.
2013   *Race and Ethnicity: The Key Concepts.* New York: Routledge.

Antoun, R. T.
2008   *Understanding Fundamentalism: Christian, Islamic, and Jewish Movements,* 2nd ed. Lanham, MD: AltaMira.

Appadurai, A.
1990   Disjuncture and Difference in the Global Cultural Economy. *Public Culture* 2(2): 1-24.
1991   Global Ethnoscapes: Notes and Queries for a Transnational Anthropology. In *Recapturing Anthropology: Working in the Present,* R. G. Fox, ed. pp. 191-210. Santa Fe: School of American Research Advanced Seminar Series.

Appiah, K. A.
1990   Racisms. In *Anatomy of Racism,* David Theo Goldberg, ed. pp. 3-17. Minneapolis: University of Minnesota Press.

Arens, W.
1981   Professional Football: An American Symbol and Ritual. In *The American Dimension: Cultural Myths and Social Realities,* 2nd ed., W. Arens and S. P. Montague, eds. pp. 1-10. Sherman Oaks, CA: Alfred.

Ariens, C.
2017   Jornal Nacional Is the Flagship Program of Brazil's Globo TV. *Adweek,* August 29. http://www.adweek.com/tv-video/this-tv-news-show-gets-more-viewers-than-the-academy-awards-and-it-does-every-night/.

Arnold, J. E., et al.
2012   *Life at Home in the Twenty-First Century: 32 Families Open Their Doors.* Los Angeles: Cotsen Institute of Archaeology Press.

Arrighi, G.
2010   *The Long Twentieth Century: Money, Power, and the Origins of Our Times,* new and updated ed. New York: Verso.

Asad, T.
2008   (orig. 1983) The Construction of Religion as an Anthropological Category. In *A Reader in the Anthropology of Religion,* M. Lambek, ed., pp. 110-226. Malden, MA: Blackwell.

Ashcroft, B., G. Griffiths, and H. Tiffin
2013   *Postcolonial Studies: The Key Concepts,* 3rd ed. New York: Routledge, Taylor and Francis.

Askew, K. M., and R. R. Wilk, eds.
2002   *The Anthropology of Media: A Reader.* Malden, MA: Oxford, Blackwell.

Atkinson, W.
2020   *The Class Structure of Capitalist Societies. Volume 1, A Space of Bounded Variety.* New York: Routledge.

Atran, S.
2016   The Devoted Actor: Unconditional Commitment and Intractable Conflict across Cultures. *Current Anthropology* 57 (Supplement 13): S192-S203.

Atran, S., et al.
2014   The Devoted Actor, Sacred Values, and Willingness to Fight: Preliminary Studies with ISIL Volunteers and Kurdish Frontline Fighters. University of Oxford, United Kingdom: ARTIS Research. http://johnjayresearch.org/ct/files/2015/05/The-Devoted-Actor-Sacred-Values-and-Willingness-to-Fight.pdf.

Bachman, J. ed.
2019   *Cultural Genocide: Law, Politics, and Global Manifestations.* New York: Routledge.

Baer, H. A., and M. Singer
2018   *The Anthropology of Climate Change: An Integrated Critical Perspective* New York: Routledge/Taylor & Francis Group.

Baer, H. A., M. Singer, and I. Susser
2013   *Medical Anthropology and the World System,* 3rd ed. Santa Barbara, CA: Praeger.

Bailey, R. C., et al.
1989   Hunting and Gathering in Tropical Rain Forests: Is It Possible? *American Anthropologist* 91: 59–82.

Ball, C. A., ed.
2016   *After Marriage Equality: The Future of LGBT Rights.* New York: New York University Press.

Banton, M.
2015   *What We Now Know about Race and Ethnicity.* New York: Berghahn Books.

Barfield, T. J.
2010   *Afghanistan: A Cultural and Political History.* Princeton, NJ: Princeton University Press.

Barnard, A. J.
2019   *Bushmen: Kalahari Hunter-Gatherers and Their Descendants.* New York: Cambridge University Press.

Baron, D. E.
2009   *A Better Pencil: Readers, Writers, and the Digital Revolution.* New York: Oxford University Press.
2015   Singular They Is Word of the Year. The Web of Language, November 19. University of Illinois. https://illinois.edu/blog/view/25/280996.

Barth, F.
1968   (orig. 1958) Ecologic Relations of Ethnic Groups in Swat, North Pakistan. In *Man in Adaptation: The Cultural Present,* Yehudi Cohen, ed., pp. 324–331. Chicago: Aldine.
1969   *Ethnic Groups and Boundaries: The Social Organization of Cultural Difference.* London: Allen and Unwin.

Beck, S., and C. A. Maida, eds.
2013   *Toward Engaged Anthropology.* New York: Berghahn Books.
2015   *Public Anthropology in a Borderless World.* New York: Berghahn Books.

Beckerman, S., and P. Valentine
2002   *Cultures of Multiple Fathers: The Theory and Practice of Partible Paternity in Lowland South America.* Gainesville: University of Florida Press.

Bee, R. J.
2020   Climate Change and the Global Order., pp. 7-18. *Great Decisions: 2020 Edition.* New York: Foreign Policy Association.

Beeman, W.
1986   *Language, Status, and Power in Iran.* Bloomington: Indiana University Press.

Bellah, R. N.
1978   Religious Evolution. In *Reader in Comparative Religion: An Anthropological Approach,* 4th ed., W. A. Lessa and E. Z. Vogt, eds., pp. 36–50. New York: Harper & Row.
2011   *Religion in Human Evolution: From the Paleolithic to the Axial Age.* Cambridge, MA: Belknap Press of Harvard University Press.

Benedict, R.
1946   *The Chrysanthemum and the Sword.* Boston: Houghton Mifflin.
1959   (orig. 1934) *Patterns of Culture.* New York: New American Library.
2019   (orig. 1940) *Race, Science and Politics.* Athens: University of Georgia Press.

Bennett, J. W.
1969   *Northern Plainsmen: Adaptive Strategy and Agrarian Life.* Chicago: Aldine.

Berger, P.
2010   Pentecostalism—Protestant Ethic or Cargo Cult? Peter Berger's blog, July 29. http://blogs.the-american-interest.com/berger/2010/07/29/pentecostalism-%E2%80%93-protestant-ethic-or-cargo-cult/.

Beriss, D.
2004   *Black Skins, French Voices: Caribbean Ethnicity and Activism in Urban France.* Boulder, CO: Westview Press.

Berlin, B. D., and P. Kay
1991   *Basic Color Terms: Their Universality and Evolution,* 2nd ed. Berkeley: University of California Press.
1999   *Basic Color Terms: Their Universality and Evolution.* Stanford, CA: Center for the Study of Language and Information.

Bernard, H. R.
2018   *Research Methods in Anthropology: Qualitative and Quantitative Methods,* 6th ed. Lanham, MD: Rowman & Littlefield.
2013   *Social Science Research Methods: Qualitative and Quantitative Approaches,* 2nd ed. Los Angeles: Sage.

Bernard, H. R., and C. G. Gravlee, eds.
2014   *Handbook of Methods in Cultural Anthropology,* 2nd ed. Lanham, MD: Rowman & Littlefield.

Bernard, H. R., A. Wutich, and G. W. Ryan
2017   *Analyzing Qualitative Data: Systematic Approaches,* 2nd ed. Los Angeles: SAGE.

Bertram, G. W.
2019   *Art as Human Practice: An Aesthetics,* translated from the German by N. Ross. London: Bloomsbury.

Besnier, N., and S. Brownell
2016   The Untold Story behind Fiji's Astonishing Gold Medal. *SAPIENS,* August 19. http://www.sapiens.org/culture/fiji-rugby-racial-sexual-politics/.

Bielo, J. S.
2015   *Anthropology of Religion: The Basics.* New York: Routledge.

Bilefsky, D.
2006   Polygamy Fosters Culture Clashes (and Regrets) in Turkey. *New York Times,* July 10.

Bilgrami, A.
2016   *Beyond the Secular West.* New York: Columbia University Press.

Bjuremalm, H.
1997   Rättvisa kan skipas i Rwanda: Folkmordet 1994 går att förklara och analysera på samma sätt som förintelsen av judarna. *Dagens Nyheter* [06-03-1997, p. B3].

Black, J.
2015   *The British Empire: A History and a Debate.* Burlington, VT: Ashgate.

Blackwood, E.
2010   *Falling into the Lesbi World: Desire and Difference in Indonesia.* Honolulu: University of Hawaii Press.

Blewitt, J.
2018   *Understanding Sustainable Development,* 3rd ed. New York: Routledge, Taylor & Francis.

Blommaert, J., and D. Jie
2020   *Ethnographic Fieldwork: A Beginner's Guide,* 2nd ed. Blue Ridge Summit: Multilingual Matters.

Boas, F.
1966   (orig. 1940) *Race, Language, and Culture.* New York: Free Press.

Boddy, J., and M. Lambek, eds.

2014   *A Companion to the Anthropology of Religion.* Hoboken, NJ: Wiley.

Bodley, J. H.

2012   *Anthropology and Contemporary Human Problems,* 6th ed. Lanham, MD: AltaMira.

2015   *Victims of Progress,* 6th ed. Lanham, MD: Rowman & Littlefield.

2017   *Cultural Anthropology: Tribes, States, and the Global System,* 6th ed. Lanham, MD: Rowman & Littlefield.

Boellstorff, T.

2015   *Coming of Age in Second Life: An Anthropologist Explores the Virtually Human.* Princeton, NJ: Princeton University Press.

Boellstorff, et al.

2012   *Ethnography and Virtual Worlds: A Handbook of Method.* Princeton, NJ: Princeton University Press.

Bohannan, P.

1971   Artist and Critic in an African Society. In *Anthropology and Art: Readings in Cross-Cultural Aesthetics,* C. Otten, ed., pp. 172–181. Austin: University of Texas Press.

Bonvillain, N.

2016   *The Routledge Handbook of Linguistic Anthropology.* New York: Routledge.

2020   *Language, Culture, and Communication: The Meaning of Messages,* 8th ed. Lanham, MD: Rowman & Littlefield.

2021   *Women and Men: Cultural Constructs of Gender,* 5th ed. Lanham, MD: Rowman & Littlefield.

Borjian, M.

2017   *Language and Globalization: An Autoethnographic Approach.* New York: Routledge.

Borneman, J., and L. K. Hart

2015   The Institution of Marriage Our Society Needs: Anthropological Investigations over the Last Century Have Shown That Marriage Is an Elastic Institution. *Aljazeera America,* July 12. http://america.aljazeera.com/opinions/2015/7/the-institution-of-marriage-our-society-needs.html.

Borofsky, R.

2000   Public Anthropology: Where To? What Next? *Anthropology Newsletter* 41(5): 9–10.

Borofsky, R., and S. Hutson

2016   Maybe "Doing No Harm" Is Not the Best Way to Help Those Who Helped You. *Anthropology News* 57(1–2): 29.

Bouckaert, R., et al.

2012   Mapping the Origins and Expansion of the Indo-European Language Family. *Science* 337: 957–960.

Bourdieu, P.

1977   *Outline of a Theory of Practice.* Translated by Richard Nice. Cambridge, UK: Cambridge University Press.

1982   *Ce Que Parler Veut Dire.* PaFris: Fayard.

1984   *Distinction: A Social Critique of the Judgment of Taste.* Translated by R. Nice. Cambridge, MA: Harvard University Press.

Bourque, S. C., and K. B. Warren

1987   Technology, Gender and Development. *Daedalus* 116(4): 173–197.

Bowen, J. R.

2017   *Religion in Practice: An Approach to Anthropology of Religion,* 7th ed. New York: Routledge.

Boyer, P.

2018   *Minds Make Societies: How Cognition Explains the World Humans Create.* New Haven, CT: Yale University Press.

Brace, C. L.

2005   *"Race" Is a Four-Letter Word: The Genesis of the Concept.* New York: Oxford University Press.

Bradley, D., and M. Bradley

2019   *Language Endangerment.* New York: Cambridge University Press.

Braudel, F.

1981   *Civilization and Capitalism, 15th–18th Century.* Volume I: *The Structure of Everyday Life: The Limits.* Translated by S. Reynolds. New York: Harper & Row.

1982   *Civilization and Capitalism, 15th–18th Century.* Volume II: *The Wheels of Commerce.* New York: Harper Collins.

1992   *Civilization and Capitalism, 15th–18th Century.* Volume III: *The Perspective of the World.* Berkeley: University of California Press.

Brekhus, W. H., and G. Ignatow

2019   *The Oxford Handbook of Cognitive Sociology.* New York: Oxford University Press.

Brettell, C. B., and C. F. Sargent, eds.

2017   *Gender in Cross-Cultural Perspective,* 7th ed. New York: Routledge.

Briggs, C. L.

2005   Communicability, Racial Discourse, and Disease. *Annual Review of Anthropology* 34: 269–291.

Briody, E. K., and R. T. Trotter II.

2008   *Partnering for Organizational Performance; Collaboration and Culture in the Global Workplace.* Lanham, MD: Rowman & Littlefield.

Brookings Institution

2010   *State of Metropolitan America: On the Front Lines of Demographic Transition.* The Brookings Institution Metropolitan Policy Program. http://www.brookings.edu/˜/media/Files/Programs/Metro/state_of_metro_america/metro_america_report1.pdf.

Brower, B.,and B. R. Johnston

2007   *Disappearing Peoples? Indigenous Groups and Ethnic Minorities in South and Central Asia.* Walnut Creek, CA: Left Coast Press.

Brown, A.

2001   Communism. *International Encyclopedia of the Social & Behavioral Sciences,* pp. 2323–2326. New York: Elsevier.

Brown, M. F.

2003   *Who Owns Native Culture?* Cambridge, MA: Harvard University Press.

Brown, P. J., and S. Closser

2016   *Understanding and Applying Medical Anthropology: Biosocial and Cultural Approaches,* 3rd ed. Walnut Creek, CA: Left Coast Press.

Brownstein, R.

2010   The Gray and the Brown: The Generational Mismatch. *National Journal,* July 24. http://www.nationaljournal.com/njmagazines/cs_20100724_3946php.

Bruno, D.

2018   Was I Part British, Part Dutch, a Little Bit Jewish? The Oddness of DNA Tests. *Washington Post,* November 3. https://www.washingtonpost.com/national/health-science/was-i-part-british-part-dutch-a-little-bit-jewish-the-oddness-of-dna-tests/2018/11/02/.

Buettner, E.

2016   *Europe after Empire: Decolonization, Society, and Culture.* Cambridge, UK: Cambridge University Press.

Burbank, J., and F. Cooper

2010   *Empires in World History: Power and the Politics of Difference.* Princeton, NJ: Princeton University Press.

Burbank, V. K.

1988   *Aboriginal Adolescence: Maidenhood in an Australian Community.* New Brunswick, NJ: Rutgers University Press.

Burdick, J.

1993   *Looking for God in Brazil: The Progressive Catholic Church in Urban Brazil's Religious Arena.* Berkeley: University of California Press.

1998   *Blessed Anastácia: Women, Race, and Popular Christianity in Brazil.* New York: Routledge.

Bures. F.

2016   *The Geography of Madness: Penis Thieves, Voodoo Death, and the Search for the Meaning of the World's Strangest Syndromes.* Brooklyn, NY: Melville House.

Burling, R.

1970   *Man's Many Voices: Language in Its Cultural Context.* New York: Harcourt Brace Jovanovich.

Burn, S. M.

2019   *Women across Cultures.* New York: McGraw-Hill Education.

Burridge, K., and A. Bergs

2017   *Understanding Language Change.* New York: Routledge.

Burt, B.

2013   *World Art: An Introduction to the Art in Artefacts.* New York: Bloomsbury.

Butler, J.

1988   Performative Acts and Gender Constitution: An Essay in Phenomenology and Feminist Theory. *Theatre Journal* 40(4): 519–531.

1990   *Gender Trouble: Feminism and the Subversion of Identity.* New York: Routledge.

2015   *Notes toward a Performative Theory of Assembly.* Cambridge: Harvard University Press.

Cairns, M. F.

2015   *Shifting Cultivation and Environmental Change: Indigenous People, Agriculture and Forest Conservation.* New York: Routledge.

Caldararo, N. L.

2014   *The Anthropology of Complex Economic Systems: Inequality, Stability, and Cycles of Crisis.* Lanham, MD: Lexington Books.

Caldas-Coulthard, C. R.

2020   *Inovations and Challenges: Women, Language and Sexism.* New York: Routledge.

Candea, M.

2019   *Comparison in Anthropology: The Impossible Method.* New York: Cambridge University Press.

Carey, B.

2007   Washoe, a Chimp of Many Words Dies at 42. *New York Times,* November 1.

Carneiro, R. L.

1956   Slash-and-Burn Agriculture: A Closer Look at Its Implications for Settlement Patterns. In *Men and Cultures,* Selected Papers of the Fifth International Congress of Anthropological and Ethnological Sciences, pp. 229–234. Philadelphia: University of Pennsylvania Press.

1968   (orig. 1961) Slash-and-Burn Cultivation among the Kuikuru and Its Implications for Cultural Development in the Amazon Basin. In *Man in Adaptation: The Cultural Present,* Y. A. Cohen, ed., pp. 131–145. Chicago: Aldine.

1970   A Theory of the Origin of the State. *Science* 69: 733–738.

1990   Chiefdom-Level Warfare as Exemplified in Fiji and the Cauca Valley. In *The Anthropology of War,* J. Haas, ed., pp. 190–211. Cambridge, UK: Cambridge University Press.

1991   The Nature of the Chiefdom as Revealed by Evidence from the Cauca Valley of Colombia. In *Profiles in Cultural Evolution,* A. T. Rambo and K. Gillogly, eds., *Anthropological Papers* 85, pp. 167–190. Ann Arbor: University of Michigan Museum of Anthropology.

Carneiro, R. L., et al., eds.

2017   *Chiefdoms: Yesterday and Today.* Clinton Corners, NY: EWP, Eliot Werner Publications.

Carrier, J. G., ed.

2012   *A Handbook of Economic Anthropology.* Cheltenham, UK: Edward Elgar.

2016   *After the Crisis: Anthropological Thought, Neoliberalism and the Aftermath.* New York: Routledge.

Carrier, J. G., and D. Kalb, eds.

2015   *Anthropologies of Class: Power, Practice, and Inequality.* Cambridge, UK: Cambridge University Press.

Casanova, J.

2001   Religion, the New Millennium, and Globalization. *Sociology of Religion* 62: 415–441.

Castellanos, M. B., ed.

2019   *Detours: Travel and the Ethics of Research in the Global South.* Tucson: University of Arizona Press.

Cefkin, M., ed.

2009   *Ethnography and the Corporate Encounter: Reflections on Research in and of Corporations.* New York: Berghahn Books.

Cernea, M. M., ed.

1991   *Putting People First: Sociological Variables in Rural Development,* 2nd ed. New York: Oxford University Press (published for the World Bank).

Ceuppens, B., and P. Geschiere

2005   Autochthony: Local or Global? New Modes in the Struggle over Citizenship and Belonging in Africa and Europe. *Annual Review of Anthropology* 34: 385–407.

Chagnon, N. A.

2013a   *Yanomamö,* 6th ed. Australia: Wadsworth Cengage.

2013b   *Noble Savages: My Life among Two Dangerous Tribes—The Yanomamo and the Anthropologists.* New York: Simon & Schuster.

Chambers, E.

1987   Applied Anthropology in the Post-Vietnam Era: Anticipations and Ironies. *Annual Review of Anthropology* 16: 309–337.

Chibnik, M.

2011   *Anthropology, Economics, and Choice.* Austin: University of Texas Press.

Chicchelli, V., et al., eds.

2020   *Aesthetic Cosmopolitanism and Global Culture.* Leiden: Koninklijke Brill NV.

Chomsky, N.

1955   *Syntactic Structures.* The Hague: Mouton.

Christiansen, B., and O. Karnaukhova, eds.

2021   *Handbook of Research on Modern Economic Anthropology.* Hershey: Information Science Reference.

Church, A. T., ed.

2017   *The Praeger Handbook of Personality across Cultures.* Santa Barbara, CA: Praeger.

Cilluffo, A., and D. Cohn

2017   10 Demographic Trends Shaping the U.S. and the World in 2017. Pew Research Center, April 27. http://www.pewresearch.org/fact-tank/2017/04/27/10-demographic-trends-shaping-the-u-s-and-the-world-in-2017/.

Clark, G.

2010   *African Market Women: Seven Life Stories from Ghana.* Indianapolis: Indiana University Press.

Coates, J.

2016 *Women, Men, and Language: A Sociolinguistic Account of Gender Differences in Language.* New York: Routledge.

Coburn, N.

2011 *Bazaar Politics: Power and Pottery in an Afghan Market Town.* Stanford, CA: Stanford University Press.

Codding, B. F., and K. L. Kramer, eds.

2016 *Why Forage? Hunters and Gatherers in the Twenty-first Century.* Albuquerque: University of New Mexico Press and School of Advanced Research Press.

Cody, D.

1998 British Empire. http://www.victorianweb.org/.

Cohen, J. H.

2015 *Eating Soup without a Spoon: Anthropological Theory and Method in the Real World.* Austin: University of Texas Press.

Cohen, R.

1967 *The Kanuri of Bornu.* New York: Harcourt Brace Jovanovich.

Cohen, Y. A.

1974 Culture as Adaptation. In *Man in Adaptation: The Cultural Present,* 2nd ed., Y. A. Cohen, ed., pp. 45–68. Chicago: Aldine.

Colbourne, R., and R. B. Anderson, eds.

2020 *Indigenous Wellbeing and Enterprise: Self-Determination and Sustainable Economic Development.* New York: Routledge.

Coleman, S., and R. I. J. Hackett, eds.

2015 *The Anthropology of Global Pentecostalism and Evangelicalism.* New York: New York University Press.

Coles, R. L.

2016 *Race and Family: A Structural Approach,* 2nd ed. Lanham, MD: Rowman & Littlefield.

Colson, E., and T. Scudder

1988 *For Prayer and Profit: The Ritual, Economic, and Social Importance of Beer in Gwembe District, Zambia, 1950–1982.* Stanford, CA: Stanford University Press.

Cooper, F.

2014 *Africa in the World: Capitalism, Empire, Nation-State.* Cambridge, MA: Harvard University Press.

2019 *Africa since 1940: The Past of the Present,* 2nd ed. Cambridge, MA: Harvard University Press.

Cooper, F., and A. L. Stoler

1997 *Tensions of Empire: Colonial Cultures in a Bourgeois World.* Berkeley: University of California Press.

Cornwall, A., and N. Lindisfarne, eds.

2017 *Dislocating Masculinity: Comparative Ethnographies,* rev. ed. New York: Routledge, Taylor & Francis.

Council of Economic Advisers

2014 Nine Facts about American Families and Work. Executive Office of the President of the United States. https://www.whitehouse.gov/sites/default/files/docs/nine_facts_about_family_and_work_real_final.pdf.

Crenson, M.

2000 Music—from the Heart or from the Genes. http://www.cis.vt.edu/modernworld/d/musicgenes.html.

Crewe, E., and R. Axelby

2013 *Anthropology and Development: Culture, Morality and Politics in a Globalised World.* Cambridge, UK: Cambridge University Press.

Crosby, A. W., Jr.

2003 *The Columbian Exchange: Biological and Cultural Consequences of 1492.* Westport, CT: Praeger.

2015 *Ecological Imperialism.* New York: Cambridge University Press.

Cultural Survival Quarterly

1989 Quarterly journal. Cambridge, MA: Cultural Survival.

Cummings, V., P. Jordan, and M. Zvelebil, eds.

2014 *The Oxford Handbook of the Archaeology and Anthropology of Hunter-Gatherers.* Oxford, UK: Oxford University Press.

Dagne, T. W.

2015 *Intellectual Property and Traditional Knowledge in the Global Economy: Translating Geographical Indications for Development.* New York: Routledge.

DaMatta, R.

1991 *Carnivals, Rogues, and Heroes: An Interpretation of the Brazilian Dilemma.* Translated from the Portuguese by John Drury. Notre Dame, IN: University of Notre Dame Press.

D'Andrade, R.

1984 Cultural Meaning Systems. In *Culture Theory: Essays on Mind, Self, and Emotion,* R. A. Shweder and R. A. Levine, eds., pp. 88–119. Cambridge, UK: Cambridge University Press.

Danesi, M.

2020 *Language, Society, and New Media: Sociolinguistics Today,* 3rd. ed. New York: Routledge.

Darwin, H.

2017 Doing Gender Beyond the Binary: A Virtual Ethnography. Symbolic Interaction. https://onlinelibrary.wiley.com/doi/abs/10.1002/symb.316.

Das, V., and D. Poole, eds.

2004 *Anthropology in the Margins of the State.* Santa Fe, NM: School of American Research Press.

Davenport, C., and J. Haner

2015 The Marshall Islands Are Disappearing. *New York Times,* December 1. http://www.nytimes.com/interactive/2015/12/02/world/The-Marshall-Islands-Are-Disappearing.html.

Davis, A. K.

2020 Bathroom Battlegrounds: How Public Restrooms Shape the Gender Order. Oakland: University of California Press.

Day, E.

2015 #BlackLivesMatter: The Birth of a New Civil Rights Movement. *The Guardian,* July 19. http://www.theguardian.com/world/2015/jul/19/blacklivesmatter-birth-civil-rights-movement.

Degler, C.

1970 *Neither Black nor White: Slavery and Race Relations in Brazil and the United States.* New York: Macmillan.

de la Peña, G.

2005 Social and Cultural Policies toward Indigenous Peoples: Perspectives from Latin America. *Annual Review of Anthropology* 34: 717–739.

De Leon, J.

2015 *The Land of Open Graves: Living and Dying on the Migrant Trail.* Oakland: University of California Press.

Denny, R. M., and P. L. Sunderland, eds.

2014 *Handbook of Anthropology in Business.* Walnut Creek, CA: Left Coast Press.

Dentan, R. K.

1979 *The Semai: A Nonviolent People of Malaya,* fieldwork edition. New York: Harcourt Brace.

2008 *Overwhelming Terror: Love, Fear, Peace and Violence among the Semai of Malaysia.* Lanham, MD: Rowman & Littlefield.

DeSalle, R., and I. Tattersall

2018 *Troublesome Science: The Misuse of Genetics and Genomics in Understanding Race.* New York: Columbia University Press.

Descartes, L., and C. P. Kottak
2009   *Media and Middle-Class Moms.* New York: Routledge.

Desmond, M., and M Emirbayer
2020   *Race in America.* New York: W. W. Norton.

del Valle, I., et al., eds.
2020   *Iberian Empires and the Roots of Globalization.* Nashville: Vanderbilt University Press.

Diamond, J. M.
2017   (orig. 1997) *Guns, Germs, and Steel: The Fates of Human Societies,* 20th anniversary ed. New York: W. W. Norton.

Di Leonardo, M., ed.
1991   *Gender at the Crossroads of Knowledge: Feminist Anthropology in the Postmodern Era.* Berkeley: University of California Press.

Di Liberto, T.
2017   Reviewing Hurricane Harvey's Catastrophic Rain and Flooding. *Climate.gov.* September 18.https://www.climate.gov/news-features/event-tracker/reviewing-hurricane-harveys-catastrophic-rain-and-flooding.

Divale, W. T., and M. Harris
1976   Population, Warfare, and the Male Supremacist Complex. *American Anthropologist* 78: 521–538.

Dolan, P., and J. Connolly, eds.
2018   *Sport and National Identities: Globalization and Conflict.* New York: Routledge.

Domingues, V. R., and B. M. French
2020   *Anthropological Lives: An Introduction to the Profession of Anthropology.* New Brunswick, NJ: Rutgers University Press.

Donnelly, S.
2019   *The Lie of Global Prosperity: How Neoliberals Distort Data to Mask Poverty and exploitation .* New York: Monthly Review Press.

Donovan, J. M.
2007   *Legal Anthropology: An Introduction.* Lanham, MD: Rowman & Littlefield.

Dorward, D. C., ed.
1983   *The Igbo "Women's War" of 1929: Documents Relating to the Aba Riots in Eastern Nigeria.* Wakefield, UK: East Ardsley.

Dos Santos, M., and J-F. Pelletier
2018   *The Social Constructions and Expressions of Madness.* Leiden, Netherlands: Koninklijke Brill, NV.

Douglas, M.
1970*a*   *Natural Symbols: Explorations in Cosmology.* London: Barrie and Rockliff, The Crescent Press.
1970*b*   *Purity and Danger: An Analysis of Concepts of Pollution and Taboo.* Harmondsworth, UK: Penguin.

Dove, M. R., P. E. Sajise, and A. A. Doolittle, eds.
2011   *Beyond the Sacred Forest: Complicating Conservation in Southeast Asia.* Durham, NC: Duke University Press.

Downey, D., I. Kinane, and E. Parker, eds.
2016   *Landscapes of Liminality: Between Space and Place.* Lanham, MD: Rowman & Littlefield.

Doyle, C. M.
2015   *Indigenous Peoples, Title to Territory, Rights, and Resources: The Transformative Role of Free Prior and Informed Consent.* New York: Routledge.

Drahos, P.
2014   *Intellectual Property, Indigenous People, and Their Knowledge.* Cambridge, UK: Cambridge University Press.

Dresch, P., and H. Skoda
2012   *Legalism: Anthropology and History.* Oxford, UK: Oxford University Press.

Dresser, S.
2020   The Life and Meaning of Margaret Mead. *SAPIENS* February 11. https://www.sapiens.org/culture/mead-freeman/.

Duffield, M., and V. Hewitt, eds.
2009   *Empire, Development, and Colonialism: The Past in the Present.* Rochester, NY: James Currey.

Dunn, J. S.
2000   *The Impact of Media on Reproductive Behavior in Northeastern Brazil.* Ph.D. dissertation, Department of Anthropology, University of Michigan, Ann Arbor.

Duranti, A., ed.
2009   *Linguistic Anthropology: A Reader.* Malden, MA: Wiley-Blackwell.

Durkheim, E.
1951   (orig. 1897) *Suicide: A Study in Sociology.* Glencoe, IL: Free Press.
2001   (orig. 1912) *The Elementary Forms of the Religious Life.* Translated by Carol Cosman. Abridged with an introduction and notes by Mark S. Cladis. New York: Oxford University Press.

Dürr, E., and R. Jaffe, eds.
2010   *Urban Pollution: Cultural Meanings, Social Practices.* New York: Berghahn Books.

Earle, T. K.
1987   Chiefdoms in Archaeological and Ethnohistorical Perspective. *Annual Review of Anthropology* 16: 279–308.
1997   *How Chiefs Come to Power: The Political Economy in Prehistory.* Stanford, CA: Stanford University Press.

Eckert, P.
1989   *Jocks and Burnouts: Social Categories and Identity in the High School.* New York: Teachers College Press, Columbia University.
2000   *Linguistic Variation as Social Practice: The Linguistic Construction of Identity in Belten High.* Malden, MA: Blackwell.
2018   *Meaning and Linguistic Variation:The Third Wave in Sociolinguistics.* New York: Cambridge University Press.

Eckert, P., and S. McConnell-Ginet
2013   *Language and Gender,* 2nd ed. Cambridge, UK: Cambridge University Press.

Eckert, P., and N. Mendoza-Denton
2002   Getting Real in the Golden State. *Language,* March 29. http://www.pbs.org/speak/seatosea/americanvarieties/californian/.

Edelman, M., and A. Haugerud
2005   *The Anthropology of Development and Globalization: From Classical Political Economy to Contemporary Neoliberalism.* Malden, MA: Blackwell.

Egloff, B. J.
2019   *Archaeological Heritage Conservation and Management.* Oxford: Archaeopress.

Ellen, R., S. J. Lycett, and S. E. Johns, eds.
2013   *Understanding Cultural Transmission in Anthropology: A Critical Synthesis.* New York: Berghahn.

Eller, J. D.
2015   *Introducing Anthropology of Religion,*2nd ed. New York: Routledge.

Ellick, C. J., and J. E. Watkins
2011   *The Anthropology Graduate's Guide: From Student to a Career.* Walnut Creek, CA: Left Coast Press.

Ember, M., and C. R. Ember
1997   Science in Anthropology. In *The Teaching of Anthropology: Problems, Issues, and Decisions,* C. P. Kottak, J. J. White, R. H. Furlow, and P. C. Rice, eds., pp. 29–33. Mountain View, CA: Mayfield.

Erickson, J.
2016 Minority, Low-Income Neighborhoods Targeted for Hazardous Waste. University of Michigan, *The University Record,* January 20.

Erickson, P. A., and L. D. Murphy
2017 *A History of Anthropological Theory,* 5th ed. Toronto: University of Toronto Press.

Eriksen, T. H.
2014 *Globalization: The Key Concepts,* 2nd ed. New York: Bloomsbury Academic.

Errington, F., and D. Gewertz
1987 *Cultural Alternatives and a Feminist Anthropology: An Analysis of Culturally Constructed Gender Interests in Papua New Guinea.* New York: Cambridge University Press.

Ervin, A. M.
2014 *Cultural Transformations and Globalization: Theory, Development and Social Change.* Boulder, CO: Paradigm.

Escobar, A.
2012 *Encountering Development: The Making and Unmaking of the Third World.* Princeton, NJ: Princeton University Press.

Evans-Pritchard, E. E.
1940 *The Nuer: A Description of the Modes of Livelihood and Political Institutions of a Nilotic People.* Oxford: Clarendon Press.
1970 Sexual Inversion among the Azande. *American Anthropologist* 72: 1428–1433.

Fearon, J. D.
2003 Ethnic and Cultural Diversity by Country. *Journal of Economic Growth* 8(2): 195–222.

Fedorak, S.
2014 *Global Issues: A Cross-Cultural Perspective.* Toronto: University of Toronto Press.

Ferguson, D.
2015 First Black Player on PGA Tour Dies. *Associated Press, Post and Courier.* Charleston, SC, February 5.

Ferguson, R. B.
1995 *Yanomami Warfare: A Political History.* Santa Fe, NM: School of American Research Press.

Ferraro, G. P., and E. K. Briody
2017 *The Cultural Dimension of Global Business,* 8th ed. New York: Routledge, Taylor & Francis.

Feuer, J.
2012 The Clutter Culture, *UCLA Magazine Online,* July 1. http://magazine.ucla.edu/features/the-clutter-culture/.

Fikentscher, W.
2016 *Law and Anthropology.* München, Germany: C. H. Beck.

Fillitz, T., and P. van der Grijp
2017 *An Anthropology of Contemporary Art: Practices, Markets and Collectors.* New York: Bloomsbury Academic.

Finnan, C.
2016 Residential Schooling Brings Opportunity to India's Poorest Indigenous Children. *SAPIENS,* October 12. http://www.sapiens.org/culture/india-indigenous-education.

Finnstrom, S.
1997 Postcoloniality and the Postcolony: Theories of the Global and the Local. http://www.postcolonialweb.org/.

Fiske, J.
2011 *Reading the Popular,* 2nd ed. New York: Routledge.

Fiske, J., and J. Hartley
2003 *Reading Television,* 2nd ed. New York: Routledge.

Fleisher, M. L.
2000 *Kuria Cattle Raiders: Violence and Vigilantism on the Tanzania/Kenya Frontier.* Ann Arbor: University of Michigan Press.

Ford, C. S., and F. A. Beach
1951 *Patterns of Sexual Behavior.* New York: Harper Torchbooks.

Fortes, M.
1950 Kinship and Marriage among the Ashanti. In *African Systems of Kinship and Marriage,* A. R. Radcliffe-Brown and D. Forde, eds., pp. 252–284. London: Oxford University Press.

Fortier, J.
2009 The Ethnography of South Asian Foragers. *Annual Review of Anthropology* 39: 99–114.

Foster, G. M.
1965 Peasant Society and the Image of Limited Good. *American Anthropologist* 67:293–315.

Foster, G. M., and B. G. Anderson
1978 *Medical Anthropology.* New York: McGraw-Hill.

Foucault, M.
1979 *Discipline and Punish: The Birth of the Prison.* Translated by Alan Sheridan. New York: Vintage Books, University Press.
1990 *The History of Sexuality,* Volume 2, *The Use of Pleasure.* R. Hurley (trans.). New York: Vintage.

Fountain, H., N. Popovich
2020 2019 Was the Second-Hottest Year Ever, Closing Out the Warmest Decade. *The New York Times.* January 15. https://www.nytimes.com/interactive/2020/01/15/climate/hottest-year-2019.html

Fourshey, C., et al.
2018 *Bantu Africa: 3500 BCE to Present.* New York: Oxford University Press.

Fouts, R.
1997 *Next of Kin: What Chimpanzees Have Taught Me about Who We Are.* New York: William Morrow.

Fowler, C. S., and D. D. Fowler, eds.
2008 *The Great Basin: People and Place in Ancient Times.* Santa Fe, NM: School for Advanced Research Press.

Fox, S.
2020 *Culture and Psychology.* Los Angeles: SAGE.

Free Dictionary
2004 Honorific (definition of). http://encyclopedia.thefreedictionary.com/Honorific.

Freston, P., ed.
2008 *Evangelical Christianity and Democracy in Latin America.* New York: Oxford University Press.

Frey, W. H.
2019 Less than Half of US Children under 15 Are White, Census Shows. Brookings Institution, June 24. https://www.brookings.edu/research/less-than-half-of-us-children-under-15-are-white-census-shows/

Fricke, T.
1994 *Himalayan Households: Tamang Demography and Domestic Processes,* 2nd ed. New York: Columbia University PressCo.

Fried, M. H.
1960 On the Evolution of Social Stratification and the State. In *Culture in History,* S. Diamond, ed., pp. 713–731. New York: Columbia University Press.
1967 *The Evolution of Political Society: An Essay in Political Anthropology.* New York: McGraw-Hill.

Friedan, B.
1963 *The Feminine Mystique.* New York: W. W. Norton.

Friedl, E.
1962 *Vasilika: A Village in Modern Greece:* New York: Holt, Rinehart, and Winston.
1975 *Women and Men: An Anthropologist's View.* New York: Harcourt Brace Jovanovich.

Gal, S.
  1989   Language and Political Economy. *Annual Review of Anthropology* 18: 345–367.

Galbraith, J. K.
  2016   *Inequality: What Everyone Needs to Know.* New York: Oxford University Press.

Galman, S. C.
  2019   *Shane, The Lone Ethnographer.* Lanham, MA: Rowman & Littlefield.

Garate, D.
  2018   Solving a Riddle about the Dawn of Art. *SAPIENS,* January 16. https://www.sapiens.org/archaeology/atxurra-cave-art-spain/.

Garcia, O., Flores, N., and M. Spotti, eds..
  2017   *The Oxford Handbook of Language and Society.* New York: Oxford University Press.

Garcia Canclini, N.
  2014   *Art beyond Itself: Anthropology for a Society without a Story Line.* Durham, NC: Duke University Press.

Gardner, R. A., B. T. Gardner, and T. E. Van Cantfort, eds.
  1989   *Teaching Sign Language to Chimpanzees.* Albany: State University of New York Press.

Garsten, C., and A. Nyqvist, P., eds.
  2013   *Organisational Anthropology: Doing Ethnography in and among Complex Organisations.* London: Pluto Press.

Geertz, C.
  1973   *The Interpretation of Cultures.* New York: Basic Books.
  1983   *Local Knowledge.* New York: Basic Books.

Gell-Mann, M., and M. Ruhlen
  2011   The Origin and Evolution of Word Order. *Proceedings of the National Academy of Sciences* 108(42): 17290–17295. http://www.pnas.org/content/early/2011/10/04/1113716108.

Gevorkyan, A. V.
  2018   *Transition Economies: Transformation, Development, and Society in Eastern Europe and the Former Soviet Union.* New York: Routledge.

Giddens, A.
  1981   *The Class Structure of the Advanced Societies,* 2nd ed. London: Hutchinson.

Gilmore, D. D.
  1987   *Aggression and Community: Paradoxes of Andalusian Culture.* New Haven, CT: Yale University Press.

Gimpel, J.
  1988   *The Medieval Machine: The Industrial Revolution of the Middle Ages,* 2nd ed. Aldershot, Hants, UK: Wildwood House.

Ginsburg, F. D., L. Abu-Lughod, and B. Larkin, eds.
  2002   *Media Worlds: Anthropology on New Terrain.* Berkeley: University of California Press.

Giordano, C., F. Ruegg, and A. Boscoboinik, eds.
  2014   *Does East Go West? Anthropological Pathways through Postsocialism.* Zurich, Switzerland: Lit Verlag.

Giugale, M.
  2017   *Economic Development: What Everyone Needs to Know,* 2nd ed. New York: Oxford University Press.

Gmelch, G.
  1978   Baseball Magic. *Human Nature* 1(8): 32–40.
  2006   *Inside Pitch: Life in Professional Baseball.* Lincoln: University of Nebraska Press.

Gmelch, G., and D. A. Nathan, eds.
  2017   *Baseball beyond our Borders: An International Pastime.* Lincoln: University of Nebraska Press.

Goldstein, A. D.
  2017   *Janesville: An American Story.* New York: Simon & Schuster.

Golash-Boza, T. M.
  2019   *Race & Racisms: A Critical Approach,* 2nd ed. New York: Oxford University Press.

Goleman, D.
  1992   Anthropology Goes Looking for Love in All the Old Places. *New York Times,* November 24, 1992, p. B1.

Golub, A.
  2017   What You Can REALLY Do with an Anthropology Degree. *Savage Minds,* September 8. https://savageminds.org/2017/09/08/what-you-can-really-do-with-an-anthropology-degree/.

Goodale, J., and J. D. Koss
  1971   The Cultural Context of Creativity among Tiwi. In *Anthropology and Art: Readings in Cross-Cultural Aesthetics,* C. Otten, ed., pp. 182–203. Austin: University of Texas Press.

Goodale, M.
  2017   *Anthropology and Law: A Critical Introduction.* New York: New York University Press.

Goodman, A. H., et al.
  2020   *Race: Are We So Different?* 2nd ed. Hoboken, NJ: Wiley-Blackwell.

Gören, E.
  2013   Economic Effects of Domestic and Neighbouring Countries' Cultural Diversity. March. https://www.etsg.org/ETSG2013/Papers/042.pdf.

Gotkowitz, L., ed.
  2011   *Histories of Race and Racism: The Andes and Mesoamerica from Colonial Times to the Present.* Durham, NC: Duke University Press.

Gough, E. K.
  1959   The Nayars and the Definition of Marriage. *Journal of Royal Anthropological Institute* 89: 23–34.

Gould, T. H. P.
  2016   *Global Advertising in a Global Culture.* Lanham, MD: Rowman & Littlefield.

Graber, M., and J. Atkinson
  2012   Business Anthropology Unlocks Opportunities. *Memphis Daily News* 127(185), September 21. https://www.memphisdailynews.com/news/2012/sep/21/business-anthropology-unlocks-opportunities/.

Graburn, N. H. H., J. Ertle, and R. K. Tierney, eds.
  2008   *Multiculturalism in the New Japan: Crossing the Boundaries Within.* New York: Berghahn Books.

Graca, L. da, and A. Zingarelli, eds.
  2015   *Studies on Pre-capitalist Modes of Production.* Boston: Brill.

Graef, D. J.
  2017   Natural Disasters Are Social Disasters. *SAPIENS,* December 13. https://www.sapiens.org/column/the-climate-report/hurricane-harvey-inequality/.

Gramsci, A.
  1971   *Selections from the Prison Notebooks.* Edited and translated by Quenten Hoare and Geoffrey Nowell Smith. London: Wishart.

Grasmuck, S., and P. R. Pessar
  1991   *Between Two Islands : Dominican International Migration.* Berkeley: University of California Press.

Gravlee, C.
  2009   How Race Becomes Biology: Embodiment of Social Inequality. *American Journal of Physical Anthropology* 139(1): 47–57.

Green, P.
  1999   Mirror, Mirror; The Anthropologist of Dressing Rooms. *The New York Times,* May 2.

http://www.nytimes.com/1999/05/02/style/mirror-mirror-the-anthropologist-of-dressing-rooms.html.

2006   Archaeologist Makes the Case for Burying Dominant Theory of First Americans. Austin: University of Texas Research. http://www.utexas.edu/research/impact/collins.html.

Gremaux, R.
1993   Woman Becomes Man in the Balkans. In *Third Sex Third Gender: Beyond Sexual Dimorphism in Culture and History,* G. Herdt, ed. Cambridge: MIT Press.

Griffin, P. B., and A. Estioko-Griffin, eds.
1985   *The Agta of Northeastern Luzon: Recent Studies.* Cebu City, Philippines: University of San Carlos.

Grimshaw, A., and A. Ravetz
2009   *Observational Cinema: Anthropology, Film, and the Exploration of Social Life.* Bloomington: Indiana University Press.

Gu, S.
2012   *Language and Culture in the Growth of Imperialism.* Jefferson, NC: McFarland.

Gudeman, S. F.
2016   *Anthropology and Economy.* New York: Cambridge University Press.

Gudeman, S. F., and C. Hann, eds.
2015   *Economy and Ritual: Studies of Postsocialist Transformations.* New York: Berghahn Books.

Gupta, A., and J. Ferguson
1997   Beyond "Culture": Space, Identity, and the Politics of Difference. In *Culture, Power, Place: Explorations in Critical Anthropology,* A. Gupta and J. Ferguson, eds., pp. 33–51. Durham, NC: Duke University Press.

Gupta, A., and J. Ferguson, eds.
1997a   *Anthropological Locations: Boundaries and Grounds of a Field Science. Anthropology.* Berkeley: University of California Press.
1997b   *Culture, Power, Place: Explorations in Critical Anthropology.* Durham, NC: Duke University Press.

Gusterson, H.
2020   What's Wrong with "The Chinese Virus"? *SAPIENS,* March 23. https://www.sapiens.org/column/conflicted/coronavirus-name/.

Ha, K. O.
n.d. Anthropologists Dig into Business: Researchers Observe Consumer Habits to Design New Products. *Mercury News.* http://www.antropologi.info/antromag/corporate/kopi/business.html.

Haapala, A.
1998   Literature: Invention of the Self. *Canadian Aesthetics Journal* 2. https://www.uqtr.ca/AE/vol_2/haapala.html.

Haenn, N., R. R. Wilk, and A. Harnish, eds.
2016   *The Environment in Anthropology: A Reader in Ecology, Culture, and Sustainable Living.* New York: New York University Press.

Hallowell, A. I.
1955   *Culture and Experience.* Philadelphia: University of Pennsylvania Press.

Hampton, K., et al.
2011   Social Networking Sites and Our Lives. Pew Research Center, Internet and American Life Project, June 16. http://www.pewinternet.org/2011/06/16/social-networking-sites-and-our-lives/.

Hankins, J. D.
2014   *Working Skin: Making Leather, Making a Multicultural Japan.* Oakland: University of California Press.

Hann, C., and K. Hart
2011   *Economic Anthropology: History, Ethnography, Critique.* Malden, MA: Polity Press.

Hann, C., and K. Hart, eds.
2009   *Market and Society: The Great Transformation Today.* New York: Cambridge University Press.

Hansen, K. V.
2005   *Not-So-Nuclear Families: Class, Gender, and Networks of Care.* New Brunswick, NJ: Rutgers University Press.

Hanzel, I.
2017   *50 Years of Language Experiments with Great Apes.* New York: Peter Lang Edition.

Harris, M.
1964   *Patterns of Race in the Americas.* New York: Walker.
1970   Referential Ambiguity in the Calculus of Brazilian Racial Identity. *Southwestern Journal of Anthropology* 26(1): 1–14.
1974   *Cows, Pigs, Wars, and Witches: The Riddles of Culture.* New York: Random House.
1978   *Cannibals and Kings.* New York: Vintage. Walnut Creek, CA: AltaMira.
2001a   (orig. 1979) *Cultural Materialism: The Struggle for a Science of Culture.* Walnut Creek, CA: AltaMira.
2001b   (orig. 1968) *The Rise of Anthropological Theory.* Walnut Creek, CA: AltaMira.

Harris, M., and C. P. Kottak
1963   The Structural Significance of Brazilian Racial Categories. *Sociologia* 25: 203–209.

Harris, R., and R. Pease
2015   *Pieces of the Musical World: Sounds and Culture.* New York: Routledge.

Harrison, G. G., W. L. Rathje, and W. W. Hughes
1994   Food Waste Behavior in an Urban Population. In *Applying Anthropology: An Introductory Reader,* 3rd ed., A. Podolefsky and P. J. Brown, eds., pp. 107–112. Mountain View, CA: Mayfield.

Harrison, K. D.
2007   *When Languages Die: The Extinction of the World's Languages and the Erosion of Human Knowledge.* New York: Oxford University Press.
2010   *The Last Speakers: The Quest to Save the World's Most Endangered Languages.* Washington, DC: National Geographic.

Hart, C. W. M., A. R. Pilling, and J. C. Goodale
1988   *The Tiwi of North Australia,* 3rd ed. Fort Worth: Harcourt Brace.

Harvey, D. J.
1980   French Empire. *Academic American Encyclopedia,* vol. 8, pp. 309–310. Princeton, NJ: Arete.

Haugerud, A., M. P. Stone, and P. D. Little, eds.
2011   *Commodities and Globalization: Anthropological Perspectives.* Lanham, MD: Rowman & Littlefield.

Hayes, M.
2019   *John Maynard Keynes.* Malden, MA: Polity Press.

Heinrich, P., and Y. Ohara, eds.
2019   *Routledge Handbook of Japanese Sociolinguistic.* New York: Routledge. Helliwell, J., R. Layard, and J. Sachs
2019   *World Happiness Report 20197.* New York: Sustainable Development Solutions Network. https://worldhappiness.report/ed/2019/.

Henry, J.
1955   Docility, or Giving the Teacher What She Wants. *Journal of Social Issues* 2: 33-41.
1972   *Jules Henry on Education.* New York: Random House.

Herdt, G.
2006   *The Sambia: Ritual, Sexuality, and Change in Papua New Guinea.* Belmont, CA: Thomson/Wadsworth.

Herdt, G. H., ed.
1984   *Ritualized Homosexuality in Melanesia.* Berkeley: University of California Press.

Herdt, G. H., and N. Polen-Petit
2021   *Human Sexuality: Self, Society, and Culture,* 2nd ed. New York: McGraw-Hill.

Herzog, T.
2015   *Frontiers of Possession: Spain and Portugal in Europe and the Americas.* Cambridge, MA: Harvard University Press.

Hess, E.
2008   *Nim Chimsky: The Chimp Who Would Be Human.* New York: Bantam Books.

Hewitt, B. L., ed.
2020   *The Secret Lives of Anthropologists: Lessons from the Field.* New York: Routledge.

Hickel, J.
2017   *The Divide: A Brief Guide to Global Inequality and its Solutions.* London: William Heinemann.

Hill, J. H.
1978   Apes and Language. *Annual Review of Anthropology* 7: 89–112.
2017   A Linguist Walks into a Mexican Restaurant. *Edible Baja Arizona 5(25).* http://ediblebajaarizona.com/linguist-walks-mexican-restaurant.

Hill, K. R., et al.
2011   Co-residence Patterns in Hunter-Gatherer Societies Show Unique Human Social Structure. *Science* 331: 1286–1289.

Hill-Burnett, J.
1978   Developing Anthropological Knowledge through Application. In *Applied Anthropology in America,* E. M. Eddy and W. L. Partridge, eds., pp. 112–128. New York: Columbia University Press.

Hinton, A. L., and K. L. O'Neill, eds.
2009   *Genocide: Truth, Memory, and Representation.* Durham, NC: Duke University Press.

Hobhouse, L. T.
1915   *Morals in Evolution,* rev. ed. New York: Holt.

Hock. H. H.
2019   *Language History, Language Change, and Language Relationship: An Introduction to Historical and Comparative Linguistics.* Berlin de Gruyter.

Hodgson, D. L.
2016   *The Gender, Culture, and Power Reader.* New Brunswick, NJ: Rutgers University Press.

Hoebel, E. A.
1954   *The Law of Primitive Man.* Cambridge, MA: Harvard University Press.
1968   (orig. 1954) The Eskimo: Rudimentary Law in a Primitive Anarchy. In *Studies in Social and Cultural Anthropology,* J. Middleton, ed., pp. 93–127. New York: Crowell.

Hogan, B., N. Li, and W. H. Dutton
2011   *A Global Shift in the Social Relationships of Networked Individuals: Meeting and Dating Online Comes of Age* (February 14). Oxford Internet Institute, University of Oxford. doi:10.2139/ssrn.1763884.

Hornborg, A., B. Clark, and K. Hermele, eds.
2011   *Ecology and Power: Struggles over Land and Material Resources in the Past, Present and Future.* New York: Routledge.

Hornborg, A., and C. L. Crumley, eds.
2007   *The World System and the Earth System: Global Socioenvironmental Change and Sustainability since the Neolithic.* Walnut Creek, CA: Left Coast Press.

Horton, R.
1963   The Kalabari Ekine Society: A Borderland of Religion and Art. *Africa 33:* 94–113.
1993   *Patterns of Thought in Africa and the West: Essays on Magic, Religion, and Science.* New York: Cambridge University Press.

Hosseini, S. A. H., et al., eds.
2020   *Routledge Handbook of Transformative Global Studies.* New York: Routledge.

Hyde, J. S., and J. D. DeLamater
2019   *Understanding Human Sexuality,* 14h ed. New York: McGraw-Hill Education.

Ignatius, D.
2007   Summer's Escape Artists. *Washington Post,* July 26. http://www.washingtonpost.com/wp-dyn/content/article/2007/07/25/AR2007072501879.html.

Ikeya, K., and R. K. Hitchcock, eds.
2016   *Hunter-Gatherers and Their Neighbors in Asia, Africa, and South America.* Suita, Osaka: National Museum of Ethnology.

Ingold, T.
2013   *Making: Anthropology, Archaeology, Art and Architecture.* New York: Routledge.

Inhorn, M. C., and E. A. Wentzell, eds.
2012   *Medical Anthropology at the Intersections: Histories, Activisms, and Futures.* Durham, NC: Duke University Press.

Iqbal, S.
2002   A New Light on Skin Color. *National Geographic Online Extra.* http://magma.nationalgeographic.com/ngm/0211/feature2/online_extra.html.

Isto É
1984   *Olimpíadas,* August 8.

Ivison, D.
2020   *Can Liberal States Accommodate Indigenous Peoples?* Malden, MA: Polity Press.

Jablonski, N. G.
2006   *Skin: A Natural History.* Berkeley: University of California Press.
2012   *Living Color: The Biological and Social Meaning of Skin Color.* Berkeley: University of California Press.

Jablonski, N. G., and G. Chaplin
2000   The Evolution of Human Skin Coloration. *Journal of Human Evolution 39:* 57–106.

Jackson, J., and K. B. Warren
2005   Indigenous Movements in Latin America, 1992–2004: Controversies, Ironies, New Directions. *Annual Review of Anthropology 34:* 549–573.

Jaffe, R., and A. De Koning
2016   *Introducing Urban Anthropology.* New York: Routledge, Taylor & Francis.

Jankowiak, W. R., ed.
1995   *Romantic Passion: A Universal Experience?* New York: Columbia University Press.
2008   *Intimacies: Love and Sex across Cultures.* New York: Columbia University Press.

Jankowiak, W. R., and E. F. Fischer
1992   A Cross-Cultural Perspective on Romantic Love. *Ethnology* 31(2): 149–156.

Jaschik, S.
2015   Embedded Conflicts. Army Shuts down Controversial Human Terrain System, Criticized by Many Anthropologists, July 7. *Inside Higher Ed.* https://www.insidehighered.com/news/2015/07/07/army-shuts-down-controversial-human-terrain-system-criticized-many-anthropologists.

Jenks, A.

2016   Teaching Race: Provocation. Correspondence, *Fieldsights*, July 11. Society for Cultural Anthropology. https://culanth.org/fieldsights/teaching-race-provocation.

Jodoin, S.

2017   *Forest Preservation in a Changing Climate: REDD+ and Indigenous and Community Rights in Indonesia and Tanzania.* New York: Cambridge University Press.

Johnson, A. W., and T. Earle

2000   *The Evolution of Human Societies: From Foraging Group to Agrarian State,* 2nd ed. Stanford, CA: Stanford University Press.

Johnston, B. R.

2005   Chixoy Dam Legacy Issues Study. http://www.centerforpoliticalecology.org/chixoy.html.

2010   *Life and Death Matters: Human Rights, Environment and Social Justice,* 2nd ed. Walnut Creek, CA: Left Coast Press.

Jones, A.

2017   *Genocide: A Comprehensive Introduction.* New York: Routledge, Taylor & Francis.

Joralemon, D.

2010   *Exploring Medical Anthropology,* 3rd ed. Boston: Pearson.

Jordan, A.

2013   *Business Anthropology,* 2nd ed. Long Grove, IL: Waveland.

Jordan, B., ed.

2013   *Advancing Ethnography in Corporate Environments: Challenges and Emerging Opportunities.* Walnut Creek, CA: Left Coast Press.

Joyce, R.

2015   Aztec Marriage: A Lesson for Chief Justice Roberts. *Psychology Today,* June 26. https://www.psychologytoday.com/blog/what-makes-us-human/201506/aztec-marriage-lesson-chief-justice-roberts.

Jurafsky, D.

2014   *The Language of Food: A Linguist Reads the Menu.* New York: W. W. Norton.

Kalberg, S.

2017   *Social Thought of Max Weber.* Los Angeles: Sage.

Kamrava, M.

2013   *The Modern Middle East: A Political History since the First World War,* 3rd ed. Berkeley: University of California Press.

Kan, S.

1986   The 19th-Century Tlingit Potlatch: A New Perspective. *American Ethnologist* 13: 191–212.

2016   *Symbolic Immortality: The Tlingit Potlatch of the Nineteenth Century,* 2nd ed. Seattle: University of Washington Press.

Kaneshiro, N. K.

2009   Intersex. *Medline Plus.* National Institutes of Health, U.S. National Library of Medicine. http://www.nlm.nih.gov/medlineplus/ency/article/001669.htm.

Kaplan, H. R.

2014   *Understanding Conflict and Change in a Multicultural World.* Lanham, MD: Rowman & Littlefield.

Kapovic, M.

2017   *The Indo-Eurpean Languages,* 2nd ed. New York: Routledge.

Karrebæk, M. S., K. C. Riley, and J. R. Cavanaugh

2018   Food and Language: Production, Consumption, and Circulation of Meaning and Value. *Annual Review of Anthropology* 47:17–32.

Kaufman, S. R., and L. M. Morgan

2005   The Anthropology of the Beginnings and Ends of Life. *Annual Review of Anthropology* 34: 317–341.

Kelly, R. C.

1976   Witchcraft and Sexual Relations: An Exploration in the Social and Semantic Implications of the Structure of Belief. In *Man and Woman in the New Guinea Highlands,* P. Brown and G. Buchbinder, eds., pp. 36–53. Special Publication, no. 8. Washington, DC: American Anthropological Association.

Kelly, R.

2013   *The Lifeways of Hunter-Gatherers: The Foraging Spectrum.* New York: Cambridge University Press.

Kennedy, M. D.

2015   *Globalizing Knowledge: Intellectuals, Universities, and Publics in Transformation.* Stanford, CA: Stanford University Press.

Kent, S.

1996   *Cultural Diversity among Twentieth-Century Foragers: An African Perspective.* New York: Cambridge University Press.

Kent, S., ed.

2002   *Ethnicity, Hunter-Gatherers, and the "Other": Association or Assimilation in Africa.* Washington, DC: Smithsonian Institution Press.

Kent, S., and H. Vierich

1989   The Myth of Ecological Determinism: Anticipated Mobility and Site Organization of Space. In *Farmers as Hunters: The Implications of Sedentism,* S. Kent, ed., pp. 96–130. New York: Cambridge University Press.

Keynes, J. M.

1927   *The End of Laissez-Faire.* London: L. and Virginia Woolf.

1936   *General Theory of Employment, Interest, and Money.* New York: Harcourt Brace.

Khan, N.

2017   *Mental Disorder.* Toronto: University of Toronto Press.

King, E.

2012   Stanford Linguists Seek to Identify the Elusive California Accent. *Stanford Report,* August 6. http://news.stanford.edu/news/2012/august/california-dialect-linguistics-080612.html.

King, T. F., ed.

2011   *A Companion to Cultural Resource Management.* Malden, MA: Wiley-Blackwell.

Kinsey, A. C., W. B. Pomeroy, and C. E. Martin

1948   *Sexual Behavior in the Human Male.* Philadelphia: W. B. Saunders.

Kirman, P.

1997   An Introduction to Ethnomusicology. Inside World Music. http://www.insideworldmusic.com/library/weekly/aa101797.htm.

Kirner, K., and J. Mills

2020   *Introduction to Ethnographic Research: A Guide for Anthropology.* Los Angeles: Sage.

Kirsch, S.

2018   *Engaged Anthropology: Politics beyond the Text.* Oakland: University of California Press.

Kluckhohn, C.

1944   *Mirror for Man: A Survey of Human Behavior and Social Attitudes.* Greenwich, CT: Fawcett.

Kohrt, B., and E. Mendenhall, eds.

2015   *Global Mental Health: Anthropological Perspectives.* Walnut Creek, CA: Left Coast Press.

Konopinski, N., ed.

2014   *Doing Anthropological Research: A Practical Guide.* New York: Routledge.

Kontopodis, M., C. Wulf, and B. Fichtner, eds.
2011 *Children, Development, and Education: Cultural, Historical, and Anthropological Perspectives.* New York: Springer.

Koonings, K., D. Kruijt, and D. Rodgers. eds.
2019 *Ethnography as Risky Business; Field Research in Violent and Sensitive Contexts.* Lanham, MD: Lexington Books.

Kottak, C. P.
1980 *The Past in the Present: History, Ecology, and Social Organization in Highland Madagascar.* Ann Arbor: University of Michigan Press.
1990a *Prime-Time Society: An Anthropological Analysis of Television and Culture.* Belmont, CA: Wadsworth.
1990b Culture and Economic Development. *American Anthropologist* 92(3): 723–731.
1991 When People Don't Come First: Some Lessons from Completed Projects. In *Putting People First: Sociological Variables in Rural Development,* 2nd ed., ed. M. Cernea, pp. 429–464. New York: Oxford University Press.
1999 The New Ecological Anthropology. *American Anthropologist* 101(1): 23–35.
2004 An Anthropological Take on Sustainable Development: A Comparative Study of Change. *Human Organization* 63(4): 501–510.
2007 Return to Madagascar: A Forty Year Retrospective. *General Anthropology: Bulletin of the General Anthropology Division of the American Anthropological Association* 14(2): 1–10.
2009 *Prime-Time Society: An Anthropological Analysis of Television and Culture,* updated ed. Walnut Creek, CA: Left Coast Press.
2018 *Assault on Paradise: The Globalization of a Little Community in Brazil,* 4th ed. Long Grove, IL: Waveland.

Kottak, C. P., and K. A. Kozaitis
2012 *On Being Different: Diversity and Multiculturalism in the North American Mainstream,* 4th ed. New York: McGraw-Hill.

Kottak, N. C.
2002 *Stealing the Neighbor's Chicken: Social Control in Northern Mozambique.* Ph.D. dissertation. Department of Anthropology, Emory University, Atlanta, GA.

Kotz, D. M.
2015 *The Rise and Fall of Neoliberal Capitalism.* Cambridge, MA: Harvard University Press.

Kozaitis, K.
2021 *Indebted: An Ethnography of Despair and Resilience in Greece's Second City.* New York: Oxford University Press.

Kozlowski, K.
2016 Virginia Tech Expert Helped Expose Flint Water Crisis. *Detroit News,* January 24. http://www.detroitnews.com/story/news/politics/2016/01/23/virginia-tech-expert-helped-expose-flint-water-crisis/79251004/.

Kroeber, A. L.
1944 *Configurations of Cultural Growth.* Berkeley: University of California Press.
1987 (orig. 1952) *The Nature of Culture.* Chicago: University of Chicago Press.

Krogstad, J. M.
2017 U.S. Hispanic Population Growth Has Leveled Off. Pew Research Center, August 3. http://www.pewresearch.org/fact-tank/2017/08/03/u-s-hispanic-population-growth-has-leveled-off/.

Kulick, D.
1998 *Travesti: Sex, Gender, and Culture among Brazilian Transgendered Prostitutes.* Chicago: University of Chicago Press.

Labov, W.
1972a *Language in the Inner City: Studies in the Black English Vernacular.* Philadelphia: University of Pennsylvania Press.
1972b *Sociolinguistic Patterns.* Philadelphia: University of Pennsylvania Press.
2006 *The Social Stratification of English in New York City.* New York: Cambridge University Press.
2012 *Dialect Diversity in America: The Politics of Language Change.* Charlottesville: University of Virginia Press.

Laine, A-K.
2018 *Practicing Art and Anthropology: A Transdisciplinary Journey .* New York: Bloomsbury Academic. Lambek,M., ed.
2008 *A Reader in the Anthropology of Religion.* Malden, MA: Blackwell.

Lakoff, R. T.
2004 *Language and Woman's Place.* New York: Harper & Row.
2017 *Context Counts: Papers on Language, Gender, and Power.* New York: Oxford University Press.

Lakoff, G. P., and G. Duran
2018 Trump Has Turned Words into Weapons. And He's Winning the Linguistic War. *The Guardian,* June 13. https://www.theguardian.com/commentisfree/2018/jun/13/how-to-report-trump-media-manipulation-language.

Lange, P. G.
2019 *Thanks for Watching: An Anthropological Study of Video Sharing on YouTube.* Louisville: University Press of Colorado.

Lange, M.
2009 *Lineages of Despotism and Development: British Colonialism and State Power.* Chicago: University of Chicago Press.
2017 *Killing Others: A Natural History of Ethnic Violence.* Ithaca, NY: Cornell University Press.

Lassiter, L. E.
1998 *The Power of Kiowa Song: A Collaborative Ethnography.* Tucson: University of Arizona Press.

Leach, E. R.
1955 Polyandry, Inheritance and the Definition of Marriage. *Man* 55: 182–186.
1961 *Rethinking Anthropology.* London: Athlone Press.
1970 (orig. 1954) *Political Systems of Highland Burma: A Study of Kachin Social Structure.* London: Athlone Press.

Lechner, F. J., and J. Boli, eds.
2019 *The Globalization Reader,* 6th ed. Hoboken, NJ: Wiley-Blackwell.

Lederman, R.
2015 Big Man, Anthropology of. *International Encyclopedia of the Social & Behavioral Sciences,* 2nd ed., pp. 567-573. New York: Elsevier.

Lee, R. B.
2012 The !Kung and I: Reflections on My Life and Times with the Ju/'hoansi. *General Anthropology* 19(1): 1–4.
2013 *The Dobe Ju/'hoansi.* 4th ed. Belmont, CA: Wadsworth Cengage.
2018 Hunter-Gatherers and Human Evolution: New Light on Old Debates. *Annual Review of Anthropology* 47:513–531.

Lee, R. B., and R. H. Daly, eds.
1999 *The Cambridge Encyclopedia of Hunters and Gatherers.* New York: Cambridge University Press.

Lemke, A. K., ed.
2018 *Foraging in the Past: Archaeological Studies of Hunter-Gatherer Diversity.* Louisville: University Press of Colorado.

Lenski, G.

    1966   *Power and Privilege: A Theory of Social Stratification.* New York: McGraw-Hill.

Lentin, A.

    2020   *Why Race Still Matters.* Malden, MA: Polity Press.

Lerman, S., Ostrach, B., and M. Singer. eds.

    2017   *Foundations of Biosocial Health: Stigma ad Illness Interactions.* Lanham, MD: Lexington Books.

Levine, P.

    2020   *The British Empire: Sunrise to Sunset,* 3rd ed. New York: Routledge.

Levinson, B. A. U., and M. Pollock, eds.

    2011   *A Companion to the Anthropology of Education.* Malden, MA: Blackwell.

Lévi-Strauss, C.

    1963   *Totemism.* Translated by R. Needham. Boston: Beacon Press.

    1967   *Structural Anthropology.* New York: Doubleday.

    1969   (orig. 1949) *The Elementary Structures of Kinship.* Boston: Beacon Press.

Levy, J. E., with B. Pepper

    1992   *Orayvi Revisited: Social Stratification in an "Egalitarian" Society.* Santa Fe, NM: School of American Research Press; Seattle: University of Washington Press.

Lewellen, T. C.

    2010   Groping toward Globalization: In Search of Anthropology without Boundaries. *Reviews in Anthropology* 31(1): 73–89.

Lewin, E., and L. M. Silverstein, eds.

    2016   *Mapping Feminist Anthropology in the Twenty-First Century.* New Brunswick, NJ: Rutgers University Press.

Lim, L., and U. Ansaldo

    2016   *Languages in Contact.* New York: Cambridge University Press.

Lima, E. C.

    2012   As Evangelicals Gain, Catholics on Verge of Losing Majority in Brazil. *National Catholic Reporter.* February 20. https://www.ncronline.org/news/parish/evangelicals-gain-catholics-verge-losing-majority-brazil.

Lindenbaum, S.

    1972   Sorcerers, Ghosts, and Polluting Women: An Analysis of Religious Belief and Population Control. *Ethnology* 11: 241–253.

Lindquist, G., and D. Handelman, eds.

    2013   *Religion, Politics, and Globalization: Anthropological Approaches.* New York: Berghahn Books.

Lock, M., and V.-K. Nguyen

    2018   *An Anthropology of Biomedicine.* Hoboken, NJ: Wiley.

Lockwood, W. G.

    1975   *European Moslems: Economy and Ethnicity in Western Bosnia.* New York: Academic Press.

Lockwood, Y. R.

    1983   *Text and Context: Folksong in a Bosnian Muslim Village.* Columbus, OH: Slavica.

Loomis, W. F.

    1967   Skin-Pigmented Regulation of Vitamin-D Biosynthesis in Man. *Science* 157: 501–506.

López, A. A.

    2011   New Questions in the Immigration Debate. *Anthropology Now* 3(1): 47–53.

Loveday, L.

    1986   Japanese Sociolinguistics: An Introductory Survey. *Journal of Pragmatics* 10: 287–326.

    2001   *Explorations in Japanese Sociolinguistics.* Philadelphia: J. Benjamins.

Lowie, R. H.

    1961   (orig. 1920) *Primitive Society.* New York: Harper & Brothers.

Lowrey, A.

    2013   The Rich Get Richer through the Recovery. *New York Times,* September 13. http://economix.blogs.nytimes.com/2013/09/10/the-rich-get-richer-through-the-recovery/?_r=0.

Lucas, R.

    2020   *Anthropology for Architects: Social Relations and the Built Environment.* New York: Bloomsbury.

Lugo, A.

    1997   Reflections on Border Theory, Culture, and the Nation. In *Border Theory: The Limits of Cultural Politics,* S. Michaelsen and D. Johnson, eds., pp. 43–67. Minneapolis: University of Minnesota Press.

    2008   *Fragmented Lives, Assembled Parts: Culture, Capitalism, and Conquest at the U.S.-Mexico Border.* Austin: University of Texas Press.

Lugo, A., and B. Maurer

    2000   *Gender Matters: Rereading Michelle Z. Rosaldo.* Ann Arbor: University of Michigan Press.

Lule, J.

    2018   *Globalization and Media: Global Village of Babel,* 3rd ed. Lanham, MA: Rowman & Littlefield.

Lundberg, C. and V. Ziakis, eds.

    2019   *Routledge Handbook of Popular Culture and Tourism.* New York: Routledge.

Lupton, D.

    2012   *Medicine as Culture: Illness, Disease, and the Body,* 3rd ed. Los Angeles: Sage.

Lyons, A. P., and H. D. Lyons, eds.

    2011   *Sexualities in Anthropology: A Reader.* Malden, MA: Blackwell.

Madsbjerg, C., and M. B. Rasmussen

    2014   An Anthropologist Walks into a Bar. *Harvard Business Review,* March. https://hbr.org/2014/03/an-anthropologist-walks-into-a-bar.

Maguire, M., C. Frois, and N. Zurawski, eds.

    2014   *The Anthropology of Security: Perspectives from the Frontline of Policing, Counter-terrorism, and Border Control.* Sterling, VA: Pluto Press.

Malefyt, T. de W., and M. McCabe, eds.

    2020   *Women, Consumption, and Paradox.* New York: Routledge.

Malinowski, B.

    1927   *Sex and Repression in Savage Society.* London and New York: International Library of Psychology, Philosophy and Scientific Method.

    1929   Practical Anthropology. *Africa* 2: 23–38.

    1944   *A Scientific Theory of Culture and Other Essays.* Chapel Hill: University of North Carolina Press.

    1961   (orig. 1922) *Argonauts of the Western Pacific.* New York: Dutton.

    1978   (orig. 1931) The Role of Magic and Religion. In *Reader in Comparative Religion: An Anthropological Approach,* 4th ed., W. A. Lessa and E. Z. Vogt, eds., pp. 37–46. New York: Harper & Row.

Malkki, L. H.

    1995   *Purity and Exile: Violence, Memory, and National Cosmology among Hutu Refugees in Tanzania.* Chicago: University of Chicago Press.

Manderson, L., Cartwright, E., and A. Hardon, eds.

    2016   *The Routledge Handbook of Medical Anthropology.* New York: Routledge.

Manjapra, K.
2020 *Colonialism in Global Perspective.* New York: Cambridge University Press.

Mann, C. C.
2012 *1493: Uncovering the New World Columbus Created.* New York: Vintage Books.

Månsson, M., et al., eds.
2020 *Routledge Companion to Media and Tourism.* New York: Routledge.

Maquet, J.
1986 *The Aesthetic Experience: An Anthropologist Looks at the Visual Arts.* New Haven, CT: Yale University Press.

Marcus, G. E., and M. M. J. Fischer
1986 *Anthropology as Cultural Critique: An Experimental Moment in the Human Sciences.* Chicago: University of Chicago Press.

Marger, M. N.
2015 *Race and Ethnic Relations: American and Global Perspectives,* 10th ed. Stamford, CT: Cengage.

Margolis, M.
2000 *True to Her Nature: Changing Advice to American Women.* Prospect Heights, IL: Waveland.
2013 *Goodbye, Brazil: Emigrés from the Land of Soccer and Samba.* Madison: University of Wisconsin Press.
2020 *Women in Fundamentalism: Modesty, Marriage and Motherhood.* Lanham, MD: Rowman & Littlefield.

Marks, J. M.
2016 Teaching Race: Translation. Correspondence, *Fieldsights,* July 11. Society for Cultural Anthropology. https://culanth.org/fieldsights/teaching-race-translation.
2017 *Is Science Racist?* Malden, MA: Polity Press.

Marks, R.
2020 *The Origins of the Modern World: A Global and Environmental Narrative from the Fifteenth to the Twenty-First Century,* 4th ed. Lanham, MD: Rowman & Littlefield.

Marshall, A.
2020 This Art Was Looted 123 Years Ago. Will It Ever Be Returned? *The New York Times,* January 26. https://www.nytimes.com/2020/01/23/arts/design/benin-bronzes.html.

Martin, D.
1990 *Tongues of Fire: The Explosion of Protestantism in Latin America.* Cambridge, MA: Blackwell.

Martin, K., and B. Voorhies
1975 *Female of the Species.* New York: Columbia University Press.

Martin, S. M.
1988 *Palm Oil and Protest: An Economic History of the Ngwa Region, South-Eastern Nigeria, 1800–1980.* New York: Cambridge University Press.

Marx, K., and F. Engels
1976 (orig. 1848) *Communist Manifesto.* New York: Pantheon.

Mathur, H. M.
2019 *Development Anthropology: Putting Culture First.* Lanham, MD: Lexington Books.

Matias, D.
2019 New Report Says Women Will Soon Be Majority of College-Educated U.S. Workers. NPR, June 20. https://www.npr.org/2019/06/20/734408574/new-report-says-college-educated-women-will-soon-make-up-majority-of-u-s-labor-f.

Matsumoto, D. R., and L. Juang
2019 *Culture and Psychology.* 2nd ed. New York: Oxford University Press.

Maugh, T. H., III
2007 One Language Disappears Every 14 Days; about Half of the World's Distinct Tongues Could Vanish This Century, Researchers Say. *Los Angeles Times,* September 19.

Maybury-Lewis, D.
2002 *Indigenous Peoples, Ethnic Groups, and the State,* 2nd ed. Boston: Allyn & Bacon.

Maybury-Lewis, D., T. Macdonald, and B. Maybury-Lewis, eds.
2009 *Manifest Destinies and Indigenous Peoples.* Cambridge, MA: David Rockefeller Center for Latin American Studies and Harvard University Press.

Mba, N. E.
1982 *Nigerian Women Mobilized: Women's Political Activity in Southern Nigeria, 1900–1965.* Berkeley: University of California Press.

McAllester, D. P.
1954 *Enemy Way Music: A Study of Social and Esthetic Values as Seen in Navaho Music.* Cambridge, MA: Peabody Museum of American Archaeology and Ethnology, Papers 41(3).

McCabe, M., ed.
2017 *Collaborative Ethnography in Business Environments.* New York: Routledge, Taylor & Francis.

McConnell-Ginet, S.
2020 Words Matter: Meaning and Power. New York: Cambridge University Press.

McConvell, P., I. Keen, and R. Hendery, eds.
2013 *Kinship Systems: Change and Reconstruction.* Salt Lake City: University of Utah Press.

McElroy, A., and P. K. Townsend
2014 *Medical Anthropology in Ecological Perspective,* 6th ed. Boulder, CO: Westview Press.

McGee, R. J., and R. L. Warms
2017 *Anthropological Theory: An Introductory History,* 6th ed. Lanham, MD: Rowman & Littlefield.

McGregor, W.
2015 *Linguistics: An Introduction.* New York: Bloomsbury Academic.

McLaughlin, E. C.
2016 5 Things to Know about Flint's Water Crisis. CNN, January 21. http://www.cnn.com/2016/01/18/us/flint-michigan-water-crisis-five-things/.

McManamon, F. P., ed.
2017 *Perspectives in Cultural Resource Management.* New York: Routledge.

McNeil, D. G., Jr..
2019 Scientists Were Hunting for the Next Ebola. Now the U.S. Has Cut Off Their Funding. *The New York Times,* October 25. https://www.nytimes.com/2019/10/25/health/predict-usaid-viruses.html.

McWhorter, J. H.
2014 *The Language Hoax: Why the World Looks the Same in Any Language.* New York: Oxford University Press.
2017 *Talking Back, Talking Black: Truths about America's Lingua Franca.* New York: Bellevue Library Press.
2018 The Unmonitored President. Trump Is the First President Who, Rather Than Striding Forward and Speaking, Just Gets Up and Talks. *The Atlantic,* July 20. https://www.theatlantic.com/ideas/archive/2018/07/trump-speech/565646/.

Mead, M.
1937 *Cooperation and Competition among Primitive Peoples.* New York: McGraw-Hill.
1950 (orig. 1935) *Sex and Temperament in Three Primitive Societies.* New York: New American Library.

1961   (orig. 1928) *Coming of Age in Samoa.* New York: Morrow Quill.

1977   Applied Anthropology: The State of the Art. In *Perspectives on Anthropology, 1976.* Washington, DC: American Anthropological Association.

Meigs, A., and K. Barlow

2002   Beyond the Taboo: Imagining Incest. *American Anthropologist* 104(1): 38–49.

Meneley, A.

2018   Consumption. *AnnualReviewof Anthropology* 47: 117–132.

Menzies, C. R., ed.

2006   *Traditional Ecological Knowledge and Natural Resource Management.* Lincoln: University of Nebraska Press.

Merriam-Webster

2016   Art (definition of). *Merriam-Webster's Collegiate Dictionary,* 11th Edition (www.Merriam-Webster.com).

Methenitis, D.

2019   *Globalization, Modernity, and the Rise of Religious Fundamentalism: The Challenge of Religious Resurgence against the End of History (Deus Ex Machina).* New York: Routledge.

Meyer, B.

1999   *Translating the Devil: Religion and Modernity among the Ewe in Ghana.* Trenton, NJ: Africa World Press.

Meyerhoff, M.

2019   *Introducing Sociolinguistics,* 3rd ed. New York: Routledge/Taylor & Francis.

Miller, B. D.

1997   *The Endangered Sex: Neglect of Female Children in Rural North India.* New York: Oxford University Press.

Mintz, S. W.

1985   *Sweetness and Power: The Place of Sugar in Modern History.* New York: Viking Penguin.

2007   *Caribbean Transformations.* New Brunswick, NJ: Aldine Transaction.

Moberg, M.

2019   *Engaging Anthropological Theory: A Social and Political History,* 2nd ed. New York: Routledge.

Mohai, P., and R. Saha

2015   Which Came First, People or Pollution? Assessing the Disparate Siting and Post-Siting Demographic Change Hypotheses of Environmental Injustice. *Environmental Research Letters* 10: 1–17. http://iopscience.iop.org/article/10.1088/1748-9326/10/11/115008/pdf.

Montague, S., and R. Morais

1981   Football Games and Rock Concerts: The Ritual Enactment. In *The American Dimension: Cultural Myths and Social Realities,* 2nd ed., W. Arens and S. B. Montague, eds., pp. 33–52. Sherman Oaks, CA: Alfred.

Mooney, A., and B. Evans, eds.

2019   *Language Society and Power: An Introduction,* 5th ed.New York: Routledge.

Moore, J. D.

2019   *Visions of Culture: An Introduction to Anthropological Theories and Theorists,* 5th ed. Lanham, MD: AltaMira.

Morency, J-D., E. C. Malenfant, and S. MacIsaac.Morency, J-D., E. C. Malenfant, and S. MacIsaac.

2017   Immigration and Diversity: Population Projections for Canada and its Regions, 2011 to 2036. Statistics Canada, January 25. https://www150.statcan.gc.ca/n1/pub/91-551-x/91-551-x2017001-eng.htm.

Morgan, L. H.

1963   (orig. 1877) *Ancient Society.* Cleveland, OH: World Publishing.

1966   (orig. 1851) *League of the Ho-dé-no-sau-nee or Iroquois.* New York: B. Franklin.

Morin, R.

2013   The Most (and Least) Culturally Diverse Countries in the World. Pew Research Center, July 18. http://www.pewresearch.org/fact-tank/2013/07/18/the-most-and-least-culturally-diverse-countries-in-the-world/.

Mosse, D., ed.

2011   *Adventures in Aidland: The Anthropology of Professionals in International Development.* New York: Berghahn Books.

Motseta, S.

2006   Botswana Gives Bushmen Tough Conditions. *Washington Post,* December 14. http://www.washingtonpost.com/wp-dyn/content/article/2006/12/14/AR2006121401008.html.

Mukhopadhyay, C. C., R. Henze, and Y. T. Moses

2014   *How Real Is Race? A Sourcebook on Race, Culture, and Biology,* 2nd ed. Lanham, MD: AltaMira.

Mullaney, T.

2011   *Coming to Terms with the Nation: Ethnic Classification in Modern China.* Berkeley: University of California Press.

Murchison, J. M.

2010   *Ethnography Essentials: Designing, Conducting, and Presenting Your Research.* San Francisco: Jossey Bass.

Murdock, G. P., and C. Provost

1973   Factors in the Division of Labor by Sex: A Cross-Cultural Analysis. *Ethnology* 12(2): 203–225.

Murray, S.O., and W. Roscoe, eds.

1998   *Boy-Wives and Female Husbands: Studies in African Homosexualities.* New York: St. Martin's Press.

Myers, S. L.

2020   China's Markets Are in the Eye of a Lethal Outbreak Once Again. New York Times. January 25. https://www.nytimes.com/2020/01/25/world/asia/china-markets-coronavirus-sars.html2020.

Myers-Moro, P. A., and J. E. Myers

2012   *Magic, Witchcraft, and Religion: A Reader in the Anthropology of Religion,* 9th ed. New York: McGraw-Hill.

Nahm, S., and C. Hughes Rinker, eds.

2016   *Applied Anthropology: Unexpected Spaces, Topics, and Methods.* New York: Routledge.

Nanda, S.

1996   Hijras: An Alternative Sex and Gender Role in India. In *Third Sex Third Gender: Beyond Sexual Dimorphism in Culture and History,* G. Herdt, ed., pp. 373–418. New York: Zone Books.

1998   *Neither Man nor Woman: The Hijras of India.* Belmont, CA: Thomson/Wadsworth.

2014   *Gender Diversity: Crosscultural Variations,* 2nd ed. Long Grove, IL: Waveland.

Naples, N. A., ed.

2020   *The Wiley Blackwell Companion to Sexuality Studies.* Hoboken, NJ: Wiley.

Narayan, K.

2016   *Everyday Creativity: Singing Goddesses in the Himalayan Foothills.* Chicago: University of Chicago Press.

Nardi, B. A.

2010   *My Life as an Elf Priest: An Anthropological Account of World of Warcraft.* Ann Arbor: University of Michigan Press.

Nayar, P. K., ed.

2016   *Postcolonial Studies: An Anthology.* Malden, MA: Wiley.

Nicholas, G.

2018 Protecting Heritage Is a Human Right. *The Conversation,* September 9. https://theconversation.com/protecting-heritage-is-a-human-right-99501.

Nolan, R.

2017 *Using Anthropology in the World: A Guide to Becoming an Anthropological Practitioner.* New York: Routledge.

Nonini, D. M. ed.

2014 *A Companion to Urban Anthropology.* Malden, MA: Wiley-Blackwell.

Nonini, D. M. and I. Susser

2020 *The Tumultuous Politics of Scale: Unsettled States, Migrants, Movements in Flux.* New York: Routledge.

Northwestern University in Qatar

2017 Overview: Media Use in the Middle East, 2017. http://mideastmedia.org/survey/2017/overview/.

Nunn, N., and N. Qian

2010 The Columbian Exchange: A History of Disease, Food, and Ideas. *Journal of Economic Perspectives* 24(2): 163–188.

O'Brien, J., et al., eds.

2021 *Sport, Globalisation and Identity: New Perspectives on Regions and Nations .* New York: Routledge.

Ochs, E. and T. Kremer-Sadlik, eds.

2013 *Fast-forward Family: Home, Work, and Relationships in Middle-Class America.* Berkeley: University of California Press.

O'Connor, K.

2015 *The Never-Ending Feast: The Anthropology and Archaeology of Feasting.* New York: Bloomsbury Academic.

Omohundro, J. T.

2001 *Careers in Anthropology,* 2nd ed. New York: McGraw-Hill.

O'Neil, P. H.

2018 *Essentials of Comparative Politics.* New York: W. W. Norton.

Ong, A.

1987 *Spirits of Resistance and Capitalist Discipline: Factory Women in Malaysia.* Albany: State University of New York Press.

1989 Center, Periphery, and Hierarchy: Gender in Southeast Asia. In *Gender and Anthropology: Critical Reviews for Research and Teaching,* S. Morgen, ed., pp. 294–312. Washington, DC: American Anthropological Association.

2010 *Spirits of Resistance and Capitalist Discipline: Factory Women in Malaysia,* 2nd ed. Albany: State University of New York Press.

Ontario Consultants on Religious Tolerance

2011 Religions of the World: Number of Adherents of Major Religions, Their Geographical Distribution, Date Founded, and Sacred Texts. http://www.religioustolerance.org/worldrel.htm.

Oriji, J. N.

2000 Igbo Women from 1929–1960. *West Africa Review* 2: 1.

Ortner, S. B.

1984 Theory in Anthropology since the Sixties. *Comparative Studies in Society and History* 126(1): 126–166.

Osborne, R., and J. Tanner, eds.

2007 *Art's Agency and Art History.* Malden, MA: Blackwell.

Pace, R., and B. P. Hinote

2013 *Amazon Town TV: An Audience Ethnography in Gurupá, Brazil.* Austin: University of Texas Press.

Pace, R., ed.

2018 *From Filmmaker Warriors to Flash Drive Shamans: Indigenous Media Production and Engagement in Latin America.* Nashville: Vanderbilt University Press.

Pagden, A.

2015 *The Burdens of Empire: 1539 to the Present.* New York: Cambridge University Press.

Paine, R.

2009 *Camps of the Tundra: Politics through Reindeer among Saami Pastoralists.* Oslo: Instituttet for sammenlignende kulturforskning.

Parker, K., and G. Livingston

2017 6 Facts about American Fathers. FactTank. Pew Research Center. http://www.pewresearch.org/fact-tank/2017/06/15/fathers-day-facts/

Parrillo, V. N.

2016 *Understanding Race and Ethnic Relations,* 5th ed. Boston: Pearson.

2019 *Strangers to These Shores: Race and Ethnic Relations in the United States,* 12th ed. New York: Pearson.

Patterson, F.

1978 Conversations with a Gorilla. *National Geographic,* October, pp. 438–465.

1999 *Koko-love! Conversations with a Signing Gorilla.* New York: Dutton.

Paul, R.

1989 Psychoanalytic Anthropology. *Annual Review of Anthropology* 18: 177–202.

Payne, K.

2018 *Anthropology of Religion.* Valley Cottage, NY: Socialy Press.

Pearce, C.

2009 *Communities of Play: Emergent Cultures in Multiplayer Games and Virtual Worlds.* Cambridge, MA: MIT Press.

Peletz, M.

1988 *A Share of the Harvest: Kinship, Property, and Social History among the Malays of Rembau.* Berkeley: University of California Press.

2009 *Gender Pluralism; Southeast Asia since Early Modern Times.* New York: Routledge.

Pelto, P. J.

2013 *Applied Ethnography: Guidelines for Field Research.* Walnut Creek, CA: Left Coast Press.

Perrin, A., and Anderson, M.

2019 Share of U.S. Adults Using Social Media, Including Facebook Is Mostly Unchanged since 2018. Pew Research Center, April 10. https://www.pewresearch.org/fact-tank/2019/04/10/share-of-u-s-adults-using-social-media-including-facebook-is-mostly-unchanged-since-2018/

Pertierra, A. C.

2018 *Media Anthropology for the Digital Age.* Malden, MA: Polity Press.

Petraglia-Bahri, D.

1996 Introduction to Postcolonial Studies. http://www.emory.edu/ENGLISH/Bahri/.

Pew Research Center

2011 The Pew Forum on Religion and Public Life. http://www.pewforum.org/uploadedFiles/Topics/Religious_Affiliation/Christian/Evangelical_Protestant_Churches/Global%20Survey %20of%20Evan.%20Prot.%20Leaders.pdf.

2015a America's Changing Religious Landscape. Pew Research Center: Religion & Public Life, May 12. http://www.pewforum.org/2015/05/12/americas-changing-religious-landscape/.

2015b The Changing Global Religious Landscape. Demographic Study, April 5. http://www.pewforum.org/

2017/04/05/the-changing-global-religious-landscape/#global-population-projections-2015-to-2060.

2015c The Future of World Religions: Population Growth Projections, 2010-2050. Pew Research Center: Religion & Public Life, April 2. http://www.pewforum.org/files/2015/03/PF_15.04.02_ProjectionsFullReport.pdf.

2017a The Changing Global Religious Landscape. April 5. https://www.pewforum.org/2017/04/05/the-changing-global-religious-landscape/

2017b Four-in-Ten Countries Have Official State Religions or Preferred Religions. October 3. http://www.pewforum.org/2017/10/03/many-countries-favor-specific-religions-officially-or-unofficially/pf_10-04-17_statereligions-00/.

2019 In U.S., Decline of Christianity Continues at Rapid Pace. October 17. https://www.pewforum.org/2019/10/17/in-u-s-decline-of-christianity-continues-at-rapid-pace/.

Piddocke, S.
1969 The Potlatch System of the Southern Kwakiutl: A New Perspective. In Environment and Cultural Behavior, A. P. Vayda, ed., pp. 130–156. Garden City, NY: Natural History Press.

Piemmons, D., and A. W. Barker, eds.
2015 Anthropological Ethics in Context: An Ongoing Dialogue. Walnut Creek, CA: Left Coast Press.

Piketty, T.
2020 Capital and Ideology, translated by A. Goldhammer. Cambridge, MA: Harvard University Press.

Pink, S., and S. Abram
2015 Media, Anthropology and Public Engagement. New York: Berghahn Books.

Pink, S., V. Fors, and T. O'Dell, eds.
2017 Theoretical Scholarship and Applied Practice. New York: Berghahn Books.

Pipatti, O.
2019 Morality Made Visible: Edward Westermarck's Moral and Social Theory. New York: Routledge.

Pirie, F.
2013 Anthropology of Law. Oxford, UK: Oxford University Press.

Plessner, H.
2018 Political Anthropology, translated from the German by N. F. Schott. Evanston, IL: Northwestern University Press.

Podolefsky, A., and P. J. Brown, eds.
1992 Applying Anthropology: An Introductory Reader, 2nd ed. Mountain View, CA: Mayfield.

Polanyi, K.
1968 Primitive, Archaic and Modern Economies: Essays of Karl Polanyi. G. Dalton, ed. Garden City, NY: Anchor Books.

Pospisil, L.
1978 The Kapauku Papuans of West New Guinea, 2nd ed. New York: Holt, Rinehart, and Winston.

Potash, B., ed.
1986 Widows in African Societies: Choices and Constraints. Stanford, CA: Stanford University Press.

Prasad, I.
2016 Teaching Race: Deviation. Correspondence, Fieldsights, July 11. Society for Cultural Anthropology. https://culanth.org/fieldsights/teaching-race-deviation.

Price, D.
2000 Anthropologists as Spies. Nation, November 20, 24–27.

Price, R., ed.
1973 Maroon Societies. New York: Anchor Press, Doubleday.

Qian, Z.
2013 Divergent Paths of American Families. September 11. Brown University, US2010. http://www.s4.brown.edu/us2010/Data/Report/report09112013.pdf.

Qian, Z., and S. Huo, eds.
2018 Political Anthropology. Valley Cottage, NY: Socialy Press.

Radcliffe-Brown, A. R.
1952 (orig. 1924) The Mother's Brother in South Africa. In A. R. Radcliffe-Brown, Structure and Function in Primitive Society, pp. 15–31. London: Routledge & Kegan Paul.
1965 (orig. 1962) Structure and Function in Primitive Society. New York: Free Press.

Radin, J.
2018 Ethics in Human Biology: A Historical Perspective on Contemporary Challenges. Annual Review of Anthropology 47: 263-278.

Ramos, A. R.
1995 Sanumá Memories : Yanomami Ethnography in Times of Crisis. Madison: University of Wisconsin Press.

Random House College Dictionary
1982 Art (definition of). New York, Random House.

Ranger, T.O.
1996 Postscript. In Postcolonial Identities, R. Werbner and T. O. Ranger, eds. London: Zed.

Ransby, B.
2017 Black Lives Matter Is Democracy in Action. New York Times, October 21. https://www.nytimes.com/2017/10/21/opinion/sunday/black-lives-matter-leadership.html.

Rapoza, K.
2012 Disturbing Trend for Putin, Russian Poverty Rising. Forbes, April 12. http://www.forbes.com/sites/kenrapoza/2012/04/12/disturbing-trend-for-putin-russian-poverty-rising/.

Rappaport, R. A.
1974 Obvious Aspects of Ritual. Cambridge Anthropology 2: 2–60.
1999 Holiness and Humanity: Ritual in the Making of Religious Life. New York: Cambridge University Press.

Rathje, W. L., and C. Murphy
2001 Rubbish!: The Archaeology of Garbage. Tucson: University of Arizona Press.

Rathus, S. A., J. S. Nevid, and J. Fichner-Rathus
2018 Human Sexuality in a Changing World. Hoboken, NJ: Pearson Higher Education.

Reagan, T.
2018 Non-Western Educational Traditions: Local Approaches to Thought and Practice, 4th ed. New York: Routledge.

Reardon, S.
2015 Psychologists Seek Roots of Terror: Studies Raise Prospect of Intervention in the Radicalization Process. Nature 517 (421). http://www.nature.com/polopoly_fs/1.16756!/menu/main/topColumns/topLeft-Column/pdf/517420a.pdf.

Redfield, R., R. Linton, and M. Herskovits
1936 Memorandum on the Study of Acculturation. American Anthropologist 38: 149–152.

Reich, D, Reiter, R., ed.
1975 Toward an Anthropology of Women. New York: Monthly Review Press.

Renfrew, C.
1987 Archaeology and Language: The Puzzle of Indo-European Origin. London: Pimlico.

Reyburn, S.
2015 Chris Ofili's "The Holy Virgin Mary" to Be Sold. New York Times, May 28. http://www.nytimes.com/

2015/05/29/arts/design/chris-ofilis-the-holy-virgin-mary-to-be-sold.html?_r=0.

Reyhner, J., ed.
2015 *Teaching Indigenous Students: Honoring Place, Community, and Culture.* Norman: University of Oklahoma Press.

Rhodes, R. A. W., and P. `t Hart
2014 *The Oxford Handbook of Political Leadership.* Oxford, UK: Oxford University Press.

Riach, J.
2013 Golf's Failure to Embrace Demographics across Society Is Hard to Stomach. *The Guardian,* May 22. http://www.theguardian.com/sport/blog/2013/may/22/uk-golf-clubs-race-issues.

Rice, T.
2014 *Ethnomusicology: A Very Short Introduction.* New York: Oxford University Press.

Rich, M.
2018 In U.S. Open Victory, Naomi Osaka Pushes Japan to Redefine Japanese. New York Times, September 9. https://www.nytimes.com/2018/09/09/world/asia/japan-naomi-osaka-us-open.html.

Rickford, J. R.
1997 Suite for Ebony and Phonics. http://www.stanford.edu/~rickford/papers/SuiteForEbonyandPhonics.html (also published in *Discover,* December 1997).
2019 *Variation, Versatility, and Change in Linguistics and Creole Studies.* New York: Cambridge University Press.

Rickford, J. R., and R. J. Rickford
2000 *Spoken Soul: The Story of Black English.* New York: Wiley.

Risman, B. J.
2018 *Where the Millennials Will Take Us: A New Generation Wrestles with the Gender Structure.* New York: Oxford University Press.

Robbins, Jim
2012 The Ecology of Disease. *New York Times,* July 14. https://www.nytimes.com/2012/07/15/sunday-review/the-ecology-of-disease.html.

Robbins, Joel
2004 The Globalization of Pentecostal and Charismatic Christianity. *Annual Review of Anthropology* 33: 17–143.

Robbins, R.
2014 *Global Problems and the Culture of Capitalism,* 6th ed. Boston: Pearson.

Robertson, J.
1992 Koreans in Japan. Paper presented at the University of Michigan Department of Anthropology, Martin Luther King Jr. Day Panel, January. Ann Arbor: University of Michigan Department of Anthropology (unpublished).

Robson, D.
2013 There Really Are 50 Eskimo Words for Snow. *Washington Post,* January 14. http://articles.washingtonpost.com/2013-01-14/national/36344037_1_eskimo-words-snow-inuit.

Rommen, T. et al.
2020 *Critical Themes in World Music: A Reader for Excursions in World Music,* 8th. ed. New York: Routledge.

Root, D.
1996 *Cannibal Culture: Art, Appropriation, and the Commodification of Difference.* Boulder, CO: Westview Press.

Roothaan, A.
2019 *Indigenous, Modern and Postcolonial Relations to Nature: Negotiating the Environment.* New York: Routledge/Taylor & Francis Group.

Roque, R., and K. A. Wagner, eds.
2011 *Engaging Colonial Knowledge: Reading European Archives in World History.* New York: Palgrave Macmillan.

Rosaldo, M. Z.
1980a *Knowledge and Passion: Notions of Self and Social Life.* Stanford, CA: Stanford University Press.
1980b The Use and Abuse of Anthropology: Reflections on Feminism and Cross-Cultural Understanding. *Signs* 5(3): 389–417.

Roscoe, W.
1991 *Zuni Man-Woman.* Albuquerque: University of New Mexico Press.
1998 *Changing Ones: Third and Fourth Genders in Native North America.* New York: St. Martin's Press.

Rothstein, E.
2006 Protection for Indian Patrimony That Leads to a Paradox. *The New York Times,* March 29.

Royal Anthropological Institute of Great Britain and Ireland
1951 *Notes and Queries on Anthropology,* 6th ed. London: Routledge and K. Paul.

Ruhlen, M.
1994 *The Origin of Language: Tracing the Evolution of the Mother Tongue.* New York: Wiley.

Ryan, S.
1990 *Ethnic Conflict and International Relations.* Brookfield, MA: Dartmouth.

Ryang, S., and J. Lie
2009 *Diaspora without Homeland: Being Korean in Japan.* Berkeley: University of California Press.

Rylko-Bauer, B., M. Singer, and J. Van Willigen
2006 Reclaiming Applied Anthropology: Its Past, Present, and Future. *American Anthropologist* 108(1): 178–190.

Saenz, R.
2020 Children of Color Projected to Be Majority of U.S. Youth This Year. January 9. PBS News Hour. https://www.pbs.org/newshour/nation/children-of-color-projected-to-be-majority-of-u-s-youth-this-year.

Sahlins, M. D.
1968 *Tribesmen.* Englewood Cliffs, NJ: Prentice Hall.
2013 *What Kinship Is—And Is Not.* Chicago: University of Chicago Press.
2017 (orig. 1972) *Stone Age Economics.* New York: Routledge Classics.

Salazar, C., and J. Bestard, eds.
2015 *Religion and Science as Forms of Life: Anthropological Insights into Reason and Unreason.* New York: Berghahn Books.

Salzman, P. C.
1974 Political Organization among Nomadic Peoples. In *Man in Adaptation: The Cultural Present,* 2nd ed., Y. A. Cohen, ed., pp. 267–284. Chicago: Aldine.
2004 *Pastoralists: Equality, Hierarchy, and the State.* Boulder, CO: Westview Press.
2008 *Culture and Conflict in the Middle East.* Amherst, NY: Humanity Books.
2012 *Classic Comparative Anthropology: Studies from the Tradition.* Long Grove, IL: Waveland.

Salzmann, Z.
2012 *Linguistic Anthropology: A Short Introduction.* Prague, Czech Republic: Nezavisle centrum pro studium politiky.

Salzmann, Z., J. Stanlaw, and N. Adachi
2015 *Language, Culture, and Society: An Introduction to Linguistic Anthropology,* 6th ed. Boulder, CO: Westview.

Samuels, D. J.
2021 *Comparative Politics,* 2nd ed. Hoboken, NJ: Pearson.

Sanday, P. R.

1974 Female Status in the Public Domain. In *Woman, Culture, and Society,* M. Z. Rosaldo and L. Lamphere, eds., pp. 189–206. Stanford, CA: Stanford University Press.

2002 *Women at the Center: Life in a Modern Matriarchy.* Ithaca, NY: Cornell University Press.

2003 Public Interest Anthropology: A Model for Engaged Social Science. http://www.sas.upenn.edu/anthro/CPIA/PAPERS/SARdiscussion%20paper.65.html.

Sanjek, R.

2004 Going Public: Responsibilities and Strategies in the Aftermath of Ethnography. *Human Organization* 63(4): 444–456.

2014 *Ethnography in Today's World: Color Full before Color Blind.* Philadelphia: University of Pennsylvania Press.

Sanjek, R., and S. W. Tratner, eds.

2016 *eFieldnotes: The Makings of Anthropology in the Digital World.* Philadelphia: University of Pennsylvania Press.

Sansi-Roca, R.

2015 *Art, Anthropology and the Gift.* New York: Bloomsbury Academic.

Sapir, E.

1931 Conceptual Categories in Primitive Languages. *Science* 74: 578–584.

1956 (orig. 1928) The Meaning of Religion. In E. Sapir, *Culture, Language and Personality: Selected Essays.* Berkeley: University of California Press.

Schaefer, R.

2013 *Race and Ethnicity in the United States,* 7th ed. Upper Saddle River, NJ: Prentice Hall.

Schaeffer, K.

2019 The Most Common Age among Whites in the U.S. is 58–More than Double that of Racial and Ethnic Minorities. July 30. Pew Research Center. https://www.pewresearch.org/fact-tank/2019/07/30/most-common-age-among-us-racial-ethnic-groups/.

Scheidel, W.

1997 Brother-Sister Marriage in Roman Egypt. *Journal of Biosocial Science* 29(3): 361–371.

Schneider, A.

2017 *Alternative Art and Anthropology: Global Encounters.* New York: Bloomsbury Academic.

Schneider, A., and C. Pasqualino, eds.

2014 *Experimental Film and Anthropology.* New York: Bloomsbury Academic.

Schneider, A., and C. Wright, eds.

2013 *Anthropology and Art Practice.* New York: Bloomsbury Academic.

Schneider, D. M., and K. Gough

1961 *Matrilineal Kinship.* Berkeley: University of California Press.

Schumacher, S., and N. Kent

2020 8 Charts on Internet Use around the World as Countries Grapple with COVID-19. April 2. Pew Research Center. Https://www.pewresearch.org/fact-tank/2020/04/02/8-charts-on-internet-use-around-the-world-as-countries-grapple-with-covid-19/.

Schwanhäusser, A., ed.

2016 *Sensing the City: A Companion to Urban Anthropology.* Gütersloh: Bauverlag.

Schwartz, M. J., V. W. Turner, and A. Tuden, eds.

2011 *Political Anthropology.* New Brunswick, NJ: Aldine Transaction.

Scott, J. C.

1985 *Weapons of the Weak.* New Haven, CT: Yale University Press.

1990 *Domination and the Arts of Resistance.* New Haven, CT: Yale University Press.

2009 *The Art of Not Being Governed: An Anarchist History of Upland Southeast Asia.* New Haven, CT: Yale University Press.

2017 *Against the Grain: A Deep History of the Earliest States.* New Haven, CT: Yale University Press.

Scott, S., and C. Duncan

2004 *Return of the Black Death: The World's Greatest Serial Killer.* Hoboken, NJ: Wiley.

Scudder, T., and E. Colson

1980 *Secondary Education and the Formation of an Elite: The Impact of Education on Gwembe District, Zambia.* London: Academic Press.

Scupin, R.

2012 *Race and Ethnicity: The United States and the World,* 2nd ed. Upper Saddle River, NJ: Prentice Hall.

Sèbe, B., and M. G. Stanard, eds.

2020 *Decolonising Europe?: Popular Responses to the End of Empire.* New York: Routledge. Sebeok,T. A., and J. Umiker-Sebeok, eds.

1980 *Speaking of Apes: A Critical Anthropology of Two-Way Communication with Man.* New York: Plenum Press.

Semega, J. L., K. R. Fontenot, and M. A. Kollar

2019 *Income and Poverty in the United States: 2018.* U.S. Census Bureau, Current Population Reports, P60-266. Washington, DC: U.S. Government Printing Office. https://www.census.gov/content/dam/Census/library/publications/2019/demo/p60-266.pdf.

Service, E. R.

1962 *Primitive Social Organization: An Evolutionary Perspective.* New York: McGraw-Hill.

1966 *The Hunters.* Englewood Cliffs, NJ: Prentice Hall.

Shaffer, L.

2019 Is a More Generous Society Possible? *Scientific American.* February 23. https://www.scientificamerican.com/article/is-a-more-generous-society-possible/.

Shannon, T. R.

1996 *An Introduction to the World-System Perspective,* 2nd ed. Boulder, CO: Westview Press.

Shapiro, W.

2009 *Partible Paternity and Anthropological Theory: The Construction of an Ethnographic Fantasy.* Lanham, MD: University Press of America.

Sharma, A., and A. Gupta, eds.

2006 *The Anthropology of the State: A Reader.* Malden, MA: Blackwell.

Sharpley, R., and D. J. Teller, eds.

2015 *Tourism and Development; Concepts and Issues.* Buffalo, NY: Channel View Publications.

Shih, C.-K.

2010 *Quest for Harmony: The Moso Traditions of Sexual Union and Family Life.* Stanford, CA: Stanford University Press.

Shivaram, C.

1996 Where Women Wore the Crown: Kerala's Dissolving Matriarchies Leave a Rich Legacy of Compassionate Family Culture. *Hinduism Today* 96(2). http://www.hinduism-today.com/archives/1996/2/1996-2-03.shtml.

Shore, C., S. Wright, and D. Però, eds.

2011 *Policy Worlds: Anthropology and the Analysis of Contemporary Power.* New York: Berghahn Books.

Shryock, A.

1988 Autonomy, Entanglement, and the Feud: Prestige Structures and Gender Values in Highland Albania. *Anthropological Quarterly* 61(3): 113–118.

Sidky, H.
2015 *Religion: An Anthropological Perspective.* New York: Peter Lang Publishing.

Siegel, R.
2020 Women Outnumber Men in the American Workforce for Only the Second Time. *Washington Post,* January 10. https://www.washingtonpost.com/business/2020/01/10/january-2020-jobs-report/.

Simpson, A.
2019 *Language and Society: An Introduction.* New York: Oxford University Press.

Simpson, P., A. Mayer, and S. Statham
2019 *Language and Power: A Resource Book for Students,* 2nd ed. New York: Routledge.

Sims, C.
2016 Academics in Foxholes: The Life and Death of the Human Terrain System. *Foreign Affairs,* February 4. https://www.foreignaffairs.com/articles/afghanistan/2016-02-04/academics-foxholes.

Singer, M.
2015 *The Anthropology of Infectious Disease.* Walnut Creek, CA: Left Coast Press.
2019 *Climate Change and Social Inequality: The Health and Social Costs of Global Warming.* New York: Routledge/Taylor & Francis Group.

Singer, M., H. Baer, D. Long, and A. Pavlotski
2020 *Introducing Medical Anthropology: A Discipline in Action,* 3rd ed. Lanham, MD: Rowman & Littlefield.

Slaughter, A-M.
2013 Women Are Sexist, Too: If Women Are Equal at the Office, Why Can't Men Be Equal at Home? http://time.com/women-are-sexist-too/.
2015 *Unfinished Business: Men, Women, Work, Family.* New York: Random House.

Smitherman, G.
1986 *Talkin and Testifyin: The Language of Black America.* Detroit: Wayne State University Press.

Snowden, F. M., Jr.
1970 *Blacks in Antiquity: Ethiopians in the Greco-Roman Experience.* Cambridge, MA: Belknap Press of Harvard University Press.
1995 Europe's Oldest Chapter in the History of Black White Relations. *In Racism and Anti-Racism in World Perspective,* B. P. Bowser, ed., pp. 3–26. Thousand Oaks, CA: Sage.

Solway, J., and R. Lee
1990 Foragers, Genuine and Spurious: Situating the Kalahari San in History (with CA treatment). *Current Anthropology* 31(2): 109–146.

Sotomayor, S.
2009 (orig. 2001) A Latina Judge's Voice. The Judge Mario G. Olmos Memorial Lecture, delivered at the University of California, Berkeley, School of Law in 2001; published in the spring 2002 issue of the *Berkeley La Raza Law Journal,* republished by *The New York Times* on May 14, 2009.

Spickard, P., ed.
2013 *Multiple Identities: Migrants, Ethnicity, and Membership.* Bloomington: Indiana University Press.

Spooner, B., ed.
2015 *Globalization: The Crucial Phase.* Philadelphia: University of Pennsylvania Museum of Archaeology and Anthropology.

Srivastava, J., N. J. H. Smith, and D. A. Forno
1999 *Integrating Biodiversity in Agricultural Intensification: Toward Sound Practices.* Washington, DC: World Bank.

Stack, C. B.
1975 *All Our Kin: Strategies for Survival in a Black Community.* New York: Harper Torchbooks.

Starn, O.
2011 *The Passion of Tiger Woods: An Anthropologist Reports on Golf, Race, and Celebrity Scandal.* Durham, NC: Duke University Press.

Statistics Canada
2010 Study: Projections of the Diversity of the Canadian Population. http://www.statcan.gc.ca/daily-quotidien/100309/dq100309a-eng.htm.

Staudt, K. A.
2018 *Border Politics in the Global Era: Comparative Perspectives.* Lanham, MD: Rowman & Littlefield

Stearns, P. N.
2019 *Globalization in World History,* 3rd ed. New York: Routledge/Taylor & Francis.

Stein, R. L., and P. L. Stein, eds.
2017 *The Anthropology of Religion, Magic, and Witchcraft,* 4th ed. New York: Routledge.

Steward, J. H.
1955 *Theory of Culture Change.* Urbana: University of Illinois Press.
1956 *The People of Puerto Rico: A Study in Social Anthropology.* Urbana: University of Illinois Press.

Stimpson, C. R.,and G. H. Herdt, eds.
2014 *Critical Terms for the Study of Gender.* Chicago: University of Chicago Press.

Stoler, A.
1977 Class Structure and Female Autonomy in Rural Java. *Signs* 3: 74–89.
2002 *Carnal Knowledge and Imperial Power: Race and the Intimate in Colonial Rule.* Berkeley: University of California Press.
2009 *Along the Archival Grain: Epistemic Anxieties and Colonial Common Sense.* Princeton, NJ: Princeton University Press.
2013 *Imperial Debris: On Ruins and Ruination.* Durham: Duke University Press.

Stoler, A. L., C. McGranahan, and P. C. Perdue, eds.
2007 *Imperial Formations.* Santa Fe, NM: School for Advanced Research Press.

Stone, L., and D. E. King
2019 *Gender and Kinship: An Introduction,*6th ed. New York: Routledge.

Storey, R., and G. R. Storey
2017 *Rome and the Classic Maya: Comparing the Slow Collapse of Civilizations.* New York: Routledge/Taylor & Francis.

Streets-Salter, H., and T. Getz
2016 *Empires and Colonies in the Modern World: A Global Perspective.* New York: Oxford University Press.

Stryker, R., and R. J. Gonzalez, eds.
2014 *Up, Down, and Sideways: Anthropologists Trace the Pathways of Power.* New York: Berghahn Books.

Sullivan, M.
2012 Trouble in Paradise: UCLA Book Enumerates Challenges Faced by Middle-Class L.A. Families. UCLA Newsroom, June 19. http://newsroom.ucla.edu/portal/ucla/trouble-in-paradise-new-ucla-book.aspx.

Sunstein, B. S., and E. Chiseri-Strater
2012 *Fieldworking: Reading and Writing Research,* 4th ed. Boston: Bedford/St. Martin's.

Suttles, W.
1960 Affinal Ties, Subsistence, and Prestige among the Coast Salish. *American Anthropologist* 62: 296–395.

Svoboda, E.
   2017   Life and Death after the Steel Mills. *SAPIENS*,
   October 18. https://www.sapiens.org/culture/
   postindustrial-world-chicago-steel/.

Talbot, M. M.
   2019   *Language and Gender,* 3rd. ed. Malden, MA: Polity
   Press.

Tamai, L. A. Y. W., et al., eds.
   2019   *Shape-Shifters: Journeys across Terrains of Race and
   Identity.* Lincoln: University of Nebraska Press.

Tanaka, J.
   2014   *The Bushmen: A Half-Century Chronicle of
   Transformations in Hunter-Gatherer Life and Ecology.*
   Kyoto, Japan: Kyoto University Press.

Tannen, D.
   1990   *You Just Don't Understand: Women and Men in
   Conversation.* New York: Ballantine.
   2017   *You're the Only One I Can Tell Inside the Language
   of Women's Friendships.* New York: Ballantine.

Tannen, D., and A. M. Trester, eds.
   2013   *Discourse 2.0: Language and New Media.*
   Washington, DC: Georgetown University Press.

Tattersall, I., and R. De Salle
   2011   *Race? Debunking a Scientific Myth.* College Station:
   Texas A&M University Press.

Taylor, P., et al.
   2012   When Labels Don't Fit: Hispanics and Their
   Views of Identity. Pew Research Hispanic Center,
   April 4. http://www.pewhispanic.org/2012/04/04/
   when-labels-dont-fit-hispanics-and-their-views-of-identity.

Tehan, M.
   2017   *The Impact of Climate Change Mitigation on
   Indigenous and Forest Communities: International, National,
   and Local Law Perspectives on REDD+.* New York:
   Cambridge University Press.

Telegraph, The
   2005   Third Sex Finds a Place on Indian Passport
   Forms. *The Telegraph,* March 10. http://infochangeindia.
   org/humanrights/news/third-sex-finds-a-place-on-
   indianpassport-forms.html.

Terrace, H. S.
   1979   *Nim.* New York: Knopf.
   2019   *Why Chimpanzees Can't Learn Language and Only
   Humans Can.* New York: Columbia University Press.

Thomas, M., and A. Harris, eds.
   2018   *Expeditionary Anthropology: Teamwork, Travel, and
   'The Science of Man'.* New York: Berghahn.

Thompson, T., ed.
   2015   *Same-Sex Marriage.* Farmington Hills, MI:
   Greenhaven Press.

Titiev, M.
   1992   *Old Oraibi: A Study of the Hopi Indians of Third
   Mesa.* Albuquerque: University of New Mexico Press.

Toossi, M., and T. L. Morisi
   2017   Women in the Workforce before, during, and after
   the Great Recession. U.S. Bureau of Labor Statistics.
   https://www.bls.gov/spotlight/2017/women-in-the-
   workforce-before-during-and-after-the-great-recession/pdf/
   women-in-the-workforce-before-during-and-after-the-great-
   recession.pdf

Tougher, S.
   2008   *The Eunuch in Byzantine History and Society.* New
   York: Routledge.

Toyosaki, S., and S. Eguchi, eds.
   2017   *Intercultural Communication in Japan: Theorizing
   Homogenizing Discourse.* New York: Routledge.

Trehub, S. E.
   2001   Musical Predispositions in Infancy. *Annals of the
   New York Academy of Sciences* 930(1): 1–16.

Tremlett, P.-F., G. Harvey, and L. T. Sutherland, eds.
   2017   *Edward Burnett Tylor, Religion, and Culture.*
   New York: Bloomsbury Academic.

Trevathan, W., and K. R. Rosenberg, eds.
   2016   *Costly and Cute: Helpless Infants and Human
   Evolution.* Santa FE, NM: School for American Research
   Press.

Trivedi, B. P.
   2001   Scientists Identify a Language Gene.
   National Geographic News, October 4. http://news.
   nationalgeographic.com/news/2001/10/1004_
   TVlanguagegene.html.

Trosper, R. L.
   2009   *Resilience, Reciprocity and Ecological Economics:
   Northwest Coast Sustainability.* New York: Routledge.

Trouet, V.
   2020   *Tree Story: The History of the World Written in Trees.*
   Baltimore: Johns Hopkins University Press.

Trudgill, P.
   2010   *Investigations in Sociohistorical Linguistics: Stories
   of Colonisation and Contact.* New York: Cambridge
   University Press.

Turnbull, C.
   1965   *Wayward Servants: The Two Worlds of the African
   Pygmies.* Garden City, NY: Natural History Press.
   1972 *The Mountain People.* New York: Simon and
   Schuster.

Turner, V. W.
   1967   *The Forest of Symbols: Aspects of Ndembu Ritual.*
   Ithaca, NY: Cornell University Press.
   1995   (orig. 1969) *The Ritual Process.* Hawthorne, NY:
   Aldine.

Tusting, K. ed.
   2020   *Routledge Handbook of Linguistic Ethnography.*
   New York: Routledge.

Tylor, E. B.
   1889   On a Method of Investigating the Development
   of Institutions: Applied to Laws of Marriage and
   Descent. *Journal of the Royal Anthropological Institute* 18:
   245–269.
   1958   (orig. 1871) *Primitive Culture.* New York: Harper
   Torchbooks.

Underhill, P.
   2009   *Why We Buy? The Science of Shopping.* New York:
   Random House.

United Nations, Department of Economic and Social Affairs,
   Population Division
   2014. World Urbanization Prospects, The 2014 Revision.
   https://esa.un.org/unpd/wup/publications/files/wup2014-
   highlights.pdf.
   2018a   68% of the World Population Projected to Live in
   Urban Areas by 2050, Says UN.
   https://www.un.org/development/desa/en/news/
   population/2018-revision-of-world-urbanization-prospects.html
   2018b   The World's Cities in 2018—Data Booklet (ST/
   ESA/ SER.A/417). https://www.un.org/en/events/
   citiesday/assets/pdf/the_worlds_cities_in_2018_data_
   booklet.pdf.

U.S. Bureau of Labor Statistics
   2020 Union Members Summary. Economic News Release.
   January 22. https://www.bls.gov/news.release/union2.
   nr0.htm#:~:text=The%20number%20of%20wage%20
   and,were%2017.7%20million%20union%20workers.

Valentine, P., et al.
2017 *The Anthropology of Marriage in Lowland South America: Bending and Breaking the Rules.* Gainesville: University of Florida Press. Vallegia, C. R., and J. J. Snodgrass
2015 Health of Indigenous Peoples. *Annual Review of Anthropology* 44: 117–135.

Van Allen, J.
1971 *"Aba Riots" or "Women's War"?: British Ideology and Eastern Nigerian Women's Political Activism.* Waltham, MA: African Studies Association.

Van Cantfort, T. E., and J. B. Rimpau
1982 Sign Language Studies with Children and Chimpanzees. *Sign Language Studies* 34: 15–72.

Vannini, P.
2019 *Doing Public Anthropology: How to Create and Disseminate Ethnographic and Qualitative Research to Wide Audiences.* New York: Routledge.
2020 *The Routledge International Handbook of Ethnographic Film and Video.* New York: Routledge.

Vayda, A. P.
1968 (orig. 1961) Economic Systems in Ecological Perspective: The Case of the Northwest Coast. In *Readings in Anthropology,* 2nd ed., vol. 2, M. H. Fried, ed., pp. 172–178. New York: Crowell.

Veblen, T.
1934 *The Theory of the Leisure Class: An Economic Study of Institutions.* New York: The Modern Library.

Veja
1984a *Olimpíadas,* August 8, pp. 36–50.

Velupillai, V.
2015 *Pidgins, Creoles, and Mixed Languages: An Introduction.* Philadelphia: John Benjamins.

Ventkatesan, S., and T. Yarrow, eds.
2014 *Differentiating Development: Beyond an Anthropology of Critique.* New York: Berghahn Books.

Verdery, K.
2001 Socialist Societies: Anthropological Aspects. *International Encyclopedia of the Social & Behavioral Sciences,* pp. 14496–14500. New York: Elsevier.

Vespa, J., D. M. Armstrong, and L. Medina
2020 Demographic Turning Points for the United States: Population Projections for 2020 to 2060. February. U.S. Census Bureau, Current Population Reports, P25-1144. Washington, DC: U.S. Government Printing Office. https://www.census.gov/library/publications/2020/demo/p25-1144.html.

Vigil, J. D.
2010 *Gang Redux: A Balanced Anti-gang Strategy.* Long Grove, IL: Waveland.
2012 *From Indians to Chicanos: The Dynamics of Mexican-American Culture,* 3rd ed. Boulder, CO: Westview Press.

Vinyeta, K., and K. Lynn
2013 *Exploring the Role of Traditional Ecological Knowledge in Climate Change Initiatives.* Portland, OR: U.S. Department of Agriculture, Forest Service, Pacific Northwest Research Station.

Vivanco, L. A.
2017 *Field Notes: A Guided Journal for Doing Anthropology.* New York: Oxford University Press.

Vogels, E. A.
2020a 10 Facts about Americans and Online Dating. Pew Research Center, February 6.https://www.pewresearch.org/fact-tank/2020/02/06/10-facts-about-americans-and-online-dating/.
2020b About Half of Never-married Americans have Used an Online Dating Site or App. Pew Research Center, March 24. https://

www.pewresearch.org/fact-tank/2020/03/24/the-never-been-married-are-biggest-users-of-online-dating/.

Wade, B. C.
2013 *Thinking Musically: Experiencing Music, Expressing Culture,* 3rd ed. New York: Oxford University Press.
2020 *Global Music Cultures: An Introduction to World Music.* New York: Oxford University Press.

Wade, P.
2010 *Race and Ethnicity in Latin America,* 2nd ed. New York: Pluto Press.
2015 *Race: An Introduction.* New York: Cambridge University Press.
2017 *Degrees of Mixture, Degrees of Freedom: Genomics, Multiculturalism, and Race in Latin America.* Durham, NC: Duke University Press.

Wallace, A. F. C.
1966 *Religion: An Anthropological View.* New York: McGraw-Hill.

Wallace, S.
2016 Dodging Wind Farms and Bullets in the Arctic. *National Geographic,* March 1. http://news.nationalgeographic.com/2016/03/160301-arctic-sami-norway-reindeer/.

Wallerstein, I. M.
2004 *World-Systems Analysis: An Introduction.* Durham, NC: Duke University Press.

Wallerstein, I. M., et al.
2013 *Does Capitalism Have a Future?* New York: Oxford University Press.

Walley, C. J.
2013 *Exit Zero: Family and Class in Postindustrial Chicago.* Chicago: University of Chicago Press.

Walton, D., and J. A. Suarez, eds.
2016 *Culture, Space, and Power: Blurred Lines.* Lanham, MD: Lexington Books.

Wang, A-L., ed.
2020 *Redefining the Role of Language in a Globalized World.* Hershey: Information Science Reference.

Ward, M. C., and M. Edelstein
2014 *A World Full of Women,* 6th ed. Upper Saddle River, NJ: Pearson.

Warne, A. D., ed.
2015 *Ethnic and Cultural Identity: Perceptions, Discrimination, and Social Challenges.* Hauppauge, NY: Nova Science.

Wasson, C., M. O. Butler, and J. Copeland-Carson, eds.
2012 *Applying Anthropology in the Global Village.* Walnut Creek, CA: Left Coast Press.

Watters, E.
2010 The Americanization of Mental Illness. *New York Times,* January 8. http://www.nytimes.com/2010/01/10/magazine/10psyche-t.html.

Weber, M.
1968 (orig. 1922) *Economy and Society.* Translated by E. Fischoff et al. New York: Bedminster Press.
2011 (orig. 1904) *The Protestant Ethic and the Spirit of Capitalism.* New York: Oxford University Press.

Weiner, M.
2009 *Japan's Minorities: The Illusion of Homogeneity,* 2nd ed. New York: Routledge.

Weston, G. M., and N. Djohari
2020 *Anthropological Controversies: The "Crimes" and Misdemeanors That Shaped a Discipline.* New York: Routledge.

White, L. A.
1949 *The Science of Culture: A Study of Man and Civilization.* New York: Farrar, Strauss.

1959 *The Evolution of Culture: The Development of Civilization to the Fall of Rome.* New York: McGraw-Hill.
2009 *Modern Capitalist Culture,* abridged ed. Walnut Creek, CA: Left Coast Press.

White, R. G., et al., eds.
2017 *The Palgrave Handbook of Sociocultural Perspectives in Global Mental Health.* New York: Palgrave Macmillan.

Whiting, J. M.
1964 Effects of Climate on Certain Cultural Practices. In *Explorations in Cultural Anthropology: Essays in Honor of George Peter Murdock,* W. H. Goodenough, ed. pp. 511–544. New York: McGraw-Hill.

Whorf, B. L.
1956 A Linguistic Consideration of Thinking in Primitive Communities. In *Language, Thought, and Reality: Selected Writings of Benjamin Lee Whorf,* J. B. Carroll, ed., pp. 65–86. Cambridge, MA: MIT Press.

Whyte, M. F.
1978 Cross-Cultural Codes Dealing with the Relative Status of Women. *Ethnology* 17(2) 211–239.

Widlok, T.
2017 *Anthropology and the Economy of Sharing.* New York: Routledge.

Wiley, A. S., and J. S. Allen
2017 *Medical Anthropology: A Biocultural Approach,* 3rd ed. New York: Oxford University Press.

Wilk, R. R.
2006 *Fast Food/Slow Food: The Cultural Economy of the Global Food System.* Lanham, MD: AltaMira.

Wilk, R. R., and L. Barbosa
2012 *Rice and Beans: A Unique Dish in a Hundred Places.* New York: Berg.

Wilkinson-Weber, C. M., and A. O. DeNicola, eds.
2016 *Critical Craft: Technology, Globalization, and Capitalism.* New York: Bloomsbury Academic.

Williams, L. M., and D. Finkelhor
1995 Paternal Caregiving and Incest: Test of a Biosocial Model. *American Journal of Orthopsychiatry* 65(1): 101–113.

Wilmsen, E. N.
1989 *Land Filled with Flies: A Political Economy of the Kalahari.* Chicago: University of Chicago Press.

Wilson, J., and K. Stierstorfer, eds.
2018 *The Routledge Diaspora Studies Reader.* New York: Routledge.

Winzeler, R. L.
2012 *Anthropology and Religion,* 2nd ed. Lanham, MD: Rowman & Littlefield.

Wittfogel, K. A.
1957 *Oriental Despotism: A Comparative Study of Total Power.* New Haven, CT: Yale University Press.

Wodak, R, and B. Forchtner, eds.
2018 *The Routledge Handbook of Language and Politics.* New York: Routledge.

Wolf, A. P.
2014 *Incest Avoidance and the Incest Taboos: Two Aspects of Human Nature.* Stanford, CA: Stanford Briefs.

Wolf, E. R.
1966 *Peasants.* Englewood Cliffs, NJ: Prentice Hall.
1982 *Europe and the People without History.* Berkeley: University of California Press.

Wolf, E. R., with S. Silverman
2001 *Pathways of Power: Building an Anthropology of the Modern World.* Berkeley: University of California Press.

Wolfram W., and R. Fasold
1974 *The Study of Social Dialects in American English.* Englewood Cliffs, NJ: Prentice-Hall.

Worsley, P.
1985 (orig. 1959) Cargo Cults. In *Readings in Anthropology* 85/86. Guilford, CT: Dushkin.

Wortham, J.
2018 On Instagram, Seeing between the (Gender) Lines. *New York Times Magazine,* November 16. https://www.nytimes.com/interactive/2018/11/16/magazine/tech-design-instagram-gender.html.

Wright, H. T.
1977 Recent Research on the Origin of the State. *Annual Review of Anthropology* 6: 379–397.
1994 Prestate Political Formations. In *Chiefdoms and Early States in the Near East: The Organizational Dynamics of Complexity,* G. Stein and M. S. Rothman, eds., *Monographs in World Archaeology* 18: 67–84. Madison, WI: Prehiet al.story Press.

Wuebbles, D. J., et al., eds.
2017 Executive Summary. *Climate Science Special Report: Fourth National Climate Assessment,* 1: 12–34. Washington, DC: U.S. Global Change Research Program.

Xygalatas, D.
2020 Explaining the Emergence of Coronavirus Rituals. *SAPIENS,* April 1. https://www.sapiens.org/culture/coronavirus-rituals/.

Yamashiro, J. H.
2017 *Redefining Japaneseness: Japanese Americans in the Ancestral Homeland.* New Brunswick, NJ: Rutgers University Press.

Yaneva, A.
2020 *Crafting History: Archiving and the Quest for Architectural Legacy.* Ithaca, NY: Cornell University Press.

Yetman, N., ed.
1991 *Majority and Minority: The Dynamics of Race and Ethnicity in American Life,* 5th ed. Boston: Allyn & Bacon.

Young, A.
2000 *Women Who Become Men: Albanian Sworn Virgins.* New York: Berg.

Zapotosky, M.
2017 Grandparents, Other Extended Relatives Exempt from Trump Travel Ban, Federal Judge Rules. *Washington Post,* July 14. https://www.washingtonpost.com/world/national-security/grandparents-other-extended-relatives-exempt-from-trump-travel-ban-federal-judge-rules/2017/07/14/ce67aa72-6888-11e7-8eb5-cbccc2e7bfbf_story.html.

Zhang, Y.
2016 *Trust and Economics: The Co-evolution of Trust and Exchange Systems.* New York: Routledge.

Zimmer-Tamakoshi, L.
1997 The Last Big Man: Development and Men's Discontents in the Papua New Guinea Highlands. *Oceania* 68(2):107–122.

Zimring, C. A., ed.
2012 *Encyclopedia of Consumption and Waste: The Social Science of Garbage.* Thousand Oaks, CA: Sage Reference.

Zukin, S., P. Kasinitz, and X. Chen
2016 *Global Cities, Local Streets: Everyday Diversity from New York to Shanghai.* New York: Routledge.

NAME INDEX

Page number followed by f (e.g., 216f) references a figure; page number followed by t (e.g., 170t) references a table.

Maugh, T. H., III, 99
Maurer, B., 180
Maxwell, L.A., 124
Maybury-Lewis, B., 33
Maybury-Lewis, D., 33, 318
Mba, N. E., 174
McAllester, D. P., 270
McCabe, M., 75, 76, 142
McCain, J., 124, 156
McConnell-Ginet, S., 88, 93
McConvell, P., 212
McElroy, A., 73
McGee, R. J., 47
McGranahan, C., 289
McGregor, W., 85
McLaughlin, E. C., 288
McNeil, D. G., Jr., 313
McWhorter, J. H., 87, 95
Mead, M., 13, 37, 47, 51, 52f, 56t, 57,
    64, 157f, 172, 179
Medina, L., 125f
Meigs, A., 222, 223
Melia, B., 99f
Mendenhall, E., 71
Mendoza-Denton, N., 91-92
Menely, A., 299
Menzies, C. R., 139
Mercader, J., 23, 24
Methenitis, D., 255
Meyer, B., 253, 254
Meyerhoff, M., 88
Michelangelo, 263, 263f
Middleton, C., 5
Miller, B., 184
Mills, J., 38
Mintz, S., 55, 55f, 56t
Mintz, S. W., 284
Mitani, J. C., 24
Moberg, M., 47
Mohai, P., 289
Mohanty, A., 187t, 190, 190t, 287t
Monet, C., 266
Monroe, M., 264
Montague, S., 276
Mooney, A., 88, 94, 95
Moore, J. D., 37, 47
Morais, R., 276
Morency, J-D., 69
Morgan, L. H., 47-49, 51, 56t, 57, 63, 223
Morgan, L. M., 74
Morin, R., 120
Mosse, D., 65
Motseta, S., 136, 158
Mukhopadhyay, C. C., 105
Mullaney, T., 114
Murchison, J. M., 41
Murdock, G. P., 181t
Murphy, C., 10
Murphy, L. D., 47
Murray, S. O., 195, 226
Myers, J. E., 240
Myers, S. L., 312
Myers-Moro, P. A., 240

Noah, J., 113f
Noah, Z., 113f
Nolan, R., 78
Nonini, D. M., 70
Nyqvist, A., 75

Prado, R., 279
Prasad, I., 105
Presley, E., 260
Price, D., 74
Price, R., 172
Provost, C., 181t

Sahlins, M. D., 141, 145, 148, 210
Sajise, P. E., 139
Salazar, C., 241
Salzman, P. C., 140, 163
Salzmann, Z., 50, 82
Samuels, D., 156
Sanday, P. R., 77, 181, 183f
Sanders, B., 33, 288, 299
Sanjek, R., 42, 77, 272
Sansi-Roca, R., 271
Santos-Dumont, A., 53
Sapir, E., 87, 240
Sargent, C. F., 179
Schaeffer, K., 104
Schaik, C. V., 23
Scheidel, W., 223
Schneider, A., 265, 268, 271
Schneider, D. M., 53, 210
Schumacher, S., 274, 275
Schwanhäusser, A., 70
Schwartz, M. J., 156
Scott, J. C., 170, 172
Scudder, T., 42
Sears, D. A., 86f
Sèbe, B., 293
Sebeok, T. A., 83
Semega, J. L., 104, 187, 187t, 190, 190t, 287t
Service, E. R., 148, 157-158
Shaffer, L., 150
Shakespeare, W., 265
Shannon, T. R., 283, 300f
Shapiro, W., 211
Sharma, A., 167
Sharpley, R., 314
Shih, C.-K., 202
Shirazi, S., 10f
Shivaram, C., 202
Shore, C., 158, 170
Shryock, A., 193
Sidky, H., 239
Siegel, R., 22
Sifford, C., 116
Silva, R., 278f
Silva family, 223f
Silverman, S., 157
Silverstein, L. M., 179
Simpson, A., 88
Simpson, P., 94
Sims, C., 47
Singer, M., 70, 71, 309
Slaughter, A.-M., 189
Smith, A., 293-294, 294f
Smith, N. J. H., 139
Smitherman, G., 95
Snead, S., 117
Snodgrass, J., 71
Snowden, F., Jr., 106
Snyder, R., 288
Soleimani, Q., 30
Solway, J., 134
Sorkin A., 274
Sotomayor, S., 113
Spencer, D., 5
Spickard, P., 103, 104
Spitz, M., 238
Spooner, B., 32
Spotti, M., 81
Srivastava, J., 139
Stack, C. B., 203
Standard, M. G., 293
Starn, O., 117
Staudt, K. A., 33
Stearns, P. N., 289
Stein, P. L., 239, 240, 241
Stein, R. L., 239, 240, 241

Steward, J., 51, 52, 55, 56t
Stierstorfer, K., 316
Stimpson, C. R., 179
Stoler, A., 56t, 57, 293
Stoler, A. L., 289
Stone, L., 182, 210
Stone, M. P., 32
Streep, M., 265
Streets-Salter, H., 293
Stryker, R., 157
Suarez, J. A., 156, 174
Sullivan, M., 208, 209
Sunderland, P. L., 77
Sunstein, B. S., 41
Susser, I., 70, 71
Suttles, W., 152
Svoboda, E., 298-299

T

Talbot, M. M., 88, 93
Tamai, L. A. Y. W., 103
Tanaka, J., 158
Tannen, D., 84, 85, 88, 93
Tanner, J., 263
Tattersall, I., 105, 106
Taylor, P., 104
Taylor, T. L., 44
Tehan, M., 308
Teller, D. J., 314
Terrace, H. S., 83, 84
Thomas, M., 42
Thompson, T., 226
Tierney, R. K., 116
Tiffin, H., 293
Titiev, M., 231
Tolkien, J. R. R., 44
Tougher, S., 192
Townsend, P. K., 73
Toyosaki, S., 116
Tratner, S. W., 272
Trehub, S., 267
Tremlett, P.F., 240
Trester, A. M., 85
Trivedi, B. P., 84
Trosper, R. L., 152
Trotter, R. T., II, 74
Trump, D., 30, 33, 95, 96, 116, 123-124, 156, 296, 299
Tuden, A., 156
Turnbull, C., 134, 150
Turner, V., 53, 56t
Turner, V. W., 156, 243, 244t
Tusting, K., 81
Tylor, E., 19-20
Tylor, E. B., 47-49, 51, 56t, 224, 240

U

Umiker-Sebeok, J., 83
Underhill, P., 76

V

Valdez, I., 61f
Valentine, P., 211
Valeggia, C., 71
Van Allen, J., 174
Van Cantfort, T. E., 83
van der Grijp, P., 261, 272
Vannini, P., 63, 77, 268
Varner, H., III, 117
Vayda, A., 152
Veblen, T., 152
Velupillai, V., 86
Venkatesan, S., 65
Verdery, K., 296
Vespa, J., 125, 125f

Victoria (Queen of England), 290
Vierich, H., 158
Vigil, J. D., 70, 124
Vinyeta, K., 309
Vivanco, L. A., 38
Vogels, E., 234
Voorhies, B., 183
Vucetic, D., 63f
Wade, B. C., 97, 98, 266
Wade, P., 105, 120, 121
Wagner, K. A., 56
Wallace, A. F. C., 238-239, 248
Wallace, A. R., 53
Wallace, S., 318
Wallerstein, I. M., 283, 289
Walley, C., 298-299
Walters, L., 288, 289f
Walton, D., 156, 174
Wang, A.-L., 82
Ward, M. C., 179
Warhol, A., 263-264
Warms, R. L., 47
Warne, A. D., 103, 104
Warren, K. B., 179, 320
Wasson, C., 62, 311
Watkins, J. E., 78
Watson, D. K., 215
Watters, E., 14
Weber, M., 52, 167, 167t, 248, 249, 285, 286, 286f
Weiner, M., 116
Wentzell, E. A., 73
Weston, G. M., 47
White, L. A., 20, 51, 52, 53, 56t, 224, 286
White, R. G., 72
Whiting, J. M., 14
Whorf, B. L., 87
Whyte, M. F., 181, 182t
Widlok, T., 135, 149, 151
Wiley, A. S., 70
Wilford, J. N., 266
Wilk, R. R., 152, 273, 315
Wilkinson-Weber, C. M., 268, 272
William (Prince of England), 5
Williams, L. M., 223
Williams, S., 117
Wilmsen, E., 158
Wilson, J., 316
Winzeler, R. L., 240
Wodak, R., 94
Wolf, A. P., 222
Wolf, E. R., 7, 55, 55f, 56t, 141, 145, 157, 289
Wolfram, W., 93
Woods, T., 114, 116-117, 116f
Worsley, P., 250
Wortham, J., 192, 193, 195
Wright brothers, 53
Wright, C., 265
Wright, S., 158
Wuebbles, D. J., 307, 308
Wulf, C., 69
Wutich, A., 16

X

Xygalatas, D., 245

Y

Yamashiro, J. H., 117
Yaneva, A., 263
Yarrow, T., 65
Yeltsin, B., 296
Yetman, N., 114
Young, A., 193
Yousafzai, M., 184, 184f, 186

SUBJECT INDEX

Page number followed by f (e.g., 216f) references a figure; page number followed by t (e.g., 170t) references a table.

cassava, 139
caste
  endogamy, 225
  untouchable (India), 224f
catharsis, 269
cattle, Hindus and, 246, 246f
Caucasoid people, 106
cave art, Paleolithic, 266
cell phones, 33
censorship, 171
Center on Everyday Lives of Families
    (CELF, UCLA), 208–209
ceremonial fund, 145
chiefdoms
  defined, 157, 165
  economic basis and political regulation, 168t
  political and economic systems, 165–166
  redistribution, 166
  status systems, 166–167
  stratification, 167
child rearing
  enculturation and, 51
  siblings' role in, 201f
children
  enculturation and, 20–21
  German, skin color and, 110f
  Indian boy at livestock fair, 107f
  indigenous Australian, 108f
  Samburu girls (Kenya), 109f
chimpanzees
  language and, 82–83
  same-sex sexual activity, 197
  similarities with humans, 24
  toolmaking by, 23–24, 25f
China
  censorship system in, 171
  energy consumption in, 306t
  female swimmers in, 6
  industrialization, 298
  rice terraces (Guangxi province), 139f
"Chinese virus," 96, 113, 123
Chixoy Dam (Guatemala), 65
Christianity
  fundamentalist, 255
  Islam vs., 126
  as monotheistic, 248
  Pentecostal/charismatic, 254
  as revitalization movement, 250
  as state religion, 249–250
  in U.S., 251–252
  as world religion, 249
chromosomes
  intersex, 192
  X and Y, 178–180
Cinderella, 54
circumcision, 29
cisgender, 191
cities
  development of, 10
  population in, 69–70
  urban anthropology, 69–70
Civilization and Capitalism, 15th-18th Century
    (Braudel), 283
Civil Rights Act of 1964, 195
clans, 207–209
class
  multiple negation according to, 93t
  subculture and, 28
class consciousness, 286
classical economic theory, 145
climate change
  global, 306–309
  global warming vs., 307
  indigenous peoples and, 318–319
clitoridectomy, 29

cloning, 22
Coca-Cola Company, 62
cocoteros, 203f
code of ethics
  American Anthropological Association
    (AAA), 46–47
  social control and, 247
collateral household, 203
collateral relatives, 213
Colombia
  chiefdoms in, 165
  indigenous population, 320
  same-sex marriage in, 226
colonialism, 121
  British, 290, 291, 291f
  cultural, 129
  defined, 289–292
  French, 282f, 290–292
  identity and, 292
  postcolonial studies, 293
  Spain and Portugal, 289–290
  West African nations created by, 292f
Columbian exchange, 284
Coming of Age in Samoa (Mead), 51
communication. See also language
  art and, 268–269
  nonverbal, 84–86
  skills, political success and, 156
communism, 296
Communism, 296
communitas, 244
complex societies, 45
CONASUPO, 295
concierge medicine, 72
configurationalism, 51
conflict resolution, 159
connectivity, 274–276
conscience collectif, 53
conspicuous consumption, 152, 299
consumption culture, 315–316
Contagion (movie), 312
contagious magic, 241
contemporary functionalism, 50–51
conversation (ethnography), 38–39
cooperatives, 67
core countries, 283
core values, 23
coronavirus. See also COVID-19
  Americans flee Europe during, 317f
  art inspired by, 269f
  effects on rituals and religion, 245
  as emerging disease, 311
  naming, 96
  online meditation during, 276f
correlations, 136
cosmology, 246
Costa Rica, same-sex marriage in, 226
cousins
  cross, 220–221
  parallel, 220
Covenant on Civil and Political Rights
    (UN), 30
Covenant on Economic, Social and
    Cultural Rights (UN), 30
COVID-19. See also coronavirus
  drive-thru testing site (New York), 312f
  as emerging disease, 311
  globalization and, 306
  ground zero for, 312, 312f
  recession and, 287
Creation of Adam, The (Michelangelo), 263f
cremation ceremony (Bali), 26f
creole language, 86
CRM. See cultural resource management
cross cousins, 220–221

cross-cultural test, 2
Cuba
  cocoteros in, 203f
  as Communist state, 296
  Internet service in, 171
  religious activities in, 250, 253
  Santeria shrine, 252f
  as Spanish colony, 290
cultivation continuum, 138–139
cultural adaptation, 4t
cultural anthropology, 7, 13
cultural appropriation, 29f
cultural change, opposition to, 124
cultural colonialism, 129
cultural consultants, 39–40
cultural determinism, 52–53
cultural diffusion, 28, 32
cultural diversity
  anthropological scrutiny of, 37–38
  art appreciation and, 264
  cultural anthropology and, 7
  ethical issues and, 46
  ethnocentrism vs., 29
  gender roles and, 179
  indigenous people and, 320
  language loss and, 99
  perception and motivation changes and, 146
  transnational migration and, 304
cultural ecology, 52, 152, 246
cultural generalities, 49
cultural generation gap, 124
cultural heritage, 30–31
cultural imperialism, 313–314
cultural learning, 20. See also enculturation
culturally appropriate marketing, 74–75
culturally specific syndromes, 13
cultural materialism, 52
cultural relativism, 29
cultural resource management (CRM)
  applied anthropology and, 64–65
  defined, 12
cultural rights, 30–31
cultural transmission, 83
culture
  adaptability of, 23
  as all-encompassing, 22
  anthropological theory, 56–57
  bathroom habits, 22
  change mechanisms, 32
  core values of, 23
  cultural relativism, 29
  cultural rights, 30–31
  defined, 3, 28
  ethnocentrism, 29
  evolutionary basis of, 23–25
  expressive, 261–262
  generalities, 25–26
  globalization and, 32–33
  human rights, 30
  ideal culture, 28
  individuals and, 27–32
  as instrumental, 23
  as integrated, 22–23
  international culture, 28
  international level of, 28f
  language and, 86–88, 98–99
  as learned, 20
  levels of, 28–29
  media and, 272–276
  national culture, 28
  nature and, 21–22
  particularities of, 26–27
  popular, 272
  real culture, 28
  representations of, 268

climate change and, 307
resource depletion and, 306
industrialization, 284-287
alienation and, 143-145
energy consumption and, 305-306
family organization and, 202-203, 205-206
Industrial Revolution, 284-285
industrial stratification, 285-287
medical anthropology and, 73-74
infibulation, 29
informants, 39
informed consent, 46
Inka empire, Spain and, 289
innovation
culturally appropriate, 62
indigenous models, 68-69
overinnovation, 66-67
underdifferentiation, 67-68
Instagram, 21, 193, 275
Intel corporation, 76f
intellectual property rights (IPR), 31
intensive agriculture, 139
Inter-American Development Bank, 294
interethnic contact, 313-316
consumption culture, 315-316
cultural imperialism, 313-314
indigenization, 314-315
media, 315
international culture, 28
International Labor Organization (ILO), 320
International Monetary Fund (IMF), 32,
33, 294
International Organization for Migration
(IOM), 169
International Wall (Belfast), 264f
Internet
Americans' use of, 275
Brazilians' use of, 274-275
criticism via, 266
ethnic and national identities and, 315
as gateway, 193, 195
global economy and, 144
globalization and, 33
international spread of, 274-275
linguistic diversity and, 88
maintaining connections through, 23
medical information via, 72-73
nonusers, 275
online dating, 234
restricted access to, 171
role in world system, 300
interpretive anthropology, 53-54
intersex, 192, 193
intervention philosophy, 293
interview schedule, 39
interviewing, 38-39
intrinsic racism, 117
Inuit people
foraging by, 134, 159-160, 182, 182f
gender stratification among, 182f
location, 159f
IPR. See intellectual property rights
Iran
cultural sites, 30
energy consumption in, 306t
location of, 164f
Mesopotamian state in, 165
nomadic groups in, 141
U.S. travel ban and, 215
Iraq
cultural sites, 30
Human Terrain System program and, 47
location of, 164f
Mesopotamian state in, 165
refugees from, 169

religious radicalization in, 255
Ireland
British empire and, 290
International Wall (Belfast), 264f
same-sex marriage and, 226
single-parent households in, 190
irrigation, 138
Islam. *See also* Muslims
as common state religion, 249
religious radicalization, 255-256
spread of, 254-255
Islamic state (IS), 126
destruction of ruins by, 30-31
Jihad militants, 256f
as religious extremist group, 255-256
Italy
bocci in, 28
COVID-19 in, 245
Sistine Chapel (Rome), 263f
Ivory Coast, Adjeme Market vendor, 225f

J

Japan
energy consumption in, 306t
industrialization, 298
race in, 116-119
Tokyo Rainbow Pride Parade, 193f
Jeopardy (TV show), 273
jobs, gender and, 188
Judaism, 249
judiciary, 168

K

Kalabari people, 264-265, 265f
Kalahari Desert
foraging in, 134, 136f
San ("Bushmen") of, 134
Kalinga Institute of Social Sciences (KISS),
8-9
Kanuri people, 232-233
Kapauku Papuans
"big man," 161-162
location, 161f
Kennewick Man, 31
key cultural consultants, 39
key informants, 39
khan, 164
Khasi ethnic group (India), 202f
Kibale National Park (Uganda), 24
kin terms, 93-94
kin-based mode of production, 141
kin-based societies, 39
kinesics, 85
kings, divine right of, 240
kinship
bilateral, 212
changes in North American, 203, 205-206
chiefdoms and, 166
"close family members" definition, U.S., 215
exogamy and, 25
genealogical kin types, 211
kin terms, 211-212
kinship calculation (classification), 210-212
social security and, 204
symbols and genealogical type notation, 211f
kinship terminology, 212-394
bifurcate collateral, 214, 214f
bifurcate merging, 213-214, 213f
generational, 214, 214f
lineal, 213
social and economic correlates, 216t
Klinefelter's syndrome, 192
koro, 13
Kuikuru people, 137, 139
"Kung Flu," 123

Kurds, 126
Kwakiutl people, 49, 151
Kwashiorkor Rehabilitation Facility (Haiti), 14f

L

labor, 142
labor-force participation rate, 188, 191t
labor unions, U.S., 300
lacross, 48f
Lakher people, 222, 222f
land, 142
language
call systems *vs.,* 84t
cultural transmission and, 83
defined, 81-82
evolution of word order, 98f
focal vocabulary, 87-88
historical linguistics, 97-99
Homo sapiens and, 20-21
meaning, 88
nonhuman primate communication,
82-84
nonverbal communication, 84-86
origin of, 84
Sapir-Whorf hypothesis, 86-87
sociolinguistics, 88-97
status position and, 93-94
structure of, 85-86
subculture and, 28
thought, culture and, 86-88
words of the year, 90-91
Language of Food, The (Jurafsky), 92
languages
creole, 86
daughter, 97
Indo-European (IE), 97
loss of, 99
pidgin, 32
Proto-Indo-European (PIE), 97-98, 97f
relationship between, 98-99
Romance, 97
Latin America
government officials in, 68
indigenous people in, 320
susto illness in, 71
Latinxs, 104
law
defined, 159
scientific, 14, 15t
law of supply and demand, 148
League of the Ho-de'-no-sau-nee or Iroquois
(Morgan), 47
learning, cultural (*See* cultural learning;
enculturation)
legends, 271
Lesbos, 169f
Les Misérables, 271
less-developed countries (LDCs)
underdifferentiation fallacy, 67
urbanization in, 70
levirate, 231, 231f
lexicon, 85, 87
LGBTQ, 195, 234
life-cycle events, universal, 26f, 27
Life at Home in the Twenty-First Century
(Arnold), 208-209
life history, 40
liminality
defined, 243
normal social life *vs.,* 244f
lineage, 207, 208-209
lineal kinship terminology, 213, 213f
lineal relative, 213
linguistic anthropologists, 82
linguistic anthropology, 6-7, 11, 63

linguistic displacement, 83
linguistic diversity, 88–91
   California, 89–92
   language of food, 92
   regional variation, 89
   Southwestern Spanglish, 92–93
   words of the year, 90–91
linguistic relativity, 94
linguistics. *See also* sociolinguistics
   descriptive, 85
   historical, 97–99
LinkedIn, 23, 275
livestock, as lobola, 229, 230f
Living Anthropologically blog, 77
lobola gifts, 229, 230f
local descent group, 208
locally based demand, 62
longitudinal studies, 42–43
Lord of the Rings, The (Tolkien), 44
love, romantic, marriage and, 227–228
Lyme disease, 311

M

*M*A*S*H* (TV show), 260
Maasai people
   reciprocity and, 150
   warriors' rites of passage, 243f
macaques, 24
Madagascar
   assault on *ombiasa* autonomy, 310
   colonialism and, 282
   deforestation, 310–311
   descent groups, 68
   erosion in, 311f
   rice production in, 142f
   Vezo girls fishing, 135f
magic
   baseball and, 238, 242f
   cargo cults and, 251, 254
   defined, 241
   emotional solace and, 241–242, 245
   ombiasa, 310
   religion and, 241
   rites of passage and, 243
   shamanic healing, 71, 248
maize, NAFTA's effects on, in Mexico,
   294–296
Major League Baseball, 5, 260
majority groups, 104
Makua people, 172–173, 173f, 210
mal de ojo, 14
maladaptive traits, 23
Malagasy people
   descent groups, 68
   environmental degradation and, 310–311
   French colonialism and, 282
malaria, 71
Malay peasants, 172
Malaysia
   circuit board factory, 143f
   industrial alienation in, 143–145
malnutrition, in indigenous populations, 71
mana, 241
Manchester school, 50
manioc, 139
manspreading, 84, 84f
Maori people, haka, 29f
marginality, foraging economies and, 134
market principle, 148
market research, 75–76
marketing
   culturally appropriate, 74–75
   mass media and, 260
   smartphone and, Middle East, 316
   social, 273–274

West African women and, 183f
marriage
   Americans' reasons for, 228
   arranged, 227
   ceremony, Betsileo people, 27
   childless, 229
   defining, 220
   divorce and, 231–232
   durable alliances, 230–231
   endogamy, 224–225
   exogamy, 220–222
   genealogical method and, 39
   gifts at, 228–230
   human mating and, 25
   online market, 233–234
   plural, 220, 232–233
   romantic love and, 227–228
   same-sex, 226–227
   sibling, 223
   Thai wedding, 26f
Masai people, 163, 163f
Masters golf tournament, 116–117
mating, humans *vs.* other primates, 25
matriarchy, 183
matrifocal household, 203
matrilateral skewing, 212
matrilineal descent
   defined, 182, 207
   five generations, 207f
   parallel and cross cousins, 221, 221f
   residence rules and, 208–209
matrilineal-matrilocal societies, 182–183, 231
matrilocality, 183, 209
Mbuti pygmy, 151
McDonald's
   culturally appropriate marketing and, 62,
   74–75
   Ho Chi Minh City, 315f
means of production, 142–143
media
   consumption culture and, 316
   culture and, 272–276
   globalization and, 32–33
   interethnic contact and, 315
   online access and connectivity, 274–276
   as social cement, 273
   television's effects, 273–274
   using, 272–273
medical anthropology, 62, 70–74
   disease-theory systems, 71–72
   globalization and, 73–74
   industrialization and, 73–74
   scientific *vs.* Western medicine, 72–73
medical care, indigenous populations and, 71
Medicare, 125
Melanesia
   cargo cults of, 250, 251f
   location of, 250f
   mana, 241
melanin, 110
Merina state, 68
mestizaje, 320
mestizos, 320
Mexico
   invention of agriculture in, 32
   NAFTA and, 294–296
Middle East
   Arab Spring and social media, 316
   female genital modification in, 29
   invention of agriculture in, 32
   Islam in, 249
migration
   to cities, 70
   illegality industry and, 169
   multiculturalism and, 122–123

Millennials, online dating and, 234
Minangkabau people, 183
minimal pairs, 85
minority groups
   environmental hazards and (U.S.), 288–289
   linguistic insecurity and, 95
   stratification and, 104–105, 105t
   toxic waste exposure and, 288
Missing Migrants Project (MMP), 169
mission civilisatrice, 291, 293
MMP. *See* Missing Migrants Project
modern world system, 282. *See also* world
   system
modes of production, 141–145
   alienation in industrial economies, 143–145
   defined, 141
   means of production, 142–143
   nonindustrial societies, 142
moiety, 220–221
Moken people, 38f
Mongoloid people, 106
monkeys
   capuchin, use of tools, 24
   learning by, 24
monocrop production, 284
monotheism, 240, 248
Mormons, 185
morphemes, 85
morphology, 85
Moso people, 202
Mount Olympus, 248
Mountain People, The (Turnbull), 150
movimento, 69
moxibustion, 72f
multiculturalism, 122–123
   backlash to, 123–124
multilinear evolution, 52
multinational corporations, 33
multisited ethnography, 43
multitimed ethnography, 43
Mundugumor people, 179
music
   biological roots of, 267
   carcaba (Morocco), 267f
   comparative study of, 266–268
   global consumption culture and, 316
   as social art, 267f
   traditional Navajo, 270
   young students, 271f
Muslims. *See also* Islam
   ethnic conflicts and, 126
   pilgrimage to Mecca, 28f
   public singing, 268
   western Bosnia, *zadrugas,* 201
Myanmar
   location of, 222f
   political organization, Kachin Hills, 55
Myst Online: Uru Live (online environment), 44
myths, 271

N

NAACP. *See* National Association for the
   Advancement of Colored People
NAFTA. *See* North American Free Trade
   Agreement
NAGPRA. *See* Native American Graves
   Protection and Repatriation Act
nation(s)
   defined, 120
   ethnic groups and, 120–121
   linguistic diversity within, 88–91
   nationalities without, 121
National Association for the Advancement of
   Colored People (NAACP), 115
national culture, 28

National Endowment for the Arts, 269
National Football League, 260
nationalism, 121
nationalities
    defined, 121
    ethnic groups and, 120–121
    without nations, 121
National Weather Service, 308
nation-state
    defined, 120
    foragers in, 134
Native American Graves Protection and
    Repatriation Act (NAGPRA), 31
Native Americans
    early studies, 7
    faith healers, 247
    federal judge, 231f
    female boat makers (Hidatsa group), 180
    first, land bridge crossing, 105
    foraging by, 134–135
    gender-variant, 192–193
    Great Plains, buffalo hunting, 163f
    horses and, 140
    Iroquois tribes, early ethnography on, 47–48,
        48f
    Kwakiutl people, 49
    Navajo music, 270
    negative reciprocity example, 149
    New Age religions and, 252
    pantribal sodalities, 162–163
    redistribution example, 148
    Seneca Iroquois study (19th century), 63
    skin color of, 107, 110
    time concept for, 87
    totemic carvings, 246
    "Two-Spirit," 226
    U.S. Census categories, 114–115
    village head of Yanomami, 160–161
Native Australians. See also aboriginal peoples;
        Australian aborigines
    New Age religions and, 252
    religion, 239
    totemic carvings, 246
native taxonomy, 212
natural disasters, 22
naturalistic disease theories, 71
natural selection, skin color and, 109–112
nature, culture and, 21–22
Navajo people, 270f
Nayar people, 201–202
Nazis, Holocaust genocide, 128
Ndembu people (Zambia), 243
négritude, 121
need-based transfer, 150
needs functionalism, 50
negative equity impact, 66
negative reciprocity, 149
Negroid people, 106
neoliberalism, 293–296
neolocality, 203
Netherlands
    female swimmers in, 6
    flower parade festival, 264f
    same-sex marriage in, 226
neural tube defects (NTDs), 112
New Age religions, 252
new media.
    anthropological knowledge via, 77
    globalization and, 33
    maintaining connections through, 23
    political role of, 171
    sharing opinions on, 21
New York City
    Big Apple Job Fair, 101f
    gender-free store in, 177f

Indigenous Peoples rally, 157f
Museum of Modern Art, 264
non-binary rights demonstration, 192f
pronunciation of *r* in, 94t
Whitney Museum of American Art, 270f
New York Times dialect quiz, 81
New Zealand
    labor-force participation rate, 191t
    location of, 250f
    Maori haka and Kiwis rugby team, 29f
    same-sex marriage in, 226
NGOs. *See* nongovernmental organizations
Nigeria
    Igbo "Women's War" in, 174–175, 174f
    Kalabari people, 265f
    as nonsettler country, 293
    as periphery nation, 283
    polygyny among Kanuri people in, 232–233
    rape in, 184
    religious sculptures (Kalabari people), 264
    word for "art" (Yoruba people), 261
Nilote people, 108
Nipah virus, 312, 313
Nobel Peace Prize, Malala Yousafzai, 184, 184f,
    186
nomadic politics, 163–165
nomadism, pastoral, 140, 164f
nonbinary gender, 192
nongovernmental organizations (NGOs), 157
nonhuman primate communication
    call systems, 82
    sign language, 82–83
nonindustrial societies, 142
nonverbal communication, 84–86
norms, 159
North Africa
    bifurcate collateral kinship in, 214
    Evangelicals in, 253
    in French empire, 291f
    Islam in, 249
    pastoral nomads in, 141
North America
    anthropology subfields in, 7
    in British empire, 290, 291f
    exchange principles in, 151
    family organization in, 202–203, 205–206
    gender speech contrasts, 93
    HIV/AIDS in, 312
    kin terms in, 211–212
    kinship bonds in, 205
    meal preferences, 21–22
    NAFTA and, 295
    Native Americans in (*See* Native Americans)
    parental gift giving in, 149
    political organization in, 157
    polygyny in, 232f
    religion in, 249, 253–254
    same-sex marriage in, 227
    serial monogamy in, 232
North American Free Trade Agreement
    (NAFTA), 294–296
Norway
    female labor-force participation in, 191
    same-sex marriage in, 227
    Sami people in, 140, 318–319
Notes and Queries on Anthropology, 220
NTDs. *See* neural tube defects
nuclear family
    defined, 201
    descent group *vs.,* 206
    neolocal American, 212f
    traditional American, 26
Nuer people
    cross-cousin marriages, 229
    focal vocabulary example, 88

paternity, 220
    same-sex marriages, 220, 226
    structural societal principles, 50
Nuer, The (Evans-Pritchard), 50

O
Obergefell v. Hodges, 228
observation, 38
Occupy movement, 33
oceans, climate change and, 307
office, 166
Ojibwa people, 222–223
Olympian gods, 248
Olympic Games
    media coverage of, 5, 277
    summer (2016), 6f, 72f, 194, 194f, 277, 278f
    winter (2018), 259f
ombiasa, 310
online dating, 234–235, 235f
online ethnography, 44–45
opposable thumbs, 23
osteology, 11
osteoporosis, 111
outsourcing jobs, 283f, 284
overinnovation, 66–67

P
paganism, 240
paleoanthropologists, 11
paleoecology, 10
paleontologists, 11
pandemics
    COVID-19 (*See* coronavirus; COVID-19)
    defined, 312
    geographic naming, 96
    globalization of risk and, 306
    HIV/AIDS, 73
    rituals during, 245
pantheons, 248
pantribal sodalities, 162–163
Papua New Guinea
    "big man," 162f
    cargo cults of, 250
    Mead's study of gender roles in, 179
    Parliament building (Port Moresby), 155f
    patrilineal-patrilocal complex, 184, 184f
    sexual relations in, 195–197
parallel cousins, 220
parents. *See also* family(ies)
    bifurcate collateral terminology
        and, 214
    enculturation and, 20–21
    in foraging bands, 136
    generalized reciprocity and, 149, 151
    helicopter, 219
    immigrant, 49
    labor-force participation rate of (U.S.), 188
    marriage approval and, 227
    media images of, 273
    North American kinship and, 205–206, 209,
        211, 213
    in nuclear family, 26
    religion of, 252
    work–family time bind and, 133
participant observation, 38
particularities, 25–27
Pashtun ethnic group, 185
pastoral nomadism, 140
pastoralism, 139–141, 141f
pater, 220
paternity, 220
patriarchy
    defined, 183, 184
    fundamentalist communities, 185
    violence and, 184, 186

patrilineal descent
  defined, 183, 207
  divorce and, 231
  five generations, 207f
  identity and incest among Lakher, 222f
  lobola gifts, 229
  parallel and cross cousins, 221, 221f
  residence rules and, 208
patrilineal-patrilocal complex, 183-184
patrilocality, 208
patrilocal societies, 183
Patterns of Culture (Benedict), 51
peasants, 148
Pentagon's Human Terrain System (HTS), 47
Pentecostalism, 253-254
People of Puerto Rico, The (Steward), 55
periphery
  countries on, 283
  living on American, 288-289
personal diary, 38
personalistic disease theories, 71
Peru
  Andes of, chiefdoms in, 165
  Andes of, high altitudes and, 4
  constitutional reforms in, 320
  horticulture in, 137
  outdoor market, 18f
  royal endogamy in ancient, 226
  in Spanish empire, 289
petroglyphs, 87f
Pew Research Center
  Americans' social media use, 276
  on Internet access, 274
  marriage reasons (in U.S.), 228, 228f
  online dating survey, 234-235
  Religious Landscape Studies, 251-252
  world religions survey, 249f
PGA. *See* Professional Golfers' Association of
    America
phenotype
  Brazilian racial classification by, 119-120,
    119f
  defined, 106
  racial classification by, 106-109
Phoenicians, 289
phoneme
  defined, 85
  in Standard American English, 86f
phonemics, 86
phonetics, 86
phonology, 85
physical features. *See* phenotype
physician-patient dialogue research, 77
pidgin language, 32, 86
Pinterest, 21, 275
plural marriages, 220, 232-233
plural society, 122
political economy, 55-56
political organization, 55, 157
political regulation, 157
political systems
  adaptive strategies and, 157
  bands and tribes, 158-165 (*See also* band(s);
    tribe(s))
  chiefdoms, 165-167
  Communism, 296
  social control and, 170-175 (*See also* social
    control)
  state systems, 167-170
  types and trends, 157-158
Political Systems of Highland Burma (Leach), 55
politics
  art and, 269-270
  globalization concept and, 32
pollution

economic inequality and, 288
  fossil fuel use and, 308, 309f
  industrial, 309
  urban slums and, 70
polyandry
  fraternal, 220, 233, 233f
  multiple husbands, 181, 232-233
polydactylism, 223f
polygamy, 185, 232
polygyny, 181, 186, 232-233
Polynesia
  chiefdoms, 165-166, 166f
  feminine men in, 193
  interactions and social status, 85
  mana in, 241
  skin color of people in, 106-107, 107f
Polynesian Triangle, 107f
polytheism, 240, 240f
popular culture, 272
population(s)
  capacities for culture, 20
  control of, state systems and, 167-168
Portugal
  climate change rally in, 303f
  colonialism and, 289-290
  same-sex marriage in, 227
postcolonial studies, 293
postmarital residence rule, 210f
postmodern, 317
postmodernism, 317
postmodernity, 317
postpartum taboo, 14-16
postsocialist societies, 296-297
potlatch, 152-153
potsherds, 9-10
pottery. *See* potsherds
poverty
  feminization of, 190
  in Flint, Michigan, 289
  as focus of anthropology, 8, 64, 70
  illness and, 73
  as liminal feature, 244
  in Madagascar, 310
  postsocialist Russia and, 297
  reducing, 7, 9, 65
  in Russia, 307
  single-parent households and, 203
power
  anthropological theory, 56-57
  defined, 156
  as social stratification dimension, 167
practical anthropology, 64
practice theory, 28, 54-55
PREDICT program, 312-313
prejudice, ethnic conflict and, 126-127
prestige, 160, 167
Pride and Prejudice (Austen), 273
primates
  characteristics of, 23-24
  differences from humans, 25
primatologists, 11
primatology, 11
Primitive Culture (Tylor), 19-20, 49
Primitive Religion (Tylor), 49
private-public contrast, 182
problem-oriented ethnography, 41-42
production
  domestic system of, 285, 285f
  Longfellow's vision of, 144
productivity, linguistic, 83
Professional Golfers' Association of America
    (PGA), 116-117
profit motive, 145
Project Nim (documentary film), 84
proletariat, 286

*Protestant Ethic and the Spirit of Capitalism,
    The* (Weber), 248
Protestantism
  evangelical, 253-254
  in U.S., 251-252
  values of, capitalism and, 248-249
Proto-Indo-European (PIE) languages,
    97-98, 97f
protolanguage, 97
psychological anthropology, 13-14
public anthropology, 77
public archaeology, 12
public events, symbolic acts at, 27f
public interest anthropology, 77

Q

Qashqai people, 164, 164f
questionnaire, 39
questions, inflection changes with, 86

R

race
  ascribed *vs.* achieved status, 103
  in Brazil, 119-120
  classification problems, 105-106
  as cultural category, 105
  defined, 105
  ethnicity and, 112-113
  human biological diversity and, 105-112
  in Japan, 116-119
  no biological distinctions among, 106-109
  social construction of, 113-120
Race, Language, and Culture (Boas), 49
Race, Language, and Politics (Boas), 49
racial classification, 105
  government and, 114
  by phenotype, 106-109
  by physical features, 108
  by skin color, 106-108
racism
  defined, 105-106
  intrinsic, 117
random sample, 45
rapport, 38
real culture, 28
reciprocity, 148-151
  defined, 148
  human survival and, 150
  need-based transfer, 150
  types of, 148-149
reciprocity continuum, 149
redistribution
  chiefly, 166
  defined, 148
refugees
  "caravan" of, 317f
  Central American, 317f
  climate change, 318
  defined, 129
  in Europe, 169
  NAFTA's economic, 294-295
  religious radicalization of, 255
  study of, 43
  in U.S., 296
  Uru (virtual world), 44
region(s)
  ethnic diversity by, 120-121
  subculture and, 28
regulation, political, 157
reindeer
  food products, 140f
  Sami domestication of, 140
religion. *See also entries for individual religions*
  antimodernism, 255
  art and, 262-263

burnt offering, 239f
change and, 250–253
changes in U.S., 251–252
cultural ecology and, 246
cultural globalization and, 253–256
defined, 238
deities, 248
effects of coronavirus on, 245
ethnic conflicts and, 126
evangelicals, 253–254
expressions of, 240–246 (*See also* religious expressions)
fundamentalism, 255
homogenization, 254
hybridization, 254
indigenization, 254
as international culture level, 28f
Islam, spread of, 254–255
kinds of, 247–249
new and alternative movements, 252–253
Protestant values, 248
radicalization, 255–256
religious specialists, 248
revitalization movements, 250–251
Russian Orthodox, 248f
secular rituals, 256–257
social control and, 247
subculture and, 28
symbols and, 20
verbal manifestations, 239–240
what is?, 238–240
world, 249–250, 249f
Religion: An Anthropological View (Wallace), 238
religious expressions
magic, 241
powers and forces, 241
rites of passage, 243–244
rituals, 242–243
spiritual beings, 240–241
totemism, 244–246
uncertainty, anxiety, solace, 241–242
rent fund, 146
replacement fund, 145
research
survey, 45–46
team, 42–43
virtual, 44
resistance
to social control, 171–172
"weapons of the weak," 172
resources, differential access to, 157
respondents, 45
retail anthropologist, 76
revitalization movements, 250–251
rickets, 111
risk, globalization of, 306
rites of intensification, 244–246
rites of passage
art and, 263
as religious expressions, 243–244
rituals
baseball, 242f
defined, 242
effects of coronavirus on, 245
Marine Corps haircuts, 242f
as religious expressions, 242–243
secular, 256–257
universal life-cycle events, 26f, 27
Roman Catholicism
in Brazil, 253
international culture and, 28
Protestantism *vs.,* 248f
symbols in, 20
in U.S., 251–252
Romance languages, 97

Roman Empire
imperialism and, 289
marriage in, 228
romantic love, marriage and, 227–228
Rosie the Riveter, 187f
Royal Anthropological Institute, 220
royal endogamy, 225–226
Russia
energy consumption in, 306t
market-oriented reform in, 296
Rwandan genocide, 128, 292, 318

S
Salish people, 151
Samburu people, 109f
same-sex marriage, 226–227
countries allowing (2020), 226t
legalization of, U.S., 195, 228–229
society's recognition of, 220
Sami people
as pastoralists, 140
threats to, 318–319
sample, 45
San ("Bushmen") of southern Africa
foraging by, 134, 136, 136f, 158–159
location of, 149f
skin color of, 108, 108f
sanitary citizens, 73
Santeria religion, 252f, 253
Sapir-Whorf hypothesis, 86–87
SARS (severe acute respiratory syndrome), 311, 312
Sat-mar Hasidim people, 185
Saudi Arabia
energy consumption in, 306t
location of, 164f
pilgrimage to Mecca, 28f
savagery, stages of, 48
Scandinavia
language in, 97
preparations against Russian incursion, 319
Scandinavian people
female swimmers, 6
racial classification and, 108
schistosomiasis, 73
schools. *See also* education
floating one-room, 69f
Kalinga Institute of Social Sciences (KISS), 8–9
patriarchies and attendance in, 184
study of elementary classroom (U.S.), 69
transmission of culture via, 8–9
science
defined, 12
value and limitations of, 16
scientific medicine, 72–73
scientific method, 14–16
case study: postpartum taboo, 14–16
steps in, 15t
theories, associations, explanations, 14, 15t
scientific theory. *See* theory
Search of the Hamat'sa: A Tale of Headhunting (film), 48f
Second Life (online environment), 44
secret societies, 163
secular rituals, 256–257
Semai people, 149
semantics, 88
semiperiphery countries, 283
serial monogamy, 232
sex, gender and, 179–180
sexual dimorphism, 179
sexual orientation, 195–197
Sex and Temperament in Three Primitive Societies (Mead), 51, 179

shaman
as curer, 71
defined, 248
in foraging societies, 136
shame, social control and, 173–174
Shan (political form), 55
shifting cultivation, 137
Shiites, 126
Shoshoni people, 206f
Shrek (film), 268
sibling marriage, 223, 225–226
siblings
in extended families, 202–203
incest and, 223
kin terms for, 211, 213–214
in nuclear families, 201
role in child-rearing, 201f
Sicily, ancient amphitheater, 272f
sign language, nonhuman primate, 82–83
"silent trade," 151
simultaneity of discovery, 53
"sitting on a man," 174
situational negotiation of social identity, 102, 104
skin color
advantage/disadvantages, 111t
melanin and, 110–111
natural selection and, 109–112
racial classification by, 106–108
slash-and-burn cultivation, 137, 137f
slavery
in ancient Rome, 106
trans-Atlantic trade, demand for sugar and, 284f
slave ships, clues from sunken, 10
smartphones
age and use of, 275, 275f
Middle East marketing and, 316
online access through, 275
ownership of, 274, 275
as shopping tool, 76
smelting
as male activity, 181t
upper barbarism and, 48
Snapchat, 21, 275
Snow White (film), 268
soap operas, 273
social control
defined, 170
hegemony, 170–171
Igbo women's war, 174–175, 174f
religion and, 247
resistance to, 171–172
shame and gossip, 172–174
"weapons of the weak," 172
social distancing
online dating and, 234
pandemic and, 245
traffic sign reminder, 89f
social facts, 53
social fund, 145
social identity, situational negotiation of, 102, 104
social indicators, 45
socialism, 296
socialist internationalism, 129
sociality, subsistence *vs.,* 133
social marketing, 273–274, 274f
Social Network, The (film), 274
social networks. *See* new media;
social paternity, 220
social relations with economic aspects, 143
social security, kinship and, 204
Social Security, 125